PRAISE FOR
WHY GLOBAL HEALTH MATTERS

Chris Stout's latest publication provides a wealth of resources for practitioners, researchers, academics, leaders, individuals, and groups who are interested in addressing the complexities of global health. The wide range of contributors provides a rich background for grasping the scale of what we need to address as we learn to live together. As they integrate physical health and emotional well-being, the authors map our way forward using sustainable solutions. We now have a practical approach to examining the scope of the global health problems and opportunities, and a clear case for community-based solutions.

— *Breeda McGrath, PhD, Dean of Academic Affairs, The Chicago School of Professional Psychology*

Why Global Health Matters addresses some of the most important issues facing humanity today. Not only does it provide an insightful description of global health problems, but the book focuses on important, sustainable solutions. An insightful and eye-opening read that will challenge you to engage.

— *Greg Martin, MD, Chief Editor at Globalization and Health, Board of Directors at Irish Forum for Global Health*

Why Global Health Matters offers a blueprint for creating successful humanitarian projects in a complex, multi-disciplinary world. Its strength is in the diversity of viewpoints it brings together to detail global health trends and the mechanisms for improvement around the world. The book masterfully gets at the true collaborative nature of global health — which is not a strictly medical field. This is an excellent resource for the doers trying to create change in global health and is also a good introduction to rising practitioners in the field.

— *Jaclyn Schiff, journalist and consultant*

Global health is a flourishing area of research, practice, training, and advocacy. Edited by Dr. Chris Stout, *Why Global Health Matters* features chapters by internationally renowned experts who recognize that global health is multiply determined and calls for innovative, yet feasible policies and programs designed by all stakeholders. The diverse sections of the book share a core message: a multidisciplinary, multisectoral, and multicultural approach is essential for understanding, improving, and sustaining global health. *Why Global Health Matters* is a font of information

i

drawn from contemporary research and fieldwork and is an indispensible benchmark resource for academics, practitioners, and students. *Why Global Health Matters* is an inspiration to anyone interested in socially responsible action aimed at improving the well-being of at-risk or suffering individuals and communities.

— Michael Stevens, PhD, DHC,
International Psychology Program at The Chicago School of Professional Psychology,
Past-President of the APA Division of International Psychology

Why Global Health Matters is not the only book out there that highlights global health issues; however, this book, edited by Chris Stout, aims to illustrate how seemingly disparate disciplines intersect to work towards health for all. Through a broad mental health lens, the book draws upon the humanitarian aspects of work experts have been doing in their field. The World Health Organization defines health as "a state of complete physical, mental, and social well-being and not merely the absence of disease or infirmity." However one defines it, the achievement of health is multifaceted, complicated, and not a guarantee. There are a multitude of biomedical, cultural, and socioeconomic factors that impede its path. To work towards health and make a difference requires a holistic approach. No one person can accomplish it alone. This book excels in highlighting the various ways and means of what people have done and people can do to tackle seemingly impossible challenges and solve them.

— Janet Lin, MD, MPH, Associate Professor, Emergency Medicine
(College of Medicine) and Community Health Sciences (School of Public
Health), Director of Health Systems Development (Center for Global
Health), University of Illinois at Chicago

That the world is effectively both shrinking and yet remaining unstable seems clear. Psychology has much to offer in regard to the manifestations of this instability, perhaps especially to health and mental health concerns. We can learn from each other, from our research, our practices, and our successes. I know no one more qualified and more expert in world mental health than Chris Stout, and he has brought together an amazing team to discuss global health and mental health issues and their interaction. This volume can actually help make the world a better, healthier place.

— Kurt F. Geisinger, PhD,
Meierhenry Distinguished University Professor and Director, Buros Center for Testing,
The University of Nebraska-Lincoln

The world is increasingly facing natural and man-made humanitarian disasters that negatively impact the health and well-being of the world's most vulnerable populations. In this current political and environmental climate, it is even more essential to reengage and act in a responsible, sustainable, feasible, and effective manner to "make the world a better place." Chris Stout has compiled an incredible cadre of humanitarian activists, scholars, and scientists from a wide range of academic spheres to share insights on why global health matters and lessons learned from the field. These diverse global health practitioners help shed light on the complexities, scope, and interrelated nature of this work, with an emphasis on understanding the importance of mental health in overall well-being. This book will no doubt serve to inspire a new generation to embrace this meaningful calling, as well as encourage and inform those of us making our way in this essential and complex field of study.

— Valerie Dobiesz, MD, MPH, FACE, Director of External Programs: STRATUS Center for Medical Simulation, Brigham & Women's Hospital, Harvard Humanitarian Initiative, Harvard Medical School

CHRIS E. STOUT

Why Global Health Matters:

How to (*Actually*) Make the World a Better Place

EDITED BY

CHRIS E. STOUT

DEDICATION

To those committed to making global health matter.

TABLE of CONTENTS

PART II – Approaches and Clinical Solutions

PART III – Approaches and Structural Solutions

FOREWORD

Jody Williams, Nobel Peace Laureate

In October of 1992, my colleagues and I launched the International Campaign to Ban Landmines (ICBL). At that time, landmines plagued more than eighty countries. Every twenty minutes, someone somewhere would fall victim to these relentless, indiscriminate killers. Unlike other weapons of war, after a conflict ended, landmines remained in the ground, ready to kill or maim any civilian unfortunate enough to detonate them. Landmines recognize no peace accord. They continued to kill for generations.

In 1997, the ICBL's goal for an international treaty banning antipersonnel landmines was achieved. Today 162 nations are part of the treaty and it is considered to be one of the most effective disarmament treaties in the world. Its provisions have resulted in more than three dozen countries being completely cleared of landmines. More than 58 million mines have been destroyed in stockpiles. This has resulted in new victims dropping from 20,000 to 4,000 a year. Of course, that's still 4,000 too many, but this is a success story nonetheless.

In many ways, the success of the mine ban movement must be measured beyond the Mine Ban Treaty itself and the changes it has brought about. Our movement demonstrated that when ordinary people come together in common cause, we can create extraordinary change. When we work together with like-minded governments and international institutions, we can help to make the world a better place for everyone and contribute to world peace.

This book is an example of one such collaboration. The contributing authors, who are from around the world and represent many different professions, have pooled their knowledge about global health issues to share with others. Here they address mental health, poverty, HIV/AIDS, dementia, and PTSD. They tackle tough questions like how to act for change, how to start an NGO, how to establish and build global health curriculums, and how to make continual, sustainable, global improvement.

Issues pertaining to global health are not just medical in nature. Global health is a vast topic, full of interrelated crises. It is affected by disasters of disease, of nature, and of war, and problems are further aggravated by lack or misuse of resources. Health care professionals are needed, but so are financial analysts, engineers, political scientists, agriculturists, volunteer coordinators, and so many others. In other words, regardless of your field of expertise, you can make a difference

It is my hope, and that of the authors and editors involved, that this book will inspire new projects and improve existing ones as people reading it are motivated to identify problems and work together to solve them.

4

ACKNOWLEDGEMENTS
Chris E. Stout

First and foremost, I want to thank the amazing group of contributing authors that have made this book such a success. When one stops for a moment to realize that many of the authors herein are responsible for changing/saving many lives had it not been for their work and passion. Period. Full stop. It is their zeal that has so inspired me to take on this project. My thanks to each of you for taking the time to craft the chapters that have become this book. I am fortunate to be able to call each of you my friend, and the world is blessed to have you. I hold a great and abiding respect for all of those working in global health in all of its varied forms. The world is in your debt.

I was fortunate to gain valuable help in organizing and managing this project with the amazing skill-set of Gracie Wang, who from the start displayed not only a keen sense of organization of the myriad of complexities that this project involved, but also demonstrated a wonderful balance of professionalism blended with an amazing editorial ability that benefitted all manuscripts herein. She's also responsible for the subtitle. All of this is an incredible feat by an incredible person, tip-o'-the-hat to you, Gracie.

The support of my wife, Karen, is always invaluable, whether I am writing or not. And a special thanks to my son, Grayson, who volunteered to provide an ever-sharp review of many of the first drafts of what now appear herein. Thanks also to my daughter, Annika, who became quite good at tolerating my innumerable, longwinded, overly-animated discourses about the incredible work of the contributing authors. I thank and love you all.

Chris E. Stout
Naperville, IL

Care to do more yourself? Please do! Here's how…

1. Visit CenterForGlobalInitiatives.org for more information on projects you can support. If you don't see something that you think we can help with, email me at <u>DrChrisStout@gmail.com</u> and I may be able to connect you to another organization that can help, or we may be able to initiate a new project.
2. Proceeds from this book goes to support the work of the Center for Global Initiatives, so please share with your friends and colleagues, recommend for graduate course adoption, and spread the word!
3. Consider suggesting **Why Global Health Matters** to others and start a viral buzz! Think of all your contacts who may be interested

in this book. Send them the link, WhyGlobalHealthMatters.org and they can learn more and order the book.

4. Inquire if your local or university library has **Why Global Health Matters** in its collection, or on order. If you recommend it to them and they may add it and others can read it as well.

5. Request a presentation at your local college, university, public library, high school, church, mosque, synagogue, book seller, coffee shop, service organization (Rotary, Lyons, etc.), or book club by emailing a request to DrChrisStout@gmail.com or by calling 847.550.0092.

6. Request an interview by a broadcast, cable, or internet television program, radio, podcast, newspaper or magazine reporter. Media kits are also available by request via DrChrisStout@gmail.com or by calling 847.550.0092.

INTRODUCTION
Chris E. Stout and Gracie Wang

As the subtitle notes, we hope this book will inform and inspire readers in bringing new and novel approaches to making the world a better place by learning from some of the greatest minds, thought leaders, and ambitious workers in the field. We are in awe of the work of the contributing authors herein. They are indeed an inspiration and demonstrate such brilliance in their work and approaches.

It seems there is a growing interest in such matters as well. In Chicago, the top three medical schools, University of Illinois (where CES is on faculty and serves as an advisor to their center), Northwestern University, and University of Chicago all have centers for global health. In fact, many other health care training programs include global health as either part of their curriculum or provide actual clinical experience. Back to the University of Illinois at Chicago as an example, the schools of nursing, dentistry, public health, and medicine all have such involvements.

Graduate programs have developed with some overlapping aspects to global concerns, many of which include health matters. For example, the University of Denver offers a master's degree in international disaster psychology. The Chicago School of Professional Psychology offers a Ph.D. program in international psychology. There is a disaster mental health program at the University of South Dakota. Brandeis University offers master's level training in conflict and coexistence. There is an international trauma studies program at New York University, and Lehigh University has programs in both international counseling psychology and comparative and international education. State University of New York at New Paltz has the Institute for Disaster Mental Health, a free-standing institute that offers two academic programs: an undergraduate minor in disaster studies and a graduate certificate in trauma and disaster mental health. My (CES) Center for Global Initiatives (CGI) offers a certificate program in a variety of global health aspects.

The overlap with global health matters and humanitarian relief are obviously great. Disasters of nature as well as of war and conflict lead to subsequent illness and increased morbidity and mortality. Such events have displaced more than 60 million people today — on par with World War II (VanRooyen, 2016). While there are many significant problems in the processes of providing humanitarian aid as noted by Hancock (1989), Polman (2010), Stout, Olweean, Wang, and Adeniji (2015), and VanRooyen (2016), in contrast, we are encouraged by the smaller-in-scale but larger-in-results leverage of the work and programs discussed herein.

The book is rather organically derived as it has four sections. First, we set a context for the various problems in global health, along with a bit of background and current trends. Next, we delve into solutions. This is divided into distinct (but overlapping) categories of those that are clinical and therapeutic, and those that are focused on structural solutions involving education and training, peacebuilding, and other such approaches as applied to global health. The fourth and final area is that of sustainability — moving forward with solutions as well as leadership to maintaining gains and momentum.

As readers will see, it is a difficult task to differentiate these chapters as most all of these topics have a great deal of overlap. This also speaks to the complexity of what is involved in working in the sphere of global health.

As an old friend and World Economic Forum pal, Joshua Cooper Ramo, said in his book, *The Age of the Unthinkable* (2009):

...we are now tied to one another in ways we can't see, through webs of finance or disease or information, and — here's the dangerous paradox — the more closely we're bound, the less resilient we become. (And) as they become more densely linked, they also become less resilient; networks after all, propagate and even amplify disturbances. Worse, the more efficient these networks are, the faster they spread those dangers.

Interconnections such as the ties between brokers and banks or between the health of every passenger on a long-distance airplane flight are vehicles for sharing risk and triggering hysteresis. (p.198)

Thankfully, there is a growing number of experts focusing their work on dealing with these complexities, and the world owes them a debt of gratitude.

Global health represents an interesting integration of multi-causal problems being worked on by a diverse set of professions and humanitarian actors. This has also served as a draw to me (CES) in my work. Global health concerns can span not only healthcare, per se, but also political science, engineering (clean water plants), health sciences (labs), agricultural sciences, military intervention, veterinary medicine, and policy (to name a few). All such factors are considered with the connecting thread of sustainability.

The difficulty of sustainability is amplified and destabilization leads to a self-perpetuating cycle of state-instability, poverty, and illness. "Of the forty nations at the bottom of the UN's Human Development Index — a statistical measure of life expectancy, education, income, and other factors — 65 percent have experienced recurrent war and disaster" (VanRooyen, 2016, p. 38). These "complex humanitarian emergencies" all involve health and illness aspects. The impact on civilians and displaced refugees also worsens as food or water become scarce and contagious and infectious diseases spread in iatrogenic mini-epidemics.

As VanRooyen (2016) notes, humanitarian intervention is not just bringing in bags of grain and bottles of medication, but rather a tool of diplomacy. Global health matters as it straddles the fields of emergency humanitarian intervention and development work. Global health concerns involve the building of the dam – not only for access to a potable water source for drinking and agriculture, but also as a prevention from the disaster of flooding and subsequent cholera outbreaks. It is very difficult to distinguish or differentiate such overlap. Likewise was our challenge in the organization of this book. And that is as it should be in our opinion.

My (CES) personal path to working in global health – starting the non-profit CGI and co-founding the Consortium for Humanitarian Intervention – has all been somewhat of a wonderful accident. I've frequently written and presented on my being an "Accidental Humanitarian" and my goal to open-source humanitarian intervention. I think there is a remarkable amount of innovation in the non-profit/non-governmental organization (NGO) arena. Much of this opinion is informed by other projects such as The New Humanitarians: Inspiration, Innovations, and Blueprints for Visionaries (Stout, 2008), and this optimism continues as new projects unfold and other NGOs proceed with their work.

As to our work at the CGI, it is our mission to create self-sustaining programs that improve access to health care in underserved communities throughout the world. We believe in the "power of the small project," wherein generally we do this by:

- Serving as an incubator for new initiatives that creatively solve health care inequities throughout the world,
- Acting as a collaborator with individuals and organizations in developing and launching projects that address the needs of medically impoverished populations,
- Functioning as a facilitator in directing public and private resources towards programs aimed at improving health, and
- Working as an educator to provide new information and tools to empower others.

We suspect readers can thus see the overlap with the authors herein. While my (CES) career has been quite varied, I believe that such variation has provided a helpful platform of education, experience, and contacts to do the work I do today — and to draw together a group of contributing authors that appear in this work.

Part 1: Trends and Background

Lori Holleran, Maryke Van Zyl, and Bruce Bongar

These authors consider the influence of mental health disorders among the global population. Through the utilization of indicators such as disability adjusted life-years, years of life lost, and activity impairment, the authors highlight how mental and substance use disorders are notable contributors to the global burden of disease.

Furthermore, Holleran, Van Zyl, and Bongar consider treatment of mental health issues across settings, specifically highlighting discrepancies between developed and developing regions. They compare global responses to highly prevalent disorders (e.g., mood and anxiety disorders) and high impact mental health issues (e.g., psychosis and suicidality). They also consider how culture and stigma influence care.

Finally, Holleran, Van Zyl, and Bongar contemplate the future of global mental health by reflecting on the influence of the Millennium Development Goals on the field, and by examining how the Sustainable Development Goals are expected to influence global progress and response regarding mental health.

Falu Rami and Kathleen Davis

Rami and Davis discuss the proliferation of global conflicts (war, terrorism, and political instability) and their immediate, chronic consequences on the mental and physical health of impacted populations, including disease, injury, substance abuse, and posttraumatic stress.

Rami and Davis hold that these global crises are not limited to particular regions in the world, but rather are prevalent in all contexts. Furthermore, most regions show either deteriorating or no improvements. Finally, they recognize the significant dearth of research pertaining to this subject due to lack of access to affected populations. Therefore, the authors address the need for a unified, concerted effort in order to identify solutions.

Anjhula Mya Singh Bais

Bais considers South and Southeast Asia, a region comprised of countries with some of the fastest-growing economies and densest populations in the world. With that in mind, global health concerns lie squarely in the forefront of enquiry. In particular, Bais examines Sri Lanka, Malaysia, and Singapore because of their geo-political and historical backdrops. For example, despite many similarities between Indian and Sri Lankan health systems, Sri Lanka boasts of impressive maternal mortality rates, while India struggles significantly in women's and reproductive health. In addition, Singapore, despite having splintered off from Malaysia less than sixty years ago, now has the most advanced global health standard in Asia, while Malaysia ricochets between second- and third-world status.

Bais considers how health concerns, research, and outcomes are navigated and disseminated in these countries through an intersectional analysis of ideas and actions such as freedom of press, draconian laws, and post-colonial conflict, which both aid and clamp down on global health activism.

Furthermore, Bais discusses how identity, locations of war, religion, and socio-cultural attitudes affect the priority and understanding bestowed on global health in South and Southeast Asia. She holds that addressing major global health concerns begins with realizing a significant level of peace and that interconnectedness between countries is paramount in surmounting the unprecedented level of human suffering in the 21st century.

Shufang Sun, William T. Hoyt, and Ryan P. Westergaard

Sun, Hoyt, and Westergaard discuss the human immunodeficiency virus/acquired immunodeficiency syndrome (HIV/AIDS) through the lens of minority stress theory, a theoretical perspective of understanding health-related issues among minority populations which argues that minority status as a social identity is a chronic and social stressor that causes adverse mental, behavioral, and physical health outcomes for gender, sexual, and racial minorities (e.g., Meyer, 2003).

After introducing the global HIV/AIDS epidemiology as well as the populations disproportionately affected by HIV/AIDS, the authors review the theoretical framework and offer a minority stress perspective in understanding psychosocial factors contributing to vulnerability to HIV/AIDS and treatment barriers. Finally, they provide recommendations on research investigations, health policies, and education programs targeting HIV prevention and treatment with vulnerable populations globally.

Kathy Sexton-Radek and Alissa Rubinfeld

Sexton-Radek and Alissa Rubinfeld consider a common presentation problem in the medical community: sleep disturbances. Recent evidence suggests that disruption in the sleep cycle not only negatively impacts general functioning (e.g., lower grades in school, absentees, and industrial errors), but also exacerbates medical conditions such as diabetes, cardiovascular disease, and depression. Sexton-Radek and Rubinfeld address the extent of sleep disturbances globally and indicate representative treatments aimed at reducing the impact of poor sleep quality on general functioning. They specifically focus on the prevalence of sleep disturbances by country as well as representative medical and psychological treatment interventions.

Octavio A. Santos and Caroline D. Bergeron

Santos and Bergeron consider dementia, a condition identified by the World Health Organization in 2012 as a threat to global health, affecting over 47 million people worldwide. In particular, Santos and Bergeron stress the importance of formal neuropsychological assessment in patients with suspected or known cognitive deficits for early detection, diagnosis, and treatment of mild cognitive impairment or dementia.

Santos and Bergeron address the cognitive domains frequently examined during a neuropsychological assessment of dementia, appropriate referral situations and realistic expectations of these assessments, common barriers faced by the global public health community in the utilization of neuropsychological services for dementia assessment and, finally, lifestyle changes shown to decrease the risk of developing dementia.

Steve Olweean and Myron Eshowsky

Olweean and Eshowsky discuss the Syrian crisis, and report that the damage has been catastrophic, with over half a million people seriously injured, nearly as many killed, and countless more traumatized. Over 200,000 are missing, fighting, or in detention subjected to torture. At least half of the homes are damaged, and nearly half of all Syrians displaced, the majority of whom are children and women. As refugees, they are crammed into insecure camps, dilapidated buildings, or the streets. However, psychological damage is even more severe, harder to repair, and sorely neglected. Without adequate healing, it is difficult to imagine how Syrian society can be put back together after years of hatred, violence, and profound trauma at all levels.

Olweean and Eshowsky hold that international humanitarian efforts historically tend to focus on food, shelter, and clothing. Despite widespread acknowledgement of high levels of traumatization within displaced populations in the past and present, including Syrian society, there is a lack of awareness and understanding of large-scale psychological wounds as a global health issue.

The authors determine that in the face of old, ineffective models of intervention, new models are needed for addressing communal trauma, building communal resiliency, adapting culturally specific methods for healing, local capacity building skills training at the grassroots and professional levels for treating mass traumatization, and strategic collaboration amongst humanitarian response groups.

Neena S. Jain and A. Maya Casagrande

These authors, with emBOLDen Alliances, evaluate their practice and paradigm. They hold that for international aid to deliver on the promise of supporting positive economic, social, and political change, they must reevaluate the very basic terms they use to define success and failure as well as their roles and responsibilities as students, individual donors, community members, emergency responders, and global citizens. They write that compassion alone is not enough, but compassion coupled with the power and practice of specific skills and proven models leads to meaningful, durable impact.

Part 2: Approaches and Clinical Solutions

Daria Diakonova-Curtis, Ani Kalayjian, and Loren Toussaint

These authors consider humanitarian aid approaches and methodologies. In particular, they discuss Meaningfulworld, a relief organization that has worked in over 45 countries and over 25 states in the U.S. The primary focus of Meaningfulworld is to transform trauma and promote healing through forgiveness and meaning-making, as well as empowerment and emotional intelligence (EQ) for promoting inner peace, health, well-being, and harmony. The model is utilized during workshops to promote healing in the community, transforming generational as well as individual traumas, and in so doing, building the mental health care delivery system.

Brandon A. Knettel and Shay E. Slifko

Knettel and Slifko consider the rise of community health workers (CHWs), lay people who provide basic health interventions. They outline CHW programs in three nations: a training program in Haiti, implementation in U.S. refugee communities, and the impact of a behavioral health program in Tanzania.

Haiti suffers from an extreme deficit in health care providers and infrastructure, needs that have drawn a flood of foreign aid including training programs for CHWs. Knettel and Slifko examine one such venture by a U.S.-based NGO and the pitfalls and successes of their efforts. In addition, the issue of refugee resettlement has taken center stage due to mass migrations stemming from global crises. The authors describe a group of case aids in Philadelphia tasked with assisting fellow refugees while taking their own steps toward independence. Lastly, in Tanzania, providers in a fledgling mental health system are identifying major shortcomings in behavioral health, including substance abuse, sexual violence, and serious mental illness.

Knettel and Slifko evaluate the impact of CHWs in addressing these concerns via a program aimed at educating teachers to provide basic mental health screening and counseling.

Samara Lipsky and Marissa Vishnu Mack

Lipsky and Vishnu Mack discuss a global treatment program that will utilize the biopsychosocial model to assist in the prevention of chronic diseases while promoting global health. Specifically, they address biological, psychological, and social factors that contribute to an individual's health and well-being, including smoking, alcohol consumption, nutrition, exercise, and compliance with physician orders.

Amy Nitza, Kerrie Fineran, and Lidija Hurni

Nitza, Fineran, and Hurni discuss promoting global health through counselor education. They hold that despite increasing recognition of the relationship of mental health to overall health around the world, gains in mental health have not kept pace with those in other areas of global health, particularly in lower-resource settings. Furthermore, in many of the lower-resource settings that are in greatest need of mental health support, there is a major shortage of mental health service providers as well as a shortage (or complete absence) of mental health training programs.

Counselor education programs prepare master's-level clinicians in the United States and increasingly, in other countries around the world. Nitza, Fineran, and Hurni review the current status of global mental health as it relates to the counseling profession, including the role of mental health in global health guiding documents. They also propose a set of best practices for training counselors in global mental health and give special attention to the role of cultural competence and social justice in counselor preparation.

Kenneth H. Kessler

Kessler considers post-traumatic stress disorder (PTSD) in Ugandan refugees. These refugees typically reach their would-be safe-haven without a job, knowledge of the language, or support systems. Quite often, they show symptoms of PTSD as a result of torture, rape, severe physical abuse, child abuse, or rebel wars. The lucky ones connect with NGOs that strive to help them learn skills necessary for survival and success in Uganda.

One such NGO is Hope of Children and Women Victims of Violence (HOCW). HOCW asked Rosalind Franklin University of Medicine and Science to assist them in establishing a psychologically-based treatment program for refugees with PTSD. Kessler delineates how a global health partnership can be formed between university in a first-world country and an NGO operating in a third-world country.

Kate Hudgins

Hudgins considers the Therapeutic Spiral Model (TSM), a method of experiential change to prevent and treat trauma that has been used in therapy, education, community building, and cultural activism over the past 25 years. Specifically, Hudgins describes the ways that TSM has contributed to the prevention and intervention of PTSD in global psychological health.

Adeyinka M. Akinsulure-Smith, Enyi Anosike, and Kenneth Nwaubani

These authors introduce Amaudo Itumbuazo, a community-based psychosocial service located in a rural setting in Southeast Nigeria. In a country with very limited mental health resources, Amaudo Itumbuazo is unique in the Nigerian mental health care system with regard to its community-based approach to service provision for the mentally-ill homeless.

This approach includes components of group treatment for residents and their families. Specific treatments include psychiatric care, psychotherapeutic treatments, and psychoeducation. These elements of treatment involve the residents, care providers, families, and the larger community. Amaudo Itumbuazo's integrative treatment approach draws on the critical roles of family and community within the sub-Saharan African cultural setting to provide psychosocial services.

Part 3: Approaches and Structural Solutions

Stephanie Benjamin

Benjamin considers international disaster response and the preparedness, coordination, and mobilization it requires. Specifically, Benjamin addresses the multitude of ethical issues that arise during a disaster response, such as recruitment of volunteers, safety of responders, respect for local customs, and utilizing health care providers-in-training like medical students and residents.

Benjamin also discusses how lay people and health care providers can get involved. She provides both a foundation for understanding disaster response and encouragement for individuals to involve themselves on an international level. She holds that greater understanding of these issues will lead to improved response times, minimize waste of resources, and enhance global health care outcomes for all victims and responders involved in future disasters.

Barbara Lutz and Nausheen Pasha-Zaidi

Lutz and Pasha-Zaidi discuss a rights-based curriculum for global mental health. In September 2015, mental health and substance abuse were included in the Sustainable Development Agenda adopted at the United Nations (UN) General Assembly. Thus psychological concerns will likely become part of international country development plans. The individuals and organizations involved in developing mental health across the world need to be prepared adequately for this task.

When training providers/strategists of international interventions to plan improvements in mental health with culturally different populations, it is important to acknowledge the limitations of a Western ethnocentric approach to mental health and to consider the historic context of colonialism. Mental health planners and practitioners need to sensitize themselves in their training to be collaborative and community-oriented, rather than dominant.

A rights-based approach creates a humanistic force to counterbalance the predominantly economical definition of globalization; however, the conceptual tools, research, and interventions in the field of mental health are often still lacking the cooperative orientation that is needed to collaborate effectively in addressing global concerns.

Tristan Hansell, Lisa M. Brown, and Robert Groelsema

These authors consider the role of peacebuilding interventions in global mental health. Conflict and war zones are proliferating worldwide at unprecedented rates. The resulting high rates of post-traumatic stress disorder, depression, and anxiety make it challenging to promote peace and rebuild communities. The mental health of those living in conflict and transitional societies, as well as those who are displaced, is complex as psychological health is influenced by the presence of pre-existing disorders, traumatic experiences, psychosocial stressors, and resource insufficiency.

The authors evaluate existing peace building and humanitarian aid interventions. They provide an overview of global mental health initiatives and current practices in order to illustrate both successful outcomes as well as instances where mismatches between the program goals and outcomes occurred. The authors hold that a review of effective interventions will provide insight to factors of resilience and offer examples of the potential value of mental health treatment on peace-building initiatives.

Aaron Hermann, Jenifer L. White, and Klara Lubej

These authors consider Project 1948, an arts-based international NGO specializing in photography, human rights, and global health. Project 1948 gives a camera and a voice to civil society in order to promote human rights and institutional change. Project 1948 holds that psychological principles should be paramount in the development of universal policies and procedures. Hermann, White, and Lubej provide details of the establishment of an arts-based global health NGO, specifically funding sourcing, structuring, reporting, administration, logistics, and recruitment.

Marlene J. Cohen and Joseph Martin Stevenson

Cohen and Stevenson detail the development of a technological infrastructure, the Virtual Academy for Overcoming Global Poverty (VAOGP), which allows undergraduate and graduate students and faculty to examine global poverty online, onsite, and in class. This infrastructure would facilitate online discussions between students from various countries and enable them to conduct research and to examine methods to combat poverty.

Cohen and Stevenson hold that the issues surrounding global poverty are complex and are not likely to be resolved by one field of study, one location, or one institution. Creating a space for ongoing and dynamic, open discussion about effective, efficient, and sustainable interventions will allow for greater hope in addressing this critical, societal challenge for the voiceless, marginalized, and too-often left behind around the world.

Zohray Talib and Lalit Narayan

Talib and Narayan highlight the critical role of a robust health workforce in improving health outcomes globally. They draw on historical examples where better access to health workers led to improved health outcomes in low-resource settings. They then explain why strengthening the health workforce needs to be a priority in the decade ahead, especially in light of the looming burden of non-communicable diseases.

Talib and Narayan address the specific goals for the health workforce, namely improving the number, quality, and distribution of workers to match the needs of underserved populations. They describe health care gaps and ongoing efforts and draw from personal experiences in Africa, Central Asia, and South Asia as they worked with global experts and consulted with academic training programs in low-resource settings. Talib and Narayan then reflect on the critical challenges that face the health workforce as well as potential solutions to these challenges.

Daniel Velasco

Dr. Velasco considers global health in Japan. While many countries have taken great strides to further the field of global health by promoting relevant issues and creating educational programs, others, including Japan, struggle with promotion due to issues related to ethnocentrism. Dr. Velasco explores ethnocentrism in Japan, the challenges in establishing both global health curriculums and projects in Japan's educational institutions, and ways in which Japan and other countries may overcome these challenges.

Part 4: Sustainability

Roseanne Flores, Ayorkor Gaba, Rashmi Jaipal, Nélida Quintero, and Neal Rubin

These authors consider the role of mental health in facilitating global health. At the U.N. and within the NGO and humanitarian community, the focus on mental health as a global health issue is gaining acceptance.

The authors discuss how representatives of U.N. agencies and Member States, NGOs, and businesses might best incorporate culture-specific psychological resources into their interventions and policies in order to facilitate positive outcomes. For instance, addressing health needs along with promoting emotional well-being is integral to instilling resilience following trauma. This highly integrated view of the relationship between physical health and emotional well-being is represented in the U.N. Sustainable Development Goals.

The authors' goal is to increase awareness about mental health as a global health issue and psychology's role in enhancing resilience and emotional well-being. They address topics like youth suicide, poverty, child rights, dislocation, migration, stress, and climate change.

Genomary Krigbaum, Gretchen Johnson, and Amma Boakye

These authors discuss primary care in global health as a sustainable, integrated enterprise. They address primary and family care in the U.S. and other countries. They focus on how it can benefit not only individual health, community health, and the health care system as a whole.

Kathleen B. Harrison and John A. McNulty

Harrison and McNulty consider Project Harambee, specifically its program, PLANT A SEED, GROW A DOC (PSGD). Project Harambee is an NGO working in sub-Saharan Africa to help those affected by HIV/AIDS. PSGD has a long-term goal of improving health care services to medically underserved populations.

PSGD provides contractual, medical education scholarships to deserving candidates who have lost one or both parents to HIV and are from resource-poor areas. Six years after inception there is a 100 percent success rate: seven graduates, eight current students. This represents not only preservation of indigenous human potential, but significant societal impact reducing morbidity and mortality.

Laura Reid Marks, Madeline Stenersen, and Shondolyn D. Sanders

These authors discuss global health and HIV/AIDS. HIV/AIDS has been a global epidemic for several decades. Innovative advances in treatment and research, including new medicine, technology, and an interdisciplinary approach have increased life expectancy and the quality of life for HIV-positive individuals.

However, HIV/AIDS is still a problem. This disease impacts individuals on a physical level, but also on social and emotional levels. Therefore, the authors argue that the role of psychology in ameliorating the psychosocial impact of HIV/AIDs is critical. They provide an overview of statistics related to HIV/AIDS, the role of psychologists in treatment and research, current advances and challenges in the treatment from a psychological perspective, and future directions for psychologists working in this field.

Neena S. Jain and A. Maya Casagrande

Jain and Casagrande consider sustainable humanitarian aid. Existing methods are limited in global health and humanitarian assistance. Programs are incomplete and funding is difficult to obtain, untracked, and often wasted. More importantly, locally-based solutions are often overlooked. After decades of falling short, the local, national, and international community can no longer afford to follow the old models when lives are at risk. The stakes are simply too high.

As a registered 501(c) 3 nonprofit organization, emBOLDen Alliances (eA) serves as an "incubator" of sorts for other NGOs, specifically those embedded in their own communities throughout the developing world. Through hands-on partnerships that solve operational and programmatic challenges, eA functions as a catalyst for these locally-based partners to measure and maximize impact. eA achieves this by listening, utilizing its experience in working hand-in-hand with communities, customizing tools, adapting what eA implements, and then stepping back. Ultimately, eA closes the gaps between organizations' intentions and durable, positive impact.

Efosa Guobadia

Guobadia considers the importance of sustainable change and measuring action and impact. Guobadia shares his experience as a physical therapist serving in Guatemala and how it helped him understand the necessity of sustainable, stable change so that more communities can be improved at a greater scale as often as possible.

Tiffany Masson, Alisha DeWalt, and Philip Adu

These authors provide readers with a fundamental understanding of effective ways to develop human capacity projects that empower communities and create sustainable, long-term solutions. Masson, DeWalt, and Adu discuss the intricacies involved in developing a cultural-specific model, leveraging in-country resources for sustainability, and engaging the local community for long-term positive outcomes. Through a case study of the Global HOPE (Healing Opportunities through Purposeful Engagement) Training Initiative, readers are offered an overview of the lessons challenges, and successes in launching a human capacity building project.

We hope that after reading this book you more fully understand why global health matters, and we wish you all the best in your endeavors.

References

Hancock, G. (1989). *The lords of poverty: The power, prestige, and corruption of the international aid business.* New York, NY: Atlantic Monthly Press.

Polman, L. (2010). *The crisis caravan: What's wrong with humanitarian aid?* New York, NY: Metropolitan Books.

Ramo, J.C. (2009). *The age of the unthinkable: Why the new world disorder constantly surprises us and what we can do about it.* New York, NY: Little, Brown and Company

Stout, C. E. (2008). *The new humanitarians: Inspiration, innovations, and blueprints for visionaries.* Westport, CT: Praeger.

Stout, C.E., Olweean, S.S., Wang, G.A., & Adeniji, V.O.(2015). Economies of help: The concept behind the consortium for humanitarian intervention. *International Psychology Bulletin, 19*(2), 41- 44.

VanRooyen, M. (2016). *The world's emergency room: The growing threat to doctors, nurses, and humanitarian workers.* New York: MacMillan.

PART 1

TRENDS AND BACKGROUND

CHAPTER 1

Global Mental Health: Examining Trends Globally and among Developing Regions

Lori Holleran, Maryke Van Zyl, and Bruce Bongar

Mental health, as defined by the World Health Organization (WHO), is "a state of well-being in which every individual realizes his or her own potential, can cope with the normal stresses of life, can work productively and fruitfully, and is able to make a contribution to her or his community" (WHO, 2014a, p. 1). Although traditionally, mental health has not been considered an immediate cause for concern, specifically within Low- and Middle-Income Countries (LMICs), it is increasingly receiving more attention as the extent to which people suffer from various disorders has become apparent. As such, within this chapter, we seek to quantify and analyze the burden of mental health disorders, consider the treatment gaps regarding mental health concerns, and highlight how the global community has attempted to address inadequacies related to mental illness and the challenges that still remain. These issues will largely be considered within the context of LMICs, seeing as they account for approximately 85 percent of the world's population (Jacobs, 2007, p. 1061).

Global Burden of Disease

To quantify the magnitude of mental health conditions across the world, researchers have relied on the Global Burden of Disease (GBD) Study, which examined aspects (e.g., incidence, prevalence, duration, and fatality rates) of over 100 conditions, including mental health disorders and their consequences (Murray and Lopez, 1996). The findings were used to calculate disability-adjusted life years (DALYs), a comprehensive measure of disease burden. DALYs are essentially the sum of the years of life lost

(YLL) due to premature mortality in the population and the years lived with disability (YLD) for people living with health conditions and/or their consequences (Albert, Edelstein, Anderson, Dew, & Reynolds III, 2015). Therefore, to understand the impact of mental health as compared to other diseases, or to evaluate the burdens associated with numerous mental health conditions, one can look at related DALYs.

While the GBD Study has been widely accepted as an appropriate measuring tool for determining the impact of mental and substance use disorders, the study is not without flaw in calculating the true burden. According to more recent research, the burden of mental illness is actually underestimated by more than a third using current approaches (Vigo, Thornicroft, & Atun, 2016, p. 171). Vigo and colleagues (2016) speculate that this underestimation occurs due to an:

> ...overlap between psychiatric and neurological disorders; the grouping of suicide and self-harm as a separate category; conflation of all chronic pain syndromes with musculoskeletal disorders; exclusion of personality disorders from disease burden calculations; and inadequate consideration of the contribution of severe mental illness to mortality from associated causes. (p.171)

So, as these measures allow us to consider the impact of mental health throughout the world, it must be mentioned that the true burden is likely even greater than currently identified.

Mental Health Burden

In 1996, the GBD report, which considered the present burden in 1990 and the predicted burden through 2020, was the first to recognize mental health disorders as significant contributors to global disability (Murray and Lopez, 1996). As noted in the report, and consistently recognized today, mental health was often neglected as a significant burden based on mental health conditions often leading to disability rather than to fatality. However, the GBD measure allowed for improved consideration of disability, and subsequently, for better recognition of the impact of mental disorders. Since the first report, YLDs attributed to mental disorders have increased significantly, with mental health concerns accounting for 22.9% of YLDs, representing the leading cause of global disability (Whiteford et al., 2013, p. 1579). Further, four of the top ten independent contributors to YLDs globally were mental disorders (WHO, 2001, p. 28).

When considering the overall burden associated with mental disorders, 7.4%, or 183.9 million DALYs are accounted for by mental health concerns experienced globally (Whiteford et al., 2013, p. 1579; Murray et al., 2012, p. 2203). Further, when accounting for mental, neurological, and substance use (MNS) disorders, the global burden increases, comprising 10.4% of DALYs assessed within the 2010 GBD study (Patel et al., 2016, p. 1673).

Additionally, when considering only those aged 15-49, 18.6% of DALYs were attributed to MNS disorders. While increased attention is being placed upon the impact of mental disorders, estimates predict that the global burden associated with MNS disorders will continue to grow, reaching 14.4% by 2030 (Albert et al., 2015, p. 177). This increased burden will be particularly challenging for LMICs as 75% of the burden associated with MNS disorders is experienced in these regions (WHO, 2008a, p. 2). Moreover, when considering the effect of mental disorders, it is imperative to recognize that self-harm and suicide are reported under a separate category and do not contribute to mental health-related impact findings. Here we will consider some of the independent mental health disease burden contributors.

Mood Disorders

Depression is one of the two most prevalent disorders globally and accounts for 65.5 million DALYs (Collins et al., 2011, p. 28) or 40.5% of DALYs associated with mental health concerns (Whiteford et al., 2013, p. 1575). While anxiety disorders are more commonly experienced, depression accounts for greater burden as it comprises the largest portion of MNS-related burden globally (Collins et al., 2011). Specifically within LMICs, depression accounts for 3.1% of the total burden of disease attributable to non-communicable conditions, making it the primary neuropsychiatric cause of burden of disease (Patel and Kim, 2007, p.77). Additionally, it ranks first in YLDs within LMICs (WHO, 2008b). When considering the general global burden of disease, depression is the third highest contributor (Collins et al, 2011, p. 27) and second most prominent cause of YLDs (Vos et al., 2013, p. 2163). Moreover, the WHO has predicted that depression will be the leading contributor to the global disease burden by 2030 (WHO, 2012). Furthermore, bipolar disorder comprised 14.4 million DALYs (Collins, 2011, p. 28), accounting for 7.0% of mental health related DALYs (Whiteford et al., 2013, p. 1575). While depression is seen to peak between the ages of 10-29, bipolar disorder peaks globally among individuals 25-50 years of age, presenting increased challenges during adulthood (Whiteford et al., 2013, p. 1580).

Schizophrenia

Schizophrenia is the sixth leading cause of disability associated with mental health disorders (Whiteford et al., 2013, p. 1582), contributing to 16.8 million DALYs (Collins et al., 2011, p. 28). This represents 7.4% of the mental health-related DALYs (Whiteford et al., 2013, p. 1575). Specifically within LMICs, schizophrenia accounts for 14.8 million YLDs (WHO, 2008b, p. 37). The finding that individuals are likely to experience a gap of two years between their first episode of psychosis and receiving treatment

(Large, Farooq, Nielssen, & Slade, 2008) may be one potential factor contributing to the YLDs within these regions. Further, when considering YLDs, schizophrenia has been found to rank below other conditions, such as depression and substance use disorders (Whiteford et al., 2013); however, this should be recognized as an outcome of its low prevalence rather than an indicator of the burden placed among those suffering from schizophrenia as it assumes the greatest disability weight of all mental health concerns.

Substance Use Disorders

Alcohol use disorders accounted for 23.7 million DALYs globally, while drug use disorders comprised 8.4 million (Collins et al., 2011, p. 28). This represents 9.6%, and 10.9% of the burden attributed to mental health disorders, respectively (Whiteford et al., 2013, p. 1575). The burden associated with drug use was most prominent for those 15-29 years of age, while those 25-50 years old experienced the greatest alcohol use-related burden. While mental health concerns are often considered based on their influence on YLDs, substance use disorders contributed to approximately 7 million YLLs, 81.1% of all YLLs associated with mental health disorders (Whiteford et al., 2013, p. 1580).

It is apparent that mental illness is a significant contributor to the global burden of disease, which is not expected to diminish without intervention; however, it is also imprudent to consider mental health in a discrete manner. To fully understand the impact of mental health, one must also consider the relationship between mental health and physical health concerns.

Comorbidity

One of the many challenges present when attempting to address mental health concerns is their multidimensional relationship with physical health issues. However, it is known that suffering from a mental health condition increases one's risk for both communicable and non-communicable diseases (Prince et al., 2007). Further, experiencing physical health conditions may foster the development of mental health issues.

This latter point is illustrated in findings highlighting that depression is substantially more likely to present amongst those experiencing a medical condition than those without (Moussavi et al., 2007). Additionally, when considering those diagnosed with HIV/AIDS, mental health disorders are significantly more prevalent compared to the general population (WHO, 2008c). Yet, when an individual presents with a subsequent mental health concern, it is often not provided the same attention as their physical conditions motivate (Prince et al., 2007). However, mental health issues may worsen treatment adherence and reduce help-seeking behaviors (Prince et al., 2007), illustrating the importance of attending to mental health issues even when seemingly more important physical concerns are present.

Additionally, the presence of a mental health condition heightens the risk of experiencing a comorbid physical condition. Mental illness increases the chance that the individual will suffer from an additional chronic illness (Ngo et al., 2013) as early-onset mental conditions increase one's risk for a multitude of physical conditions (Kessler et al., 2009). Mental health issues have been found to increase rates for HIV/AIDS (WHO, 2008c), cardiovascular disease, diabetes (Prince et al., 2007; Rehm et al., 2006), cirrhosis of the liver (Rehm et al., 2006), tuberculosis, and cancer (Prince et al., 2007). Further, having comorbid psychological and physical disorders often impairs the ability of the individual to manage both illnesses effectively, leading to increased treatment costs (Naylor et al., 2012). Specifically amongst those with a mental illness and another chronic condition, costs were seen to increase by 45% (Naylor et al., 2012, p. 1). This is particularly concerning because (as we have seen) mental health issues can independently diminish help-seeking behaviors, and because 60% of excess mortality amongst those suffering with serious mental illness is attributed to physical conditions (Brown, 1997, p. 506).

Further, initial mental health conditions can motivate other mental health conditions such as depression, substance abuse, and intentional injuries (Rehm et al., 2006). Specifically within LMICs, where over three-quarters of individuals suffering from serious mental illnesses do not receive regular treatment, suicide has been recognized as an aftereffect of poorly addressed mental health issues (Chisholm, Sanderson, Ayuso-Mateos, & Saxena, 2004; Chisholm, Van Ommeren, Ayuso-Mateos, & Saxena, 2005). While depression is recognized as a potential suicide risk factor in higher-income countries, impulse-related difficulties are more predictive in LMICs (Nock, 2008). This highlights how a broad spectrum of mental health concerns may increase risk for suicide in those regions. It also presents a sequela that can be targeted with the aim of saving a substantial number of lives as 75% of the suicides globally occur within LMICs (Vijayakumar, Phillips, Silverman, Gunnell, & Carli, 2015, p. 163).

Ultimately, we recognize that MNS disorders present tremendous burdens across the globe, and that experiencing a mental disorder increases risk for subsequent physical and additional mental health concerns. Additionally, suffering from a mental health condition is reportedly experienced as more severely disabling than any comorbid physical conditions (Ormel et al., 2008) and decreases health-engagement and medical treatment compliance (Ngo et al., 2013), subsequently worsening overall health outcomes (Naylor et al., 2012). However, for mental health conditions and their sequelae to be adequately addressed, nations must recognize the economic value in such an investment.

Mental Health Economics

Even with mental disorders accounting for 7.4% of the global burden (Whiteford et al., 2013, p. 1579; Murray et al., 2012, p. 2203), LMICs overwhelmingly fail to allocate the necessary budgeting to effectively treat and attend to these issues. Considering that 75% of GBD due to MNS disorders is associated with LMICs (WHO, 2008a, p. 2), it is concerning that just 1% of the average health budget in LMICs is designated for mental health, and nearly half of all LMICs spend less than 1% of their health budget on mental health (WHO, 2005, p. 25). More specifically, low-income countries spend approximately 0.5% of their health budget on mental health-related spending, while lower-middle income countries, on average, spend 1.9% (WHO, 2011, p. 27). According to the WHO, there is a 200-fold difference in mental health expenditures between High-Income Countries (HICs) and LMICs (WHO, 2011, p. 25). Moreover, while over 80% of the world's population resides within LMICs, these countries use less than 20% of global mental health resources (Patel and Prince, 2010, p. 1976). These findings illustrate the need for increased and more equitable allocation of financial resources toward mental health, specifically within LMICs.

Cost of Inaction

The global economic burden caused by mental disorders ranked among the top ten non-communicable diseases (Collins et al., 2011) and exceeded the economic burden of diabetes, cancer, and cardiovascular diseases (Bloom et al., 2011). Additionally, when examining how health conditions impact one's daily functioning by comparing the ten most commonly occurring physical and mental conditions, it was found that in 84% of the comparisons, mental health conditions were endorsed as more impairing (Kessler et al., 2009, p. 8). Impairment experienced due to mental illness is often illustrated through absence from regular daily activities and subsequent reduced productivity. While days "out of role" have been most extensively examined within the U.S., it was projected that one-third of days missed (or billions of work days per year) within the country were due to mental health issues, with estimates of similar findings expected in other countries. When considering production levels, mental health concerns as innocuous as mild depression have been found to decrease rate of output by 30% (Lo Sasso, Rost, & Beck, 2006, p. 1149). Taking into account the effects of depression and anxiety on global productivity, it is estimated that approximately $1 trillion is lost annually (Chisholm et al., 2016, p. 419). These economic costs are expected to continue to grow over the coming decades, with mental disorders projected to contribute over half of the global economic burden associated with ten non-communicable diseases (Lo Sasso et al., 2006).

Unfortunately, the economic burden related to mental disorders reaches beyond days out of role and also reduces productivity in influencing families and communities (Collins et al., 2011). Existing literature provides multiple global examples of the cyclical relationship between mental illness and poverty. Mothers who experience maternal depression are at significantly increased risk to give birth to children who suffer developmental, emotional, and behavioral challenges (Ramchandani, Richter, Norris, & Stein, 2010; Patel, DeSouza, & Rodrigues, 2003; Koutra et al., 2013). Since it is difficult to grasp the cost of mental illness on families and communities, one of the ways that the impact can be estimated is by considering that most mental illnesses begin during childhood and young adulthood – precisely when impairment severely impacts an individual's ability to become educated and build a foundation for a career (Patel, 2007). The economic and social impact on the community of losing the productivity of these individuals due to mental illness is assumed to contribute to greater systemic strain.

Cost of Action

Adequately addressing global mental health needs requires increased resources, including both financial and improved human and governmental support. Within LMICs, there is a paucity of trained mental health workers. Estimates recognize a workforce shortage of over 1 million individuals (Kakuma et al., 2011, p. 1655). This creates a situation where the majority of those with mental health concerns go without treatment (Whiteford et al., 2013), with rates increasing up to 85% when broadening the category to consider individuals dealing with MNS disorders (Patel et al, 2010, p. 169). Yet this inadequate response is unlikely to change without governmental support. Of reporting WHO Member States, 68% have specific mental health policies, but only 15% endorse their full implementation (WHO, 2014b, p. 23). Further, 51% of responding countries recognized the presence of mental health legislation within their nation (WHO, 2014b, p. 26). When considered more closely, many of the implemented policies and laws fail to meet international human rights benchmarks. While introducing or revising these plans will likely require coordinated governmental efforts, the potential impact is arguably expansive.

Beyond enhancing national regulations and support for mental health, increased financial allocation is critical to improving care and reducing the associated burdens. Fortunately, it is also easier to assess the specific costs associated with this action. Numerous studies have considered the cost of introducing effective interventions within LMICs. Offering treatment for common mood and anxiety disorders was found to cost less than an average annual income for each DALY prevented, which is considered highly cost-effective (WHO, 2006). To adequately address 80% of the global instances of depression and anxiety, it is projected to cost $147 billion between 2016 and 2030 (Chisholm et al., 2016, p. 421). Further, even though treatment for serious mental illnesses is typically more intensive as it often requires psychopharmacotherapy, it was also found to be cost-effective, with each DALY averted requiring an investment of less than three times the average annual income (WHO, 2006). While examination of cost-effectiveness has mainly occurred with regard to depression and anxiety, the benefit-to-cost ratio, when accounting for increased productivity and improved health, ranges between 3.3-5.7 (Chisholm et al., 2016, p. 420). When considered conservatively, that illustrates a $4.00 return for every $1.00 invested. However, recognizing that investing in mental health treatment makes economic sense does not inevitably transition into improved intervention. This fact is felt acutely in LMICs.

Mental Health Treatment Gap

Mental illness, particularly depression, has frequently been viewed as an illness of affluence, implying that communities with fewer resources are too concerned with basic survival to experience mental illness to the degree that individuals in higher-income communities do (Koplewicz, Gurian, & Williams, 2009). This sentiment has been largely refuted with a relatively recent surge in cross-cultural research focusing on mental health in a range of communities with different incomes, geographic locations, and cultural backgrounds (Patel, Price, 2010). Any notion that mental illness is a Western problem has been rebutted by research showing the prevalence and impact of mental illness in LMICs.

The mental health treatment gap can be defined as the difference between the prevalence of a disorder and the number of individuals receiving treatment for that disorder, expressed as the percentage of individuals who require care but do not receive treatment (Kohn, Saxena, Levav, & Saraceno, 2004). The treatment gap has proven to be difficult to measure since it is challenging to estimate the prevalence of a disorder for which treatment is not being received. Said differently, when communities are not being provided any form of treatment, their disorders go undiagnosed, making it seemingly impossible to accurately report the prevalence of mental health disorders within those regions. Moreover, Kohn et al. (2004) point out that estimating the treatment gap involves understanding the time frame of service utilization, the prevalence period, and how representative the sample is of the population, all of which is challenging information to gather when basic mental health care needs are not being met in most of the world.

Global Gap between Disorders

The realization that mental illness has a global impact is gaining traction. This is evidenced by the growing focus on mental illness by the WHO, with the publication of the Mental Health Report in 2001 and the development of organizations like the Lancet Global Mental Health Group, which played an important part in the study and dissemination of information about global mental health (Patel, & Prince, 2010). One striking finding discussed earlier is that four of the top ten YLD contributors, according to the WHO's GBD report, were mental disorders (World Health Organization, 2001). However, while research has recognized the presence of mental illness in LMICs, the provision of mental health treatment continues to lag behind. Subsequently, there is a clear discrepancy between the varying degrees of prevalence and treatment for different disorders.

Mood Disorders

The estimated global median rate of untreated depression and dysthymia were calculated to be 53.9% and 53.5% respectively, and untreated bipolar disorders projected at 48.9% (Kohn et al., 2004, p. 861). The treatment gap for mood disorders varies between countries. For example, the United Kingdom indicates an estimated 83.9% gap for depression, compared to a 40.7% gap in the United States (Kohn et al., 2004, p. 861). This gap persists (but with a different trend) when considering the treatment gap for bipolar disorders across larger regions, with an estimated 60.2% treatment gap in the Americas, compared to a 39.9% gap in Europe (Kohn et al., 2004, p. 862).

It has been argued that with the increased use of effective antidepressants, the treatment gap associated with mood disorders (as compared between HICs and LMICs) would continue to grow (Padmavathi, Rajkumar & Srinivasan, 1998). Specifically, this growth would be motivated by a decreasing gap within HICs due to psychopharmacotherapy and a presumably unaffected gap within LMICs due to lack of availability and accessibility. In support of this assumption, Kohn et al., (2004) compare the availability of mood stabilizing medications according to the proportion of the population in each region for which primary care physicians have access to these medications. A 95.3% availability rate was identified within the Americas, compared 48.1% in Africa, which highlights critical availability concerns (Kohn et al., 2004, p. 863).

Schizophrenia and Related Psychotic Disorders

In an estimate of the global extent of the treatment gap, schizophrenia and non-mood dependent psychoses were calculated to account for 31.1% of this gap (Kohn et al., 2004, p. 861). The treatment gap for schizophrenia and related psychotic disorders was found to vary by country, as illustrated by a 5.9% gap amongst Israeli Jews, compared to a 61.5% gap amongst 21-

year old New Zealanders (Kohn et al., 2004, p. 859). In a study of treatment for different diagnoses in Belize, researchers found that 63% of individuals with schizophrenia had gone untreated (Lehtinen et al., 1990 in Kohn et al., 2004, p. 11). In sub-Saharan Africa the treatment gap for schizophrenia and other psychoses is estimated to exceed 90%, with less than 10% receiving treatment (Kebede et al., 2003, p. 627). Globally, it is estimated that one-third of individuals suffering from Schizophrenia remain untreated (Kohn et al., 2004, p. 861).

Anxiety and Related Disorders

The estimated global gap in the treatment of anxiety disorders appears to be similar for panic disorder, generalized anxiety disorder, and obsessive-compulsive disorder (OCD) (50.6%, 56.1% and 52.8% respectively) (Kohn et al., 2004, p. 861). Increased variability exists in the treatment gap when considering specific regions, with a 66.7% gap for panic disorder in Western Pacific regions (including China, Japan, New Zealand, and Australia), compared to a 47.2% gap in Europe (Kohn et al., 2004, p. 862). Differences persist when considering specific countries, with an estimated gap of 72% in the U.K. and 41.2% in the U.S. (Kohn et al., 2004, p. 861). When examining the treatment gap with regard to OCD, starker differences present, with an 82% gap within the Americas and a 24.6% gap in Europe (Kohn et al., 2004, p. 862). However, this may highlight increasing treatment discrepancies between regions within the Americas, as a treatment gap of 99% was recognized within Belize when considering general anxiety disorders (Lehtinen et al., 1990 in Kohn et al., 2004, p. 11).

Substance Use Disorders

It is estimated that 76.3 million individuals globally are diagnosed with alcohol use disorders and 15.3 million are diagnosed with disorders related to drug use (WHO, 2003, p. 22). Alcohol abuse and dependence had the largest estimated global treatment gap of 76.2% (Kohn et al., 2004, p. 861). In a comparison of the treatment gap for alcohol abuse and dependence by region, the estimated gap in Europe was found to be 92.4% compared to 71.6% in Western Pacific regions (Kohn et al., 2004, p. 862). Of note, both the U.K. and Mexico City demonstrated relatively high treatment gaps for alcohol abuse and dependence (estimated at 96%). Young Jewish adults residing in Israel demonstrated the smallest gap (exhibited at 49.4%) (Kohn et al., 2004, p. 859).

Comorbid Disorders

The treatment gap between specific disorders may be grossly underestimated, not only due to the lack accurate diagnosis, but because comorbid disorders are not accounted for in most studies of service utilization (Kohn et al., 2004). One study that looked specifically at the cost of comorbid illness found that for each person with a comorbid mental disorder and other chronic condition, treatment costs increased by 45% (Naylor et al., 2012, p. 11). There are arguably numerous factors that complicate treatment amongst individuals with comorbid disorders, but for those with a medical disorder, having an additional psychological diagnosis often impairs their ability to manage both illnesses effectively, which often leads to increased costs.

Gap between HICs and LMICs

Another gap discussed is the treatment differential between HICs and LMICs. This differential refers to the disparity in the treatment gap between HICs and LMICs. The World Health Organization's Mental Health Atlas (2003, p. 5) found that although the majority of the global burden of mental illness is centralized in LMICs, 90% of the world's mental health resources are located in HICs. More than 80% of the world's population resides in LMICs, but these countries use less than 20% of global mental health resources (Saxena, Thornicroft, Knapp, Whiteford, 2007 in Patel & Prince, 2010, p. 1). The discrepancy in treatment gap between HICs and LMICs was illustrated by the WHO (2003, p. 5), which found a treatment gap of between 44% and 70% in HICs, but up to 90% in LMICs. The gap in treatment of general mental health conditions is believed to exceed 75% in most of the world (Kohn et al., 2004 in Patel et al., 2011, p. 523) and increases to as high as 90% in some of the lowest-income countries (Alem et al., 2009, p. 651).

The discrepancy between treatment availability in HICs and LMICs becomes more apparent when one compares the number of psychiatrists in a given region. In the U.S., an estimated 50,000 psychiatrists serve a population of approximately 300 million, while in India, an estimated 4,000 psychiatrists provide for a population of over one billion (Patel, 2012, p. 8). In Africa, there are approximately 1,800 psychiatrists for 702 million people, compared to 89,000 psychiatrists in Europe for 879 million people (World Health Organization, 2005, p. 33). Further, in Tanzania, a country with a population of more than 49 million, there are only 19 psychiatrists, or 0.4 per 100,000 (African Psychological Association, 2013, p. 12). In rural South Africa, there is one psychiatrist for up to five million residents, or 0.28 per 100,000 (WHO, 2007, p. 18). The median rate of psychiatrists in LMICs is 0.05 per 100,000; however, it is 8.59 per 100,000 in HICs (WHO, 2011, p. 56). It is estimated that there are more psychiatrists in the U.S. than there are in India, China, and the entire continent of Africa combined (Patel & Thornicroft, 2009). Despite the greater population size in LMICs, community mental health care facilities are found in 51.7% of LMICs as opposed to 97.4% of HICs (WHO, 2005, p. 17).

Contributors to the Mental Health Gap

Some of the barriers to treatment commonly cited in the literature include inadequate access to care, limited resources, sparse research, cultural norms and stigma, and lack of mental health education. Direct barriers to care include limited resources and inadequate access to care, potentially experienced as lack of financial resources needed to obtain treatment, limited availability of mental health care, and inaccessibility of treatment (e.g., time and distance constraints; Cooper & Sartorius, 1996). Further, the lack of knowledge about mental disorders may translate to individuals not seeking help because they either do not acknowledge that they have a problem, or they believe that the problem will go away by itself, that they can deal with it on their own, or that treatment will be ineffective (Katz et al., 1997).

Culture and Stigma

Cultural norms and beliefs often influence if, how, and when help is sought. Stigma has been found to have a direct effect on the psyche of the person suffering from a mental illness in terms of personal acceptance or rejection, willingness to seek treatment, and feelings of self-worth and self-efficacy (Evans-Lacko, Rose, Henderson, Thornicroft, 2010). Stigma related to mental disorders often leads to under-reporting, especially in smaller rural communities where individuals experience a legitimate fear that they will be ostracized if others learn of their diagnosis (Patel, 2007). Health care providers often perpetuate stigma due to the grossly inadequate mental health training for health care providers in both LMICs and HICs (Patel, 2007).

Stigma refers to the attitudes towards individuals suffering from mental illness and those who treat them as well as the lack of governmental action. As mentioned earlier, there are very few LMIC governments that allocate any of their budgets towards mental health care (Patel, 2012), indicating that mental health is not viewed as a worthy expense. Individuals working in the mental health field often experience similar discrimination to those who suffer from mental illness. As a result, mental health professionals often become disengaged from the mental health community (Patel, 2012), which leads to a lack of providers advocating for adequate care and, ultimately, to a dearth of systemic responses aimed at addressing mental health issues.

In order to effectively address stigma, one must understand what leads to stigma and what beliefs or values lie at the core of stigma. Through their research, Pescosolido, Medina, Martin, and Long (2013) distinguished between two core causes of stigma, including lack of knowledge (ignorance or misinformation) and prejudice (rejection or devaluation). The authors dispelled the notion that increased education alone would necessarily decrease stigma. In fact, they found that the majority of the public has accepted that mental illness lies in the same realm as other illnesses and does not imply moral failure or individual weakness (Pescosolido et al., 2013). Further, while it appears as though awareness campaigns have been successful in informing public perception about the pathology of mental illness and has normalized mental illness to an extent, previously overt stigmatization may have only transitioned into implicit and more subtle prejudice (Pescosolido et al., 2013). While many communities now intellectually understand mental illness, they do not yet seem to trust individuals suffering from mental illness, know how to act around them, or want them in close proximity (Pescosolido et al., 2013). Consequently, it may then be wise to shift the focus of educational campaigns towards inclusion.

Research

While research in global mental health has been growing, there still exists a prominent research gap, with the majority of mental health research being done in Europe and North America. According to a study published in 2001, 94% of psychiatric journals publish articles concerning only 10% of the world's population, and the remaining 90% of the population is represented in 6% of psychiatric journals (Becker & Kleinman, 2012, p. 3). This illustrates how underrepresented the majority of the world is in psychiatric research and is further evidenced by the diagnostic categories and treatments generally offered, which are primarily based on Western populations (Knapp et al., 2006). Research conducted predominantly within Western populations may not be generalizable to populations with different religious and cultural beliefs or distinct political and economic circumstances.

In addition to the complications with generalizability of research, mental health care providers and clinical decision makers may not have access to the relevant research (Knapp et al., 2006). In many developing countries, clinicians often have nothing more to inform their clinical decisions than outdated textbooks (Soltani et al. 2004), which increases the likelihood of using ineffective or outdated therapeutic and medical interventions. As a result, service providers may allow their decisions to be informed by opinion, rather than evidence, thereby further contributing to misconceptions and stigma. Not only does this lack of evidence present challenges to clinical decision makers, but the lack of epidemiological data limits the ability of policy makers and those responsible for resource distribution to allocate resources according to the actual need of the population (Knapp et al., 2006).

Resources

The WHO World Mental Health Survey Consortium (2004) has found reason to believe that the mental health treatment gap is not merely due to a lack of resources but also a misallocation of resources. The WHO reported that across most of the countries considered, the majority of people in treatment were sub-threshold cases, while those with serious disorders were going untreated. In addition to the misallocation of resources, mental health resources are often centralized in institutions, rather than in communities (Knapp et al., 2006). When these resources are allocated to institutions over community programs, individuals and communities who have limited access to care are unable to engage with, and ultimately benefit from, this support. As a result, individuals who live in these underserved communities are often forced to remove themselves from their communities and families in order to benefit from these institutionalized mental health resources (Knapp et al., 2006).

Moreover, since resources are often centralized in institutions, skilled workers are scarcely found outside of these institutions. Not only are skilled workers generally financially unable to provide mental health resources in communities with limited access to institutions, but there is often a paucity of skilled workers in LMICs due to mass migration to countries able to offer higher salaries and better opportunities (Knapp et al., 2006). While policy change and increased funding have long been the focus of community advocates in underserved communities, the daunting task of systemic change and resource development has been slow and arduous. Recently, research has recognized effective programs in which non-specialist health care workers and lay community members deliver psychological treatment in a stepped-care approach that is both evidence-based and culturally sensitive (Lancet Global Mental Health Group, 2007).

Access

The scarcity of mental health care workers is often overlooked. It is estimated that only 51% of LMICs have access to community health care facilities, compared to 97.4% of HICs (Mental Health Atlas, 2005, p. 17). In LMICs, individuals tend to seek treatment from primary care doctors, either due to the stigma associated with, or limited access to, mental health care. Primary care doctors are often constrained by time and resources, which leads to low recognition rates of mental illness, misdiagnosis based on somatic symptoms, and inadequate use of medication (Patel, 2007). Primary care physicians are generally not trained to consider the social determinants of mental disorders and how these may affect a patient's presentation and treatment. Furthermore, they may not have access to updated mental health information regarding evidence-based interventions and medications (Patel, 2007). In many rural settings with limited resources, physicians are often faced with addressing mental illnesses that they have not been trained in – a problem that is exacerbated by a lack of access to evidence-based treatments (Patel, Chowdhary, Rahman, & Verdeli, 2011).

Global Goals in Mental Health

Goals towards the improvement of global mental health have evolved and gained support since the new millennium. This evolution can be seen in both the U.N., which progressed from the Millennium Development Goals in 2000 to the Sustainable Development Goals in 2015 with an increased focus on mental health, and the WHO, which advanced from the World Mental Health Report in 2001 to their operationalized Mental Health Gap Action Program in 2008. These developments illustrate how leading global organizations have been increasing their focus on mental health. Moreover, organizations such as the Lancet Series on Global Mental Health, the Movement for Global Mental Health, and the Programme for Improving Mental Health Care have been driving relevant research, developing programs for change, and working towards the goals set forth by the global mental health community.

Millennium Development Goals

In 2000, the U.N. put forth a list of eight global goals to be met by 2015. These Millennium Development Goals (MDG's) did not explicitly address non-communicable diseases, particularly mental illness, an oversight which was met with disdain from some in the mental health community (Miranda & Patel, 2006). However, others believed that disparities in mental illness were indirectly addressed by the MDGs, specifically through goals related to eradicating hunger and poverty (Sachs & Sachs, 2007).

WHO World Mental Health Report

In a significant step towards global mental health, the WHO released its Mental Health Report in 2001. In this report, the WHO highlighted the global mental health gap, or what it saw as perpetuating the problem, and provided suggestions for bridging the gap in mental health globally (WHO, 2001). The report argued for deinstitutionalization and increased utilization of community-based services, with specific recommendations for action, including increasing access to care, augmenting supportive structures, improving interdisciplinary relationships, advocating for policy change and education, as well as training health professionals.

The WHO World Mental Health Report (2001) promoted implementing a holistic approach to bridging the global mental health gap. The promotion included providing mental health treatment in primary care, offering care within the community, increasing availability of psychiatric medication, educating the public, involving the family and the community in patient care, monitoring community health, integrating other sectors, supporting more research, and establishing national policies and legislation.

This report by the WHO is viewed as a pivotal point in the development of global mental health as it lays the ground work for future developments in global mental health (Patel & Prince, 2010; Collins et al., 2013; Kohn et al., 2004).

The Lancet Series on Global Mental Health

The Lancet Series on Global Mental Health consists of two series of publications, the first published in 2007, and the most recent published in 2011 (Patel, Garrison, et al., 2008).

2007 Series

The initial series concluded with a call to action from the Lancet group, which has been credited for the genesis of several new organizations and services (Patel, Garrison, et al., 2008). The first article in the 2007 series advocated for the inclusion of mental health care in existing health care settings, asserting that there is "no health without mental health" (Prince et al., 2007). The second article highlighted the inequity of resources between LMICs and HICs, while discussing barriers to resource provision and advocating the reallocation of resources (Saxena, Thornicroft, Knapp, & Whiteford, 2007). The next addition to the series outlined strategies for the prevention and treatment of mental illness in LMIC. It advocated the use of low-cost antidepressants and community-based rehabilitation models as psychological intervention (Patel et al., 2007). The final three articles in the initial series looked at developments in global mental health to date and provided an overview of remaining barriers to bridging the global mental health gap. It ended with a call to action for governments, multilateral agencies, and stakeholders to increase resources, research, and affect policy change (Jacob et al., 2007; Saraceno et al., 2007; Lancet, 2007).

2011 Series

The first two articles of the second series examined improved economic outcomes associated with mental health interventions (Lund et al., 2011) as well as mental health needs of children and adolescents in LMICs, including disorder prevalence rates and risk and protective factors (Kieling et al., 2011), respectively. In the third article, authors conducted a meta-analysis to determine the evidence base of, funding for, and integration of psychological interventions and then offered recommendations for mental health and psychological support implementation (Tol et al., 2011). The next article explored the scalability of mental health treatment in order to decrease the treatment gap and provided an overview of barriers and recommendations for developing feasible mental health services (Eaton et al., 2011). Following the WHO's 2006 focus on the shortage of health workers globally, the authors of the penultimate article reviewed the deficient state of human resources and illustrated how implementing task shifting could effectively address this inadequacy (Kakuma et al., 2011). The final article in the second series served to emphasize the critical costs associated with the global mental health gap by highlighting the human rights violations suffered by individuals in LMICs experiencing mental illness (Drew et al., 20110).

Movement for Global Mental Health

One of the organizations that credits its inception to the 2007 Lancet Series is the Movement for Global Mental Health (MGMH), which aims to improve access to mental health care in LMICs, increase scientific evidence, and protect human rights (MGMH, 2016). Members of the MGMH collaborated to contribute to the second Lancet series published in 2011 (MGMH, 2016). The MGMH has been instrumental in the growth of the study of global mental health as evidenced by its various publications, international bi-annual summits, and membership represented in more than 200 institutions (MGMH, 2016, para. 3). In fact, following a lecture series on cognitive decline in Ujjain, Nasik, Haridwar and Prayag, India, there was a significant decrease in lost or abandoned older adults diagnosed with dementia (Kardile, 2015).

WHO Mental Health Gap Action Program

The WHO Mental Health Gap Action Programme (mhGAP) was developed in 2008 as an extension of the WHO Mental Health Global Action Programme, which was presented in 2002 at the World Health Assembly (WHO, 2008). The mhGAP was developed in an effort to address the chasm in global mental health and outlined evidence based interventions, identified countries in need of additional support, highlighted barriers to the development of mental health services, and put forth a robust action plan for the treatment of mental, neurological, and substance use disorders globally (WHO, 2008). The mhGAP has been implemented and evaluated in various countries, with generally positive outcomes. One such study, which was conducted with primary health care physicians in the Sudan, showed a positive impact on knowledge of and attitudes towards mental illness and emphasized the importance of extensive training and supervision (Ali, Saeed, & Hughes, 2012). A study conducted in Nepal showed modest success; however, it recommended that the protocol be translated and adapted for cultural differences prior to implementation (Richards, 2016). While mhGAP was received with widespread support and enthusiasm, it requires more extensive empirical evaluation to fully understand its utility (Becker & Kleinman, 2013).

The Programme for Improving Mental Health Care

The Programme for Improving Mental Health Care (PRIME), developed in 2011, is an example of an organization that is implementing and evaluating the guidelines set forth by mhGAP with the hopes of improving treatment coverage for mental illness in underserved communities (Lund et al., 2012). PRIME spans five countries in Africa and Asia and partners with the WHO as well as the U.K. government's Department for International Development (Lund et al., 2012). The hope of PRIME is to answer the call for increased access to mental health care and increased research in LMICs, specifically as it relates to the efficacy of mhGAP (Lund et al., 2012). Consistent with the ideals originally outlined in the Lancet series (Patel et al., 2007), PRIME intends to empower health care practitioners (Lund et al., 2012), and therefore the community at large, to deliver mental health services and take ownership of their well-being.

Sustainable Development Goals

In an effort to sustain and expand upon the MDG's of 2000, the U.N. presented a list of 17 Sustainable Development Goals (SDGs) to be met by 2030 (UN, 2015). Specifically, these SDG's resolve to reduce premature mortality related to non-communicable diseases by one third, to "promote mental health and well-being," and to improve the prevention and treatment of substance abuse (UN, 2015, p. 9). The inclusion of non-communicable diseases and the explicit mention of mental health implies that mental health, well-being, and the prevention and treatment of substance abuse are becoming a higher priority in the agenda of global development (WHO, 2016).

Lessons Learned

Recent research, including reports from the WHO, recommend a systemic approach beyond advocating for additional resources in order to reduce the deficits and inequities in mental health care globally (Becker, & Kleinman, 2012). Four significant elements to be incorporated to bridge global mental health care include improving access to evidence-based care, training and supervising lay community members and health care workers, employing task shifting, and integration (Van Ginneken et al., 2013). This approach would require robust empirical research aimed at increased understanding of local communities as well as incorporating known evidence-based psychotherapeutic treatments and medication.

Evidence-Based Care

Rather than accepting that there are not enough resources to provide effective treatment for current global mental health needs, we need to understand why there is a paucity of resources, what the barriers are to improving these discrepancies, and how to competently overcome these barriers in order to adequately bridge the global mental health gap (Saraceno, 2007). Globally, we must focus on expanding culturally appropriate research and introducing evidence-based care to more effectively address mental health concerns.

In order to move from theoretical goals to global implementation, the data in support of task shifting in mental health care should be increased across diverse settings (Eaton, McCay, Semrau, et al., 2011). Task shifting is still a relatively new idea (WHO, 2006b) and must be supported by evidence in order to gain the support necessary for implementation in diverse communities with high need and limited resources. Along with research to support task shifting, empirical data is needed on the adaptation and evaluation of models used for the training of lay health workers (Lewin, Dick, Pond, et al., 2005). Continued support and implementation of training models to be used with lay health workers depends on evidence showing its efficacy as well as evaluating the need for adaptation of these models.

Before any training program is initiated, research must guide the strategic planning and implementation of the program (Thornicroft, Cooper, Van Bortel, Kakuma, & Lund, 2012). A thorough understanding of the population, possible barriers, and common pitfalls experienced by similar programs would be required for efficient policy and planning prior to the implementation of a program. Similarly, screenings and assessments of the program as well as the population being served should be informed by research to ensure that it is culturally appropriate for use in the particular population (Collins, Pate, Joestl, March, Insel, Daar, 2011).

Training

Recently, research has begun to focus more specifically on how training and education can improve the provision of mental health care. For example, a study conducted in Soweto, South Africa showed that when primary care nurses were trained to discriminate between dementia and delirium, they were able to accurately refer cases of delirium to acute care, thereby preventing these cases from going untreated (Prince & Trebilco, 2005). In the West African country of Guinea-Bissau, four hours of basic training provided to primary health care workers increased their ability to correctly diagnose mental disorders by 40%. Furthermore, their ability to deliver appropriate prescription of medication for these disorders increased from 0% to 75%. This supports the sentiment that mental health service delivery could be greatly enhanced for minimal cost. It was estimated that 50 residents of Guinea-Bissau could be served for every dollar spent (De Jong, 1996, p. 98).

Another study assessed the outcome of increasing education on mental health in schools in Rawalpindi, Pakistan. This initiative increased the use of antenatal clinics, rates of immunization, use of primary health care, and detection of mental health problems (Rahman, Mubbashar, Gater, & Goldberg, 1998). As a result, the Pakistani government assigned specific funding for mental health care. Furthermore, in the Ugandan provinces of Masaka and Rakai, a study was conducted in which community members with no prior mental health education were intensively trained for two weeks to lead group psychotherapy with individuals of similar cultural background diagnosed with Major Depressive Disorder. This program decreased depression to 6.5%, compared to over 50% in the control group – an effect that was sustained at 6-month follow-up (Bass et al., 2006, p. 569).

The limited resources in LMICs call for innovative approaches to training non-specialist health care workers. Trained mental health specialists would have to be prepared to teach what they have learned and provide consultation and supervision throughout the process to ensure that mental health interventions and assessments are practiced to a high standard of care. Above the anticipated financial and human resource benefits and increased access to care, training health workers as well as lay community members may provide the opportunity for mental health care to be combined with the existing indigenous responses that are culturally accepted and effective in their own way (McKenzie et al. 2004). Training must then incorporate the culture in which it will be practiced in order to maximize its potential use and efficiency.

Task Shifting

Task shifting refers to an approach to increasing health care resources in which tasks are redistributed among health care teams in order to address the shortage of specialist health care providers (Patel, 2012). This approach has been growing in popularity since the 2006 World Health Report advocated for the systematic delegation of specialized health care to less-specialized health care teams as well as for increased community involvement and patient self-management (WHO, 2006b). While enhancing the skills and resources of existing health care providers would be vital to bridging the global mental health gap, it is also important to realize that this strategy may still not be enough with an already-taxed global health care system.

Existing mental health care professionals would practice task shifting by taking on the vital role of training and supervising less-specialized health care workers and lay individuals and by monitoring and evaluating larger program outcomes (Patel, 2007). Due to the limited number of specialist mental health care providers, these experts would serve as consultants to help enhance the capacity of medical health care workers to provide common mental health interventions (Patel et al., 2013). Those currently in mental health care would become the mental health specialists, shifting their role to focus on training, supervision, research, and tertiary care while the majority of direct mental health service delivery would shift to community workers and primary care professionals (Patel, 2009). Similar models of task shifting have been effective, yet its success would rely on thorough specialized training, ongoing supervision by health care professionals, and recurring refresher training (Becker, Kleinman, 2013).

Integration

Integration is viewed as a vital part of bridging the mental health care gap since mental health resources are unlikely to be expanded to meet the needs of those suffering from mental illness globally (Cohen, 2001). Even with increased funding for mental health care in LMICs, the issue of stigma and access would not be addressed. Generally, patients with mental illnesses prefer to seek care from their primary care physician; therefore, integrating mental health into primary care would allow for existing resources to be enhanced rather than attempting to establish new ones (Cohen, 2001). Integrated treatment programs provide the opportunity to take a holistic approach to treatment in which health care providers are able to treat the entire person, rather than only addressing their physical or behavioral concerns (Patel et al., 2013). This patient-centered approach enables the health care worker to address all of the patient's concerns with the support of specialized mental health providers (Patel et al., 2013).

The idea of integration can be extended beyond general medical practitioners to include traditional medical practitioners, who often serve as the primary health care providers in many African and Eastern regions. In Southern Africa for example, the sangoma is consulted regardless of the type or severity of an ailment, despite the fact that sangomas traditionally do not receive any medical training (Ngoma, Prince, & Mann, 2003). Traditional healers form part of the cultural fabric of their local community and have considerable influence over health practices, making them potentially powerful agents of change when trained in the provision of mental health care. However, one of the many challenges to this approach is to develop an evidence-based generalized method to assessing diagnostic criteria, prescribing psychiatric medication, and practicing simple psychological interventions while incorporating traditional ways of healing (McKenzie, Patel, Araya, 2004).

Yet while there are challenges, integrated care programs are able to provide more accessible mental health interventions alongside general health care, which would improve the efficiency of care in general (Patel, 2013). Further, these settings are often more attractive to patients and their families who are concerned with the stigma associated with typical, institutionalized mental health settings.

Moving Forward

Shifting the focus from policy and fundraising to integrative care and research may, in turn, facilitate bidirectional growth and inform policy and advocacy (Collins et al., 2013). Provided the conditions for task shifting, training, and supervision are met, the potential human resource for mental health care delivery may be extended to include practically any member of the community. In the future, research could examine the potential of peers, volunteers, and spiritual leaders to assist in mental health care.

A great deal can be learned through knowledge-sharing about improving access to mental health care in LMICs and HICs. There is a mounting evidence base in HICs on improving access to psychotherapy for ethnic minority groups who have traditionally been underrepresented in mental health care service utilization (Miranda et al., 2005). Many of the lessons learned from such studies parallel the experiences described in LMICs and point towards some universal certainties about adapting psychotherapy across health systems and cultures (Patel et al., 2011).

While some components of psychotherapy have been shown to be effective universally, others require substantial adaptation in order to be used in a different contexts and to incorporate the cultural practices. Future work should describe the extent to which such adaptations may influence the original theoretical model at the core of psychotherapy and the extent to which elements common to many brief, structured psychotherapies may outweigh the differences between these interventions. It is reasonable to believe that these common elements may be the most cost-effective interventions to improving access to mental health care in communities with limited resources.

References

African Psychological Association. (August, 2013). Tanzania Mental Health Profile. Retrieved from http://psychologyinafrica.com/profiles/2013/8/13/tanzania-mental-health-profile

Albert, S. M., Edelstein, O. E., Anderson, S. J., Dew, M. A., & Reynolds, C. I. (2015). Global priorities and possibilities. In O. I. Okereke, O. I. Okereke (Eds.), *Prevention of late-life depression: Current clinical challenges and priorities* (pp. 171-183). New York, NY, US: Springer Science + Business Media.

Alem, A., Kebede, D., Fekadu, A., Shibre, T., Fekadu, D., Beyero, T., &... Kullgren, G. (2009). Clinical course and outcome of schizophrenia in a predominantly treatment-naive cohort in rural Ethiopia. *Schizophrenia Bulletin, 35*(3), 646-654.

Ali, S., Saeed, K., & Hughes, P. (2012). Evaluation of a mental health training project in the republic of the Sudan using the Mental health Gap action Programme curriculum. *Guest editorial, 9*(2), 43.

UN General, Department of Economic and Social Affairs. (2015). Transforming our world: The 2030 Agenda for Sustainable Development. *Report of the UN General Assembly.*

Retrieved from
https://sustainabledevelopment.un.org/post2015/transformingourworld

Bale, T. L., Baram, T. Z., Brown, A. S., Goldstein, J. M., Insel, T. R., McCarthy, M. M., ... & Nestler, E. J. (2010). Early life programming and neurodevelopmental disorders. *Biological psychiatry, 68*(4), 314-319.

Bass, J., Neugebauer, R., Clougherty, K. F., Verdeli, H., Wickramaratne, P., Ndogoni, L., ... & Bolton, P. (2006). Group interpersonal psychotherapy for depression in rural Uganda: 6-month outcomes. The British Journal of Psychiatry, 188(6), 567-573.

Becker, A. E., & Kleinman, A. (2012). Introduction an agenda for closing resource gaps in global mental health: Innovation, capacity building, and partnerships. Harvard review of psychiatry, 20(1), 3-5.

Becker, A. E., & Kleinman, A. (2013). Mental health and the global agenda. New England Journal of Medicine, 369(1), 66-73.

Bloom, D. E., Cafiero, E. T., Jané-Llopis, E., Abrahams-Gessel, S., Bloom, L. R., Fathima, S, ... & Weinstein, C. (2011). The Global Economic Burden of Noncommunicable Diseases. Geneva: World Economic Forum. Retrieved from https://www.hsph.harvard.edu/program -on-the-global-demography-of-aging/WorkingPapers/2012/PGDA_WP_87.pdf

Brown, S. (1997). Excess mortality of schizophrenia: A meta-analysis. *The British Journal of Psychiatry, 171*, 502-508. doi:10.1192/bjp.171.6.502

Chisholm, D., Sanderson, K., Ayuso-Mateos, J. L., & Saxena, S. (2004). Reducing the global burden of depression: Population-level analysis of intervention cost-effectiveness in 14 world regions. *The British Journal of Psychiatry, 184*(5), 393-403.

Chisholm, D., Sweeny, K., Sheehan, P., Rasmussen, B., Smit, F., Cuijpers, P., & Saxena, S. (2016). Scaling-up treatment of depression and anxiety: A global return on investment analysis. *The Lancet Psychiatry, 3*(5), 415-424.

Chisholm, D., Van Ommeren, M., Ayuso-Mateos, J., & Saxena, S. (2005). Cost-effectiveness of clinical interventions for reducing the global burden of bipolar disorder. *The British Journal of Psychiatry, 187*(6), 559-567.

Cohen, A. (2001). The Effectiveness of Mental Health Services in Primary Care: The View from the Developing World. Retrieved from http://www.who.int/mental_health/media/en/50.pdf

Collins, P. Y., Insel, T. R., Chockalingam, A., Daar, A., & Maddox, Y. T. (2013). Grand challenges in global mental health: integration in research, policy, and practice. PLoS Med, 10(4), 1-6.

Collins, P. Y., Patel, V., Joestl, S. S., March, D., Insel, T. R., Daar, A. S., ... & Glass, R. I. (2011). Grand challenges in global mental health. Nature, 475(7354), 27-30.

Cooper JE, Sartorius N. (1996). Mental disorders in China: results of the National Epidemiological Survey in 12 Areas. London: Gaskell.

De Jong, J. T. (1996). A comprehensive public mental health programme in Guinea-Bissau: a useful model for African, Asian and Latin-American countries. *Psychological Medicine, 26*(01), 97-108.

Drew, N., Funk, M., Tang, S., Lamichhane, J., Chávez, E., Katontoka, S., ... & Saraceno, B. (2011). Human rights violations of people with mental and psychosocial disabilities: an unresolved global crisis. *The Lancet, 378*(9803), 1664-1675.

Eaton, J., McCay, L., Semrau, M., Chatterjee, S., Baingana, F., Araya, R., ... & Saxena, S. (2011). Scale up of services for mental health in low-income and middle-income countries. *The Lancet, 378*(9802), 1592-1603.

Evans-Lacko, S., Rose, D., Henderson, C., & Thornicroft, G. (2010). Comment on the evaluation of the time to change anti-stigma campaign. *The Psychiatrist, 34*(12), 541-542.

Jacob, K. S., Sharan, P., Mirza, I., Garrido-Cumbrera, M., Seedat, S., Mari, J. J., & ... Saxena, S. (2007). Mental health systems in countries: where are we now?. *Lancet (London, England), 370*(9592), 1061-1077.

Kakuma, R., Minas, H., van Ginneken, N., Dal Poz, M. R., Desiraju, K., Morris, J. E., & ... Scheffler, R. M. (2011). Human resources for mental health care: Current situation and strategies for action. *The Lancet, 378*(9803), 1654-1663.

Kardile, M. (2015). Successful results – Profession specific awareness raising program regarding "Dementia". *Nasik in Mental Health Aims*. Retrieved from http://www.globalmentalhealth.org/sites/default/files/uploads/docs/Success%20of% 20Dementia%20awareness%20raising%20program%20for%20Nasik%20Police%20- %20Kumbh-Mela2015.pdf

Katz, S. J., Kessler, R. C., Frank, R. G., Leaf, P., Lin, E., & Edlund, M. (1997). The use of outpatient mental health services in the United States and Ontario: the impact of mental morbidity and perceived need for care. *American Journal of Public Health, 87*(7), 1136-1143.

Kebede, D., Alem, A., Shibre, T., Negash, A., Fekadu, A., Fekadu, D., ... & Kullgren, G. (2003). Onset and clinical course of schizophrenia in Butajira-Ethiopia. *Social psychiatry and psychiatric epidemiology, 38*(11), 625-631.

Kessler, R. C., Aguilar-Gaxiola, S., Alonso, J., Chatterji, S., Lee, S., Ormel, J., & ... Wang, P. S. (2009). The global burden of mental disorders: An update from the WHO World Mental Health (WMH) Surveys. *Epidemiologia E Psichiatria Sociale, 18*(1), 23-33.

Kieling, C., Baker-Henningham, H., Belfer, M., Conti, G., Ertem, I., Omigbodun, O., ... & Rahman, A. (2011). Child and adolescent mental health worldwide: evidence for action. *The Lancet, 378*(9801), 1515-1525.

Kohn, R., Saxena, S., Levav, I., & Saraceno, B. (2004). The treatment gap in mental health care. *Bulletin of the World health Organization, 82*(11), 858-866.

Koplewicz, H. S., Gurian, A., & Williams, K. (2009). The era of affluence and its discontents. *Journal of the American Academy of Child & Adolescent Psychiatry, 48*(11), 1053-1055.

Koutra, K., Chatzi, L., Bagkeris, M., Vassilaki, M., Bitsios, P., & Kogevinas, M. (2013). Antenatal and postnatal maternal mental health as determinants of infant neurodevelopment at 18 months of age in a mother–child cohort (Rhea Study) in Crete, Greece. *Social Psychiatry and Psychiatric Epidemiology, 48*(8), 1335-1345.

Lancet Global Mental Health Group. (2007). Scale up services for global mental health: a call for action. *The Lancet, 370* (1), 1241-52.

Large, M., Farooq, S., Nielssen, O., & Slade, T. (2008). Relationship between gross domestic product and duration of untreated psychosis in low- and middle-income countries. *The British Journal of Psychiatry, 193*(4), 272-278.

Lehtinen, V., Joukamaa, M., Lahtela, K., Raitasalo, R., Jyrkinen, E., Maatela, J., & Aromaa, A. (1990). Prevalence of mental disorders among adults in Finland: basic results from the Mini Finland Health Survey. *Acta Psychiatrica Scandinavica, 81*(5), 418-425.

Lo Sasso, A. T., Rost, K., & Beck, A. (2006). Modeling the Impact of Enhanced Depression Treatment on Workplace Functioning and Costs: A Cost-Benefit Approach. *Medical Care, 44*(4), 352-358

Lund, C., De Silva, M., Plagerson, S., Cooper, S., Chisholm, D., Das, J., ... & Patel, V. (2011). Poverty and mental disorders: breaking the cycle in low-income and middle-income countries. *The Lancet, 378*(9801), 1502-1514.

Lund, C., Tomlinson, M., De Silva, M., Fekadu, A., Shidhaye, R., Jordans, M., ... & Thornicroft, G. (2012). PRIME: A programme to reduce the treatment gap for mental disorders in five low-and middle-income countries. *PLoS Med,9*(12), e1001359.

McKenzie, K., Patel, V., Araya, R. (2004). Learning from low income countries: mental health. *British Medical Journal, 329*(1), 1138–1140.

Meffert, S. M., Neylan, T. C., Chambers, D. A., & Verdeli, H. (2016). Novel implementation research designs for scaling up global mental health care: Overcoming translational challenges to address the world's leading cause of disability. *International Journal of Mental Health Systems, 10*(19).

Miranda, J. J., & Patel, V. (2006). Achieving the Millennium Development Goals: Does mental health play a role? *PLoS Med, 2*(10), e291.

Moussavi, S., Chatterji, S., Verdes, E., Tandon, A., Patel, V., & Ustun, B. (2007). Depression, chronic diseases, and decrements in health: results from the World Health Surveys. *Lancet (London, England), 370*(9590), 851-858.

Murray, C. J. L., Lopez, A. D., (Eds.). (1996). The global burden of disease: a comprehensive assessment of mortality and disability from diseases, injuries, and risk factors in 1990 and projected to 2020. Cambridge, MA: Harvard University Press.

Murray, C. J., Vos, T., Lozano, R., Naghavi, M., Flaxman, A. D., Michaud, C., ... & Aboyans, V. (2012). Disability-adjusted life years (DALYs) for 291 diseases and injuries in 21 regions, 1990–2010: A systematic analysis for the Global Burden of Disease Study 2010. *The Lancet, 380*(9859), 2197-2223.

Naylor, C., Parsonage, M., McDaid, D., Knapp, M., Fossey, M., & Galea, A. (2012). *Long-term conditions and mental health: The cost of co-morbidities.* The King's Fund – Centre for Mental Health. Retrieved from https://www.kingsfund.org.uk/sites/files/kf/field/field_ publication _file/long-term-conditions-mental-health-cost-comorbidities-naylor-feb12.pdf

Ngo, V. K., Rubinstein, A., Ganju, V., Kanellis, P., Loza, N., Rabadan-Diehl, C., & Daar, A. S. (2013). Grand challenges: Integrating mental health care into the non-communicable disease agenda. *Plos Medicine, 10*(5), 1-5.

Ngoma, M.C., Prince, M., Mann, A. (2003) Common mental disorders among those attending primary health clinics and traditional healers in urban Tanzania. *The British Journal of Psychiatry, 183*(4), 349-355.

Ormel, J., Petukhova, M., Chatterji, S., Aguilar-Gaxiola, S., Alonso, J., Angermeyer, M. C., & ... Kessler, R. C. (2008). Disability and treatment of specific mental and physical disorders across the world. *The British Journal of Psychiatry, 192*(5), 368-375.

Patel, V. (2001) Poverty, inequality and mental health in developing countries. In: Leon D, Walt G (Eds.) *Poverty, Inequality and Health.* Oxford: Oxford University Press, 247–262.

Patel, V. (2012). Global mental health: from science to action. *Harvard Review of Psychiatry, 20*(1), 6-12.

Patel, V., Chisholm, D., Parikh, R., Charlson, F. J., Degenhardt, L., Dua, T., & ... Whiteford, H. (2016). Addressing the burden of mental, neurological, and substance use disorders: key messages from Disease Control Priorities, 3rd edition. *Lancet (London, England), 387*(10028), 1672-1685.

Patel, V., Chowdhary, N., Rahman, A., & Verdeli, H. (2011). Improving access to psychological treatments: Lessons from developing countries. *Behaviour Research and Therapy, 49*(9), 523-528.

Patel, V., & Kim, Y-R. (2007). Contribution of low and middle-income countries to research published in leading psychiatry journals, 2002-2004. *British Journal of Psychiatry, 190*(1), 77-8.

Patel, V., DeSouza, N., & Rodrigues, M. (2003). Postnatal depression and infant growth and development in low income countries: a cohort study from Goa, India. *Archives of Disease in Childhood, 88*(1), 34-37.

Patel, V., Maj, M., Flisher, A. J., De Silva, M. J., Koschorke, M., & Prince, M. (2010). Reducing the treatment gap for mental disorders: a WPA survey. *World Psychiatry: Official Journal of the World Psychiatric Association (WPA), 9*(3), 169-176.

Patel, V., & Prince, M. (2010). Global mental health: a new global health field comes of age. *Journal of the American Medical Association, 303*(19), 1976-1977.

Patel, V., & Thornicroft, G. (2009). Packages of care for mental, neurological, and substance use disorders in low-and middle-income countries: PLoS Medicine Series. *PLoS Med, 6*(10), e1000160.

Pescosolido, B. A., Medina, T. R., Martin, J. K., & Long, J. S. (2013). The "backbone" of stigma: identifying the global core of public prejudice associated with mental illness. *American Journal of Public Health, 103*(5), 853-860.

Prince, M., Patel, V., Saxena, S., Maj, M., Maselko, J., Phillips, M. R., & Rahman, A. (2007). No health without mental health. *Lancet (London, England), 370*(9590), 859-877.

Prince, M., & Trebilco, P. (2005). Mental health services for older people: A developing countries perspective. *Psychogeriatric Service Delivery. Oxford University Press, Oxford*, 33-54.

Rahman, A., Mubbashar, M. H., Gater, R., & Goldberg, D. (1998). Randomised trial of impact of school mental-health programme in rural Rawalpindi, Pakistan. *The Lancet, 352*(9133), 1022-1025.

Ramchandani, P. G., Richter, L. M., Norris, S. A., & Stein, A. (2010). Maternal prenatal stress and later child behavioral problems in an urban South African setting. *Journal of the American Academy of Child & Adolescent Psychiatry, 49*(3), 239-247.

Rehm J, Chisholm D, Room R, Lopez A. Alcohol. In: Jamison D, Breman J, Measham A, Alleyne G, Evans D, Jha P, et al., (Eds.). (2006). Disease control priorities in developing countries. 2nd ed. New York: Oxford University Press; p. 887–906.

Richards, H. (2016). *Documenting the Contextualization and Implementation of mhGAP-HIG in Post-earthquake Nepal* (Doctoral dissertation).

Sachs, S. E., & Sachs, J. D. (2007). Mental health in the millennium development goals: Not ignored. *PLoS Med, 4*(1), e56.

Saraceno, B. (2007). Mental health systems research is urgently needed. *International journal of mental health systems, 1*(1), 1.

Saxena, S., Thornicroft, G., Knapp, M., & Whiteford, H. (2007). Resources for mental health: scarcity, inequity, and inefficiency. *The Lancet, 370*(9590), 878-889.

Tol, W. A., Barbui, C., Galappatti, A., Silove, D., Betancourt, T. S., Souza, R., ... & Van Ommeren, M. (2011). Mental health and psychosocial support in humanitarian settings: linking practice and research. *The Lancet, 378*(9802), 1581-1591.

Vigo, D., Thornicroft, G., & Atun, R. (2016). Estimating the true global burden of mental illness. *The Lancet Psychiatry, 3*(2), 171-178.

Vijayakumar, L., Phillips, M., Silverman, M., Gunnell, D., Carli, V., (2015). Suicide in low and middle income countries. In: Patel V, Chisholm D, Dua T, Laxminarayan R, Medina-Mora ME. (Eds.). (2015). Disease Control Priorities, vol. 4. 3rd ed. Mental, neurological and substance use disorders. Washington, DC: World Bank; p. 163–81.

Vos, T., Flaxman, A. D., Naghavi, M., Lozano, R., Michaud, C., Ezzati, M., ... & Abraham, J. (2013). Years lived with disability (YLDs) for 1160 sequelae of 289 diseases and injuries 1990–2010: a systematic analysis for the Global Burden of Disease Study 2010. *The Lancet, 380*(9859), 2163-2196.

Whiteford, H. A., Degenhardt, L., Rehm, J., Baxter, A. J., Ferrari, A. J., Erskine, H. E., & ... Vos, T. (2013). Global burden of disease attributable to mental and substance use disorders: Findings from the Global Burden of Disease Study 2010. *The Lancet, 382*(9904), 1575-1586.

World Health Organization. (2001) The World Health Report 2001: *Mental health: New Understanding, New Hope.* Geneva: World Health Organization

World Health Organization. (2003). *Investing in mental health.* Geneva: World Health Organization. Retrieved from http://www.who.int/mental_health/media/investing_mnh.pdf

World Health Organization. (2004). World Mental Health Survey Consortium: Prevalence, severity and unmet need for treatment of mental disorders in the World Health Organization World Mental Health Surveys. *Journal of the American Medical Association, 291*(1), 2581–90.

World Health Organization. (2005) Mental Health Atlas 2005. Retrieved from http://www.who.int/mental_health/evidence/atlas/global_results.pdf

World Health Organization. (2006a). Dollars, DALYs, and decisions: economic aspects of the mental health system, 2006. Retrieved from http://www.who.int/mental_health/evidence/dollars_dalys_and_decisions.pdf .

World Health Organization. (2006b). The world health report 2006: *Working together for health*. Geneva: World Health Organization

World Health Organization. (2007). AIMS report on mental health system in South Africa. Cape Town, South Africa: World Health Organization. Retrieved from http://www.who.int/mental_health/evidence/south_africa_who_aims_report.pdf

World Health Organization. (2008a) *mhGAP: mental Health Action Programme: scaling up care for mental, neurological, and substance use disorders.* Geneva: World Health Organization; 2008. Retrieved from http://www.who.int/mental_health/mhGAP_flyer.pdf

World Health Organization. (2008b) The global burden of disease: 2004 update 37. Retrieved from http://www.who.int/healthinfo/global_burden_disease/GBD_report _2004update_full.pdf.

World Health Organization. (2008c). OMS. VIH/ y Salud Mental. 124.a reunión del Consejo Ejecutivo, enero 2009 (EB124/6). Ginebra, 2008. Retrieved from http://www.who.int/gb/ebwha/pdf_ les/EB124/B124_6-sp.pdf.

World Health Organization. (2011) Mental Health Atlas 2011. Geneva: WHO. Retrieved from http://apps.who.int/iris/bitstream/10665/44697/1/9799241564359_eng.pdf

World Health Organization. (2012). Global Burden of Mental Disorders and the Need for a Comprehensive, Coordinated Response from Health and Social Sectors at the Country Level. Report by the Secretariat to the World Health Organization Sixty-Fifth World Health Assembly provisional agenda item 13.2. Geneva: World Health Organization.

World Health Organization. (2014a). Retrieved from http://www.who.int/features/factfiles/ mental_health/en/ 2014.

World Health Organization. (2014b). Mental Health Atlas 2014. Retrieved from http://apps.who.int/iris/bitstream/10665/178879/1/9789241565011_eng.pdf?ua=1& ua=1.

CHAPTER 2

Global Health Impact of War, Terrorism, Conflict, and Political Instability

Falu Rami and Kathleen Davis

The proliferation of global conflicts involving war, terrorism, and political instability have immediate and chronic consequences on the mental and physical health of impacted populations. Physical ailments include infectious and non-communicable diseases and injury. Effects on mental health include substance abuse, posttraumatic stress, anxiety, and mood and somatic symptoms. Currently 1.2 billion people are affected by ongoing violence or political insecurity, though accurate figures are difficult to obtain given the protracted nature of the conflicts and limited access to regions immersed in current crises. Additionally, in 2014, it was reported that 59.5 million people are refugees, stateless people, internally displaced persons, or asylum seekers in over 180 countries – and these figures are rapidly escalating (United Nations High Commission for Refugees [UNHCR], 2016, p. 5). These global crises are not limited to particular regions in the world and are prevalent in all contexts. Most regions show deteriorating or no improvements in resolution of the conflict. This chapter will provide a comprehensive literature review and draw further attention to the necessity of implementing a unified, concerted effort in order to identify solutions to the devastating impact on vulnerable groups. There is a significant dearth of research pertaining to this subject matter due to lack of access to affected populations that are barricaded by armed conflict or blocked from humanitarian aid (including medical and psychological services). Furthermore, in many cases, key infrastructures providing public health care have been destroyed or are severely limited in their ability to deliver basic aid.

Introduction

Since World War II and the subsequent development of the Universal Declaration of Human Rights, there has been an alarming increase in armed conflicts and genocide. Since 1948, there have been 248 armed conflicts in 153 locations. Thirty-seven of the recorded conflicts in 2011 have been in Africa and the Middle East (Tol, Song, & Jordans, 2013, p. 445). The year 2015 marks the largest increase in forced displacement of individuals since World War II (UNHCR, 2016). The latest figures record 65.3 million displaced people due to persecution, generalized violence, conflict, and human rights violations (UNHCR, 2016, p.2). Compared to the prior year, this number is an increase of 5.8 million. Furthermore, children under 18 constitute half of the forcibly displaced population (UNHCR, 2016, p.2).

Individuals can be displaced within the borders of their country or flee to other countries, usually neighboring regions to seek solace and protection. Refugees make up one-third of the displaced population at 21.3 million, and two thirds of internally displaced people [IDP] at 40.8 million (UNHCR, 2016, p.2). The lowest figures are asylum seekers at 3.2 million people (UNHCR, 2016, p.1 and p.3). This places a strain on already-sparse resources as 86% of refugees under the UNHCR mandate are hosted by low- and middle-income countries (UNHCR, 2016, p.2).

Multiple studies show the increased prevalence of mental health symptoms in populations impacted by war, terrorism, conflict, and political instability (Cardoza, Bilukha, Crawford, Shaikh, Wolfe, Gerber & Anderson, 2004; De Jong, Komproe, & Ormerl, 2003; Dyer & Bhadra, 2013; Kessler, Aguilar-Gaxiola, Alonso, Chatterji, Yanling, Heeringa, Lee & Ormerl, 2013). Despite the incidence of mental health in conflict-affected areas, the majority of studies and surveys have been conducted in regions where the World Health Organization (WHO) has offices (Kesller et. al, 2013) or in industrialized countries (WHO, 2009). Countries that face humanitarian crises relating to war, conflict, terrorism, and political instability lack data or research on the influence of conflicts on global health. Individual country reports have been conducted by other agencies in Iraq, Afghanistan, and Syria (Cardoza et al., 2004; WHO, 2009). These provide pertinent data but also demonstrate a lack of a standardized approach to collecting accurate statistics in countries and regions that are difficult to access due to conflict and humanitarian emergencies. Similarly, it is difficult to ascertain the existence of psychiatric services and providers in many of the contexts in this chapter, and several of the mental health surveys conducted are dated and do not reflect accurate prevalence rates given the protractive nature of various conflicts. Additionally, most of the research evaluates the impact of armed conflict on soldiers or veterans even though it is widely recognized that civilians suffer the overwhelming majority of war casualties. (Bell, Mendez, Martinez, Palma, & Bosch, 2012).

Studies have focused on increased risk factors that lead to the development of posttraumatic symptoms or diagnosis in armed conflict, but there is little exploration of how social and economic consequences are related to development of posttraumatic symptoms or diagnosis. Research has primarily focused on studying the mental health impacts of conflict after its resolution, but for regions still embroiled in ongoing conflict, there are limited studies. Mental health implications of war and conflict are much more prevalent in the research, though physical manifestations of injury, disease, and disability affect millions. Health care concerns place a strain on the resources in countries with limited or declining infrastructure, like the Democratic Republic of the Congo, Afghanistan, Pakistan, and regions controlled by the Islamic State also known as Daesh, ISIS, or ISIL.

Definitions and Key Terms

War: Armed conflict between and within nation states. Alternative definitions of war expand the term to include armed actions taken by groups against the government (Sidel & Levy, 2003).

Terrorism: Violence or the threat of it that is committed against civilians to invoke fear, and that is politically motivated (Sidel & Levy, 2003). Schmid (2011) reports the lack of consensus around the definition of terrorism.

Disability: Limited functioning, restriction, or inability to participate or perform an activity performed with ease by others (Cardoza et. al, 2003).

Refugee: A person that has fled their country due to fear of persecution because of race, religion, nationality, membership in a special social group, or having particular political opinions (Dyer & Bhadra, 2013).

Infectious Diseases: Microorganism pathogens such as parasites, fungi, bacteria or viruses that are spread from one person to another, either through direct or indirect contact (World Health Organization [WHO], 2016, para. 1)

Non-communicable Diseases: A medical condition that cannot be passed from one person to another, and includes four main types: cardiovascular, cancers, chronic respiratory diseases, and diabetes (WHO, 2015).

Injury: Due to inconsistency with the definition of injury from the World Health Organization, United Nations, and Centers for Disease Control it will be defined as: Harm or damage to the body. Langley and Brenner (2004) reported if there is no tissue damage, sexual assault will be classified as a psychological injury. The ICD-10 classifies Sexual Abuse, Confirmed as Non-Billable/Non-Specific Code (ICD-10Data.com, 2016). Sexual violence will be defined separately from injury due to the complex and interconnected dynamics.

Sexual Violence: Any actual, attempted, or unsolicited sexual act, advance or comment, or trafficking, against a person's sexuality using manipulation or force by any person including those who have a casual or intimate relationship with the victim (WHO, 2004).

Conflict Background

There are many more inter- and intra-country conflicts other than those listed in this chapter. The countries represented are those who have had chronic conflict, political instability, terrorism, war, and displacement.

Political Instability

Columbia

The Colombian conflict is not connected to ethnic or religious cleavages, but centers around economic, political, and military factors (Restrepo, Spagat, & Vargas, 2004). Colonization had a direct impact on development of the conflict because campesinos (peasant farmers) were in a constant state of relocation by the Colombian government. Unlike other colonized Latin American countries, Colombia did not execute agrarian restructuring to reallocate land ownership (González, 2004). Spanish colonization marginalized groups like poor whites, mestizos (people of Spanish and indigenous heritage), Afro-Colombians, and biracial groups and forced them into isolated areas while local elites controlled wealthy territories (González, 2004). This contributed to ongoing conflicts by several peasant guerilla groups for centuries. The two largest military groups are the Armed Revolutionary Forces of Colombia (FARC), and the National Liberation Army (ELN) (Restrepo et al., 2004). During the La Violencia period (1946-66), Columbia was split into liberal and conservative parties (Restrepo et al., 2004). During the last 51 years of armed conflict, over 7.6 million victims were registered, and over 6 million people were uprooted, making this the second-largest number of internally displaced peoples (United States Institute of Peace [USIP], 2016, para. 2). In June 2016, an accord was reached between the Columbian government and FARC. This ended the 51-year civil war (Friedman-Rudovsky, 2016). Columbia now has the massive burden of reconciliation.

Myanmar

Myanmar, formerly called Burma, has been embroiled in armed conflict and civil war with the Karen National Union since 1949, a year after its independence from colonial rule (Nilsen, 2013). During this period, the country was also involved in rebellions spurred by the Communist Party of Burma and some Arakanese groups. Karen communities that live in mountainous regions bordering Thailand are in direct crossfire of armed conflict (South, 2011). Despite the ceasefire of insurgency and counterinsurgency incidents in many of the Karen communities, residents are vulnerable to acts of violence and devastation of poverty. Large numbers of civilians were internally displaced in Burma, and about two million fled to Thailand as migrants under vulnerable conditions with limited protections (South, 2011, p.10). Under the new constitution in 2008, the country was divided into seven states, which were mainly of homogenous ethnic groups, and seven majority Burman regions.

Although Myanmar has begun transitioning to a democratic government as of 2010, peaceful co-existence is questionable unless the country addresses inter-group conflicts, such as the clash between the Myanmar Army in Shan and Kachin States as well as the conflict between the Buddhist majority and the Rohingya Muslim minority. The latter caused riots in Rakhine State in 2012, resulting in 160 deaths and the displacement of over 100,000 (Nilsen, 2013, p. 116). Additional attacks on Muslims occurred in central Myanmar during riots in 2013.

War

Syria

A comprehensive understanding of the war in Syria requires some foundational understanding of the history of colonialism, the Arab Spring, and the religious and ethnic makeup of the country (Dalacoura, 2012; Fildis, 2011). In addition, the Syrian War, now in its fifth year, is further complicated by geopolitical factors, regional conflicts, and the involvement of global actors and their support or opposition to pro-government forces or rebel groups (Byman, 2013; Frontline, 2014; Hove & Mutanda, 2014).

The decisions to divide regions of the Ottoman Empire and dissolve it both during and after World War I are identified as some of the most crucial factors contributing to current conflicts and turmoil in the Middle East (Chatty, 2015; Fildis, 2011). These decisions have resulted in multiple displacements over the past 150 years. Prior to this period, most Arab countries came under the auspices of the Ottoman Empire, which served to protect them against European rule. The primary countries that have been impacted include Iraq, Lebanon, and Syria. The French Mandate of 1920 of Lebanon and Syria divided these regions along regional and sectarian lines.

France divided the country along sectarian lines to maintain the balance of power, to serve private sector and religious interests, and to preserve the countries' national interests. The consequences of this ethnic, religious, and sectarian division are now manifesting in complex ways within Syria, other regional countries, and global powers.

The Arab Spring in December 2010 involved multiple Arab countries (Dalacoura, 2012). These movements either resulted in the overthrow of or protests against the governments in these regions, or they were quickly contained by government response. Mubarak's resignation in Egypt led to protests in Libya against Qadhafi. These protests escalated to violence, which claimed thousands of civilian lives and resulted in the death of Qadhafi in 2011.

Following the removal of Ben Ali in Tunisia, increased protests in Yemen demanded removal of President Ali Saleh, and a civil war started in 2015. In March 2011, Syrians amplified pro-democracy protests against the regime of President Bashar al-Assad in response to the arrest and torture of a group of teenagers who had drawn revolutionary slogans on a wall and the killing of protesters by security forces (BBC, 2016). These events quickly escalated to war.

Furthermore, the war in Syria has taken on sectarian undertones, resulting in a conflict between Sunni majorities and Shia Alawite minorities. In addition, sectarian groups in neighboring countries like Iran, Turkey, and Lebanon have become involved.

Global intervention from the United States, Jordan, Qatar, Turkey, Saudi Arabia, United Kingdom, and France assists Syrian rebel forces (BBC, 2016; Byman, 2013). The rise of ISIS has increased the complexity of the conflict, leading to the establishment of a caliphate and the recruitment of jihadists from various countries. This has resulted in increased terrorist incidents in many countries including Turkey, France, Brussels, the United States, and Germany. Finally, the increased support provided to Kurdish forces by the United States in Syria and Iraq has amplified the conflict between the Turkish government and military forces against the Kurds. The Syrian War has given rise to the largest humanitarian and refugee crisis reported since World War II and has caused half of the population of Syria to be internally displaced or to seek refuge in neighboring countries or Europe.

Terrorism

Nigeria

Nigeria achieved its independence in 1960, but has unresolved ethno, religious, and political conflict since its civil war in 1967, which resulted in the loss of three million lives (Khan & Hamidu, 2015). A sectarian conflict of significant intensity has been increasing in Nigeria for several years due to numerous insurgent and militant groups, most notably, Boko Haram. Through the leadership of Mallam Lawan, Boko Haram was developed with the primary goal of preaching and practicing Islam. The term Boko Haram is translated as "Western and non-Islamic education is sin." Ironically, Lawan left the group to continue his studies, and it became a violent sect under Muhammed Yusuf's leadership in 2009 (Dabkana, Bunu, Na'aya, Tela, & Adamu, 2015). After Yusuf's death in 2009, the group became increasingly violent under the leadership of Abubakar Shekau and declared jihad against the Nigerian government and the U.S. in 2010. The goal of the group is to establish an Islamic state in a country divided into a Christian south and a Muslim north (Council on Foreign Relations [CFR], 2016). Since 2011, Boko Haram increased terrorist attacks on local police, military, religious, and political groups, and civilians (CFR, 2016).

International attention and outrage temporarily shined a spotlight on Nigeria in 2014 when Boko Haram kidnapped more than 275 Chibok schoolgirls and threatened to sell them into slavery or force them into marriage (Kahn & Hamidu, 2015, p. 25). That same year, Boko Haram was reported to be the world's deadliest terrorist group, having caused 7,492 deaths (Institute for Economics & Peace [IEP], 2015, p. 41). The nature of terrorism in Nigeria differs from that of Iraq and Afghanistan as Nigerian terrorist groups typically use tactics and weapons commonly associated with gangs, like assault rifles and knifes. Sixty-seven percent of Boko Haram deaths were caused by firearms. Boko Haram does employ suicide bombings, although less frequently than other terrorist groups do (CFR, 2016). Dabkana et al. (2015) indicates that hospitals are woefully understaffed and understocked. Human rights violations are rife in Nigeria and will no doubt have long-lasting impact on the population's physical and mental health.

Afghanistan and Pakistan

The history of the war in Afghanistan can be traced to the overthrow of King Zahir Shah by Mohammed Daoud Khan in 1978. Khan had served as Prime Minister, promoting economic reform and emancipation of women. Pakistan was threatened by this move and encouraged Islamic leaders to fight against the regime. Daoud Khan was killed in 1978. The Soviet Union invaded a year later, which promoted the organization of rebel leaders, resulting in a civil war that lasted until 2001 (British Broadcasting Corporation, 2016a). The Taliban formed in the early 1990s following the fall of the Soviet Union in northern Pakistan by the Mujahedeen and Pashtun tribesmen and came to prominence in 1994 in Afghanistan (BBC, 2016b). The Taliban was religiously motivated by adherence to Islamic law (Fleetwood, 2014).

The United States has been at war with Afghanistan since October 7, 2001, just after the 9/11 terrorist attacks on U.S. soil. Initially, the goal was to capture Osama bin Laden, the leader of Al-Qaeda who reported to be in Afghanistan when the 9/11 attacks were ordered. The Taliban refused to hand-over bin Laden so the U.S. declared war on Afghanistan. The Taliban had control of Afghanistan until 2001, but was overthrown by a U.S.-led invasion. They regrouped in Pakistan, and insurgency movements continue to this day in Afghanistan (Institute for Economics and Peace, 2015). Bin Laden hid at a stronghold in Pakistan until U.S. military troops found and killed him in May 2011. The U.S. declared that most of the troops would be withdrawn in 2014, but the war against the Taliban continues in both Afghanistan and Pakistan (Crawford, 2015).

The Taliban has roots in both Afghanistan and Pakistan. British colonization of India led to splitting India into a predominantly Hindu India and a predominantly Muslim Pakistan. The partition was uncompleted in Kashmir, and both Pakistan and India have been embroiled in an ongoing territorial dispute since then. Sectarian and ethnic violence have been a part of Pakistan since 1947, and there are numerous interconnected armed conflicts (Peace Direct, 2016). To further complicate matters, the U.S. has been fighting militants associated with al-Qaeda and the Taliban in northwest Pakistan, and at the same time, Pakistani Security Forces are fighting militants connected with several armed groups. Civilians often get caught in the crossfire. Pakistan has placed itself precariously between retaining ally ties with the U.S. (who is supplying them with arms to fight the Taliban and other groups) and backing militant factions in Afghanistan in an attempt to ally itself with this bordering country. Unfortunately, this has increased U.S. strikes in Pakistan (Peace Direct, 2016).

ISIS/ISIL

The Islamic State was constructed by al Qaeda in Iraq and is also known as ISIL or ISIS (Glenn, 2016). Founded by Abu Masab al Zaqawi in 2004, its existence remained obscure due to the surge of U.S. troops in Iraq. ISIS was driven out of Baghdad into Diyali in 2007, and a portion of their control is limited to the area of Mosul in Iraq. However, a year later in Iraq, increased attacks against Sunni leaders by Prime Minister Maliki amplified both sectarian tensions in the country and support for ISIS in tribal areas (Frontline, 2014; Glenn, 2016).

ISIS reemerged in 2011, following the withdrawal of U.S. troops from Iraq (Frontline, 2014). The Islamic State capitalized on the instability in Iraq and Syria and expanded measures to gain power. Offensives were launched in the cities of Mosul and Inkrit in June 2014 (Glenn, 2016). A caliphate was established by the leader, Abu Bakr al Baghdadi, from Aleppo, Syria through Diyala, Iraq. The U.S. began airstrikes in Iraq in 2014 and expanded the attacks to Syria in an attempt to stem the growth of the Islamic State. Though the airstrikes helped Iraq recapture control of some of its cities, ISIS still had control over parts of Syria.

In 2015, ISIS expanded its operations to eight other countries including Egypt, Yemen, and Libya and exerted authority beyond its established caliphate (Glenn, 2016). There were many notable events of ISIS including taking control of Qaddafi, Libya in May 2015 and increasing affiliation in Yemen. Other events in 2015 included both ISIS's Egypt affiliate shooting down a Russian plane and killing 224 people and the Paris attacks, which claimed 130. Many other attacks occurred in countries such as Egypt, Libya, Tunisia, Saudi Arabia, Turkey, Bangladesh, Yemen, the U.S., Indonesia, the Netherlands, and Germany.

Conflict

Congo

The conflict in the mineral-rich Congo can be traced to colonization. Shortly after being declared the Republic of the Congo (DRC) in 1960, the country descended into a civil war that continues to this day (Peace Direct, 2009). From the 1960s-1980s, rulers splintered the country into "city-states," wherein people became increasingly isolated from one another and transportation and communication infrastructures collapsed (Peace Direct, 2009, para. 3). During the Rwandan genocide, the situation in DRC worsened as Tutsi refugees fleeing from the Hutus and Hutu soldiers and militia crossed into the country. After the Rwandan genocide, the Tutsi-dominated government invaded Congo (known then as Zaire) to bring the Hutu génocidaires to justice.

The Second Congolese War began in 1998 when 11 African countries declared war on Larent-Désiré Kabila, the DRC President. The war lasted until 2002 (Peace Direct, 2009). Since then, skirmishes erupt between multiple armed Burundian, Ugandan, Rwandan, and Mai-Mai (community-based militia groups) factions who terrorize civilians and inhibit peace (Eastern Congo Initiative, 2016). Similar to the Jewish Holocaust, over 6 million Congolese have been killed since the Second Congolese War; however, unlike the Holocaust, this genocide has received very little media attention, even though 45,000 civilians die each month from violence, poverty, disease, and famine (World without Genocide, 2016, para. 11). Children and women are particularly vulnerable. Rape and sexual violence in DRC is among the worst in the world. As of 2009, 1.92 million Congolese women had been raped during their lifetime, and 462,293 within the previous year (Dranginis, 2014, p. 4). Children in DRC have been recruited as soldiers and 30,000 (or one in ten children) between the ages of 12 and 17 were recruited since 1998 (Eastern Congo Initiative, 2016, para.

1; Johannessen & Holgersen, 2014, p. 56).

Iraq

Iraq has faced decades of instability and conflict related to various events which caused insecurity, internal displacement of people, forced displacement of refugees to neighboring countries like Syria, and political instability. These incidents have caused prolonged stress and volatility in the region, which makes the true prevalence rates of global health difficult to assess. There is limited data of prevalence rates of psychiatric disorders in the region prior to 2009 (WHO, 2009). Iraq has been involved in an eight-year war with Iran as well as the infiltration of Kuwait. The Gulf War began in 1991, followed by thirteen years of imposed sanctions, which deteriorated conditions in the country. In 2003, a regime invasion caused increased insecurities in the region and subsequently resulted in an influx of refugees to Syria in 2006 (Quosh, Eloul, & Ajlani, 2013). Additional complex humanitarian emergencies related to the war in Syria in 2011 occurred due to multiple factors such as the Arab Spring, the rise of ISIS, and an increase in terrorism and fighting. The ongoing war in Syria has resulted in an exodus of refugees into neighboring countries, including Iraq. Furthermore, the rise of ISIS has resulted in an establishment of a caliphate and recruitment of jihadists from around the world.

Ukraine

Several preceding events contributed to the Ukrainian conflict. For example, in November 2013, President Viktor Yanukovych suspended talks to sign a trade agreement and political deal with the European Union (EU) (Thompson, 2016). President Yanukovych is reported to have stalled talks due to pressure from Russia, which objected to Ukraine having closer ties with the EU. Thousands of protesters took to the streets, reflecting the deep divide between the pro-European West and those loyal to Russia in the East. Since its beginning in April 2015, approximately 9,500 people have been killed, and more than 22,600 have been injured (as of March 3, 2016) (Thompson, 2016, para. 17). It has been reported to be the most violent conflict in Europe since the wars in Yugoslavia in the 1990s.

The weeks-long escalation of violence between the police and protesters in Kiev resulted in an incident on February 20, 2014 that left dozens of people dead. (Thompson, 2016). Shortly after, in March 2015, reportedly pro-Russian military troops entered Crimea. Two weeks later, this region was annexed through a referendum that Ukraine and many other countries consider unlawful. On April 15, 2014, the government of Kiev activated military involvement in Eastern Ukraine to regain control of areas and buildings that pro-Russian rebels seized (Thompson, 2016). The new president, Petro Poroshenko, signed the EU association agreement on June

27, 2014. Less than a month later, violence escalated as rebels shot down a Malaysian airplane that flew over rebel-held territory in Eastern Ukraine, killing 298 people (Thompson, 2016, p. 10). An agreement was signed for a ceasefire in February 2015; however, violence ensued shortly after. On June 22, 2015, the European Union sanctioned Russia for its actions in Crimea and Eastern Ukraine. The violence has continued, and as of March 2016, millions of Ukrainian and Crimean people are reported to live in conflict areas (Thompson, 2016, p. 16).

Physical Effects of War, Conflict, or Terrorism
and Barriers to Recovery

Physical implications for people who reside in areas of conflict or political instability include significant increases in injuries and both infectious and non-communicable diseases (Puvacic & Weinberg, 1994). Injuries sustained from vehicular collisions, poisoning, falls, burns, drownings, and violence from assault or acts of war comprise 9% of global mortality (WHO, 2016, para. 1). Infectious and non-communicable diseases and injury affect over a billion people globally (WHO, 2015b, para. 1). In areas of conflict, disability notably contributes to vulnerability for women, who tend to be more vulnerable to physical and sexual violence (Samararatne & Soldatic, 2015). Additionally, diseases that have been minimized or eradicated in developed parts of the world (e.g., polio and tuberculosis) tend to be high in areas with ongoing conflict and instability (Akil & Ahmad, 2016; Sahloul et al., 2016). This was true during the Bosnian War, when toxinfectio alimentaris (a severe diarrheal disease with fever), scabies, tuberculosis, and Hepatitis A increased significantly (Puvacic & Weinberg, 1994), in Iraq, with outbreaks of respiratory infection, measles, mumps, and typhoid, and in Pakistan and Syria, with a proliferation of polio cases (Akil & Ahmad, 2016; Sahloul et al., 2016).

People injured by direct-war violence comprise a large portion of the population in Afghanistan and Pakistan, countries in which ongoing conflict has affected over 126,000 people (Crawford, 2015, p. 1). It is estimated that the number of injured civilians was 10 times the number of those killed as a result of terrorist bombings (Crawford, 2013, p. 2). Since the crisis began in Syria in 2011, it is estimated that at least 250,000 have died from non-communicable diseases, and harsh living conditions and lack of access to medical care in refugee camps have attributed to increased mortality from infectious diseases, like pneumonia and bronchiolitis (Sahloul et al., 2016, p. 150). Despite the history of the Colombian conflict, health infrastructure remains strong – over 98% of the population has access to health care services. However, major inequities exist for rural citizens and ethnic minority populations (World Health Organizations, 2014, p. 1). Up to 30% of the 6 million IDPs lack access to government-funded health services (Webster, 2012, para 3). Statistics on chronic disease are difficult to access; however, the Center of Development Projects at Pontificia Universidad Javeriana in Bogotá estimated that the total burden of chronic disease increased by 40% between 1995 and 2005 (Webster, 2012b, para. 3).

Like Colombia, amputee injuries are common in Afghanistan due to the use of bombs and landmines. Of the 6,849 injured in 2014, 19% (1,318) were amputees, patients who likely need long-term health care and rehabilitation (Crawford, 2015, p. 2). In developed countries, there is a 40-60% chance that lower-extremity amputees will die within two years of their surgery (Rybarczyk, Behel, and Szymanksi, 2010, p. 29). In a war-torn country, the likelihood of mortality from these injuries is much higher. According to the National Disability Survey in Afghanistan, war-related disability comprised 17% of all disability, (Crawford, 2015, p. 7). Though over 5.8 million refugees have returned to Afghanistan since 2002, the UNHCR noted that shelter remains an issue for returnees (Crawford, 2015, p. 8), making them vulnerable to potential injury or death by insurgent attacks, exposure to the elements, and lack of stability. IDPs and refugees are more vulnerable to disease and have less access to health care (Crawford, 2015). War has a devastating impact on health systems and infrastructure. During it, the population becomes vulnerable to disease, malnutrition, lack of access to safe drinking water, and injury from landmines (Crawford, 2015).

Pakistan has been one of the main targets of the controversial U. S. drone project instituted in 2004. Drones have caused somewhere between 2,499 and 4,001 deaths and have injured between 1,161 and 1,744 civilian Pakistani (Bureau of Investigative Journalism, 2016). The Pakistani Security Forces also sometimes inadvertently injure or kill civilians (Crawford, 2011). However, the greatest source of injury and death in Pakistan stems from the Taliban, al-Qaeda, and other militant organizations who use bombs, suicide attacks, and ambushes to kill civilians.

Like Afghanistan, Pakistan's main populace and internal refugees lack access to appropriate medical or psychological care (Crawford, 2011). Injuries in Pakistan are similar to those in Afghanistan and Colombia, as many are injured by ordnance (weapons, ammunition, and combat vehicles), landmines, and bombings (Muazzam & Xiang, 2008). People aged 5-44 in Afghanistan and Pakistan are most vulnerable to these types of injuries, and men and children are more susceptible (Surrency, Graitcer, & Henderson, 2007, p. 199). Landmines contribute to significant disabling injuries including foot or leg amputations. Ordnance tends to cause injuries to the head or arms. Victims of both devices tend to have the highest rates of unemployment, which indicates that the injury significantly limits their ability to work (Surrency et al., 2007). People in drone-combat areas exhibit symptoms of daily anxiety because Unmanned Air Vehicles [UAV] buzz overhead. Living in this terror-based environment produces extreme anxiety related to a fear of leaving home, limited social contact due to paranoia of being associated with a potential target, and not attending important religious and social functions such as weddings or funerals (Brave New Foundation, 2012; Stanford International Human Rights and Conflict Resolution, & Global Justice Clinic, 2012). Pervasive worry and anticipatory anxiety are common effects of those living in war zones, and many civilians in the targeted areas of Pakistan have post- and on-going traumatic stress (Stanford International Human Rights and Conflict Resolution, & Global Justice Clinic, 2012). It also has a devastating impact on children, who are often angry and anxious and live in constant fear of the drones. Long-term psychological effects may be likely in children who are raised in this type of dysfunctional and threatening environment. The U.S. should revisit its policy on the use of drones, which appear to be a weapon of questionable accuracy as 90% of those killed by UAVs were not the target (Currier & Maass, 2015, para. 7).

In the Democratic Republic of the Congo, infectious diseases (e.g., malaria, diarrheal disease, lower respiratory infections, and HIV) are some of the primary causes of death (CDC, 2015, p. 2). Rape continues to be used as a weapon of war in DRC (Dranginis; 2014). Additionally, physical implications are rarely addressed. Short-term physical effects of rape may include bleeding vaginally or anally, sexually-transmitted diseases, bruising, broken bones, and pregnancy. Some long-term effects can be HIV/AIDS, hepatitis, vaginal/anal pain or problems, musculoskeletal pain, genital/urinary difficulties, problems with normal bowel movements, and in women, gynecological or menstrual problems (Orange County Rape Crisis Center, 2016). War-related injuries/disabilities and sexually transmitted diseases are high among child soldiers, as is psychopathology (Johannessen & Holgersen, 2014). The number of human rights atrocities committed by various groups in DRC is staggering, as is their effects on both physical and mental health.

In a five-year review of 1,339 injury cases in Nigeria by Dabkana et al. (2015), 91.3% of the victims were male and 8.7% were females. Ages ranged from 1-80 years, and 59.4% of victims were in the 21-40 age brackets. Gunshot wounds accounted for 91.8% of injuries, bomb blasts for 6.7%, and knife slashes and wounds accounted for 0.3%. Body parts most affected by these injuries were the extremities (54.8%), torso (31.6%), multiple injuries (6.9%), and head and neck (6.6%). Gunshot wounds may have contributed to a myriad of complications, depending on severity and placement of wound. Human rights violations are rife in Nigeria and will have long-lasting implications on physical and mental health (p. 115-116).

Rape is used as a weapon of war, child suicide bombers are employed, and there is a food and malnutrition crisis (Searcey, 2016).

War, Age, and Gender

War and conflict affect women, men, and children differently. Infants and young children are most at-risk to the consequences of war because they dehydrate more quickly than adults, exsanguinate much faster, and are more vulnerable to both bio- and chemical weapons used in war and long-term mental and physical trauma (Sahloul et al., 2016).

Children in war-torn countries are especially vulnerable to injury and mortality from land mines (U.N., 2003). An analysis of 12,484 child deaths in Syria revealed that 75% were the result of airstrikes and shelling, which cause severe bodily damage and limb loss (Sahloul et al., 2016, p. 151). For children who do survive such trauma, acute rehabilitation may be necessary for years, and they are likely to be permanently disabled or disfigured.

Women are greatly affected in times of conflict due to their protective role as mothers, their susceptibility to sexual and physical assault, and their vulnerability to human trafficking and prostitution as a means of supporting their children or receiving protection. In Columbia, it is estimated that over 1.5 million people were displaced by the decades-long conflict, and nearly 80% were women and children (Rehn & Honshon-Sirleaf, 2002, p. 22). Additionally, adolescent girls are vulnerable to sexual exploitation and teen pregnancy. In fact, teen pregnancies are reported to be as high as 50% in some refugee camps (Rehn & Honshon-Sirleaf, 2002, p. 36). As rape has been used as a "weapon of war" in conflicts in Liberia, the Democratic Republic of the Congo, Sudan, Sierra Leone, Rwanda, and other parts of the world, women and girls are susceptible to HIV/AIDS (Aginam, 2012). Maternal and infant mortality increase significantly during conflict as a result of the destruction of medical facilities, which affects both the quality and availability of maternal and reproductive health services (Chi, et al., 2015). While recently, there has been more attention placed on women's health and the movement to end rape during war, the laws contribute to confusion and lack of prosecution. For a rape to be considered a war crime, the actual rape itself is diminished. Furthermore, it must have occurred in certain circumstances, such as a genocide or ethnic war, and must meet the legal definition of a war crime (Fiske & Shackel, 2014).

Women and children receive a great deal of attention as victims of war, but how does war affect civilian men? There appears to be a dearth of research in this respect, insinuating that men are able to protect and care for themselves against violent acts. This not only contributes to insufficient data relating to violence against men during wartime, but negates the importance of men in family structures, most notably in patriarchal societies where many of the violent conflicts occur. During the Holocaust, men were targeted first; they were sent to concentration camps, forced into labor, or murdered (Yad Vashem, 2016). Other ways of humiliation include psychological abuse and torture (Yad Vashem, 2016). Men are often forced to watch as their families are attacked, raped, beaten, or killed (Hamblen & Schnurr, 2016).

Numbers at a Glance

During times of war or political instability, health care infrastructures and tools such as hospitals, laboratories and medical records can be destroyed, which makes finding accurate statistics difficult (Puvacic & Weinberg, 1994). Table 1 (Appendix A*) provides overall injury statistics. Death counts are in Figure 1 (Appendix B), refugees and internally displaced persons are tallied in Figure 2 (Appendix C).

Mental Health Effects of War, Conflict, or Terrorism

De Jong, Kamproe, and Ommeron (2003) conducted a study in four post-conflict settings in developing countries that showed an increase in frequency of mental disorders where survivors of armed conflict reside. The disorders were organized into the following categories: Post-Traumatic Stress Disorder (PTSD), Mood Disorder, Anxiety Disorder, Somatoform Disorder, and Any Disorder. Prevalence rates were much higher in post-conflict countries than lifetime prevalence rates in other countries. Stressful experiences and events related to conflicts and crises have been reported to attribute to an increase of 1% for severe mental disorders, and mild or moderate disorders like PTSD could increase by 5-10% above the baseline. Other studies have reported that children residing in disaster- or conflict-prone areas could experience a prevalence of PTSD up to 75%, though most do recover from these symptoms (Dyer & Bhadra, 2013, p. 179-180).

The impact of more than two decades of war in Afghanistan has resulted in devastating human suffering and the displacement of Afghan people. In 2002, the CDC conducted a quantitative study in Afghanistan to measure the impact of conflict on the mental health of the general population. Surveys were conducted with 799 adults aged fifteen and older, 699 of whom were identified as nondisabled and 100 of whom were identified as disabled (Cardoza, Bilukah, Crawford, Shaikh, Wolfe, Gerber, & Anderson, 2004, p. 575). The following table depicts the results of the surveys (Cardoza et al., 2004).

---

* Appendices for this chapter can be found at: http://tinyurl.com/wghm-attachments

Table 2: National Population-Based Mental Health Survey in Afghanistan

Total Surveyed N = 799 Adults	Depression	Anxiety	PTSD
Nondisabled	67.7%	72.2%	42.1%
Disabled	71.7%	84.6%	42.2%

The Iraq Mental Health Survey (IMHS) was conducted in 2006 and 2007. It consisted of an initial sample of 10,080 households of adults aged 18+, 99% of whom participated (WHO, 2009, p. 36). According to the IMHS data, over half of the respondents reported symptoms of feeling nervous, tense, or worried in the prior 30 days. 3.5% reported having thoughts of wanting to end their lives within the prior 30 days, and 7.8% reported feeling worthless (WHO, 2009, p. 42). Lifetime prevalence rates of mental health disorders were higher overall among women than men. Overall prevalence of any mental disorder was 16.56% for men, showing an incidence of 13.69%, whereas women showed a prevalence rate of 19.46%. Of all the mental disorders, the most commonly reported were anxiety disorders (11.58%, followed by any affective disorder (7.82%). The incidence of substance abuse disorders was recorded to be only 0.92% (WHO, 2009, p. 43). In addition, there were higher incidences of disorders for any significant disorder in urban versus rural settings. Subjects that met criteria for psychiatric disorders had an overall rate of experiencing any war-related trauma at 64.95%, whereas the rate for those that did not meet criteria was 44.82% (WHO, 2009, p. 58). Respondents that met criteria for psychiatric disorders experienced any events of trauma at a lifetime prevalence rate of 74.78%, and subjects that did not meet criteria for psychiatric disorders experienced any trauma at 52.3% (WHO, 2009, p. 58). Men experienced significantly higher rates of trauma events in comparison to women, except in regards to domestic violence. The surveys conducted in the twelve months showed significantly higher incidence for traumatic events such as internal displacement, shooting, being exposed to a bomb blast, or witnessing a killing.

Sociodemographic variables showed higher rates of prevalence of psychiatric disorders in those that have fewer years of education. Widowed, divorced, or separated women showed greater prevalence rates of psychiatric disorders over those that were married (WHO, 2009). Finally, there were significant differences in occurrence rates for affective disorders between those that were employed versus those that were unemployed.

Little research has been conducted in Latin America, where there has been increased armed conflict. In Columbia, there has been armed conflict since 1964 (Bell et al., 2012), which has resulted in increased human rights abuses. Columbia hosts the world's largest number of internally displaced persons (IDPs), which was recorded to be up to 3.3-4.9 million people (Bell et al., 2012, p. 3). Although some research has been conducted in areas not currently in conflict, little data has been collected on mental health statistics for people that still reside in conflict zones. Studies in countries with high rates of human rights abuses, however, show an increase in psychopathology. A study in Tolima (Bell et al., 2012) revealed a 30% prevalence rate of common mental disorders for populations that were displaced to slum areas and were then residing in cities unaffected by violence (p. 2). Data also showed that 80% of those that had been displaced had experienced violence due to armed conflict (Bell et al., 2012, p. 2.). Finally, according to Bell et al. (2012), three studies with adults and one study with children showed an increase in prevalence rates of PTSD and anxiety for people who had been displaced as a result of violence.

Medecins Sans Frontieres, one of the few non-governmental organizations that provides services in regions of ongoing conflict, conducted a study in the South of Columbia in the rural departments of Caqueta, Cauca, Valle de Cauca, Narino, and Putumayo (Bell et al., 2012). Participants were aged 16 and older, and surveys were collected from 6,353 patients. Clinicians that conducted the interviews documented up to three symptoms from assessments and identification of up to four risk factors. Three clusters of risks were identified: violence that was directly related to the violence, personal violence that was not related to the violence, and personal hardship. There was a clear distinction between gender and the types of symptoms that were exhibited. Males exhibiting increased substance abuse, weeping, and suicidal ideation/attempts. Females reported experiencing more intrusive thoughts, fears of/feelings of threat, and sleep disorder symptoms. Other distinctions showed a link between anxiety-related symptoms like fear, feelings of threat, and sleep disorder symptoms and conflict-related violence. Violence not related to conflict was associated with increased impulsivity such as suicidal ideation/attempts, aggression, or substance abuse. Finally, symptoms of depression and increased suicidal ideation/attempts were equally represented in all categories of risks. This study shows that ongoing armed conflict impacts the surrounding population, both in terms of mental health and increased health burdens. This issue requires further research.

The Syrian crisis that started in March of 2011 has resulted in the largest displacement of refugees since World War II. This war continues to be destructive and has resulted in the displacement of half of the population – 8 million within Syria and over 4 million in neighboring countries (Hassan, Ventevogel, Jefee-Bahloul, Barkil-Oteo, & Kirmayer, 2016, p.2). Many factors influence mental health in affected Syrians including familial, material, and emotional loss. There are reports of increased stress symptoms due to the questionable safety of family members. The lack of social support, adaptation to new regions, and multiple displacements related to this war have been especially problematic. In addition, there has been increased hopelessness due to the protraction of the war and the lack of a foreseeable end to it. Economic losses along with lack of access to key resources impact mental health. Refugees have experienced increased discrimination, isolation, and social tensions that also impact mental health. Symptoms have been divided into five categories: emotional, cognitive, physical, social, and behavioral (Hassan et al., 2016). The reported symptoms include: sadness, grief, despair, anger, anxiety, and frustration. Other vulnerable groups such as children, the elderly, victims of torture, LGBTI individuals (lesbian, gay, bisexual, transgendered, and intersex), and victims of gender-based violence are increasingly at risk for mental health impacts.

Syrian victims of torture are increasingly vulnerable to developing psychological issues such as depression, increased panic attacks, posttraumatic stress reactions, suicidal thoughts and behaviors, increased pain, and increased somatic symptoms that are not linked to medical issues (Hassan et al., 2016). More than 50% of the displaced population are children, and over 75% are under the age of twelve (Hassan et al., 2016, p.4). Many of these children have been wounded as a result of the war, have been victims of physical or sexual abuse, or have witnessed incidents of violence. These children are increasingly at risk for being recruited by armed forces which further jeopardizes their physical and emotional safety. Child marriage, particularly for female children, introduces additional risk factors including loss of education, health risks, and domestic violence. Older children are also vulnerable due to lack of access to education or exploitation for child labor. Older refugees have their own unique challenges due to health problems and loss of social support. Studies that have been conducted with older refugees have reported the following symptoms: 41% have anxiety, 25% suffer from depression, 24% feel unsafe, and 23% feel lonely (Hassan et al., 2016, p. 5). Those with increased medical and health concerns are more vulnerable to these symptoms. LGBTI individuals are increasingly at risk in Syria for being persecuted, discriminated against, and isolated. In Syria, same sex acts are illegal, and there are overt forms of discrimination towards these groups.

Quosh, Eloul, and Ajlani (2013) demonstrate further complex dynamics related to mental health impact on refugees in Syria due to the war in Iraq in 2006 and the war in Syria. The war in Iraq resulted in an influx of refugees into Syria from neighboring regions, including 750,000 Iraqi refugees, up to half a million refugees from Palestine, and thousands of refugees from Sudan, Somalia, and Afghanistan as of census and data reported in 2010 (Quosh, Eloul, & Ajlani, 2013, p. 276). This influx of refugees into Syria resulted in a burden on infrastructures within the country. The Syrian War in 2011 resulted in an internal displacement of half of its population and an exodus to neighboring regions. Iraqi refugees that were residing in Syria as of 2006 were already living in precarious conditions due to lack of occupational or educational opportunities. More than 43.1% of Iraqi refugees were reported to be at high risk and required specific needs as of 2013 (Quosh, Eloul, & Ajlani, p. 277). In addition, it was documented that one in three Syrians required assistance as of 2013. The complex humanitarian situation in Syria also resulted in many people being displaced within the country multiple times prior to fleeing the region into neighboring countries.

As a result of these interconnected and complex dynamics, an overwhelming number of Iraqi refugees report being a victim or a witness of multiple traumatic events. Iraqi refugees in Jordan and Syria reported symptoms of depression and anxiety (42% in Jordan and 80% in Syria) (Quosh, Eloul, & Ajlani, 2013, p. 283). Mental health surveys conducted on IDP Syrians reported high levels of fatigue, fear and loss of control, increased feelings of distress, anxiety, and depressed mood. Tens of thousands of children have been reported to be victims of torture. Increased recruitment of child soldiers, sexual violence, child labor/killing/maiming, and witnessing atrocities of the war have deleterious impacts on a child's functioning. Syrians who fled to Lebanon and resided in border regions reported similar mental health impacts. A study conducted in Turkey with Syrian children residing in a camp in Southern Turkey documented that 3 of 4 children had lost a loved one, more than 60% had experiences where they felt their lives were in danger, and 50% of the children had more than six or more traumatic events (Quosh, Eloul, & Ajlani, 2013, p. 287). Reports of mental health symptoms documented a prevalence rate for depression at 60%, PTSD symptoms at 45%, aggression at 22%, and 65% had psychosomatic symptoms that significantly impacted their functioning. Despite these adverse events, the study also highlighted the resilience and support the children were able to identify and noted that 71% of girls and 60% of boys were able to identify someone that could help and support them with whom they had close relationships. Surveys of refugees residing in four camps in Southern Turkey recorded prevalence rates of PTSD at 61%, anxiety at 53%, and 54% reported symptoms of depression (Ozer, Sirin, & Oppedal, 2013, p. 36; Quosh, Eloul, & Ajlani, 2013, p. 287).

Infrastructure and Barriers to Health Care

There are many targets of war and conflict beyond individuals or specific groups (Summerfield, 2000). Those committing horrific acts of violence target what is considered the social fabric of a population. This includes infrastructures of social, economic, and cultural identity like community workers, health workers, facilities, schools, academics, human rights activists, and places of worship. Molica, Cardozo, Osofsky, Rafhael, Ager, and Salam (2004) examine complex emergencies that have catastrophic impacts on a country or the targeted populations through the destruction of political, economic, sociocultural, and health care infrastructures. Destruction of economic infrastructures includes devastation of hospitals or businesses and the displacement of impacted people to camps where there are limited opportunities for work.

After decades of armed and protracted conflict, Afghanistan has incurred significant damage to health care and mental health infrastructures (Cardoza et al., 2004). Damages include the destruction of the main psychiatric hospital in Kabul, a significant shortage of mental health professionals in Afghanistan, and limited access and functionality of one of four mental health clinics. Table 3 provides statistics of mental health providers in each region of Iraq. Table 4 (Appendix D) provides an overview of statistics on mental health providers in Syria. Table 5 (Appendix E) provides data on mental health services in Syria. Table 6 (Appendix F) provides an overview of how much money each country listed in this chapter spends on mental health services, what their access to services are, and an overview of providers in each country.

Table 3: Iraq Statistics of Mental Health Providers by Region (WHO, 2009)

Mental Health Providers	Kurdistan	South/Centre Regions
General Psychiatrists	17	?
Psychiatric Practitioners	2	27
Child and Adolescent Psychiatrists	4	?
Specialized Psychiatrists	?	86
Psychiatric Nurses	91	133
Psychologists	4	25
Social Workers	15	33
Psychotherapists	2	?

Global Health Policies and Conclusions

All of the countries covered in this chapter have mental health policies; however some lack mental health legislation (Jacob et. al, 2007). There are various recommendations made to provide mental health care services in countries with complex emergencies and in developing countries where there is both limited access to services as well as damage to health care infrastructures (Mollica et. al, 2004). For example, mental health care could be implemented in primary cares services, and physicians could be trained in mental health symptoms. Primary care physicians could treat both the physical and mental needs of patients, and this intervention could also be more culturally appropriate. Many populations are reluctant to seek mental health services due to the stigma associated with it, and the symptoms for which they seek medical treatment are often diagnosed as somatic (Mollica et. al, 2004; Summerfield, 2000). Traditional healers and their influence in local communities should also be utilized and incorporated for treatment of medical and psychiatric symptomatology.

According to the World Bank Indicators, 85% of countries are identified as low-income or middle-income countries (Jacbob et al., 2007, p. 1061). All of the countries assessed for the purposes of this chapter are considered to be in the low-income, or low-middle-income ranking (with the exception of Libya, which is listed as an upper-middle-income country). Given the current nature of conflict in these countries, this ranking may have changed as the report is from 2007. Since then, much of the infrastructure for health services may have been destroyed due to conflicts in these regions. There may be significant barriers to accessing existing services. Health care resources may be significantly overburdened due to surges of migrants and refugees into the regions.

Recommendations for providing services in complex emergencies include providing mental health services in primary care and educating and involving the public, family, and community. There are significant disparities in the amount that countries spend on mental health services as part of their Gross Domestic Expenditures. In some countries, there may be no separate allocation for these funds as mental health services are incorporated into the health care expenses.

Recommendations and Future areas of Research

Efforts to increase access to services and to build sustainability in complex humanitarian emergencies should be based on best practices and tried and true models (Dyer & Bhadra, 2013). Some of these practices and models are: IASC guidelines, Psychological First Aid, Training of Trainers, the integration of mental health care into primary care, the utilization of the Mental Health GAP, creation of child-friendly spaces, and capacity building amongst other resources. In addition, there is a dire need for research in conflict zones (Ratnayake, Degomme, Roberts, & Spiegel, 2014). Finally, standardized approaches to tracking and collecting data and tallying physical injuries would be useful in planning for medical care and rebuilding infrastructure according to the most critical need.

References

Agibiboa, D., & Maiangwa, B. (2013). Boko Haram, Religious Violence and the Crisis of National Identity in Nigeria: Towards a Non Killing Approach. *Journal of Developing Societies,* 29(4), pp. 379-403. Sage Publications.

Aginam, O. (2012, June 27). Rape and HIV as weapons of war. *United Nations University.* Retrieved from https://unu.edu/publications/articles/rape-and-hiv-as-weapons-of-war.html#info

Akil, L., & Ahmad, H. A. (2016). The recent outbreaks and reemergence of poliovirus in war and conflict-affected areas. *International Journal of Infectious Diseases, 49,* 40-46.

Al-Hamzawl, A., Buffaerts, R., Bromet, E., Alkhafaji, A., & Kessler, R. (2015). The epidemiology of major depressive episode in the Iraqi general population, *PLoS ONE,* 10(7), pp. 1-14. Retrieved from http://www.ncbi.nlm.nih.gov/pmc/articles/PMC4521818/pdf/pone.0131937.pdf on September 5, 2016.

BBC (2016, March 11). Syria: The story of the Conflict. *BBC.* Retrieved from http://www.bbc.com/news/world-middle-east-26116868

Bell, V., Mendez, F., Martinez, C., Palma, P., Bosch, M. (2012). Characteristics of the Colombian armed conflict and the mental health of civilians living in active conflict zones. *Conflict and Health, 6*(10), pp. 1-8.

Bons, S. (2015, September 25). Colombia's next challenge? A psychologically traumatized society. Interview with A. Moya. *Americas Quarterly.* Retrieved from http://www.americasquarterly.org/node/7715

Borton, C., & Rull, G. (2014, May 28). *Gunshot injuries.* Retrieved from http://patient.info/doctor/gunshot-injuries

Brave New Foundation. (2012, September 12). *Living under drones* [Video file]. Retrieved from https://www.youtube.com/watch?v=6yMOzvmgVhc&feature=youtu.be

British Broadcasting Corporation. (2016a, September 21). *Afghanistan profile: Timeline.* [Video file]. Retrieved from http://www.bbc.com/news/world-south-asia-12024253

British Broadcasting Corporation. (2016b, May 26). *Who are the Taliban?* [Video file]. Retrieved from http://www.bbc.com/news/world-south-asia-11451718

Bureau of Investigative Journalism. (2016). *Get the data: Drone wars.* Retrieved from https://www.thebureauinvestigates.com/category/projects/drones/drones-graphs/

Byman, D. (2013). Outside support for insurgent movements. *Studies in Conflict and Terrorism,* 36, pp. 981-1004.

Cardoza, B., Bilukha, O., Crawford, C., Shaikh, I., Wolfe, M., Gerber, M., & Anderson, M. (2004). Mental health, social functioning and disability in Postwar Afghanistan. *JAMA, 292*(5), pp. 575-584

CDC. (2015). CDC in the Democratic Republic of the Congo. Retrieved from http://www.cdc.gov/globalhealth/countries/drc/pdf/drc.pdf

Chatty, D. (2015). Displacement and Dispossession in the Middle East. In S. Altorik (Eds.), *A Companion to the Anthropology of the Middle East,* pp. 249-261. New York, NY: John Wiley & Sons, Inc.

Chi, P. C., Bulage, P., Urdal, H., & Sundby, J. (2015). Perceptions of the effects of armed conflict on maternal and reproductive health services and outcomes in Burundi and Northern Uganda: a qualitative study. *BMC International Health and Human Rights, 15*(7). Retrieved from http://doi.org/10.1186/s12914-015-0045-z

Council on Foreign Relations. (2016). Global Conflict Tracker: Nigeria. Retrieved from http://www.cfr.org/global/global-conflict-tracker/p32137#!/conflict/boko-haram-in-nigeria

Crawford, N. C. (2015, May 22). War-related death, injury, and displacement in Afghanistan and Pakistan 2001-2014. [Report]. *Costs of War: Watson Institute for International Studies, Brown University.* Retrieved from

http://watson.brown.edu/costsofwar/files/cow/imce/papers/2015/War%20Related
%20Casualties%20Afghanistan%20and%20Pakistan%202001-2014%20FIN.pdf

Crawford, N. C. (2013, March). Civilian death and injury in the Iraq War, 2003-2013.
[Report]. *Costs of War: Watson Institute for International Studies, Brown University.* Retrieved
from
http://watson.brown.edu/costsofwar/files/cow/imce/papers/2013/Civilian%20Deat
h%20and%20Injury%20in%20the%20Iraq%20War,%202003-2013.pdf

Currier, C., & Maass, P. (2015, October 15). Firing blind: Flawed intelligence and the limits
of drone technology. *The Intercept.* Retrieved from https://theintercept.com/drone-
papers/firing-blind/

Dabkana, T., Bunu, B., Na'aya, H., Tela, U., & Adamu, A. (2015). Pattern of injuries seen
during an insurgency: A 5-year review of 1339 cases from Nigeria. *Annals of African
Medicine, 14*(2), 114-117. doi:10.4103/1596-3519.149910

Dalacoura, K. (2012). The 2011 uprisings in the Arab Middle East: political change and
geopolitical implications. *International Affairs, 88*(1), 63-79.

Daw, M. A., El-Bouzedi, A., & Dau, A. A. (2015). Libyan armed conflict 2011: Mortality,
injury, and population displacement. *African Journal of Emergency Medicine, 5*, 101-107.

De Jong, J., Komproe, I., & Ommeron, M. (2003). Common mental disorders in
postconflict settings. *Lancet, 361*, 625-640.

Dranginis, H. (2014, March 20). Interrupting the silence: Addressing Congo's sexual violence
crisis within the Great Lakes Regional Peace Process. *The Enough Project.* Retrieved from
http://www.enoughproject.org/files/InterruptingtheSilence_AddressingCongosSexual
ViolenceCrisiswithintheGreatLakesRegionalPeaceProcess.pdf

Dyer, A., & Bhadra, S. (2013). Global disasters, war, conflict, and complex emergencies:
Caring for special popultations. In E.Sorel (Ed). *21st Century Global Mental Health,* pp.
171-209. Burlington, MA: Jones & Bartlett Learning.

Eastern Congo Initiative. (2016). *Did you know?* Retrieved from
http://www.easterncongo.org/about-drc/did-you-know

Fildis, A. (2011). The troubles in Syria: Spawned by French divide and rule. *Middle East Policy,*
Vol. XVIII (4), 1-4.

Fiske & Shackel (2014). Ending rape in war: How far have we come? *Cosmopolitan Civil
Societies: An Interdisciplinary Journal, 6*(3), 123-138.

Fleetwood, B. (2014, June 5). The Taliban is not al-Qaeda, and it's very dangerous for the
U.S. to confuse the two. *The Huffington Post.* Retrieved from
http://www.huffingtonpost.com/blake-fleetwood/the-taliban-is-not-al-
qae_b_5455252.html

Friedman-Rudovsky, J. (2016, July 28). Colombia is charting a path forward after a brutal
civil war. *Bloomberg Businessweek.* Retrieved from
http://www.bloomberg.com/news/articles/2016-07-28/colombia-is-charting-a-new-
path-forward-after-a-brutal-civil-war

Frontline (2014). The rise of ISIS. Retrieved from
http://www.pbs.org/wgbh/frontline/film/rise-of-isis/

Glenn, C. (2016, July 5). Timeline: Rise and spread of the Islamic State. Retrieved from
https://www.wilsoncenter.org/article/timeline-rise-and-spread-the-islamic-state

González, F. E. (2004). The Colombian conflict in historical perspective. *Accord, 14.*
Retrieved from
http://www.cr.org/downloads/Accord%2014_2The%20Colombian%20conflict%20in
%20historical%20perspective_2004_%20ENG.pdf

Hamblen, J., & Schnurr, P. (2016) Mental health aspects of prolonged combat stress in
civilians. *U.S. Department of Veterans Affairs.* Retrieved from
http://www.ptsd.va.gov/professional/trauma/war/combat-stress-civilians.asp

Hassan, G., Ventevogel, P., Jefee-Bahloul, H., Barkil-Oteo, A., & Kirmayer, L.J. (2016). Mental health and psychosocial wellbeing of Syrians affected by armed conflict. *Epidemiology and Psychiatric Sciences, 25(2)*, 129-141.

Horton, G. (2014, November 20). Explaining Burma's missing 9 million people: Evaporation or genocide? *The Ecologist*. Retrieved from http://www.theecologist.org/News/news_analysis/2641989/explaining_burmas_missing_9_million_people_evaporation_or_genocide.html

Hove, M., & Mutanda (2015). The Syrian Conflict 2011 to the Present: Challenges and Prospects. *Journal of Asian and African Studies, 50(5)*, 559-570.

ICD10Data. (2016). ICD-10-CM diagnosis code T74.2: Sexual abuse, confirmed. Retrieved from http://www.icd10data.com/ICD10CM/Codes/S00-T88/T66-T78/T74-/T74.2

Institute for Economics & Peace. (2015). Global terrorism index 2015: Measuring and understanding the impact of terrorism. Retrieved from http://economicsandpeace.org/wp-content/uploads/2015/11/Global-Terrorism-Index-2015.pdf

Internal Displacement Monitoring Centre. (2015). Libya IDP figures analysis. Retrieved from http://www.internal-displacement.org/middle-east-and-north-africa/libya/2015/libya-internal-displacement-as-of-march-2015

Jacob, K.S., Sharan, P., Mirza, I., Garrido-Cumbrera, M., Seedat, S., Mari, J.J., Sreenivas, V., & Saxena, S.(2007). Global Mental Health 4-Mental Health Systems in Countries: Where are we now? *The Lancet, 370*, 1061-1077.

Johannessen, S. & Holgersen, H. (2014). Former child solders' problems and needs: Congolese experiences. *Qualitative Health Research, 24*(1), 55-66.

Kessler, R., Aguilar-Gaxiola, S., Alonso, J., Chatterji, S., Yanling, H., Heeringa, S., Lee, S., & Ormerl, J. (2013). Global Mental Health Epidemiology. In E. Sorel, *21st Century Global Mental Health* (Eds.), pp. 3-52. Burlington, MA: Jones & Bartlett Learning.

Khan, A., & Hamidu, I. (2015). Boko Haram and Turmoil in Northern Nigeria. *Journal of International Relations, 19*(1), 22-42.

Koyama, J. (2014). Constructing Gender: Refugee Women working in the United States. *Journal of Refugee Studies, 28*(2), 258-275.

Langley, J., & Brenner, R. (2004). What is an injury? *Injury Prevention, 10*, 69-71. doi: 10.1136/ip.2003.003715

Latin America Working Group Education Fund. (n.d.). The human costs of the Colombian conflict. Retrieved from http://www.lawg.org/storage/documents/Col_Costs_fnl.pdf

Lawson, F. (2014). Syria's mutating civil war and its impact on Turkey, Iraq, and Iran. *International Affairs, 90*(6), pp. 1351-1364.

Mollica, R. F., Cardozo, B., Osofsky, H. J., Rafhael, B., Ager, A., & Salama, P. (2004). *Lancet, 364*, 2058-2067.

Muazzam, N., & Xiang, H. (2008, August). The epidemic of injuries in Pakistan: A neglected problem. *Journal of Pakistan Medical Association*. Retrieved from http://jpma.org.pk/full_article_text.php?article_id=1454

Nilsen, M. (2013). Will democracy bring peace to Myanmar? *International Area Studies Review, 16*(2), 115-141.

Orange County Rape Crisis Center. (2016). Rape trauma syndrome. Retrieved from http://ocrcc.org/resources/survivors/rape-trauma-syndrome/

Özer, B., Sirin, S. & Oppedal, B. (2013). Bahcesehir Study of Syrian Refugee Children in Turkey. Retrieved from https://www.fhi.no/globalassets/migrering/dokumenter/pdf/bahcesehir-study-report3.pdf

Peace Direct. (2016). Pakistan: Conflict profile. Retrieved from https://www.insightonconflict.org/conflicts/pakistan/conflict-profile/

Peace Direct. (2009). Democratic Republic of the Congo: Conflict profile. Retrieved from https://www.insightonconflict.org/conflicts/dr-congo/conflict-profile/

Puvacic & Weinberg. (1994). Impact of war on infectious disease in Bosnia-Hercegovina. *British Medical Journal, 309*(6963), p. 1207-1208.

Quosh, C., Eloul, L., & Ajlani, R. (2013). Mental Health of refugees and displaced persons in Syria and surrounding countries: a systematic review. *Intervention, 11*(3), 276-294.

Ratnayake, R., Degomme, O., Roberts, B., & Spiegel, P. (2014). Conflict and Health: seven years of advancing science in humanitarian crises. *Conflict and Health, 8*(7), 1-6.

Rehn, E., & Johnson-Sirleaf, E. (2002). Women, war and peace: The Independent Experts' Assessment on the impact of armed conflict on women and women's role in peacebuilding. *United Nations Development Fund for Women*. Retrieved from https://www.unfpa.org/sites/default/files/pub-pdf/3F71081FF391653DC1256C69003170E9-unicef-WomenWarPeace.pdf

Restrepo, J., Spagat, M., & Vargas, J. F. (2004). The dynamics of the Colombian civil conflict: A new data set. *Homo Oeconomicus, 21*(2), 396-428.

Rybarczyk, B., Behel, J., & Szymanksi, L. (2010). Limb amputation. In R. G. Frank, M. Rosenthal, & B. Caplan (Eds.), *Handbook of Rehabilitation Psychology* (2nd Ed.). Washington, D.C.: American Psychological Association.

Sahloul, M., Monla-Hassan, J., Sankari, A., Kherallah, M., Atassi, B., Badr, S., Abarra, A., & Sparrow, A. (2016). War is the enemy of health. *Annals of the American Thoracic Society, 13*(2), 147-155.

Samararatne, D. W. V. A., & Soldatic, K. (June 25, 2015). Inclusions and exclusions in law: experiences of women with disability in rural and war-affected areas in Sri Lanka. *Disability & Society, 30*(5), 759-772.

Schmid, A. (2011). The definition of terrorism. In A. P. Schmid Ed (2011). *The Routledge Handbook of Terrorism Research*, pp. 39-98. Abington, Oxon: Routledge.

Scrandis, D. A., & Watt, M. (2014, October). Child sexual abuse in boys: Implications for primary care. *The Journal for Nurse Practitioners, 10*(9), 706-713.

Searcy, D. (2016, September 22). Boko Haram rages in Nigeria, but the world's eyes are elsewhere. *The New York Times*. Retrieved from http://www.nytimes.com/2016/09/23/world/africa/boko-haram-terrorism-maiduguri-nigeria.html?_r=0

Sidel, V., & Levy, B. (2003). War, terrorism, and public health. *Journal of Law, Medicine, & Ethics, 31(4)*, 516-523.

South, A. (2011). Burma's longest war anatomy of the Karen conflict. [Report]. Transnational Institute Burma Center Netherlands.

Stanford International Human Rights and Conflict Resolution, & Global Justice Clinic. (2012). Living under drones: Death, injury and trauma to civilians from US drone practices in Pakistan. Retrieved from http://www.livingunderdrones.org/wp-content/uploads/2013/10/Stanford-NYU-Living-Under-Drones.pdf

Summerfield, D. (2000). War and mental health: a brief overview. *British Medical Journal, 321*, 232-235.

Surrency, A. B., Graitcer, P., & Henderson, A. K. (2007, June). Key factors for civilian injuries and deaths from landmines and ordnance. *Injury Prevention, 13*(3), 197. doi: 10.1136/ip.2005.011304

Thompson, N. (2016, August 11). Ukraine: Everything you need to know about how we got here. *CNN*. Retrieved from http://www.cnn.com/2015/02/10/europe/ukraine-war-how-we-got-here/index.html

Tol, W., Song, S., & Jordans, M. (2013). Annual Research Review: Resilience and mental health in children and adolescents living in areas of armed conflict- a systematic review of findings in low-and middle-income countries. *The Journal of Child Psychology and Psychiatry, 54*(4), 445-460.

U.N. (2003). *Demining*. Retrieved from http://www.un.org/en/globalissues/demining/

United Nations Assistance Mission in Afghanistan. (2016, July 25). Afghanistan: Record level of civilian casualties sustained in first half of 2016: UN report. Retrieved from http://unama.unmissions.org/afghanistan-record-level-civilian-casualties-sustained-first-half-2016-un-report

United Nations High Commissioner for Refugees (2016, September 26). Syria regional refugee response: Inter-agency information sharing portal. Retrieved from http://www.cfr.org/global/global-conflict-tracker/p32137#!/conflict/kurdish-conflict

United Nations High Commissioner for Refugees. (2015). Global trends: Forced displacement in 2015. [Report]. Retrieved from http://www.unhcr.org/en-us/statistics/unhcrstats/576408cd7/unhcr-global-trends-2015.html

United Nations Office of the Coordination of Humanitarian Affairs. (2016). Syria crisis regional overview: About the crisis. Retrieved from http://www.unocha.org/syrian-arab-republic/syria-country-profile/about-crisis

United States Institute of Peace. (2016, January 27). The current situation in Colombia. Retrieved from http://www.usip.org/publications/2016/01/27/the-current-situation-in-colombia

Webster, P. C. (2012, April 3). Health in Colombia: The chronic disease burden. *Canadian Medical Association Journal, 184*(6), E293-E294.

Webster, P. C. (2012b, April 3). Health in Columbia: Treating the displaced. *Canadian Medical Association Journal, 184*(6), 109-125.

World Health Organization. (2016). Infectious diseases. Retrieved from http://www.who.int/topics/infectious_diseases/en/

World Health Organization. (2016b). Injuries. Retrieved from http://www.who.int/topics/infectious_diseases/en/

World Health Organization. (2015, January). Noncommunicable diseases. Retrieved from http://www.who.int/mediacentre/factsheets/fs355/en/

World Health Organization. (2015b). World Health Organization global disability action plan 2014-2021: Better health for all people with disability. Retrieved from http://www.who.int/disabilities/actionplan/en/

World Health Organization. (2015). Yemen crisis: Health facility-based reported deaths and injuries, 19 March-16 October 2015. Retrieved from http://www.emro.who.int/yem/yemeninfocus/yemen-casualities.html

World Health Organization. (2014). Country Cooperation Strategy at a glance: Columbia. Retrieved from http://www.who.int/countryfocus/cooperation_strategy/ccsbrief_col_en.pdf

World Health Organization (2009). Iraqi Mental Health Survey-2006/2007. Retrieved from https://mhpss.net/?get=250/3.-WHO-Iraq-MH-survey.pdf

World Health Organization (2009). The Democratic Republic of the Congo: Quantifying the crisis. *Bulletin of the World Health Organization, 87*(1). Retrieved from http://www.who.int/bulletin/volumes/87/1/09-020109/en/#

World Health Organization. (2004). Chapter 6: Sexual violence. *Violence and Injury Prevention.* [Report]. Retrieved http://www.who.int/violence_injury_prevention/violence/global_campaign/en/chap6.pdf

World Health Organization (2002). World report on violence and health. Geneva: World Health Organization. Retrieved from http://www.who.int/violence_injury_prevention/violence/global_campaign/en/chap6.pdf

World Without Genocide. (2016). Democratic Republic of the Congo. Retrieved from http://worldwithoutgenocide.org/genocides-and-conflicts/congo

Yad Vashem. (2016). The Holocaust. Retrieved from http://www.yadvashem.org/yv/en/holocaust/about/

CHAPTER 3

A Comparative Analysis of Global Health in South and Southeast Asia (India, Sri Lanka, Malaysia, and Singapore)

Anjhula Mya Singh Bais

At A Glance: Moving Increasingly Eastward

For a significant time period in history, Asia was the beacon of a land flourishing as it led the world in trade, commerce, statesmanship, secular plurality, the arts, and military. Circa the 1500s, this influence began to wane, and Europe, with the colonising[*] tendencies of the British, Dutch, French, Portuguese, and Spaniards, took its place on the global stage (MacDonald & Lemco, 2011). A noteworthy history lesson repeats itself here: nothing is static. The tide began to change in the latter half of the twentieth century as Asia closed ranks with the Global North through economic resurgence and political power. It used to be that globalisation and the United States of America had interchangeable meaning, yet through world events of 9/11, the 2004 tsunami, the financial crisis of 2008, and the on-going global warming challenge, the world has cognised, however nascent, the need for synchronisation across platforms, institutions, and policies, especially within Asia. South and Southeast Asia in particular

---

[*] I have elected to write in British English given the global nature of this textbook. In addition to fluency, all countries that were formerly British colonies speak and write British English. Schools in most non-English speaking countries instruct their language classes predominantly in British English making British English familiar to a global majority.

comprise an estimated 33.42% of the world's population (World Bank, 2016a, Graph 2; Worldometers, 2016, Graph 1) with many overarching similarities that qualify both regions to be considered in tandem. Myanmar, the fastest growing economy (Myers, 2016) in the world, is situated squarely in this region with literal and metaphoric revolutions occurring in communication and technology, healthcare, and the public, private, and political (PPP) spheres. With upending change sprinkled liberally throughout, the imperative to gather context and implications on regional global health for healthcare and policy workers, medical professionals, politicians, and scholars alike becomes a necessity.

India

A Different Kind of War

India has waged and been immersed in less than twenty wars with one defeat since freeing itself from a long history of British colonialism and its establishment as the Republic of India in 1947. The new war India faces is a silent war in the health care of its citizens with outcomes that are often more tragic, yet the markers indicate an attractive opportunity across the health care vertical for people to provide, access, and create (Columbia University, 2012). As the second-most populous country and largest democracy in the world, the over one billion citizens of India have a life expectancy of sixty-eight years and a gender ratio of 940 females per 1000 males with 70% living in rural areas (Government of India, 2011, Item 3). In the early sixties, the "Green Revolution" that created advancements in agriculture yields coupled with advancements in medical technology created a population explosion that severely strained health capabilities (Rorabacher, 2015).

Health care reports, policy analysts, and mental health workers often cite cultural moorings as an impediment to effectively implementing accessible and affordable health care in India. The move by parliament in 2014 to invalidate its draconian 309 section of the Indian penal code by decriminalising suicide attempts has yet to materialise. The World Health Organisation (WHO) (2014a) cites India as having the highest suicide rate in 2012 with the Southeast Asia region carrying the most suicides globally at 39% (para. 20). In India, family problems include cultural phenomena such as the dowry system, livelihood struggles due to overpopulation, and sati, a form of suicide that requires the female to die, often forcibly, on her husband's funeral pyre. Statistics from the National Crime Records Bureau (NCBE) (2014) indicate illness and family problems as the most-cited reasons for suicide. Each spring, released exam results correlate with an increased spike in suicide amongst students. In 2013, there were 2,471 suicides as a result of exam failure (NCBR, 2014). India's population forces extreme competition where scoring close to perfect is not enough to gain admission to higher studies.

The government's neoliberal and paradoxical attempt at upholding the dignity of life by placing sanctions on suicide fails to account for its increasing numbers. Tellingly, the majority of suicides occur in middle-income India, which is grappling with an explosion of globalisation (NCBR, 2014). Evidence (WHO, 2016a) cites depression, alcohol, and substance abuse as the three highest factors involved in suicide. These factors are preventable and can be reduced with adequate provision of rehabilitation and service provision. Indian attitudes towards health issues like mental health, leprosy, and cancer however, carry deep stigma that complicates infectious disease and health management and also affects both patient and provider narratives. Studies (Namasivayam, Osuorah, Syed, & Antai, 2012) describe health issues as a complex multidimensional maze of variables including caste, socioeconomic status (SES), and gender, in which a lower-caste, dark-skinned woman is most likely to face poverty and its accompanying public shame, resulting in little access to already-overburdened health care systems.

Patriarchy wields its dangerous influence in a plethora of ways in a country that places strong emphasis on producing a boy child. Education opportunities and medical attention is bestowed as an inherently male right whenever rural and urban poor are forced to make a choice between a girl or boy child. Though India bans gender screening in an attempt to reverse gender ratio disparity, actual ratios bear testimony to the occurrence of illegal and dangerous abortions of female foetuses and simultaneously indicate causes behind high maternal mortality rates (Bhattacharyya, S.K., Saha, S.P., Bhattacharya, S., & Pal, R., 2011). The financial consequences of dowry and marriage plus worry about keeping a girl child safe render mothers vulnerable to attacks by in-laws and husbands, as well as a deep sense of shame. During field work, I have observed Indian activists poignantly attempting to reverse this cultural conditioning by hanging Haryanvi signs in Northern Indian villages which rhetorically ask, "If you kill the girl child, where will you find your daughters-in-law?" Lack of education amongst the populace spirals downward into misinformation on health rights and issues. Despite an estimated 45% reduction globally since the nineties (WHO, 2014b, para. 1), the maximum number of maternal deaths worldwide occur in India due to a significant lack of awareness. Patriarchy can be understood through relational, societal, and individual indices like earning prowess, autonomous decision making, age at school completion and marriage, attitudes towards domestic violence, shared labour, and menstruation, which provide insight into access to health care and dependence on men. Namasivayam et al. (2012) write, "The status of women and gender norms in a society determine to a great extent the dynamics of women's relationships with their spouses or male partners, and their place in the household" (para. 9). The combination of gender-based violence and India's rural, patriarchal society's tolerance of polygyny leaves women with little to no say in matters of their own health.

The British colonial rule of India, which was motivated by expedient economic gain, had less "Westernised" results than those of the Portuguese or French, who intently disseminated the original culture and religion of their colonies. The rigid and thousands-year-old caste system faced a relaxation in colonial times that assisted upward mobility for a new professional class of English-speaking elites such as doctors, teachers, lawyers, and industrialists. This easing of caste restrictions coalesced into a new "caste" of the urban elite. Today, with their disproportionate access and ability to pay for quality health care, the urban elite form the bulk of India's out-of-pocket health expenditure at 67%, putting India 23% higher than average for lower-middle-income countries (McKinsey&Company, 2012, p. 13). Overpopulation, one of India's most pressing humanitarian issues considering its effects on education, policy, and application, heralds back to colonial times. India's population bypassed a system of checks and balances as the British reduced local thievery on vast swaths of roads, reduced internal strife between Indian royal states, introduced the smallpox vaccination and quarantine, criminalised infanticide and sati, reduced rat infestations, and, to a small degree, minimised famine. Introducing Western medicine, training doctors, and emphasising sanitation and hygiene resulted in a population increase of two and half times between 1757 and 1947, the year of India's independence (Maddison, 1971).

Unlike neighbouring Sri Lanka's militaristic war, India grapples with a deathly war at the hands of corruption and lack of progressive legislation. A 2012 McKinsey& Company report on Indian health care cites India as missing a holistic regulatory framework and, for all its moving parts and pieces, "implementation has lagged" (p.16). The Clinical Establishments Registration Act, which sought to standardise quality of care, training, practice, assessment, and malpractice issues across India, was tedious in implementation. In its interim, rural India, which accounts for up to 70% of all communicable diseases (McKinsey&Company, 2012, p. 21), lay vulnerable to quacks, religious god men claiming curative powers, and persons insufficiently trained as 57% of allopathic doctors are not qualified (WHO, 2016b, p. 9). A high proportion of Indian nurses and medical practitioners are inactive in the formal work sphere; the density of practitioners to patients at 0.743 per 1000 indicates not only severe shortages of human resources, but unequal distribution as well (World Bank, 2011, figure 1 interactive world map).

The Lancet (2015) states, "The many new institutions set up in the past decade... encouraged by commercial incentives, have often fuelled corrupt practices and failed to offer quality education" (p. 2428). Despite government increases in medical training programs, specialists are lacking, in part because the incentive structure found in Singapore and because overarching policies for health are missing. The living conditions, apathy, and dispassionate bureaucracy all but grind progress to a halt and contribute largely to India's brain drain. Between 2000 and 2009, a 256% increase of citizens going abroad for higher studies occurred (ICEF Monitor, 2012, para. 1), and the majority of students and citizens continued to stay in their host country via highly-skilled migrant programmes. The Indian health care system has devolved into a war between medical doctors and the government which surrounds a 2015 move by the union health ministry to no longer issue no-objection certificates to doctors who want to settle abroad permanently as "it goes against the public health interests of the citizens of India" (Deshpande, 2016, para. 4). The Central Maharashtra Resident Doctors Association has challenged the attempt at increasing India's brain bank on the grounds of human rights (Deshpande, 2016).

Impediments and Inspirations

Whilst the road ahead remains long for India, it is evident that every impediment is matched by inspiration, quite often by quotidian juggad, a colloquial Hindi term meaning creative and low-cost solutions. Poverty has proven to be a great barrier in receiving equitable health care, yet a World Bank (2015) report estimates that India has reduced its poverty to 12.4% down from 21% between 2011-2012 (graph 1). A dramatic reduction of people subsisting on the global poverty line ($1.90 a day) is actually possible due to the provision of electricity to 96% of villages in India. The data indicates that regular and reliable sources of electricity have an inverse relation between poverty and health with health increasing; consequently, the fact that 69% (p. 27) of Indian homes do not have access to electricity can be considered a persistent impediment (Jain, Ray, Ganesan, Aklin, Cheng & Urpelainen, 2015). Bi-directional relationships between health and poverty is long established as Singh (2014) notes:

> If you look at the health burden, eighty percent of India's health problems can be solved at the primary level itself. We keep our homes very clean but the streets outside are very dirty. For example, 70% of India's bed capacity in health care is because of water borne diseases. (as cited in Kumar, 2014, para. 17)

Increased interest and research beginning in the economic liberalisation era of the early nineties attracted foreign entities including McKinsey & Company, The Boston Consulting Group, and Columbia University, whose collective recommendations include purifying water systems and prioritising sanitation to significantly reduce India's health burden. 2015 figures estimate 60.4% of Indians are without toilet access (WaterAid, 2015, p. 23).

The same sources states, "If all 774 million people in India waiting for household toilets were made to stand in a line, the queue would stretch from Earth to the moon and beyond" (p.7). The flummoxing results of research say that Indians have more access to TV than they do to tap water and have more access to cell phones than they do to toilets (Census of India, 2011; Hamilton, 2010). Encouragingly, New Delhi boasts more accessible water per capita than London; utilising efficient water management can leverage phenomenal health benefits whilst reducing pressure on hospital beds by 70% (Kumar, 2014, para. 18).

The needs of India as a developing country are unique; factoring in corresponding attitudes and identities based on religious and sociocultural variables leads to targeted health care results. Technological innovations are often viewed as costly sophistries that are unmanageable by the Indian rural illiterate. By considering accessibility and affordability and combining them with awareness campaigns, Intel India launched Lifephoneplus in 2015, which enables people to monitor ECG and glucose levels themselves (Pachouri, 2016). As non-communicable diseases rise across countries in the Association of Southeast Nations (ASEAN) and the South Asian Association of Regional Cooperation (SAARC), this technology capitalises on existing mobile phone consumption by utilising blue tooth capability and remotely sending reports directly to doctors. The increased implementation of telemedicine and mobile phone applications, which directly impact primary health care outcomes by connecting rural patients to qualified urban doctors, enjoys unprecedented acceptance by Indian and other South Asian governments like Bangladesh and Pakistan (Pachouri, 2016). Levelling the field of accessibility via technology begins the process of redressing India's inherently imbalanced caste system and SES. In liberal India, the economic gains of the poor plateau, and, in their culturally-accepted resignation to karma (a concept that accepts injustice at birth), they acquiesce that the rich, powerful upper castes were allowed to maintain the status quo until challenged by an idea rapidly gaining ground: universal health care.

Navigating India, a diverse country with over one thousand dialects and ancient cultural credos, proves to be a lesson in internationalising repertoires: less Western, in favour of a more nuanced and interconnected approach. Employing modern medicine as a one-size-fits-all proliferates disaster, yet the kaleidoscope of old wives tales, superstitions, parallel health systems, and deeply-entrenched beliefs and rituals have not served the average Indian well either. The impediment is the unregulated, unaccepted, and perceived unreliability of Indian Ayurveda and homeopathic health systems; however, receiving indigenous acceptance and cultural buy-in becomes crucial in streamlining what twenty-first century health care looks like in India. The rigorous upholding of fasting associated with religious festivals (Ramadan, Navratri) is thought to embody discipline and purification, yet has mixed results on its impact on bodily health. Jewellery and trinkets (e.g., sacred beads and threads) are worn to symbolise devotion, religious sacredness; however, since removal is forbidden, some individuals are reluctant to take MRI scans. Furthermore, due to India's relatively modest culture, hospitals typically decline a pap smear to unmarried women in order to leave an intact hymen, and Indians may resist reproductive examinations all together, least of all by a doctor of the opposite sex (Trepanowski & Bloomer, 2010; 'Caring for the Sikh Patient', 2016; Nene et al., 2007).

Triaging and monitoring pain levels is stymied as Hindu patients often view pain as progress on a spiritual path. For example, women are often deterred by their husbands and mothers-in-law from evoking their right to an epidural during childbirth. Mental illness carries deep stigma and is often believed to be the result of "evil eye" and of past life actions. Karmic beliefs may also be invoked during end-of-life decisions. Death is often viewed as pre-determined and part of one's destiny, so prolonging a life is unnecessary. The central government and separate ministries make concerted efforts in harmonising both the modern and traditional in India, thereby presenting a unified and integrated approach that can be adopted for global health. While lobbying the U.N. to declare an International Day of Yoga, Indian Prime Minister Narendra Modi stated at the U.N. General assembly in 2014:

> Yoga is an invaluable gift of India's ancient tradition. It embodies unity of mind and body; thought and action; restraint and fulfilment; harmony between man and nature; a holistic approach to health and well-being. It is not about exercise but to discover the sense of oneness with yourself, the world and the nature. By changing our lifestyle and creating consciousness, it can help in well-being... (United Nations, 2016, para. 1)

India suggested the twenty-first of June to be the day of yoga, noting its special meaning globally in being the longest day of the year. The International Day of Yoga came into effect in 2014 after being voted in by a record of 175 U.N. member states (United Nations, 2016).

Sri Lanka

War and Natural Disaster

The small, tear-shaped island of Sri Lanka (formerly known as Ceylon)fsri is strikingly similar to its Northern neighbour, India, in aspects of culture, language, religion, and dress; however, the psychological and physical terrains of its inhabitants speak another narrative. The ethnic civil war, fought between the majority Sinhalese and a minority Tamil faction group (Liberation Tigers of Tamil Eelam [LTTE]) for a separate and independent Tamil homeland, has the dubious distinction of being Asia's costliest civil war. It lasted from 1983-2009, and Murphy & Lakshminarayana, (2006) estimated that only 6% of the population did not experience war trauma (as cited in Sritharan & Sritharan, 2014, p.151). Since 1948, post-independence ethnic strife between the Tamils and Sinhalese has revolved around issues of social equality (Ross & Savada, 1988) and historically-rooted, familial, and generational ideology, including gender roles that began to transform during war (Thiranagama, 2011).

Conflicting reports between the Sri Lankan government and international bodies such as the U.N exacerbate the deep toll war has on human health and capital. Whilst the government puts the death toll at an estimated nine thousand people, a U.N. Secretary General report commissioned by Ban Ki Moon stated the tally to be an estimated forty thousand people (ICRtoP, 2017, para. 1; Moon, 2011, clause 137, p. 41). The lack of transparency, accountability, and explanation compounds issues of mental health, as evidenced by Sri Lanka's rank as fourth-highest country regarding suicide with deaths attributed to a complex array of psychosocial and geo-political factors (WHO, 2014a). The 2004 tsunami left over 35,000 dead (UNICEF, 2009, p. 10), exponentially compounding the extreme strain already placed on northern and eastern families located geographically at the heart of the war. As a result, female-headed households increased significantly, rates of drug and alcohol use increased, and the social fabric of the community was torn asunder (Somasundaram, 2014).

In a country beset both by manmade and natural disasters, Sri Lanka falls woefully short of the recommended mental health practitioner and client ratio, with approximately three psychologists in the government health sector (De Zoysa, 2013, p. 18) serving a population of over twenty million people (Department of Census, 2016, p. 2). The uphill challenges of rehabilitating child soldiers back into communities that are rejection-prone remain steep; post-traumatic stress disorder (PTSD) stemming from rape and sexual abuse as war tools and from enforced disappearances like the white van phenomena ("The return of the white van", 2016) goes untreated.

Trauma is complicated even further by political and geographical disputes pertaining to land-owning rights regarding property that was illegally-seized and annexed during war and livelihood that was displaced by the tsunami and replaced by militant factions. Religious institutions and cultural appropriation abound at the forefront of tensions amongst Tamils and Sinhalese; while the war is over, the fear is not.

Watters (2010) describes something akin to the gold rush phenomena in the early 2000s as international researchers flocked Sri Lanka to study PTSD in real time. According to Miller, Fernando, and Berger (2009) not only was PTSD prevalence overstated, but obvious variables thought to be behind PTSD (war and natural disaster) were found to be less damaging than the everyday stressors of poverty and lack of access to basic health care and education. The Sri Lankan education system almost came to a complete halt during the war, resulting in the burden of a non-skilled, unemployed, restless, and often violent youth demographic (Gunatilaka, Mayer, & Vodopivec, 2010). Considering the psychological distress of Sri Lankan citizens (especially children), the following are in dire need of further study: the pathologised idea of military violence and war at a societal level, the culture of impunity, and the cultural fit of Western trauma paradigms and counselling methods.

Perhaps the greatest burden of global health in the Sri Lankan context falls on those who have no home. Although Sri Lanka was once highly-esteemed by Singapore in terms of economic prosperity and quality of life, Sri Lanka's most significant loss is exemplified by the 2006 estimate of over 500,000 civilians displaced through the war (Lund & McDonald, 2015, p. 227). In both absolute terms and the proportion of those displaced, Sri Lankan ranks as having one of Asia's largest displacement crises. Humanitarian responses were inadequately prepared for ineffective cease-fires, indiscriminate bombings and killings, flying shrapnel, planted land mines, exhaustion of livelihoods, and propaganda by the state-controlled media. The U.N. was found to have failed Sri Lankans to the extent to which the outside world was left in the dark with incomplete evidence that could have mobilised desperately-needed help (U.N., 2012).

Power at best is often nebulous and abstract in form, yet its effects have real consequences on economic, social, political, local, regional, and global interests of individuals and groups. As president of Sri Lanka from 2005-2015, Mahinda Rajapaksa amended the constitution through stroke of executive power and attempted to scrap the two-term limit in order to seek an unprecedented third term (Bastians & Harris, 2014). Under the former Rajapaksa regime, health and economic concerns of ethnic groups were bypassed, military spending took precedence, and corruption robbed internal revenue, which forestalled any effort to provide for the well-being of Sri Lankans. The opposition government countered the nepotistic state of affairs and took office in 2015 by shock defeat, thereby dismantling the worldview of Sri Lanka as a corrupt and jingoistic government, as a country where its politics was one of the bullet rather than of the ballot (Transparency International, 2015).

Sibling Rivalry?

As the regional superpower, India is hard for Sri Lankans to ignore. Because the Sinhalese migrated from India to Sri Lanka in 500 B.C., the two are connected by shared ties of history, geography, and culture, and learning is a bi-directional process for both countries. The comparison of India and Sri Lanka (adjusting for geographical and population size) gives rise to a number of key observations. Attitudes toward and treatment of women in Sri Lanka are paradoxical. Whilst India lags behind in female equality beginning with the gender ratio, Sri Lanka reverses this trend and holds at around ninety-four males per one hundred females (Department of Census, 2012, p. 1). Its maternal mortality rate is the envy of South Asia - only thirty-two deaths per 100,000 women in 2015, compared to India's 174 (World Bank, 2015, Graph 2 overview). Sri Lanka boasts of the modern world's first female head of state, yet domestic violence is very much a part of the cultural landscape. Considering policy regarding universal health care, rigorous statistic and record keeping, and the implementation of free-of-cost mid-wifery from "womb until tomb", Sri Lanka appears to be well in terms of developmental markers. The cultural dictates of women as caregivers and nurturers, however, strengthen the stereotype of men as leaders and limit women's representation in a number of spheres. Research in Rajasthan and West Bengal, India has demonstrated that creating a quota for females in politics leads to "...increased investment in goods favoured by women..." (Pande & Ford, 2011, p.19). Addressing these gaps ensures that Sri Lanka maintains and increases its lead in women's overall health and participation.

Thrice colonised with the British leaving in 1948, Sri Lanka was left with outposts and institutions similar to India, including the hospital and tertiary university system. India officially recognises twenty-two languages, and Sri Lanka recognises one (Sinhala), though its sizeable minority speaks Tamil. The 1956 Sinhala Only Act replaced English as the official language and highlights how far-reaching policy considerations become. The law required setting up separate Tamil and Sinhala schools, and a generation later, with ethnicities unable to communicate, conflict predictably deepened in the form of the 1977 riots that presaged the traumatic civil war. Colonisation had become a double-edged sword; on the one hand, the implementation of the Sinhala Only Act justified an assertion of national identity after 1948, yet on the other, the Tamil minority bitterly opposed it as the defining piece of divisive legislature and ethnic discrimination. The policy effect was nothing short of drastic. Brown and Ganguly (2003) write:

> In 1956, 30 percent of the Ceylon administrative service, 50 percent of the clerical service, 60 percent of engineers and doctors, and 40 percent of the armed forces were Tamil. By 1970 those numbers had plummeted to 5 percent, 5 percent, 10 percent, and 1 percent, respectively. (p. 73)

Following this, during the 1960s, Tamils were largely unable to avail government services, forms, and paperwork. During the Rajapaksa regime, nascent steps were taken to lay a strong foundation for the re-emergence of bi-language capability, and a record number of government and public servants sat Sinhala-Tamil proficiency exams (Ivan, 2010). Such actions are targeted at naturally accumulating transparency and inspiring dialogue across ethnicities and formal cultural divides.

South Asia Brief

India, the world's largest democracy, has maintained, albeit haphazardly, a commitment to the ideals of democracy and a belief in unity in diversity. Sri Lanka's strategy in modern times is often viewed as "tolerating" and "accommodating" ethnic minorities, which calls into crisis the identity of various fourth-generation ethnic groups such as Moors, Tamils, and Burghers who feel Sri Lankan, but are not acknowledged as "pure blood". Identity politics within each country and amidst the South Asia region was a catalysing variable with which colonialists capitalised by further driving a wedge in existing tensions. Global health's upward trajectory remains perilous as the cluster of countries comprising SAARC has been dubbed a "system of States" in contrast to their counterpart ASEAN, which is likened to a "society of States" (Sridharan & Srinivasa-Raghavan, 2007, p.115). This implies inefficient machinery for the former and individuals gathered as a family for survival in the latter. Examining global health purely through health and development indicators in order to further growth and possibility is impossible without musing over the colonial legacies, military balance, and regional complexities vis-a-vis ideology and strategy. South Asia maintains one of the highest rates of intra-state conflict from a regional perspective – there's terrorism and political instability in Pakistan and Afghanistan, Maoist uprisings in Nepal, Tamil separatism in Sri Lanka, economic and ethnic violence in Bangladesh, illegal immigration pouring into Bhutan, and a weary India, constantly on its guard whilst facing cross-border terrorism. It's important to note that lack of cohesion and cooperation have created stagnation in a regional block that contains an estimated 21% of the world's population and 7% of the world's gross domestic product (GDP) (World Bank, 2016, graph 2; International Monetary Fund [IMF], 2016, p.7).

Malaysia

Translating Natural Abundance as a Force for Humanity

As the twenty-seventh largest economy in the world (IMF, 2016, p. 183), Malaysia enjoys a plethora of renewable and non-renewable natural resources such as palm oil, rubber, and timbre. The World Bank (2013) recognised Malaysia as being second to Taiwan in having the lowest poverty rates in the world at 3.8% (Graph 1). Not unlike Sri Lanka, Malaysia's health indicators paint another story underscoring GDP to be of less importance compared to political will and cultural emphasis on well-being. Malaysia has an estimated multicultural population of 30 million, which is comprised of Malays, Indigenous, Chinese, and Indians, with the opposite demographic divide of India: the majority of Indians live rurally, whereas over 70% of Malaysians live in urban areas. As in India, non-communicable diseases have leapt forth at an alarming rate as the race for Malaysia's 2020 developed nation status intensifies (Department of Statistics Malaysia, 2016, PDF 1; Economic Planning Unit, [EPU], 2016). Malaysia's health spending (4.6% of the GDP in 2009) is largely from public spending, yet despite an opened and expanding economy, growth has not kept pace with urbanisation, resulting in a severe shortage of doctors, trained nurses, and other health professionals (Jaafar, Noh, Muttalib, Othman, & Healy, 2013, p. xiii). In addition to a large dichotomy between the rich and poor, private and public hospitals, and health access between rural islands and the urban landscape, the Malaysian Department of Statistics estimates the gender division will also keep widening, with 107 males to every 100 females, compared to the world average of 101.8 (Department of Statistics Malaysia, 2016, PDF 1).

Whilst production of qualified medical and health professionals lags behind, financially better-off Malaysians pay out-of-pocket for private health care, emulating the trend in India. In turn, public hospitals with long wait times between onset and treatment, unavailability of doctors, accreditation issues, declining infrastructure, and a public perception of "lesser quality" treatment must treat a staggering, disproportionate number of poorer and sicker patients. Despite the steps the Malaysian government has taken to increase placements at medical university as well as the fact that the issue was debated at length in parliament, there is no conclusive policy on how to increase and better adapt the public health care system. The government, like that of India and Singapore, energises investments on medical tourism in order to capitalise on the lucrative global market as a key player. The private sector has received immense investment towards medical tourism; the number of tourists seeking medical care tripled between 2003-2007 (Medical Travel Growing, 2009, para. 4). The largest consumers of medical tourism are Indonesia (72%), Singapore (10%), and then India, Europe, and other countries (Jaafar, Noh, Muttalib, Othman, & Healy, 2013, p.21).

A key selling point the government puts forth is that 90% of its doctors are foreign accredited with English-speaking skills, which underscores the subtle but deeply-entrenched post- colonial influence (Health Tourism, 2016, para. 7). Disparities between the public and private sectors manifest in lack of coordination and communication between the sectors (save regarding highly lucrative and rewarding medical tourism, which calls attention to the humanitarian debate of why the right to universal and accessible health care is not available to all). Malaysia's policies on gender, ethnicity, environment, and human rights ought to be scrutinised in the context of how to further global health, both overtly and covertly. Malaysia refuses to be a signatory for the U.N. convention of refugees, despite the influx of undocumented Sri Lankans and Burmese fleeing persecution. Female political representation in Malaysia is the second-lowest in Southeast Asia at 10% (Mulakala, 2013, para. 3). Every thirty-five minutes, a female is raped (Tan, 2015). Mass graves of trafficked persons found on the Thai border serve as a stark reminder of the Malaysian female's predicament (Mulakala, 2013, para. 3; Women's Centre for Change, 2015; "Two Dozen", 2015). Endangering its very source of economic prosperity, Malaysia carries one of the highest rates of deforestation in the world. Annual smog has led to a full scale public health emergency, resulting in endemic long-term health problems like lung cancer, asthma, and breathing difficulties, especially pronounced amongst the elderly and school-aged children (Schwartz, 2015).

After years of holding at tier three in the Trafficking Persons Report (the lowest grade possible, which signifies a deplorable human trafficking record), Malaysia has been upgraded to tier two by the independent U.S. State Department office that grades worldwide efforts to curb trafficking. Trafficking drugs constitutes the automatic death penalty, oftentimes with secret executions in which one is presumed guilty until proven innocent and only clemency by a state sultan can convert a death sentence into life imprisonment (Amnesty, 2016a). Ethnic tensions continue to rise as policies that favour *bumiputras*, or sons of the soil, are maintained. *Bumiputras* make up approximately two-thirds of the population; Malaysia's ethnic Chinese and Indians bear the brunt of what is felt as state-sponsored discrimination ("A Never Ending", 2013). While Malaysia is touted as an exotic, modern, and a speedily-developing country, the aforementioned issues indicate oppression that is shielded from public consciousness at large. Much like Sri Lanka, Malaysia is indulging in parallel systems - the sunny face of tourism that the world sees and the stark debilitating realties that citizens face every day. This dissonance is in urgent need of rectification.

In every country, there is a core issue from which problems spring forth. A strong argument can be made that corruption is at Malaysia's core, and it's debilitating effects are felt across the world. In 2016, the United States Department of Justice (USDOJ) announced the "filing of and recovery of more than one billion USD in assets associated with an international conspiracy to launder funds misappropriated from the Malaysian sovereign wealth fund known as 1MDB" (para. 1). The move constitutes the largest single action in history under the Kleptocracy Asset Recovery Initiative. 96% of Malaysians enjoy connection to piped water and marked health improvements through administration of fluoride (Jaafar,

Noh, Muttalib, Othman, & Healy, 2013, p.22). However, water department officials who were involved in the approval process of projects in the state of Sarawak were arrested after funnelling an estimated RM190 million ($45,237,059) through abuse of power ("S'Wak leaders", 2016, line 30). A multinational government probe and investigation regarding citizen deaths and the whereabouts of the 2014 Malaysian Airlines Flight 370 have been criticised for poor handling, premature declaration of loss, failure of the Royal Air Force to identify an unidentified plane in Malaysian air space, subsequent implementation strategies, and lack of care and transparency (Pearson, 2014). Wesells and Dawes (2007) write:

> Macro-social interventions face daunting challenges of culture and power extending well beyond traditional discussions of the need for cultural sensitivity. Before conceptualising or launching an intervention, it is wise to reflect critically on the relationship between epistemology, power and ethics. (p. 274)

As Malaysia struggles to address its unique identity (that of not quite having a seat at the power table of developed nations and simultaneously wanting to forget that not so very long ago, it had shared in second- and third-world status), the idea of power and ethics becomes salient. Being compared to Singapore, a model developed nation that splintered off from Malaysia in 1965, further complicates Malaysia's identity. It has first-world living and third-world problems, all whilst maintaining a multi-ethnic and frontier feel.

To Tudung or not to Tudung? A Cultural and Religious Tug of War

As a federal constitutional monarchy, Malaysia declares Sunni Islam as its official religion with freedom of religion for non-Muslims. Religion is increasingly at the forefront of Malay politics, bi-directionally informing its approach to the world and defining the world's engagement with Malaysia. Historically considered a moderate and progressive Muslim country, the wearing of the tudung or hijab by Muslim women in Malaysia is not officially compulsory; however, conformity pressures and harassment compel many women to do so, often rendering it a political act. Although pork and alcohol are forbidden by Islam, they are readily available in urban cities such as Kuala Lumpur in order to cater to the multi-ethnic and expat communities. Juxtaposed with these freedoms are increasing rates of Islamisation. In 2015, a group of female Malaysian youth were threatened with arrest for hugging members of a Korean boy band as they had failed to uphold Malaysian Islamic civil law pertaining to public display of affection (AFP, 2015). Islamic scriptures stating that dogs are unclean have led to controversy over Muslims seen on social media hugging dogs; the word for "hot dog" has been called into question for the confusion it causes amongst Muslims in regards to what their ingredients (Fuller, 2014; "Hot Dogs", 2016). Similarly, Malaysians have been arrested for celebrating Valentine's

Day, Halloween, and Oktoberfest. Oktoberfest is characterised as a "planned attack" on Islam and because it is seen as a public vice "the same as mass-promoted adultery" (Fuller, 2016, para. 5).

2016 witnesses a move that tables and debates the Sharia Court Act 1965 (Criminal Jurisdiction) in order to enact a *Hudud* bill (Middleton, 2016). Islamic law (Sharia) views *Hudud* as punishments mandated by God. Currently, Malaysia has two sets of criminal law: one for Muslims and one for non-Muslims (Sharia and civil). Enabling *Hudud* law would strengthen aspects of Sharia law that include amputations for theft and flogging for adultery. Human rights activists decry the move to apply *Hudud* law to all people, especially considering Malaysia's multi-ethnic composition. Rape prosecuted under *Hudud* law requires a victim to call forth four male witnesses. Furthermore, the victim runs the risk of being charged with adultery and fornication, both of which can be met with a punishment of flogging (at minimum) or death (at maximum). Rape is a violent tool used against women and is already under-reported in Malaysia. The impending *Hudud* law debate stands to dramatically reduce rape reporting even further, which would increase the probability of a full blown women's health crisis. Cartoonist Zunar and other high profile Malaysians charged with sedition serve as reminders of the harsh penalties awaiting speech, expression, and research deemed by Malaysian authorities to be treason or sedition (Amnesty, 2016b).

Multiculturalism was a stabilising effect on Malaysia until recently. Though the current rhetoric of divisiveness shrouds Malaysia in political sensitivity, as a progressive asset, multiculturalism warrants further understanding and deeper investigation. Both Singapore and Malaysia carry common colonial legacies with parallel health systems in that both Western and ethnic medicine persist (e.g., Aboriginal [*Orang Asli*], Malay [*bomoh*, who are medicine men skilled with herbs and religious rites], Chinese [*acupuncture, qigong*], and Indian [*Ayurveda*]) (Ling, 1991). Although the British introduced Western medicine whilst carrying a disdain for ethnic medicine, it was tolerated as it eased the burden of caring for a significant proportion of the population. As they concentrated their efforts on converting the Malay populace through awareness campaigns, the British largely ignored the Chinese and Indian communities. As a result, ethnic practitioners coalesced and organised into medical associations and schools with a community and interpersonal emphasis. This gained impetus after the Indian mutiny of 1857 forced the British government to stall development programs in the Malay Peninsula. The fact this feature of the culture did not buckle under socio-economic, political, and urbanisation pressures and processes underscores ethnic medicine's continued utility to various communities.

In a trend that has continued since colonial times, Malaysia's infrastructure of roads, hospitals, and real estate (including the Petronas

Towers, which once ranked as the world's tallest buildings) suffers from an unmatched need of quality and quantity of human capital. Countless unoccupied, decrepit buildings dot the Kuala Lumpur skyline. Nearly all hospitals suffer shortages of qualified doctors and health care professionals. Colonial efforts to increase the acceptability and subsequent use of government public hospitals aided positive health outcomes by training Malay females in midwifery, a strategy that Sri Lanka has used with tremendous success. In addition, incentivising Chinese and Indian midwifes to pass Malay language tests and deemphasising the stigma attached to hospitals as places for charity cases resulted in increased acceptance of treatment in public hospitals. This trend has reversed in modern times due to both Malaysia's emphasis on elite private spending and medical tourism and to the government's efforts to divert attention away from access to universal health care (Ling, 1991).

Islam's approach to health care falls into categories of traditional, modern, or a combination of the two. Rural inhabitants rely on herbs, supplements, and recitation of Qur'anic verse for healing and often reject modern medicine outright because of lack of belief and access. Malaysian cultural mores also have implications on health For instance, Alshishtawy's (2012) research has shown that wearing a *tudung* potentially puts one at risk of vitamin D deficiency. The cultural emphasis on modesty combined with a lack of privacy in public places (including hospitals) may inhibit breastfeeding in new mothers. The traditional practice of supplementing honey for standard nutrients like breast milk may increase risk to infants. Similar to India, under-qualified and ill-equipped traditional medicine men may rely on "quack" practices and deeply-rooted superstitions that defy modern and traditional understanding and acceptance of Islamic ideas. Whilst a section of the Muslim populace in Malaysia disregards Islamic injunctions in lieu of secularism and Western medicine, many straddle both worlds and believe both have a healing role, acknowledging the strides modern medicine has made whilst also upholding *dhikr* (thought of Allah).

Singapore

Setting off Solo

In the early hours of August 9, 1965, Singapore became an independent and sovereign state by the signature of the then-Prime Minister Lee Kuan Yew. What perhaps seemed inevitable due to the political and ideological differences between the representatives of Singapore and Malaysia was nonetheless handled without the knowledge of the then-Singaporean Deputy Prime Minister and Culture Minister. An equally uninformed general public woke up to the shocking news of Singapore's independence – their introduction to a leader who took swift action whilst creating a tough and unrelenting environment in which the city-state always comes first. Importantly, Yew's vision of a non-communal Malaysia seeded mistrust with Malaysian representatives who encouraged the superiority of Malays or bumiputras. Thus, the split between the countries was hastened and became the raison d'être for Singapore's independence and for its development into one of the most prosperous in nations in the world within a period of thirty years. Singapore's health care ideology revolves around the idea that individuals are responsible for their health care, but it must be universal in nature and therefore accessible to all in a system in which both actors (individual and state) meet half way (Liu & Haseltine, 2016). According to the Ministry of Social and Family Development (MSF) (2016), in 2014, Singapore spent approximately 1.6% of its GDP on the health care system (~$6.7 billion) in the fiscal year (p.10), the gender ratio was 965 males for every 1000 females in an overall population of 5.46 million (p. 2), and citizens carried an average life span of 82.8 years (p.3). Though secular by law, a 33% majority practice Buddhism, followed by Christianity. Singapore's ethnic composition is 74% Chinese and the remaining population is split between Malay, Indian, and "other" (Department of Statistics Singapore, 2010a, p.2).

Like its Indian and Malaysian counterparts, Singapore faced the cultural ramifications of British colonisation. Due to the periods of political and economic variability of the colonial empire, peninsular Singapore bore persistent shortage of qualified health care personnel that affected the implementation of Western-style medicine. The Chinese, more so than other ethnic communities, became self-reliant in health care methods by organising their own resources, money, and influence into a system that still is in existence. In two hundred years, the health care landscape of Singapore has had a dramatic turnaround. Turnbull (2009) observed of mid-1800s colonial hospitals: "No one will enter who can crawl or beg, unless compelled by the police" (p.80). A showpiece hospital of the colonial system was built facing trash-dumping grounds where, in a one year period, one-third of the patients died (Turnbull, 2009, p. 80). When economic fortunes shifted in the first half of the twentieth century and Southeast Asia became one of the most exploited areas in the world due to rubber, tin, and other mining activities, investments were made to shield against malaria. Malaria was viewed primarily as a risk to economic productivity rather than a risk to universal health.

Singapore's strategy and political will over all aspects of governance and citizenry have been the subject of much speculation and discussion. In addition to receiving regular recognition for its ease of doing business, very low level of crime, good health indicators, and for going from third-world to first-world status in two generations, Singapore's administration and policies have become case studies. Aside from inherent advantages like geographical location, Prime Minister Lee Kuan Yew (often recognised as the founding father of Singapore) also deliberately focused on keeping the government from becoming large, which in turn helped to keep it efficient and truthful. Unlike what would be expected from neighbouring countries, these moves were welcomed and actively encouraged from the outset, underscoring the secularism and openness that precipitated the split from Malaysia.

In a 2004 speech to the Commonwealth Association of Public Administration and Management, Prime Minister Lee Hsien Loong outlined four principles of universal and local governance. Likening the small nation to a speedboat and other countries to big oil tankers, Loong emphasised Singaporeans' consideration of "leadership as key" (line 18). Agility, moral courage, preparedness, and the drive towards recruiting the best minds for public service all stem from this principle. "Anticipating change and staying relevant" (line 21) was cited as the second principle and means that assumptions must be continuously challenged. This is displayed in Singapore's active public participation campaigns and focus groups. The third principle, "reward for work and work for reward" (line 25), has Singaporeans actively fostering a sense of mission and contribution. Lastly, "A stake for everyone, and opportunities for all" (line 29) acknowledges that globalisation has levelled the playing field so that the best talent can go anywhere, do anything, and is welcomed by other nations. This principle emphasises not only economic wealth, but also the idea of pride and nation-building, in which citizens take ownership and understand their stake in the future, and in which the state has the ability to balance stronger individuals and weaker members of society (National Archives of Singapore, 2016).

An Island unto Itself

The framework of city-state's global health care has not been without criticism. In particular, Singapore's strict reproductive laws have come under fire for being archaic. As more women choose to become married or have children in their forties, Singapore's law that requires women to be married and under forty-five for in-vitro fertilisation (IVF) eligibility is considered restrictive. Given the disproportionate amount of Chinese in Singapore, the cultural desire to have a son as heir has created an exodus of single, older women going abroad to gender select and partake in IVF. In a bid to help mothers delay marriage and child bearing, the Singaporean government began subsidising up to three cycles of IVF treatments of S$3,000 each to qualified patients. Feminists denounce the absurdity of primarily male legal and political representatives setting the agenda for women's reproductive rights. Among other things, they point out that pre-implantation genetic diagnosis (PGD) is not allowed but abortion is, and is often employed once the gender is revealed during routine ultrasound check-ups at around the fourth or fifth month of pregnancy. The disavowal of PGD prevents Singaporeans from ruling out abnormalities such as Down's Syndrome and other genetic chromosomal abnormalities (Ministry of Health, 2011).

Singapore's authoritarian tone has been met with resistance and sharp criticism, particularly in regards to media censorship, human rights, and civic freedoms. Apple co-founder Steve Wozniak describes countercultures as a cornerstone for creativity and progress and says, "Apple could never have happened in a formal culture in Singapore" ("Singapore Far", 2011). Deputy Prime Minister Tharman Shanmugaratnam cites media censorship as necessary in some quarters, for instance, hate speech. Shanmugaratnam's philosophy relies on the idea that curbing certain freedoms helps in developing other freedoms and continues to be a balancing act (Chin, 2016). Singapore has legal provisions in place that criminalise demonstrations and dissent and put restrictions on advocacy, activism, and protest – the trade-off being that countries without these safeguards also tend to lack safety, efficiency, and equal opportunity.

The 2016 jailing of teen blogger Amos Yee was keenly observed by human rights groups, including Amnesty International and Human Rights Watch, and was attended by U.N. Human Rights Council members. Yee's social media postings which criticised both Christianity and Prime Minister Lee Kuan Yew after his death prompted presiding judge Ong Hian Sun to say that Yee's expression had, "deliberately elected to do harm" and that his "offensive and insulting words and profane gestures…hurt the feelings of Christians and Muslims" ("Singapore jails", 2016, para. 3). Bringing into sharp relief the delicate balance between freedom and 'order and discipline', a controversial 2016 bill outlining what constitutes contempt of court was recently passed. The fragile balance between individual rights and effective governments galvanises human rights groups to question and explore the modernisation and efficiency that Singapore prides itself on despite its citizenry often experiencing a different reality.

Singapore's mandatory death penalty for drug trafficking was amended in 2012 to allow limited discretion of judges to transmute life imprisonment sentences to caning. Transmutation occurs in tandem with the prosecution granting a certificate of cooperation, which indicates that the individual at trial had been indispensable in the investigations. This underscores Singapore's emphasis on utility as opposed to the fundamental value of right to life. The use of caning as a reformative measure is widespread in the judiciary, military, and school systems. Homosexuality is illegal (previously subsumed under the colonial umbrella of sex against the order of nature), as are appearing nude in a private place (including one's home) and the importation or selling of chewing gum (Singapore Statutes Online, 2015). The Media Development Authority of Singapore (MDA) banned the set up and use of the Ashley Madison website, which enables extra-marital dating. The MDA stated, "It is against the public interest to allow Ashley Madison to promote its website in flagrant disregard of our family values and public morality" (Sim, 2013, para. 4).

Singapore's conservative stance and global portrayal as a strictly no-nonsense city-state is squarely contradicted by its storied past as one of the British empire's key ports with a burgeoning sex industry. Whilst pimping and solicitation are illegal, prostitution is not, and in government-controlled red light areas, females from a plethora of nations are readily available. One advertisement read: "Young, energetic and intelligent girls in their 20s for S$150-$200 an hour or S$1000 a night" (Nee, 2006, para. 5), highlighting the tragic irony of Singapore's ruthless pragmatism (medical checks and health cards are mandatory for these girls) colliding with questions of dignity, human rights and quality of life. Speaking to Singapore's reputation for efficiency and strictness, Reuben Wong notes "Singapore's legalisation of the sex trade makes it a 'pragmatic' and 'unusual' exception in a region where prostitution thrives but is officially banned" (as cited in "Under Age", 2012, para. 14). The practical recognition by Singaporeans that prostitution is impossible to eradicate and increases public health risk, criminal organising, and trafficking enabled it to become strictly regulated.

One of the biggest health consequences of Singapore's laws and ethos is its ultra-low fertility rate. At 1.24% in 2015, Singapore was considerably below the 2.1% needed to stem population loss (Department of Statistics Singapore, 2010b, item 18). Ming (as cited in Leyl, 2012) discusses increased education and work opportunities as one of the reasons Singaporeans are not reproducing. This results in widely-documented, quantitative losses like the lessening of labour forces, stilted economic growth, and effects on health care costs and immigration policies. Stress, lifestyle, and the cost of education and property in Singapore are consistently mentioned as reasons to abstain from starting a family. The government has focused on fertility by investing S$1.3 billion in packages that encourage families to have children by paying S$15,000 per child, extending maternal and paternal leave, and creating tax breaks (Nandy & Asher, 2008). With plunging fertility rates, Singapore would do well to imbibe Asian Development Bank's Juzhong Zhuang's observation: "Demographic changes can provide impetus for structural reforms. It could also help push the growth model from a focus on resource accumulation to innovation, as well as driving industrial upgrades in order to improve productivity" (as cited in Khoo, 2016, para. 18).

Southeast Asia Brief

Malaysia and Singapore's rivalry extends beyond the origins of chili crabs and becomes a worldwide test study on governance. Singaporeans make it clear that the country was unwillingly axed from Malaysia. At the time, the strife between the countries was so great that the water supply was almost cut. Singapore enjoys the status of being one of the safest places in the world and regularly poaches talent from across the border. Critics cite size difference as the reason Malaysia is harder to govern, but adjusting for this demographic detail, the thought processes central to such varied outcomes between the countries still warrants further examination. Whilst both countries uphold uncompromising strictness regarding their war on drugs, their reasons diverge. Singapore aims to maximise the "good" and efficacious in society by weeding out "bad" influences. On the other hand, Malaysia focuses on expediency and religious influence via Islamic jurisprudence. Both countries fail to take into account that toughening on crime and utilizing retributive punishment as a criminal deterrent have been debunked by studies and fall overwhelmingly on "racial and ethnic minorities, the poor, and people with mental illness or intellectual disability" (Radlet, 2009; Amnesty International, 2016c, para. 4).

Globally, so long as low-SES communities remain underserved and underrepresented, a steady stream of vulnerable people will engage in crime in an attempt to make life bearable. Disparate access to basic human rights (like health care) should be addressed by the Singaporean and Malaysian governments in the form of social justice models based on human rights. Both countries have curtailed freedom of speech, advocacy, and other human rights, yet Singapore's quality of life, veneer, and success indicators buffer it from being perceived in the authoritarian light that is cast on Malaysia, which is doing the same. As Malaysia's Ringgit continues its downward trajectory against the Singapore dollar, in the final analysis, the political will to actualise a vision with everything at stake and nothing to fall back on has catapulted Singapore into another league resplendent with universal health care, low crime, and opportunity (Liau, Y.S., 2016), While Singapore's mentality elucidated by the prime minister is, "No one owes us a living" (Chia, 2015, p.148), Malaysia emphasises the inherent natural right of Malays over others.

It is worth mentioning that countries that had to fight for their independence (such as India in 1947) face different post-independence cultures than those that did not (e.g., Sri Lanka in 1948 or Singapore in 1965). Malaysia, which is reliant on natural resources, has not had to face a lack of security. On the other hand, Singapore faced a severe housing crisis as it struck out on its own. Singapore's misfortunes morphed into critical advantages, the alchemy of which forms a large part of Singapore's indomitable narrative. In turn, this fosters a sense of nation building and citizen interconnectedness, a crucial element to good health. Both countries suffer from high levels of stress and authoritarianism, in what one could argue is an over-involvement in citizen life. Yet Singapore distinguishes itself by its exemplary emphasis on championing the health and inclusiveness of all its people. In an unprecedented move, Singapore brought lawsuits against Indonesian plantation companies responsible for record-level air pollution, which resulted in the shutting down of schools. Under the 2014 Transboundary Haze Pollution Act, Singapore can fine a local or foreign company that contributes to unhealthy levels of haze pollution in the city, highlighting the fact that global health is sans boarders (Forsyth, 2014).

Synthesising for Peace

The various countries and city states subsumed under the health umbrella are subject not only to local regulations, customs, and cultures, but are exposed to urgent global matters, chief amongst them being the treatment of females. Former U.N. Secretary-General Kofi Annan spoke of this worldwide need: "Gender equality is a precondition for meeting the challenge of reducing poverty, promoting sustainable development, and building good governance" (as cited in Veneman, 2006, para. 54). Singapore's Convention on the Elimination of All Forms of Discrimination against Women, ratified in 1995, holds that in order to reach "critical mass", political representation should be at a minimum of 30% (United Nations Women, 2005, para. 10). Datuk Dr. Shad Saleem Faruqi, in reference to Malaysian female rape, asserts, "Islamic laws of evidence need to change and grow to accommodate the quest for female dignity" (as cited in Boo & Lim, 2014, para. 19). India's national health portal admits that females have significant health challenges that ultimately affect economic output, a key focus area of the Indian government. Sri Lanka's Sinhalese proverb, "Gedara gini eliyata danna epa" (home fires should not be put outside) (Rameez, 2016, para. 1) reflects legislation that made domestic violence a non-punishable offence until 2005.

Various leaders and organisations hold the opinion that peace is not only the absence of war, but also the presence of justice and equality. Millions of people in South and Southeast Asia are bereft of the simplest and most innate human rights: the right to life and the right to health. Misguided focus and subsequent economic policies that strengthen high SES and materialism have led to health corollaries across India, Sri Lanka, Malaysia, and Singapore where stress from the pursuit of external wealth have resulted in a preponderance of non-communicable diseases linked to lifestyle. The world has come a long way since history's bubonic plague and famines, yet I argue, given the leaps of super intelligence and technology, we have not moved far or fast enough. The problem of global health remains daunting and varied, but I put forth that countries should start by investing in women as numerous studies have demonstrated positive targeted results (Onarheim, 2016; Lomoy, 2010; Grepin & Klugman, &

Belohlav, 2016).

In economic terms, investing in women and girls would have a spill-over effect to several of the sectors that currently hold South and Southeast Asia's attention. A gender dividend is generated when governments tackle issues like policies on maternal leave, access to neonatal care, nutrients and basic health care in rural settings, and education and awareness campaigns for human rights, skills, and advocacy. Countries like India, which suffer from overpopulation, would benefit from contraceptive education and distribution. This could lower fertility rates and thereby also the physical demand on females, freeing them to contribute in the workforce. Countries that delimit the potential of female citizens by means of cultural, political, or legislative repression suffer in terms of their overall population health, increased violence, and lowered productivity with no road map for sustainability.

The current thought processes that go into legislation (postulating and "looking good on paper") stop short of actual and swift implementation in India, Sri Lanka, Malaysia, and Singapore. One way to influence positive outcomes in global health is to employ health professionals in affecting changes of consciousness at all levels simultaneously (grass roots, middle out, and top down) by creating necessary cultural buy-ins, something that international psychologists in particular are exquisitely poised to do given the emphasis on global inclusiveness and interdisciplinary work built into their curricula and training. This begins by recognising that isolation plays into a divisive antagonistic rhetoric and that a powerful way to overcome borderless issues like trans-nation pollution and trafficking is to actively realign levels of thinking through international dialogue and campaigning, being mindful that ethical and moral values have to be reprioritised. The more global health is addressed strongly, clearly, and visibly, in all its facets, the more issues become familiar and commonplace, thereby creating a reversal of dysfunctional normalcy (e.g., globally some sexual, domestic, career, and educational ideas rooted as commonplace in the twenty-first century were not possible two decades ago). Change invariably starts at an individual level by creating momentum on the physical, mental, emotional, spiritual, and political planes. Prolific peace activist and Buddhist leader, Daisaku Ikeda, portends, "A great human revolution in just a single individual will help achieve a change in the destiny of a nation, and, further, will enable a change in the destiny of all humankind" (Ikeda, 1998, para. 1).

Recommended Reading

Greenough, P., & Tsing, A.L. (2003). *Nature in the global south: Environmental projects in South and South-East Asia*. Telegana: Orient Blackswan.

Hashim, J., Chongsuvivatwong, V., Phua, K.H., Pocock, N., Teng, Y.M., Chhem, R.K., Wilopo, S.A., & Lopez, A. (2012, April 5). *Health and Health care Systems in Southeast Asia*.

Retrieved from https://unu.edu/publications/articles/health-and-health care-systems-in-southeast-asia.html

Hate, V., & Gannon, S. (2010). Public health in South Asia. *A Report of the CSIS Global Health Policy Center.* Retrieved from https://csis-prod.s3.amazonaws.com/s3fs-public/legacy_files/files/publication/100715_Hate_PublicHealthSouthAsia_Web.pdf

Lee, K., Pang, T., & Tan Yeling. (2013). *Asia's role in governing global health.* New York: Routledge.

Van Weel, C., Kassai, R., Qidwai, W., Kumar, R., Bala, K., Gupta, P.P., Haniffa, R., Hewageegana, N.R., Ranasinghe, T., Kidd, M., & Howe, A. (2016). Primary health care policy implementation in South Asia. *BMJ Global Health, 1*(e000057), 1-5.

References

A Never Ending Policy. (2013, April 27). *The Economist.* Retrieved from http://www.economist.com/news/briefing/21576654-elections-may-could-mark-turning-point-never-ending-policy

AFP. (2015, January 14). Malaysian girls who hugged K-pop band threatened with arrest. *Mail Online.* Retrieved from http://www.dailymail.co.uk/wires/afp/article-2910312/Malaysian-girls-hugged-K-pop-band-threatened-arrest.html

Alshishtawy, M.M. (2012). Vitamin D deficiency. *Sultan Qaboos University Medical Journal. 12*(2), 140-152.

Amnesty International. (2016a). Abolish death penalty. Retrieved from http://aimalaysia.org/AbolishDeathPenalty

Amnesty International. (2016b). Malaysia: Drop travel ban on Zunar and other government critics. Retrieved from https://www.amnesty.org/en/latest/news/2016/10/malaysia-drop-charges-against-zunar/

Amnesty International. (2016c). Broken beyond repair. Retrieved from http://www.amnestyusa.org/our-work/issues/death-penalty

Bastians, D., & Harris, G. (2014, Nov 20). Sri Lanka's president to seek unprecedented third term. *The New York Times.* Retrieved from http://www.nytimes.com/2014/11/21/world/asia/sri-lanka-president-mahinda-r ajapaksa-to-seek-third-term.html

Belohalav, K. (2016). Investing in women and girls for a gender dividend. *Population Reference Bureau.* Retrieved from http://www.prb.org/Publications/Articles/2016/investing-women-girls-gender-dividend.aspx

Bhattacharyya, S.K., Saha, S.P., Bhattacharya, S., & Pal, R. (2011). Consequences of unsafe abortion in India-a case report. *Proceedings in Obstetrics and Gynaecology, 2*(12):12.

Boo, S.L, & Lim, I. (2014, May, 3). Hudud will drive rape survivors deeper into shadows, say women's groups. *Malaymail Online.* Retrieved from http://www.themalaymailonline.com/malaysia/article/hudud-will-drive-rape-survivors-deeper-into-shadows-say-womens-groups

Brown, M.E., & Ganguly, S. (2003). *Fighting words: Language policy and ethnic relations in Asia.* Cambridge: MIT Press.

Caring for the Sikh Patient. (2016). *Ashford and St. Peter's hospitals.* Retrieved from https://www.ashfordstpeters.info/images/other/PAS18.pdf

Census of India. (2011). House listing and housing census data highlights-2011. Retrieved from http://censusindia.gov.in/2011census/hlo/hlo_highlights.html

Chia, Y.T. (2015). *Education, culture and the Singapore developmental state: "World-soul" lost and regained?* New York: PalGrave MacMillian.

Chin, C. (2016, May 31). More freedom of speech, but some restrictions necessary: DPM. *Today.* Retrieved from http://www.todayonline.com/singapore/more-freedom-speech-some-restrictions-necessary-dpm

CIA. (2016). The world factbook. Retrieved from
https://www.cia.gov/library/publications/the-world-factbook/geos/my.html#People

Columbia University. (2012). Health care in India. Retrieved from
http://assets.ce.columbia.edu/pdf/actu/actu-india.pdf

Cruz, M., Foster, J., Quillin, B., & Schellekens, P. (2015). World bank group policy research
note: Ending extreme poverty and sharing prosperity: Progress and policies. Retrieved
from
http://pubdocs.worldbank.org/en/109701443800596288/PRN03Oct2015TwinGoals.
pdf

Department Of Census And Statistics-Sri Lanka. (2012).Vital statistics. Retrieved from
http://www.statistics.gov.lk/PopHouSat/VitalStatistics/Tables.asp?Year=2012

Department Of Census And Statistics- Sri Lanka. (2016). Population and housing. Retrieved
from
http://www.statistics.gov.lk/PopHouSat/VitalStatistics/MidYearPopulation/Mid-
year%20population%20by%20district.pdf

Department of Statistic Malaysia, Official Portal. (2016). Selected demographic estimates
Malaysia 2016. Retrieved from
https://www.statistics.gov.my/index.php?r=column/cthemeByCat&cat=397&bul_id=
WVVQUnYrZkRwK1k1QXZMbEpuV1hNUT09&menu_id=L0pheU43NWJwRWVS
ZklWdzQ4TlhUUT09

Department of Statistics Singapore, 2010a. Census of population 2010 statistical release 1:
Demographic characteristics, education, language and religion. Retrieved from
papers/cop2010/census10_stat_release1

Department of Statistics Singapore, 2010b. [Item 18 Births and deaths].Births and deaths.
Retrieved from http://www.singstat.gov.sg/statistics/browse-by-theme/births-and-
deaths

Deshpande, S. (2016, April 23). Centre won't allow brain drain of docs. *The Times of India.*
Retrieved from
http://epaperbeta.timesofindia.com/Article.aspx?eid=31808&articlexml=Centre-wont-
allow-brain-drain-of-docs-23042016021022

De Zoysa, P. (2013). Clinical psychology in a medical setting in Sri Lanka. *International
Psychiatry, 10*(1), 18-19.

Economic Planning Unit (EPU). (2016). Vision 2020, 1991-2020. Retrieved from
http://www.epu.gov.my/en/development-policies/vision-2020

Forsyth, T. (2014). Public concerns about transboundary haze: a comparison of Indonesia,
Singapore, and Malaysia. *Global Environmental Change, 25*, 76-86.

Fuller, T. (2014, October 26). Want to Touch a Dog? In Malaysia, It's a Delicate Subject. *The
New York Times.* Retrieved from
http://www.nytimes.com/2014/10/27/world/asia/dog-petting-event-underlines-
malaysias-culture-wars.html?_r=0

Government of India. (2011). [Item 3 Trend of Birth rate, Death rate, Infant Mortality rate,
Total Fertility rate, Sex ratio at Birth and Sex ratio of children (0-4 age group), India].
Provisional population totals paper 1 of 2011 India series *1*. Retrieved from
http://censusindia.gov.in/2011-prov-results/prov_results_paper1_india.html

Grepin, K.A., & Klugman, J. (No Date). Investing in women's reproductive health: Closing
the deadly gap between what we know and what we do. Retrieved from
http://archive.womendeliver.org/assets/WD_Background_Paper_Full_Report. pdf

Gunatilaka, R., Mayer, M., & Vodopivec, M. (2010). World Bank: The challenge of youth
employment in Sri Lanka. Retrieved from
http://www.unicef.org/srilanka/challenge_youth_unemployment.pdf

Hamilton. (2010, April 14). Greater access to cell phones than toilets in India: UN. Retrieved
from https://unu.edu/media-relations/releases/greater-access-to-cell-phones-than-
toilets-in-india.html

Health Tourism. (2016). Medical tourism to Malaysia. Retrieved from https://www.health-tourism.com/medical-tourism-malaysia/

Hot dogs 'must be renamed' in Malaysia, says religious government body. (2016, October 19). *BBC*. Retrieved from http://www.bbc.com/news/world-asia-37700495

ICEF Monitor. (2012). Number of Indian students heading abroad increases dramatically over past decade. Retrieved from http://monitor.icef.com/2012/11/number-of-indian-students-heading-abroad-up-300-over-past-decade/

ICRtoP, (2017). Crisis in Sri Lanka. Retrieved from http://www.responsibilitytoprotect.org/index.php/crises/crisis-in-sri-lanka

Ikeda, D. (2015). A Great Human Revolution. *Soka Gakkai International (SGI)*. Retrieved from http://www.sgi.org/about-us/president-ikedas-writings/human-revolution.html

International Monetary Fund (IMF). (2016). Retrieved from https://www.imf.org/external/pubs/ft/weo/2011/02/pdf/tables.pdf

Jaafar, S., Noh, K.M., Muttalib, K.A., Othman, N.H., & Healy, J. (2013). Asia Pacific observatory on health systems and policies: Malaysia health system review. *Health Systems in Transition, 3*(1), 1-102.

Jain, A., Ray, S., Ganesan, K., Aklin, M., Cheng, C., & Urpelainen, J. (2015). Council of energy, environment & water report. Access to clean cooking energy and electricity, survey of states. Retrieved from http://ceew.in/pdf/CEEW-ACCESS-Report-29Sep15.pdf

Khoo, V. (2016, July 26). Singapore's low birth rate poses economic problems, as Asia's demographic stress rises. *CNBC ASIA ECONOMY*. Retrieved from http://www.cnbc.com/2016/07/26/singapores-low-birth-rate-poses-economic-problems-as-asias-demographic-stress-rises.html

Kumar, A. (2014, May 7). Sri Lanka, Bangladesh have beaten Indian in health care: Harpal Singh. Retrieved from http://southasia.oneworld.net/peoplespeak/sri-lanka-bangladesh-have-beaten-india-in-healthcare-harpal-singh#.WBnTqhRO_zK

Leyl, S. (2012, November 30). Singapore uses rap to try to boost birth rate. *BBC*. Retrieved from http://www.bbc.co.uk/news/business-20542156

Liau, Y.S. (2016, September 2013). Malaysian Ringgit sinks as lower oil and 1MDB saga hurt demand. *Bloomberg Markets*. Retrieved from http://www.bloomberg.com/news/articles/2016-09-13/malaysian-ringgit-sinks-as-lower-oil-and-1mdb-saga-hurt-demand

Ling, O,G., (1991). British colonial health care development and the persistence of ethnic medicine in peninsular Malaysia and Singapore. *Southeast Asian Studies, 29*(2), 158-178.

Liu, C., & Haseltine, W. (2016). The commonwealth fund: The Singaporean health care system. Retrieved from http://international.commonwealthfund.org/countries/singapore/

Lomoy, J. (2010, June 4). Investing in women and girls, the breakthrough strategy for achieving all the MDGs. Retrieved from https://www.oecd.org/dac/gender-development/45704694.pdf

Lund, M., & McDonald, S. (2015). *Across the lines of conflict: Facilitating cooperation to build peace.* Washington D.C.: Woodrow Wilson Center Press.

MacDonald, S.B., & Lemco, J. (2011). *Asia's rise in the 21st century.* Santa Barbara: Praeger.

Maddison, A. (1971). *Class structure and economic growth, India and Pakistan since the Moghuls.* New York: Routledge.

McKinsey&Company. (2012). India health care: Inspiring possibilities, challenging journey. Retrieved from http://health.economictimes.indiatimes.com/etanalytics/reports/industry/india-healthcare-inspiring-possibilities-and-challenging-journey/31

Medical Traveling Growing (2009). Retrieved from https://www.imtj.com/news/medical-travel-growing/

Middleton, R. (2016, May 31). Uproar in Malaysia as PM Najib Razak's ruling party fast tracks tabling of opposition's Hudud laws. *International Business Times.* Retrieved from http://www.ibtimes.co.uk/uproar-malaysia-pm-najib-razaks-ruling-party-fast-tracks-tabling-oppositions-hudud-laws-1562781

Miller, K.E., Fernando, G.A., & Berger, D.E. (2009). Daily stressors in the lives of Sri Lankan youth. *Intrevention, 7*(3), 187-203.

Ministry of Health. (2011). In-vitro fetilisation (IVF) in Singapore: Charges and success rates. Retrieved from https://www.moh.gov.sg/content/moh_web/home/Publications/information_papers/2004/in-vitro_fertilisationivfinsingaporechargesandsuccessrates.html

Ministry of Social and Family Development (MSF). (2016). Singapore's demographic: Sex ratio-males to females. Retrieved from httrps://app.msf.gov.sg/Research-Room/Research-Statistics/Sex-Ratio-Males-to-Females

Moon, B. (2011, Marc 31). Report of the Secretary-General's panel of experts on accountability in Sri Lanka. Retrieved from http://www.un.org/News/dh/infocus/Sri_Lanka/POE_Report_Full.pdf

Mulakala, A. (2013, March 13). Where are Malaysia's women politicians? *The Asia Foundation.* Retrieved from http://asiafoundation.org/2013/03/13/where-are-malaysias-women-politicians/

Murphy, R. S., & Lakshminarayana, R. (2006). Mental health consequences of war: a brief review of research prevalence symptoms post-traumatic stress disorder findings. *World Psychiatry, 5*(1), 25-30.

Myers, J. (2016, April, 18). Which are the world's fastest-growing economies? Retrieved from https://www.weforum.org/agenda/2016/04/worlds-fastest-growing-economies/

Namasivayam, A., Osuorah, D.C., Syed, R., & Antai, D. (2012). The role of gender inequities in women's access to reproductive health care: a population-level study of Namibia, Kenya, Nepal and India. *International Journal of Women's Health, 4,* 351-364.

Nandy, A., & Asher, M.G. (2008). Managing prolonged low fertility: The case of Singapore. ADBI discussion paper 114. Tokyo: Asian Development Bank Institute. Retrieved from http://www.adbi.org/discussion-paper/2008/08/22/2673.managing.prolonged.low.fertility/

National Archives of Singapore. (2016). Speeches and press releases. Retrieved from http://www.nas.gov.sg/archivesonline/speeches/view-html?filename=2004102401.htm

National Crime Records Bureau, Ministry of Home Affairs. (2014). Accidental deaths & suicides in India, 2014. Retrieved from http://ncrb.nic.in/StatPublications/ADSI/ADSI2014/adsi-2014%20full%20report.pdf

Nee, S.C. (2006, September 17). Smiles and paved roads aren't enough. *Singapore Window.* Retrieved from http://www.singapore-window.org/sw06/060917ST.HTM

Nene, B., Jayant, J., Arrossi, S., Shastri S., Budukh, A., Hingmire,S.,…Sankaranarayanan. (2007). Deteriminetns of women's participation in cervical cancer screening trial, Maharashtra, India. *Bulletin World Health Organization, 85(4),* 264-272.

Onarheim, K.H., Iversen, J.H., & Bloom, D.E. (2016). Economic Benefits of Investing in Women's Health: A Systematic Review. *PLOS | ONE. 11*(3), 1-23.

Pachouri, A. (2016, August 9). Innovation in health care in South Asia. [Blog]. Retrieved from http://www.asiapathways-adbi.org/2016/08/innovation-in-health-care-in-south-asia/

Pande, R., & Ford, D. (2011). World development report 2012: Gender quotas and female leadership. Retrieved from http://siteresources.worldbank.org/INTWDR2012/Resources/7778105-1299699968583/7786210-1322671773271/Pande-Gender-Quotas-April-2011.pdf

Patel, V., Parikh, R., Nandraj, S., Balasubramaniam, P., Narayan, K., Paul, V.K.,… Srinath Reddy, K. (2015). Assuring health coverage for all in India. *The Lancet, 386*(10011), 2422-2435.

Pearson, M. (2014). 6 missteps in Malaysia Flight 370 investigation. *CNN*. Retrieved from http://edition.cnn.com/2014/04/01/world/asia/malaysia-plane-missteps/

Radelet, M.L. (2009). Recent developments: Do executions lower homicide rates?: The views of leading criminologists. *The Journal of Criminal Law & Criminology, 99*(2), 489-508.

Rameez, R. (2016, July 25). Behind closed doors: The scourge of domestic violence in Sri Lanka. *Roar.lk*. Retrieved from http://roar.lk/features/behind-closed-doors-scourge-domestic-violence-sri-lanka/

Rorabacher, J. A. (2010). *Hunger and poverty in South Asia*. New Delhi: Gyan.

Ross, R. R., & Savada, A.M. (1988). *Sri Lanka, a country study*. Washington D.C.: Library of Congress.

S'Wak Leaders say integrity important, after Sabah scandal. (2016, October 11). *Free Malaysia Today*. Retrieved from http://www.freemalaysiatoday.com/category/nation/2016/10/11/swak-leaders-say-integrity-important-after-sabah-scandal/

Say, L., Chou, D., Gemmill, A., Tuncalp, O., Moller, A.B., Daniels, J.,… Alkema, L. (2014). Global causes of maternal death: a WHO systematic analysis. *The Lancet Global Health, 2*(6), 323-333.

Schwartz, A. (2015). 11 of the world's most threatened forests. *World Wildlife Fund*. Retrieved from http://www.worldwildlife.org/stories/11-of-the-world-s-most-threatened-forests

Sim, W. (2013, November 8). MDA bans extra-marital dating website Ashley Madison. *The Straits Times*. Retrieved from http://www.straitstimes.com/singapore/mda-bans-extra-marital-dating-website-ashley-madison

Singapore far too straight-laced: Apple co-founder. (2011, Dec 15). *AsiaOne*. Retrieved from http://news.asiaone.com/News/AsiaOne+News/Singapore/Story/A1Story20111215-316424.html

Singapore jails Amos Yee for religious 'insult'. (2016, September 30). *Aljazeera*. Retrieved from http://www.aljazeera.com/news/2016/09/singapore-jails-amos-yee-religious-insult-160929205613910.html

Singapore Statutes Online. (2015). *Singapore Statues Online*. Retrieved from http://statutes.agc.gov.sg/aol/home.w3p

Somasundaram, D. (2014). *Scarred communities:. Psychosocial impact of man-made and natural disasters on Sri Lankan society*. New Delhi, India: Sage Publications.

Sridharan, K., & Srinivasa-Raghavan, T.C.A. (2007). *Regional cooperation in South Asia and Southeast Asia*. Singapore: ISEAS Publishing.

Sritharan, J., Srithara, A. (2014). Post-conflict Sri Lanka: The Lack of mental health research and resources among affected populations. *International Journal of Humanities and Social Sciences, 4(3)*, 151-156.

Tan, T. (2015, April 22). One female raped every 35 mins in M'sia, study shows. *Free Malaysia Today*. Retrieved from http://www.freemalaysiatoday.com/category/nation/2015/04/22/one-female-raped-every-35-mins-in-msia-study-shows/

The return of the white van. (2016, April 28). *Sri Lanka campaign for peace & justice*. Retrieved from https://www.srilankacampaign.org/return-white-van/

Thiranagama, S. (2011). *In my mother's house: Civil war in Sri Lanka*. Philadelphia, PA: University of Pennsylvania Press.

Transparency International. (2015). Corruption perceptions index 2015. Retrieved from https://www.transparency.org/cpi2015/

Trepanowski, J.F., Bloomer, R.J. (2010). The impact of religious fasting on human health. *Nutrition Journal, 9(57)*, 1-9.

Turnbull, C.M. (2009). *A history of modern Singapore 1819-2005*. Singapore: NUS Press.

Two dozen skeletons found in Malaysian mass grave. (2015, August 23). *Al Jazeera,* Retrieved from http://www.aljazeera.com/news/2015/08/dozen-skeletons-malaysian-mass-grave-migrants-smuggling-150823052916560.html

Under-age call girl scandal shakes Singapore elite. (2012, April 28). *The Sunday Morning Herald.* Retrieved from http://www.smh.com.au/world/underage-call-girl-scandal-shakes-singapore-elite-20120428-1xrdi.html

UNICEF. (2009). Tsunami five-year report key figures. Retrieved from http://www.unicef.org.hk/upload/NewsMedia/dowload/international/Tsunami_5yr_en.pdf

United Nations (U.N.) (2012). Report of the Secretary-General's internal review panel on United Nations action in Sri Lanka. Retrieved from http://www.un.org/News/dh/infocus/Sri_Lanka/The_Internal_Review_Panel_report_on_Sri_Lanka.pdf

United Nations (U.N.). (2016). International day of yoga. (2016). Retrieved from http://www.un.org/en/events/yogaday/background.shtml

United Nations Women (U.N.W.) (2005). Equal participation of women and men in decision-making processes, with particular emphasis on political participation and leadership. Retrieved from http://www.un.org/womenwatch/daw/egm/eql-men/

United States Department of Justice (USDOJ). (2016, July 20). United States seeks to recover more than $1 Billion obtained from corruption involving Malaysian Sovereign Wealth Fund. Retrieved from https://www.justice.gov/opa/pr/united-states-seeks-recover-more-1-billion-obtained-corruption-involving-malaysian-sovereign

Veneman, A.M. (2006, July 31). Statement of UNICEF executive director Ann M. Veneman on international Women's Day. *UNICEF.* Retrieved from http://www.unicef.org/media/media_35134.html

Victor, I. (2010). President Mahinda Rajapaksa strengths and limitations. *The Sunday Leader.* Retrieved from http://www.thesundayleader.lk/2010/11/28/president-mahinda-rajapaksa-strengths-and-limitations/

WaterAid. (2015). It's no joke: The state of the world's toilets 2015. Retrieved from http://www.wateraid.org/what-we-do/our-approach/research-and-publications/view-publication?id=c8e9d0b5-3384-4483-beff-a8efef8f342a

Watters, E. (2010). *The globalization of the American psyche: Crazy like us.* New York: Simon & Schuster.

Wessells, M.G., & Dawes, A. (2007). Macro-level interventions: Psychology, social policy, and societal influence processes. In Stevens, M.J., & Gielen, U.P. (Ed.), *Towards a Global Psychology. Theory, Research, Intervention, and Pedagogy* (pp. 267-298). New Jersey: Lawrence Erlbaum Associates.

Women's Centre for Change. (2015). Statistics & research. Retrieved from http://wccpenang.org/statistic-research/

World Bank. (2011). [Figure 1 interactive world map]. Physicians (per 1,000 people). Retrieved from http://data.worldbank.org/indicator/SH.MED.PHYS.ZS?end=2011&start=2011&view=map&year=2011

World Bank. (2013).[Graph 1 Poverty headcount ratio at $1.90 a day (2011 PPP) (% of population] Poverty headcount ratio. Retrieved from http://data.worldbank.org/topic/poverty

World Bank. (2015*). Maternal mortality ratio (modeled estimate, per 100,000 live births).* Retrieved from http://data.worldbank.org/indicator/SH.STA.MMRT

World Bank. (2016). [Graph Illustration 2, clockwise, population total]. South Asia data. Retrieved from http://data.worldbank.org/region/south-asia

World Economic Forum (WEF). (2016). The travel & tourism competitiveness report 2015. Retrieved from

http://www3.weforum.org/docs/TT15/WEF_Global_Travel&Tourism_Report_2015
.pdf

World Health Organization (WHO). (2014a). First WHO report on suicide prevention. Retrieved from http://www.who.int/mediacentre/news/releases/2014/suicide-prevention-report/en/

World Health Organization (WHO). (2014b). United Nations agencies report steady progress in saving mothers' lives. Retrieved from http://www.who.int/mediacentre/news/releases/2014/maternal-mortality/en/

World Health Organization (WHO). (2016a). Suicide Data. Retrieved from http://www.who.int/mental_health/prevention/suicide/suicideprevent/en/

World Health Organization (WHO). (2016b). The health workforce in India human resources for health observer - Issue No. 16. Retrieved from http://www.who.int/hrh/resources/hwindia_health-obs16/en/

Worldometers. (2016). [Graph Illustration 1, South-Eastern Asia Population (1950 - 2016)]. South-Eastern Asia Population. Retrieved from http://www.worldometers.info/world-population/south-eastern-asia-population/

CHAPTER 4

HIV/AIDS and Global Health:
A Minority Stress Perspective

Shufang Sun, William T. Hoyt, and Ryan P. Westergaard

Since the beginning of the epidemic, approximately 79 million people have been infected by the HIV virus, and 37 million people currently live with HIV/AIDS globally (UNAIDS, 2015, p.1). Among them, men who have sex with men (MSM), transgender individuals, male and female sex workers, incarcerated individuals, racial and ethnic minorities, and people who inject drugs (PWID) have been disproportionately burdened by the HIV/AIDS epidemic. Minority stress theory is a theoretical perspective for understanding health-related issues among minority populations, arguing that minority status as a social identity is a chronic and social stressor that causes adverse mental, behavioral, and physical health outcomes for gender, sexual, and racial minorities (e.g., Meyer, 2003). Factors including *distal* (the external, objective stressful events of prejudice and discrimination) and *proximal* processes (internalized societal attitude, concealment, and mistrust) both affect high-risk HIV behaviors and treatment adherence. Studies in the U.S. and many other countries have found evidence that supports this model. In this chapter, we first introduce the global HIV/AIDS epidemiology and the populations disproportionately affected by HIV/AIDS. Then we review the theoretical framework and offer a minority stress perspective in understanding psychosocial factors contributing to vulnerability to HIV/AIDS and treatment barriers. Specifically, we highlight how minority stress factors (e.g., discrimination, homophobia, and identity concealment) affect health outcomes of people living with HIV/AIDS (PLWHA) and high-HIV-risk populations. We also highlight the health outcomes on the community or population level. Finally, we provide recommendations on research investigations, health policies, and education programs targeting HIV prevention and treatment with vulnerable populations globally.

Introduction

HIV, or the human immunodeficiency virus, is defined as the virus that can lead to Acquired Immune Deficiency Syndrome (AIDS) (Center for Disease Control and Prevention; CDC, 2015). AIDS is the most advanced stage of HIV infection, in which progressive deterioration of the immune system results in increased vulnerability to opportunistic infections, malignancies, and death (CDC, 2015). More than three decades have passed since HIV/AIDS was recognized in 1981, and it has become one of the greatest threats to global health. As of 2015, it was estimated that there were approximately 36.7 million people living with HIV/AIDS globally (UNAIDS, 2015, p. 1), and more than 35 million people have died from AIDS-related illnesses since the beginning of the epidemic (UNAIDS, 2015, p. 4).

Of the many scientific breakthroughs that have been made during the first four decades of the HIV/AIDS epidemic, none have had greater impact than the development of combination antiretroviral therapy (ART). ART has directly led to substantial declines in HIV-related mortality and morbidity and has been proven to be cost-effective (Porter et al., 2003). Antiretroviral therapy uses combinations of medications targeting specific steps in the HIV lifecycle to block viral replication in the body. Suppression of the HIV virus halts immune function decline and, when initiated early in the course of infection, effectively prevents progression to AIDS. A 20-year-old individual living with HIV on ART today in the U.S. can expect to live into their early seventies (Mascolini, 2013, p. 1), which is a life expectancy that approaches that of a 20-year-old in the general population. Among the 36.7 million people living with HIV/AIDS globally, more than 40% were receiving ART by 2015, a dramatic increase from 2% ART coverage in the year 2000 (UNAIDS, 2015, p. 3).

Certain groups have been disproportionately burdened by HIV/AIDS, meaning that HIV prevalence is significantly higher than the general population. The global HIV epidemic disproportionately affects minority and marginalized groups including men who have sex with men (MSM; e.g., Beyrer et al., 2012), transgender women (van Griensven, Na Ayutthaya, & Wilson, 2013), people who inject drugs (PWID; Cook, Phelan, Sander, Stone, & Murphy, 2016), female and male sex workers (Baral et al., 2012), and incarcerated individuals (e.g., Dolan et al., 2016). It is worth noting that there is some overlap between the groups, such as transgender women and sex workers, and MSM and PWID. Among these disproportionately affected populations, racial and ethnic minorities are often more vulnerable to HIV infection. For instance, HIV rates among MSM in the U.S. are disproportionately high among black and Latino MSM. Approximately 39% black MSM being HIV positive (CDC, 2016, p. 1). Additionally, these key affected populations living with HIV/AIDS often experience adverse health outcomes, including delayed treatment, nonadherence, and high mortality (e.g., Melendez et al., 2006).

There are no purely biological or genetic explanations for the increased risk of HIV transmission in minority and marginalized populations. Health disparities in the HIV epidemic are rather determined by psychosocial phenomena influencing behavioral HIV prevention (e.g., one's self worth, social circumstances to negotiate safe sex) and community or social network-level factors (Millett et al, 2012). In this chapter, we attempt to understand psychosocial mechanisms affecting the vulnerability to HIV infection and treatment outcomes of aforementioned populations from a minority stress framework and to provide recommendations for global HIV/AIDS prevention and treatment programs based on this theoretical approach.

Minority Stress: A Theoretical Framework

The minority stress framework is derived from a biopsychosocial model with the assumption that body, mind, and social factors are interconnected. To introduce the minority stress framework, we first review the philosophical foundation for the birth of the biopsychosocial model and how health and stress, especially chronic stress, are conceptualized to be interconnected. Minority stress theory started with this background, attempting to address whether minority status functions as a chronic social stress for individuals. We review the broader framework of minority stress and move into Meyer's minority stress model (2003) in understanding how sexual orientation affects health of LGB populations.

Stress and Health

The view that mind and emotions are separated from health and disease reflects a biological reductionism, proposing that physical health can be explained entirely by biological mechanisms. When this view was popular, human beings were seen as biological organisms to be understood by examining parts of the body using principles of physiology, biochemistry, and physics (Sullivan, 1986).

This view was later challenged by philosophers and health practitioners, especially in the context of understanding health and stress (Mehta, 2011). Bernard (1961) first noted that maintenance of life was dependent on a constant internal milieu in the face of a varying environment. Cannon (1929) used "homeostasis" to describe this. Physiologist Hans Selye coined the term "stress" in 1935 to represent the effects of anything that seriously threatens homeostasis; he later proposed the theory that diverse, non-specific, external stimuli can lead to undifferentiated physiological and mental responses that threaten homeostasis and lead to body damage and disease (Selye, 1956).

Based on the work of Cannon, Selye, and others, George Engel (1977) argued for a holistic view, or biopsychosocial model, noting that "Medicine's crisis stems from the logical inference that since 'disease' is defined in terms of somatic parameters, physicians need not be concerned with psychosocial issues that lie outside of medicine's responsibilities and authority" (p.129). This biopsychosocial model argues that one factor (biology) is not sufficient: health and illnesses are the result of the interplay between one's genetic makeup (biology), mental health and behavior (psychology, such as depression, trauma, and health behaviors), and sociocultural environment (sociology and culture, such as support systems and social discrimination). Research supports this idea, demonstrating (e.g., Segerstrom & Miller, 2004) that psychological stress negatively affects one's immune system, especially for individuals who are older and have pre-existing autoimmune diseases such as multiple sclerosis, Crohn's disease, lupus, or HIV.

In the field of stress and health studies, a substantial body of research has shown that stress, in various forms, affects physical health (Thoits, 2010). Earlier research in this area focused on more acute, temporally limited, and individual stressors, such as bereavement, divorce, job loss, and change of living situation. On a physical level, acute stress has been found to be associated with a cascade of change in the nervous, cardiovascular, endocrine, and immune systems. Furthermore, these changes, at least in the short term, might be adaptive for individuals (Selye, 1956). For instance, stress hormones such as adrenaline and corticosteroids are released to activate the immune system, increase heart rate, and elevate blood pressure to make stored energy available for the body (Schneiderman, Ironson, & Siegel, 2005).

Later research shifted attention to circumstantial and chronic stress that is enduring or recurrent and that requires individuals to adjust themselves for long periods of time. Examples of such stressors include financial stress, work-family conflict, abusive relationships, and living in an unsafe neighborhood. Chronic stress is the response to prolonged stressors over which an individual perceives that he or she has no control. While the immediate effects of stress might be beneficial in a particular situation, long-term exposure to stress creates a prolonged activation and imbalance of the immune system.

Prior to 2000, researchers primarily investigated how socioeconomic status such as poverty was associated with health and stress responses (e.g.,

Baum, Garofalo, & Yali, 1999; Turner & Lloyd, 1999). Researchers found that compared to individuals in more advantaged socioeconomic positions, those with lower income and occupational prestige had the highest morbidity, disability, mortality, and prevalence of mental disorders (e.g., Baum, Garofalo, & Yali, 1999; Elo & Preston, 1996; Lantz, House, Mero, & Williams, 2005; Turner & Lloyd, 1999).

Minority, Stress, and Health Outcomes

Findings on socioeconomic stress raised questions for researchers about the connection between minority status, socioeconomic stress, and health outcomes. Do members of minority groups suffer from adverse health outcomes because of stress caused by disadvantaged socioeconomic status? Or is being a minority member a stressor in and of itself and directly associated with health outcomes? Questions like these were the impetus for early research on minority stress.

Social norms play important roles in societies. Durkheim argued that suicide is caused by normlessness (1987) and that people need norms to regulate society and fulfill their needs and aspirations, which are also influenced by social norms. Durkheim's concept of anomie (1897), a sense of normlessness, was adapted by Merton to explain the distribution of deviant behaviors across various social groups by race, ethnicity, and class. Merton (1938) argued that society and social norms stand as constant stressors for minority persons by generating values, goals, and ways to achieve such goals that do not apply to them.

Psychologists offer an understanding of minority stress from an identity perspective. Social identity theory proposed that group affiliation has a strong impact on one's self esteem and how one constructs meaning (Tajfel & Turner, 1986). Similarly, psychologist Gordon Allport (1949) argued for important characterological consequences on one's sense of self via social identity, in the chapter titled "Traits due to Victimization" in his well-known book *The Nature of Prejudice*. His famous quote, "One's reputation, whether false or true, cannot be hammered, hammered, hammered into one's head without doing something to one's character," (p. 142) highlights the impact of social interactions on one's sense of self. Allport asserted that African Americans display vigilance after exposure to prejudice events, such as actively scanning social environment for potential threats. Such vigilance can be exhausting for individuals, as it requires both cognitive and emotional processing.

In 1999, guidelines were proposed for epidemiological investigations on how social inequality, including racism and sexism, affects people's health (Krieger, 1999). Similarly, Clark, Anderson, Clark, and Williams (1999) proposed racism as a stressor for black Americans and outlined a biopsychosocial model for perceived racism and discrimination as a guide for future health research.

For minority group members, stereotypes, marginalization, stigma, and discrimination that are associated with their identities often impact their physical and mental health. Scholars applied this perspective in understanding stress and health outcomes in various social group categories with stigmatizing characteristics, like being overweight (Miller & Myers, 1998) or having HIV/AIDS, cancer, or disability (Fife & Wright, 2000). In the U.S. and some other Western countries (e.g., New Zealand, France, Australia), researchers also incorporated this framework into understanding health and life expectancy issues of people of African descent related to segregation, prejudice experience, and perceived racism.

Empirical evidence supports the minority stress framework. Individuals who reported higher levels of racism (systematic, interpersonal, or other forms) had more adverse health outcomes (e.g., Larson, Gillies, Howard, Coffin, 2007; Paradies, 2006). Perceived discrimination, prejudice, and unfair treatment due to being members of a group were found to negatively affect individuals' mental and physical health (Pascoe & Richman, 2009; Schmitt, Branscombe, Postmes, & Garcia, 2014). Gee and Walsemann (2009) followed more than 6,000 youth (p. 1676) in a longitudinal study across countries and found that reported racial discrimination predicted health issues, yet not vice versa (health issues do not lead to subsequent reported racial discrimination). Other studies also confirmed the "delayed" effect of discrimination, noting that discrimination experiences are associated with later health related outcomes such as hypertension and cardiovascular disease – effects unobservable at the time of the discrimination events (Burton, Marshal, Chisolm, Sucato, & Friedman, 2013; Foynes, Smith, & Shipherd, 2015; Gee & Walsemann, 2009; Pavalko, Mossakowski, & Hamilton, 2003).

How does racial discrimination affect one's health? Research in both naturalistic and lab settings found that in the face of racial stressors, individuals showed increased cardiovascular reactivity associated with long-term cardiovascular risk, as well as increased disease progression and poorer immune system responses (Brondolo, Lov, Pencille, Schoenthaler, & Ogedegbe, 2011; Clark et al., 1999; Williams & Neighbors, 2001). Besides physical health, racial discrimination also affects one's mental health. Based on a recent meta-analysis, Paradies (2015) concluded that racism was associated with depression, anxiety, suicidal ideation, and traumatic stress. Williams and Williams-Morris (2000) theorized three ways that racism can affect mental health outcomes, including truncated socioeconomic mobility, physiological and psychological responses that lead to adverse changes in mental health, and unfavorable self-evaluations due to acceptance of negative stereotypes.

Besides overt racism, microaggression (Sue et al., 2007) is another form of discrimination consisting of "brief and commonplace daily verbal, behavioral, or environmental indignities, whether intentional or unintentional, that communicate hostile, derogatory, or negative racial slights and insults toward people of color" (p. 271). Experienced microaggression is significantly associated with depressive symptoms, negative affect, and adverse higher stress level (e.g., Nadal, Griffin, Wong, Hamit, & Rasmus, 2012). Besides race, scholars have studied microaggression based on gender (Capodilupo et al., 2010), sexual orientation (Nadal et al., 2011), gender identity (Chang & Chung, 2015), and religion (Nadal et al., 2012).

Minority Stress for LGB Populations: Meyer's Model

Like racial and ethnic minorities, sexual and gender minorities also experience a wide range of health disparities. For instance, gay and bisexual men in the U.S. had higher prevalence of depression, excessive drinking and smoking, psychological distress, and were at higher risk for disability compared to heterosexual men (Cochran, Sullivan, & Mays, 2003; Fredriksen-Goldsen, Kim, Barkan, Muraco, & Hoy-Ellis, 2013, p. 1802). Studies in the U.S. also found that lesbians and bisexual women had higher risk of cardiovascular disease and higher prevalence of anxiety disorders and depression (Cochran, Sullivan, & Mays, 2003, p. 53; Fredriksen-Goldsen et al., 2013, p. 1802; Koh & Ross, 2006, p. 33). Compared to the general population, transgender individuals were found to have higher risk for HIV/AIDS, depression, anxiety, suicide, and shorter life expectancy (e.g., Reisner, White, Bradford, & Mimiaga, 2014, p. 177).

To understand the excess of mental disorders in lesbians, gay men, and bisexuals (LGBs), Meyer proposed a conceptual framework on the mechanism of minority stress on LGB individuals' health outcomes, particularly mental health. Meyer's model (2003) explains how distal minority stresses (e.g., prejudice, discrimination) create a hostile and stressful environment that lead to proximal processes (e.g., internalized homophobia, anticipation of rejection), causing adverse mental health outcomes. Additionally, coping, social support, and characteristics of minority identity function as moderator variables on the effect of minority stress processes on mental health outcomes.

Meyer considers minority stressors on a continuum from distal to proximal. Specifically, distal stressors refer to the external and objective events and stressful conditions (such as violence and prejudice events) and proximal stressors are the subjective experiences (such as internalized stereotypes and expectation of interpersonal rejections) (Meyer, 2003). Internalized homophobia was defined by Meyer and Dean as gay individuals' "direction of negative social attitude toward the self" (1998, p. 161), and was considered to be the most proximal position along the continuum from the environment to the self. Meyer argued that both general stressors and minority stress processes (both distal and proximal) influence mental health outcomes for LGB individuals. Coping and social support (both on community and individual levels) and characteristics of minority identity all affect the influence of stress on health outcomes.

Most research on Meyer's minority stress model has been conducted in the U.S. and has focused on mental health among LGB individuals. Distal factors such as discriminative events were found to have long-term adverse health effects on LGBT individuals (e.g., Frost, Lehavot, & Meyer, 2015). Proximal minority processes, including expectations of rejection, perceived hostility, concealment of sexuality, and internalized homophobia, also affect LGBT individuals' health, particularly mental health. For instance, internalized homophobia among LGB individuals is associated with depression, anxiety, and suicide (Newcomb & Mustanski, 2010). In a recent meta-analysis, Goldbach, Tanner-Smith, Bagwell, and Dunlap (2014) found that the strongest risk factors for substance use disorders among LGB adolescents in the U.S. included victimization, lack of supportive environments, and negative disclosure reactions, highlighting the roles of social support and internalization of environmental attitudes. There is a lack of research on health disparities (physical and mental health) for LGBT populations in non-western countries. Still, the findings mentioned above argue for gay-affirmative psychotherapeutic interventions to address proximal risk factors and promote psychological well-being among LGB individuals.

Minority Stress Framework in Global HIV Prevention and Care

Meyer's model provided a foundation in understanding the mechanism by which minority stress processes affect mental health outcomes of LGB individuals. We argue that the minority stress framework should be expanded and applied in global HIV prevention and treatment work in order to better understand psychosocial factors (e.g., discrimination, HIV stigma, homophobia, transphobia, individual and community level coping of HIV) affecting outcomes of global HIV prevention and treatment.

In this section, from a theoretical perspective, we adapt the minority stress framework with PLWHA and groups disproportionately burdened by HIV/AIDS, including men who have sex with men (MSM), transgender women, people who inject drugs (PWID), female and male sex workers, incarcerated individuals, and racial and ethnic minorities. We review how the process of minority stress can lead to adverse health outcomes on both individual and population-wide levels for the disproportionately affected groups mentioned previously. At the end of this section, we offer cross-cultural perspectives to consider when adapting the minority stress framework with disproportionately affected populations in diverse cultures across the world.

Minority Populations and Vulnerability to HIV Infection

As mentioned above, the global HIV epidemic affects certain populations disproportionately. These high-risk populations are already highly marginalized in most societies due to their devalued social identities (e.g., being gay or bisexual, performing sex work, having a history of substance use). We argue that minority stress processes, both distal and proximal (e.g., discrimination, violence, internalized homophobia and stigmatization), make these groups vulnerable to HIV infection, which as a result adds another stigmatizing minority identity (HIV-positive) and further potential for marginalization. As having HIV/AIDS is highly stigmatizing in most societies and affects multiple aspects of one's functioning (social, occupational, and familial), we consider it a social- and health-related minority identity. Qualitative research also suggests that PLWHA go through an identity integration process, often from initial denial and catastrophizing to immersion in the HIV/AIDS community and acceptance of being positive (Baumgartner, 2012; Baumgartner & David, 2009; Tewksbury & McGaughey, 1998). Additionally, we call for a contextual and comprehensive application of the minority stress model with PLWHA and high-HIV-risk populations, as those groups often have multiple minority identities and need to navigate multi-layered discrimination and stigma.

Dual/Multiple Minority Identity

Dual or multiple minority status (e.g., being a black MSM, being an HIV-positive transgender woman, etc.) may amplify stressors leading to adverse health outcomes. Though Meyer's minority stress model (2003) specifically considers sexual orientation as a single source of minority stress for LGBs, we call for an intersectional framework in the application of minority stress theory with PLWHA and high-HIV-risk populations, as they often have more than one minority status (visible and invisible) and experience minority stress from multiple sources such as sexual orientation, gender identity, sex work, immigration, incarceration, and use of drugs.

Social identities do not exist in isolation. Social inequality and identities are interdependent and intersectional rather than additive. For example, Bowleg (2008) noted that LGB people of color experience unique and more frequent discrimination and microaggressions based on their social position (gender, race, sexual orientation) and may be marginalized in both communities (racial discrimination in LGB community and homophobia in racial/ethnic minority community). Similarly, as we discuss in more detail, discrimination, stigma, and other minority stress processes for PLWHA and high-HIV-risk populations are often intertwined, causing multifaceted adverse health outcomes.

From Distal to Proximal Minority Stress Processes

Major distal minority stress processes for high-HIV-risk populations may include discrimination and prejudice events, violent and unsafe environments, societal neglect, denial of basic human rights, and criminalization based on one's identity. Discrimination and prejudice toward high-HIV-risk populations may take various forms, including denial of health care, termination of employment, and even violence (e.g., hate crimes).

HIV/AIDS-related discrimination refers to discriminative acts against one's HIV/AIDS status, including violence, prejudice, and rejection (Parker & Aggleton, 2003). For PLWHA, discrimination and prejudice may be multifaceted; individuals often face discrimination due to their HIV status as well as their social identities (e.g., being gay, bisexual, transgender, a person of color, a person who injects drugs, a sex worker, or having history of incarceration). In some societies, discrimination and prejudice may be more overt than in others. For instance, studies in India showed that PLWHA often experience more public discrimination (e.g., denial of hospital care), and HIV-positive widows in rural areas were rejected by their deceased husbands' families and forced to return to the villages in which they were born (Pallikadavath, Garda, Apte, Freedman, & Stones, 2005). The lack of sufficient legal protection for PLWHA (e.g., confidentiality, job protection, protection for medical care) causes difficulties in reducing discrimination at societal and institutional levels.

HIV/AIDS-related discrimination could be viewed as a manifestation of HIV/AIDS-related stigma. Today, HIV/AIDS discrimination and stigma still affect PLWHA on the individual level as well as the community and societal levels. In the public, HIV/AIDS stigma has been manifested as anger, fear, and prejudice against PLWHA and high-HIV-risk populations, accompanied by violent and/or avoiding behaviors (Blendon, Donelan, & Knox,1992; Herek & Capitanio, 1999). HIV stigma can also be manifested through the misbelief that HIV can be transmitted through casual contact or that it is caused by certain societal groups like gay individuals, transgender individuals, or sex workers (Parker, 2002). Such misinformation further contributes to the marginalization of these groups.

Stigma can manifest through intrapersonal and interpersonal paths, usually measured by individual and public stigma (Berger, Ferrans, & Lashley, 2001). Earnshaw & Chaudoir (2009) conceptualized three HIV stigma types, including internalized, enacted, and anticipated HIV stigma, referring to self-stigmatization, experienced social HIV stigma, and expected mistreatment by others due to HIV status. It is conceptualized that anticipated/expected HIV stigma is based on experienced discrimination like social rejection, job loss, or violence (Earnshaw & Chaudoir, 2009). Anticipated HIV stigma was found to associate with avoidant coping such as less use of health care and avoidance of testing for sexually transmitted diseases (Earnshaw & Quinn, 2012). Under the minority stress framework, HIV stigma could also be considered on the distal to proximal continuum, from enacted and anticipated HIV stigma to internalized HIV stigma.

Much of the societal HIV/AIDS stigma is closely intertwined with prejudice against sexual and gender minorities, sex workers, those who use drugs, and people from lower social class. On a societal level, stigmatization of HIV is connected to sex (especially same-sex partnership) and drug use, which in many cultures are historically stigmatized and regarded as immoral. Categories like sexual orientation, race, gender, and social class encapsulate historical and continuing relations of political, cultural, and societal power, inequality, assigned resources, and stigma (Cohen, 1997). The global HIV-epidemic, as noted by scholars, is a representation of the dynamic of structural, community, and individual levels of inequality that place certain social groups at risk for HIV infection as well as stigma (e.g., Watkins-Hays, 2014). For instance, globally, the rate of HIV-infection among black MSM (or MSM of African descent) is much higher than among white MSM (or MSM of European descent). Compared to white MSM, black MSM were not found to engage in higher frequency of sexual risk behaviors or (reported) substance use (e.g., Millett, Peterson, Wolitski, & Stall, 2006). Potential explanations might be that structural difficulties (e.g., high rates of incarceration, lack of education, and limited socioeconomic resources) contribute to black MSMs' choice of sexual partners, access to HIV testing and treatment, and high HIV viral load in the community (Kelley et al., 2012; Millett et al., 2012). Meanwhile, the high prevalence of HIV among black MSM further reinforces the media's and public's fear and fetishization of black masculinity and sexuality (e.g., Mackenzie, 2013).

Perceived social or public stigma is related to concealment of disease, social withdrawal, depression, and avoidance of HIV testing/delayed treatment (e.g., Smith, Rossetto, & Peterson, 2008). A study with black MSM in the U.S. found that greater internalized stigma was associated with less disclosure about one's HIV status due to adverse interpersonal consequences (Overstreet, Earnshaw, Kalichman, & Quinn, 2013). In Meyer's minority stress model, he noted how concealing one's stigma is often used as a coping strategy but can be stressful for individuals and harm their psychological health in the long run due to the stress related to suppressing and hiding. Self-concealment is associated with the cognitive burden involved in preoccupation with hiding, and thus results in psychological distress (Larson, Chastain, Hoyt, & Ayzenberg, 2015). Both sexual orientation and HIV status are invisible and stigmatizing identities that can burden the individual in navigating concealment and disclosure. In many regions of the world, it may not be safe for sexual minorities to disclose their sexual identity (as it is criminalized or socially unacceptable). If so, it would certainly not be safe to disclose that they are infected by HIV through same sex conduct. This adds an extra layer of stress for many PLWHA who have more than one invisible minority status.

HIV disclosure may differ somewhat from coming out as a sexual minority both in terms of circumstances promoting the disclosure (e.g., prior to physical intimacy, being in a medical setting, etc.) and in terms of audience. In non-medical settings, PLWHA often shoulder a three-fold burden: their own vulnerability due to the disclosure of personal information, the necessity of educating the audience on HIV and safe sex behaviors, and the likelihood of facing rejection and/or discrimination as a result. Health psychology research shows that concealing stigmatized conditions, though aimed at avoiding negative consequences of stigma (e.g., shame, rejection, discrimination), might negatively affect health. For instance, nondisclosure of sexual orientation is associated with poor immune functioning (Strachan, Bennett, Russo, & Roy-Byrne, 2007) and higher risk for developing cancer and pneumonia (Cole, Kemeny, Taylor, Visscher, & Fahey, 1996). Concealment of HIV was found to be concurrent with poor physical health outcomes (e.g., immune system function; Strachan et al., 2007) and health behaviors such as inadequate service utilization (e.g., Pulerwitz, Michaelis, Lippman, Chinaglia, & Díaz, 2008), which harms individuals' health outcomes.

Although disclosure could be beneficial in a safe environment, forced disclosure can be problematic. Criminalization of non-disclosure (e.g., Canada) can result in further marginalization against PLWHA, including jeopardizing the health needs of PLWHA and barriers to linkage and retention in HIV care (Patterson et al., 2015).

Avoidance of HIV testing is another factor contributing to delayed treatment. Avoidance of HIV testing is linked to anticipated HIV stigma, and can be viewed as a reaction to public and societal HIV stigma as well as discrimination events (due to one's minority identities). It was estimated that only 54% of PLWHA globally were aware of their status (UNAIDS, 2015, p. 11), causing great difficulty in HIV prevention and timely treatment. Avoidance of HIV testing as a health behavior is related to many other minority stress factors. Avoidance of HIV testing among PLWHA in South Africa was associated with greater AIDS-related stigmas, shame, and experienced social disapproval (Kalichman & Simbayi, 2003). Research in Thailand showed that increased police presence and previous experience of being refused healthcare services were predictive of HIV test avoidance among PWID (Ti et al., 2013).

Discrimination events (e.g., rejection of housing due to one's gender identity) are also associated with higher levels of sexual risk behaviors and substance use behaviors, contributing to higher HIV risk. Homophobic events experienced by black MSM in the U.S. were found to be associated with higher sexual risk behaviors, such as unprotected anal intercourse with HIV-positive sex partners (Jeffries, Marks, Lauby, Murrill, & Millett, 2013). Research with black Americans (Kaplan, Hormes, Wallace, Rountree, & Theall, 2016; Stock, Peterson, Gibbons, & Gerrard, 2013) indicated that cumulative racial discrimination was also associated with greater HIV risk behaviors (substance use and risky sexual behaviors).

Social and public stigma and discrimination against PLWHA can lead to internalized HIV stigma (or self-stigma), one of the most proximal factors in minority stress model. In describing self-stigma, Thoits (1985) said, "role-taking abilities enable individuals to view themselves from the imagined perspective of others" (p. 222). For instance, a person with HIV may internalize public stigma of HIV and view himself or herself as dirty and unworthy. Such internalization has negative consequences on physical and mental health.

Internalized HIV stigma is associated with poor treatment adherence among PLWHA, social isolation, poor retention, lack of social support, and depression (Rintamaki et al., 2009; Sayles et al., 2009). For example, Holzemer et al. (2009) researched 726 people (p. 161) living with HIV internationally and found that internalized HIV stigma contributed significantly to individuals' lowered quality of life, even after controlling for factors including HIV-related symptoms and severity of illness.

International research with MSM also supports the effect of minority stressors on HIV risk and testing behaviors and mental health outcomes. Among MSM in Beijing, experience of stigma/discrimination predicted avoidance of HIV testing and lack of discussion of HIV/AIDS with male sexual partners (Hu et al., 2014). Logie, Newman, Chakrapani, and Shunmugam (2012) adapted the minority stress model to the MSM population in India and found that both internalized HIV stigma as well as gender non-conforming stigma were associated with depression, with social support and resilient coping moderating those effects. Similarly, Pala, Hart, and Steca (2015, p. 244) studied 120 Italian gay and bisexual men and confirmed that stigma related to sexual orientation was associated with a greater level of depression and viral load, and that internalized homophobia was associated with lower CD4+ cell counts.

As mentioned before, PLWHA and high-HIV-risk populations often have more than one minority identity and face many types of discrimination and stigmatization. Other types of stigmatization (not related to HIV, but based on other devalued social identities) may also influence health behaviors of high-HIV-risk populations. For instance, research in Brazil noted that substance use history was highly stigmatized by primary care providers (Ronzani, Higgins-Biddle, & Furtado, 2009). This stigmatization affects PWIDs' attitudes toward seeking professional health care and adopting HIV prevention behaviors.

Stigmatization is consequential and each layer of stigmatization puts the individual at a more vulnerable position. Take a transgender woman as an example: The individual may face high levels of discrimination – for instance, termination of employment. As a result, she may participate in the sex trade to earn income or get housing. The double stigmatization towards a person with transgender identity who works in the sex trade can be stressful and also cause difficulty for her to ask for safe sex, which puts her at high risk for HIV infection and other STDs. To avoid the negative interpersonal consequences of HIV stigma and discrimination, she may avoid HIV testing and then fail to disclose her status if she happened to be positive. On a community level, late treatment of HIV leads to increased community viral load, thereby exacerbating the spread of the disease.

Coping, Social Support, and Characteristics of Minority Identity

As Meyer (2003) noted, coping/social support and characteristics of minority identity, such as prominence of minority identity in the person's sense of self, may moderate the impact of stress on mental health outcomes. In Allport's *The Nature of Prejudice* (1949), he suggested members of minority group respond to prejudice with resilience. Resilience and problem-solving- oriented coping have been shown to be beneficial for minority members and PLWHA (e.g., Friedland, Renwick, & Mccoll, 2010; Moskowitz, Hult, Bussolari, & Acree, 2009). In the U.S. and many other western countries, coming out (disclosure instead of concealment) and seeking support from family and friends are considered to be important coping methods in identity formation for LGBT individuals. Research with PLWHA noted the positive roles of active, confrontational, and problem-solving-oriented coping and positive reappraisal on individuals' physical and mental health outcomes (Moskowitz, Hult, Bussolari, & Acree, 2009; Mulder, Antoni, Duivenvoorden, Kauffmann, & Goodkin, 1995).

Meyer (2003) addressed the importance of group-level resources to assist one's coping (e.g., group level social structural factors, group level barriers). Community level resilience is important and has many benefits for individuals of minority group, such as a sense of belonging, connection with others, and finding positive role models (e.g., Riggle, Rostosky, McCants, & Pascale-Hague, 2011). Meanwhile, individuals are limited by the sociocultural and political structure and resources within the community (Meyer, 2015).

For high-HIV-risk populations, the lack of support on the societal level often manifests in barriers to health care, housing, and the lack of HIV education and HIV testing resources. Populations that are criminalized in many societies (e.g., sex workers) are in lack of sufficient resources, including health care. For instance, in China (Yi et al., 2010), migrant female sex workers (FSWs) in urban cities are often from rural areas; they lack social support and experience insufficient access to health care and HIV testing. Additionally, coping may also be limited by one's socioeconomic status, setting (e.g., prison or jail for incarcerated individuals), and sociocultural norms. For example, in India and countries like it, women are expected to get married, but it is not culturally appropriate for a wife to discuss using condoms with her husband. Thus, women are not able to negotiate safe sex (e.g., Steinbrook, 2007). Poverty also affects health outcomes negatively. Many high-HIV-risk populations are socioeconomically disadvantaged and lack access to clean water, food, and access to sufficient health care (Marmot, 2005).

For PLWHA, group level resources are determinant of physical and mental health outcomes. Group level support may include social support, such as connection with other PLWHA, and structural support, like HIV education, affordable STD testing, and medical coverage for antiretroviral therapy (ART). Early initiation of ART has several public health benefits, including reduction of potential transmission of HIV and the risk of acquiring other STDs. Thus, timely diagnosis and treatment are essential group level resources that can combat the HIV epidemic. For PLWHA, after initial diagnosis, receiving HIV education, starting ART, and getting regular care are important steps in achieving successful HIV treatment and retention. On the largest community scale – the global level – nations need to work together to enhance global responsiveness and resources for PLWHA, especially in areas with high levels of immigration and human trafficking.

Identities are "parts of the self – internalized positional designations that represent the person's participation in structured role relationships" (Stryker & Serpe, 1982, p. 206). Identity prominence is another variable influencing the impact of stress on health according to Meyer's model (2003). Validation, self-acceptance, and integration of minority identity with the person's other identities are conceptualized as protective factors (Meyer, 2003). Instead of thinking of identity as solid and unchanged, researchers now often view identity as fluid and shaped by context and social interaction (Baumeister & Muraven, 1996; Crocker & Quinn, 2000). Identities that are invisible (e.g., sexual orientation, HIV status, etc.) and stigmatized may be less salient for individuals compared to identities that are at the forefront of one's daily social interactions. For instance, one's HIV status may become salient in health care settings, and if the individual is in the early stage of accepting HIV status, being in health care settings may cause psychological distress. Since HIV/AIDS is highly stigmatized in many societies, one may conceal this identity at work settings for self-protection and it may not be a salient identity at work or in other public settings.

For PLWHA and high-HIV-risk populations, integration of multiple devalued social identities (e.g., sexual and gender identity, being HIV positive) can be a long process and can require much psychological work. For PLWHA, one's identity as being HIV positive may be associated with their high-HIV-risk identity and how they got infected (i.e., via drug injection, sex, blood transfusion, etc.) Community is vital in providing support, normalization, and role modeling in this process of integration. After getting diagnosed, PLWHA may join the HIV/AIDS community, through which their HIV/AIDS status often becomes a central identity. From there, PLWHA become engaged in learning about HIV/AIDS and connecting with other PLWHA. Furthermore, community can serve as a buffer to minority stress-related events such as prejudice and discrimination, which could be meaningful for PLWHA in both identity integration and successful adherence of ART.

Minority Stress Processes on Population Health Level

We argue that from a minority stress perspective, on a societal level, the key factors driving the HIV epidemic among the disproportionately affected populations are: HIV stigma, discrimination and violence toward PLWHA and high-HIV-risk populations, homophobia, and transphobia. All of these factors create an unsafe and neglectful environment for PLWHA and minority populations that are particularly vulnerable to HIV.

Stigma could be related to one's sexual identity, race, weight, illness, or disability, and it has been theorized to be "a fundamental cause of population health inequalities" (Hatzenbuehler, Phelan, & Link, 2013; p. 813). Scholars argue that HIV stigma drives the increased prevalence of HIV/AIDS in society, as the manifestation of stigma – ignorance of the disease, fear of discrimination, avoidance of HIV testing, consequent denial for treatment, not informing sex partners of one's HIV status, poor treatment adherence – all contribute to the spread of the disease (Stangl & Grossman, 2013).

On a societal level, stigma and discrimination deactivate, silence, and segregate people based on their social group identity through social and structural means. In this process, stereotypes can be conceptualized as expectations assigned based on group status (e.g., people with HIV are dirty, black gay men have high sex drive, people who inject drugs are lazy). Those culturally shared expectations affect both daily interaction with people from minority groups and structural-level resources and barriers. For example, for transgender women, the stereotype might be that they all want to be models, showgirls, or porn stars, fitting into the majority groups' fetishism of transgender women. People may interact with them through the lens of this stereotype, and as a result, transgender women experience more sexual harassment and violence, which puts them at a higher risk of contracting HIV. On a structural level, stigma and discrimination toward PLWHA can be manifested in the restraint social and public health resources (e.g., employment, affordable ART coverage, etc.)

Thus, on a population health level, minority stress processes are enacted through intrapersonal (e.g., internalization of stigma, racism, homophobia, etc.), interpersonal (e.g., discrimination, violence, lack of disclosure of one's status, etc.), and structural interactions (e.g., health care coverage, segregation, access to HIV education and testing, incarceration), resulting in health disparities, which in turn reinforce population level disparities and stereotypes. For instance, the fact that rates of HIV prevalence are high among MSM and transgender women may reinforce public's stereotype that gay and bisexual men and transgender women are highly sexually active and promiscuous.

Cross-Cultural Considerations

In the application of minority stress theory to PLWHA and high-HIV-risk populations, we want to acknowledge many cultural factors that affect minority stress processes in the context of global health, from varied levels of acceptance of sexual minorities in different societies to cultural issues related to disclosure and confidentiality. Human rights issues regarding sexual minorities are still a great challenge globally. Same-sex sexual contact is criminalized in 75 countries and in 8 of them, being gay or bisexual is punishable by death (ILGA, 2015, p. 9). Homophobia and violence on a societal level certainly influence the proximal process for LGBT individuals. For example, for LGBT individuals in more conservative countries, coming out may not be an acceptable or culturally appropriate process, and it may look different (e.g., selective disclosure) for LGB individuals.

Disclosure of one's HIV status can also be complicated by cultural factors. In collectivistic and low- to mid-level income societies, concepts of confidentiality and privacy might be relatively difficult to apply compared to high-income countries. For instance, a review of HIV disclosure (Obermeyer, Baijal, & Pegurri, 2010) noted that PLWHA living in high-income countries have higher rates of disclosure. Research on HIV-positive men and women in South Africa also noted that more than 40% had not disclosed their HIV status to a sexual partner in the past three months, and non-disclosure is often associated with previous experience of discrimination due to disclosing HIV status (Simbayi et al., 2007, p. 29). In collectivistic cultures, image and identity of oneself is intertwined with image of one's family (e.g., Kashima et al., 1995). A study found that many Asian PLWHA do not disclose their status in an effort to protect their families from shame, to avoid burdening others, and to evade communication regarding highly personal information (Chin & Kroesen, 1999; Yoshioka & Schustack, 2004).

In addition to contextual factors in various cultures, immigration-related issues are also very relevant, though often ignored, in the current global HIV epidemic. In Western and Central Europe, a large number of new HIV infections occurred among migrants from outside the region (Nakagawa, Phillips, & Lundgren, 2014). Many countries' immigration systems (e.g., Australia, Canada, China) require HIV testing as a mandatory part of the medical examination for visa holders, and they will be rejected/expelled if they are found to have HIV/AIDS. Immigrants (especially refugees and undocumented immigrants) have limited access to health care and are often discriminated against on social and institutional levels, causing a high level of vulnerability to HIV/AIDS and high mortality among HIV-positive immigrants (e.g., Deblonde et al., 2015; the Migrants Working Group, 2015).

Implications and Recommendations for Global HIV Care

In sum, we argue the importance of the use of the minority stress framework in global HIV prevention and treatment work, and we propose an expanded and localized application of the minority stress model for PLWHA and high-HIV-risk populations. We conceptualize HIV status as a social and health-related identity and call for an intersectional approach in understanding how minority stress processes put certain minority populations, namely MSM, transgender individuals, male and female sex workers, PWID, and incarcerated individuals, at high risk for HIV. From the minority stress perspective, global HIV prevention and treatment need to focus not only on the medical outcomes of HIV/AIDS (e.g., viral load, adherence), but also the sociocultural and political aspects of this fight. Global HIV care is essentially health equity and social justice work, aiming at promoting well-being for HIV-affected and marginalized populations.

International research aiming to investigate how the minority stress perspective may be applied among disproportionately affected populations is in its initial stage. We call for more research in this area in general, but especially on LGBT health disparities. Research should investigate how various types of discriminations and stigma and one's identity as minority member affect health behaviors (e.g., sexual risk behaviors, substance use). Additionally, scholars may also want to address how sociocultural factors, such as societal attitudes toward same sex partnership and culture values like conforming to social norms, influence the relationships among key variables in the minority stress framework.

Based on the framework and findings reviewed above, we make several recommendations for global HIV prevention and treatment programs. First, there should be consistent global effort in reducing discrimination and stigma, not only related to HIV/AIDS, but also in terms of decreasing discrimination and prejudice against high HIV/AIDS-risk populations across the world. As discussed before, distal minority stressors like discrimination and prejudice place minority populations at higher risk for HIV and other STDs and marginalize them even further. Anti-discrimination work should target both overt discrimination (e.g., violence) and implicit bias and stereotypes in societies. Experts from various disciplines need to work together to achieve this goal. Nations should evaluate and discuss health equity and societal attitudes toward high HIV/AIDS-risk populations in order to learn from each other and to develop specific plans in the anti-discrimination work.

Second, global agents and health organizations need to enforce sufficient access to HIV and other STD testing for high-HIV-risk populations and to treatment plans for those who need them. It might be helpful to develop specific programs targeting particularly vulnerable populations such as sex workers and transgender individuals. In 2014, the World Health Organization Department of HIV released the Consolidated Guidelines on HIV Prevention, Diagnosis, Treatment, and Care for Key Populations and identified five vulnerable populations including MSM, PWID, people in prison and confined settings, sex workers, and transgender people. This was a great effort in addressing the needs of vulnerable populations from different regions of the world and contextualizing HIV prevention and treatment work. Global health institutes may want to collaborate with local LGBT centers, hospitals, and other related organizations to increase access to testing and treatment. Innovative policies and approaches may be developed based on the specific needs of key affected populations in the region.

Third, community support is an important group level resource as PLWHA and high-HIV-risk populations face discrimination and prejudice on multiple fronts. Global health organizations and agents may want to create international communities for PLWHA and key affected populations or fund programs that help PLWHA and high-HIV-risk populations develop their own local communities. Programs that promote HIV education for families of PLWHA and key affected populations, peer support, and psychological healthcare will also be helpful in reducing the level of stress and promoting public health benefits.

References

Allport, G. W. (1949). *The nature of prejudice.* Oxford, England: Addison-Wesley Publishing Co.

Baral, S., Beyrer, C., Muessig, K., Poteat, T., Wirtz, A. L., Decker, M. R.,..., & Kerrigan, D. (2012). Burden of HIV among female sex workers in low-income and middle-income countries: A systematic review and meta-analysis. *The Lancet, 12*(7), 538-549. doi: 10.1016/S1473-3099(12)70066-X

Baum, A., Garofalo, J. P., & Yali, A. M. (2006). Socioeconomic status and chronic stress: Does stress account for SES effects on health? *Annals of the New York Academy of Sciences, 896*, 131-144.

Baumgartner, L. M. (2012). The perceived effect of time on HIV/AIDS identity incorporation. *The Qualitative Report, 17*, 1-22.

Baumgartner, L. M., & David, K. N. (2009). Accepting being poz: the incorporation of the HIV identity into the self. *Qualitative Health Research, 19*(12), 1730-1743. doi: 10.1177/1049732309352907

Berger, B. E., Ferrans, C. E., & Lashley, F. R. (2001). Measuring stigma in people with HIV: Psychometric assessment of the HIV stigma scale. *Research in Nursing & Health, 24*(6), 518-529. doi: 10.1002/nur.10011

Bernard, C. (1961). *An introduction to the study of experimental medicine.* New York, NY: Collier Books.

Beyrer, C., Baral, S. D., Griensven, F. V., Goodreau, S. M., Chariyalertsak, S., Wirtz, A. L., & Brookmeyer, R. (2012). Global epidemiology of HIV infection in men who have sex with men. *Lancet, 380*, 367-377.

Blendon, R. J., Donelan, K., & Knox, R. A. (1992). Public opinion and AIDS: Lessons for the second decade. *Journal of the American Medical Association, 267*, 981-986.

Brondolo, E., Love, E. E., Pencille, M., Schoenthaler, A., & Ogedegbe, G. (2011). Racism and hypertension: A review of the empirical evidence and implications for clinical practice. *American Journal of Hypertension, 24*(5), 518-529.

Burton, C. M., Marshal, M. P., Chisolm, D. J., Sucato, G. S., & Friedman, M. S. (2013). Sexual minority-related victimization as a mediator of mental health disparities in sexual minority youth: A longitudinal analysis. *Journal of Youth and Adolescence, 42*(3), 394-402.

Cannon, W. B. (1929). *Bodily changes in pain, hunger, fear, and rage.* (2nd ed.). New York: Appleton.

Capodilupo, C.M., Nadal, K.L., Corman, L., Hamit, S., Lyons, O., & Weinberg, A. (2010). The manifestation of gender microaggressions. In D.W. Sue (Ed.), *Microaggressions and marginality: Manifestation, dynamics, and impact* (pp. 193-216). New York: Wiley & Sons.

Centers for Disease Control and Prevention. (2015). HIV basics. Retrieved from http://www.cdc.gov/hiv/basics/

Center for Disease Control and Prevention. (2015). HIV among gay and bisexual men. Retrieved from http://www.cdc.gov/hiv/pdf/group/msm/cdc-hiv-msm.pdf

Chang, T. K., & Chung, Y. B. (2015). Transgender microaggressions: Complexity of the heterogeneity of transgender identities. *Journal of LGBT Issues in Counseling, 9*(3), 217-234. doi: 10.1080/15538605.2015.1068146

Chin, D., Kroesen, K. W. (1999). Disclosure of HIV infection among Asian/Pacific Islander American women: Cultural stigma and support. *Cultural Diversity and Ethnic Minority Psychology, 5*(3), 222-235. doi: 10.1037/1099-9809.5.3.222

Clark, R., Anderson, N. B., Clark, V. R., & Williams, D. R. (1999). Racism as a stressor for African Americans: A biopsychosocial model. *American Psychologist, 54*, 805-816.

Crocker, J., & Quinn, D. M. (2000). Social stigma and the self: Meanings, situations, and self-esteem. In Heatherton, T. F., Kleck, R. E., Hebl, M. R., Hull, J. G. (editors). *The social psychology of stigma.* New York: Guilford Press. p. 153-183.

Cochran, S. D., Sullivan, J. G., & Mays, V. M. (2003). Prevalence of mental disorders, psychological distress, and mental health services use among lesbian, gay, and bisexual adults in the United States. *Journal of Consulting and Clinical Psychology, 71*(1), 53-61.

Cohen, C. J. (1997). Punks, bulldaggers, and welfare queens: The radical potential of queer politics. *GLQ: A Journal of Lesbian and Gay Studies, 3*, 437-466.

Cole, S. W., Kemeny, M. E., Taylor, S. E., & Visscher, B. R. (1996). Elevated physical health risk among gay men who conceal their homosexual identity. *Health Psychology, 15*(4), 243-251. doi: 10.1037/0278-6133.15.4.243

Deblonde, J., Sasse, A., Amo, J. D., Burns, F., Delpech, V., Cowan, S., ...& Noori, T. (2015). Restricted access to antiretroviral treatment for undocumented migrants: A bottle neck to control the HIV epidemic in the EU/EEA. *BMC Public Health, 15*, 1228. doi: 10.1186/s12889-015-2571-y

Dolan, K., Wirtz, A. L., Moazen, B., Ndeffo-mbah, M., Galvani, A., Kinner, S. A., ..., & Altice, F. L. (2016). Global burden of HIV, viral hepatitis, and tuberculosis in prisoners and detainees. *The Lancet, 388*(10049), 1089-1102. doi: 10.1016/S0140-6736(16)30466-4

Durkheim, E. (1897). *Suicide: A study in sociology.* Free Press: New York City.

Earnshaw, V. A., & Chaudoir, S. R. (2009). From conceptualizing to measuring HIV stigma: A review of HIV stigma mechanism measures. *AIDS & Behavior, 13*, 1160-1177. doi: 10.1007/s10461-009-9593-3

Earnshaw, V. A., Quinn, D. M. (2012). The impact of stigma in healthcare on people living with   chronic illnesses. *Journal of Health Psychology, 17*(2), 157-168. doi: 10.1177/1359105311414952

Earnshaw, V. A., Smith, L. R., Cunningham, C. O., & Copenhaver, M. M. (2015). Intersectionality of internalized HIV stigma and internalized substance use stigma: Implications for depressive symptoms. *Journal of Health Psychology, 20*(8), 1083-1089. doi: 10.1177/1359105313507964

Foynes, M. M., Smith, B. N., & Shipherd, J. C. (2015). Associations between race-based and sex-based discrimination, health, and functioning: A longitudinal study of marines. *Medical Care, 53*(4), 128-135. doi: 10.1097/MLR.0000000000000300

Friedland, J., Renwick, R., & McColl, M. (1996). Coping and social support as determinants of quality of life in HIV/AIDS. *AIDS Care, 8*(1), 15-31.

Elo, I. T., & Preston, S. H. (1996). Educational differentials in mortality: United States, 1979-1985. *Social Science and Medicine, 42*, 47-57.

Engel, G. L. (1977). The need for a new medical model: A challenge for biomedicine. *Science, 196*, 129-136.

Fife, B. L., & Wright, E. R. (2000). The dimensionality of stigma: A comparison of its impact on the self of persons with HIV/AIDS and cancer. *Journal of Health and Social Behavior, 41*, 50-67.

Fredriksen-Goldsen, K. I., Kim, H-J., Barkan, S. E., Muraco, A., & Hoy-Ellis, C. P. (2013). Health disparities among lesbian, gay, and bisexual older adults: Results from a population based study. *American Journal of Public Health, 103*(10), 1802-1809. doi: 10.2105/AJPH.2012.301110

Frost, N. M., Lehavot, K., & Meyer, I. H. (2015). Minority stress and physical health among sexual minority individuals. *Journal of Behavioral Medicine, 38*, 1-8. doi: 10.1007/s10865-013-9523-8

Gee, G., & Walsemann, K. (2009). Does health predict the reporting of racial discrimination or do reports of discrimination predict health? Findings from the national longitudinal study of youth. *Social Science & Medicine, 68*, 1676-1684.

Goldbach, J. T., Tanner-Smith, E. E., Bagwell, M., & Dunlap, S. (2014). Minority stress and substance use in sexual minority adolescents: A meta-analysis. *Prevention Science, 15*(3), 350-363. doi: 10.1007/s11121-013-0393-7

Hatzenbuehler, M. L., Phelan, J. C., & Link, B. G. (2013). Stigma as a fundamental cause of population health inequalities. *American Journal of Public Health, 103*(5), 813-821.

Herek, G. M., & Capitanio, J. P. (1999). AIDS stigma and sexual prejudice. *American Behavioral Scientist, 42*, 1126-1143.

Holzemer, W. L., Human, S., Arudo, J., Rosa, M. E., Hamilton, M. J., Corless, I., ...& Rivero-Mendez, M. (2009). Exploring HIV stigma and quality of life for persons living with HIV   infection. *Journal of the Association of Nurses in AIDS Care, 20*(3), 161-168.

Hu, Y., Lu, H., Raymond, H. F., Sun, Y., Sun, J., Jia, Y., ..., & Ruan, Y. (2014). Measures of condom and safer sex social norms and stigma towards HIV/AIDS among Beijing MSM. *AIDS & Behavior, 18*(6), 1068-1074. doi: 10.1007/s10461-013-0609-7

Huntington, D. (2012). Health systems perspectives: Infectious diseases of poverty. *Infectious Diseases of Poverty, 1*(1): 12. doi: 10.1186/2049-9957-1-12.

International Lesbian, Gay, Bisexual, Trans and Intersex Association (ILGA; 2015). A world survey of sexual orientation laws: Criminalisation, protection, and recognition. Retrieved from http://old.ilga.org/Statehomophobia/ILGA_State_Sponsored_Homophobia_2015.pdf

Jeffries, W. L., Marks, G., Lauby, J., Murrill, C. S., & Millett, G. A. (2013). Homophobia is associated with sexual behavior that increases risk of acquiring and transmitting HIV infection among black men who have sex with men. *AIDS & Behavior, 17*(4), 1442-1453. doi: 10.1007/s10461-012-0189-y

Kalichman, S. C., & Simbayi, L. C. (2003). HIV testing attitudes, AIDS stigma, and voluntary HIV counseling and testing in a black township in Cape Town, South Africa. *Sexually Transmitted Infections, 79,* 442-447.

Kaplan, K. C., Hormes, J. M., Wallace, M., Rountree, M., & Theall, K. P. (2016). Racial discrimination and HIV related risk behaviors in Southeast Louisiana. *American Journal of Health Behavior, 40*(1), 132-143. doi: 10.5993/AJHB.40.1.15

Kashima, Y., Yamaguchi, S., Kim, U., Choi, S-C., Gelfand, M. J., Yuki, M. (1995). *Journal of Personality and Social Psychology,* 69(5), 925-937. doi: 10.1037/0022-3514.69.5.925

Kelley, C. F., Rosenberg, E. S., O'Hara, B. M., Frew, P. M., Sanchez, T., Peterson, J. L., ..., & Sullivan, P. S. (2012). Measuring population transmission risk for HIV: An alternative metric of exposure risk in men who have sex with men (MSM) in the U.S. *PLoS ONE, 7*(12): e53284. doi: 10.1371/journal.pone.0053284

Koh, A. S., & Ross, L. K. (2006). A comparison of lesbian, bisexual and heterosexual women. *Journal of Homosexuality, 51*(1), 33-57.

Krieger, N. (1999). Embodying inequality: A review of concepts, measures, and methods for studying health consequences of discrimination. *International Journal of Health Services, 29*(2), 295-352.

Larson, A., Gillies, M., Howard, P.J., & Coffin, J. (2007). It's enough to make you sick: The impact of racism on the health of Aboriginal Australians. *Australian and New Zealand journal of Public Health, 31*(4), 322-329. doi: 10.1111/j.1753-6405.2007.00079.x

Larson, D. G., Chastain, R. L., Hoyt, W. T., & Ayzenberg, R. (2015). Self-concealment: Integrative review and working model. *Journal of Social and Clinical Psychology, 34*(8), 705-e774.

Lantz, P. M., House, J. S., Mero, R. P., & Williams, D. R. (2005). Stress, life events, and socioeconomic disparities in health: Results from the Americans' changing lives study. *Journal of Health and Social Behavior, 46,* 274-288.

Leclerc-Madlala, S. (2008). Age-disparate and intergenerational sex in southern Africa: the dynamics of hypervulnerability. *AIDS, 22*(4), s17-25. doi: 10.1097/01.aids.0000341774.86500.53.

Logie, C. H., Newman, P. A., Chakrapani, V., & Shunmugam, M. (2012). Adapting the minority stress model: Associations between gender non-conformity stigma, HIV-related stigma and depression among men who have sex with men in South India. *Social Science & Medicine, 74*(8), 1261-1268. doi: 10.1016/j.socscimed.2012.01.008.

Mackenzie, S. (2013). *Structural intimacies: Sexual stories in the black AIDS epidemic.* New Brunswick, NJ: Rutgers University Press.

Marmot, M. (2005). Social determinants of health inequalities. *The Lancet, 365,* 1099-1104.

Mascolini, M. (2013). Life expectancy with HIV jumps 15 years from 2000-2002 to 2006-2007 in U.S., Canada. Presentation at 7th IAS Conference on HIV Pathogenesis, Treatment and Prevention, June 30-July 3, 2013, Kuala Lumpur, Malaysia. Retrieved from http://www.natap.org/2013/IAS/IAS_43.htm

Masur, H., Michelis, M. A., Greene, J. B., Onorato, I., Stouwe, R. A. V., Holzman, R. S., ...Cunningham-Rundles, S. (1981). An outbreak of community-acquired Pneumocystis carinii Pneumonia--- Initial manifestation of cellular immune dysfunction. *The North England Journal of Medicine, 305*, 1431-1438. doi: 10.1056/NEJM198112103052402

Mehta, N. (2011). Mind-body dualism: A critique from a health perspective. *Mens Sana Monographs, 9*(1), 202-209. doi: 10.4103/0973-1229.77436

Melendez, R. M., Exner, T. A., Ehrhardt, A. A., Dodge, B., Remein, R. H., Rotheram-Borus, M-J.,...,& Hong, D. (2006). Health and health care among male-to-female transgender persons who are HIV positive. *American Journal of Public Health, 96*(6), 1034-1037. doi: 10.2105/AJPH.2004.042010

Merton, R. K. (1938). *Social theory and social structure*. New York, NY: Free Press.

Meyer, I. H. (2003). Prejudice, social stress, and mental health in lesbian, gay, and bisexual populations: Conceptual issues and research evidence. *Psychological Bulletin, 129*(5), 674-697.

Meyer, I. H. (2015). Resilience in the study of minority stress and health of sexual and gender minorities. *Psychology of Sexual Orientation and Gender Diversity, 2*(3), 209-213. doi: 10.1037/sgd0000132

Meyer, I. H., & Dean, L. (1998). Internalized homophobia, intimacy, and sexual behavior among gay and bisexual men. In Herek, G. M. (ed.). *Stigma and sexual orientation: Understanding prejudice against lesbians, gay men, and bisexuals*. Thousand Oaks, CA: Sage.

Miller, C. T., & Myers, A. M. (1998). Compensating for prejudice: How heavyweight people (and others) control outcomes despite prejudice. In Swim, J. K. & Stangor, C. (eds.). *Prejudice: The target's perspective*. New York: Academic Press.

Millett, G. A., Peterson, J. L., Flores, S. A., Hart, T. A., Jeffries, W., Wilson, P. A., ..., & Remis, R. S. (2012). Comparisons of disparities and risks of HIV infection in black and other men who have sex with men in Canada, UK, and USA: A meta-analysis. *The Lancet, 380*(9839), 341-348. doi: 10.1016/S0140-6736(12)60899-X

Millett, G. A., Peterson, J. L., Wolitski, R. J., & Stall, R. (2006). Greater risk for HIV infection of black men who have sex with men: A critical literature review. *American Journal of Public Health, 96*(6), 1007-1019. doi: 10.2105/AJPH.2005.066720

Moskowitz, J. T., Hult, J. R., Bussolari, C., Acree, M. (2009). What works in coping with HIV? A meta-analysis with implications for coping with serious illness. *Psychological Bulletin, 135*(1), 121-141. doi: 10.1037/a0014210

Mulder, C. L., Antoni, M. H., Duivenvoorden, H. J., Kauffmann, R. H., & Goodkin, K. (1995). Active confrontational coping predicts decreased clinical progression over a one-year period in HIV-infected homosexual men. *Journal of Psychosomatic Research, 39*(8), 957-965. doi: 10.1016/0022-3999(95)00062-3

Nadal, K. L., Griffin, K. E., Hamit, S., Leon, J., Tobio, M., & Rivera, D. P. (2012). Subtle and overt forms of Islamophobia: Microaggressions toward Muslim Americans. *Journal of Muslim Mental Health, 4*(2), 15-23.

Nadal, K. L., Issa, M-A., Leon, J., Meterko, V., Wideman, M., & Wong, Y. (2011). Sexual orientation microaggressions: "Death by a thousand cuts" for lesbian, gay, and bisexual youth. *Journal of LGBT Youth, 8*(3), 234-259. doi: 10.1080/19361653.2011.584204

Nakagawa, F., Phillips, A. N., & Lundgren, J. D. (2014). Update on HIV in Western Europe. *Current HIV/AIDS Reports, 11*(2), 177-185. doi: 10.1007/s11904-014-0198-8

Newcomb, M. E., & Mustanski, B. (2010). Internalized homophobia and internalizing mental health problems: A meta-analytic review. *Clinical Psychology Review, 30*(8), 1019-1029. doi: 10.1016/j.cpr.2010.07.003

Obermeyer, C. M., Baijal, P., & Pegurri, E. (2010). Facilitating HIV disclosure across diverse settings: A review. *American Journal of Public Health, 101*(6), 1011-1023.

Odinokova, V., Rusakova, M., Urada, L. A., Silverman, J. G., & Raj, A. (2014). Police sexual coercion and its association with risky sex work and substance use behaviors among female sex workers in St. Petersburg and Orenburg, Russia. *International Journal of Drug Policy, 25*(1), 96-104. doi: 10.1016/j.drugpo.2013.06.008

Operario, D., Soma, T., & Underhill, K. (2008). Sex work and HIV status among transgender women: Systematic review and meta-analysis. *Journal of Acquired Immune Deficiency Syndrome, 48*(1), 97-103. doi: 10.1097/QAI.0b013e31816e3971.

Overstreet, N. M., Earnshaw, V. A., Kalichman, S. C., & Quinn, D. M. (2013). Internalized stigma and HIV status disclosure among HIV-positive black men who have sex with men. *AIDS Care, 25*(4), 466-471. doi: 10.1080/09540121.2012.720362.

Pala, A. N., Hart, R. P., Steca, P. (2015). Minority stress, depression and HIV-progression biomarkers: An exploratory study on a sample of Italian HIV-positive gay and bisexual men. *Journal of Gay & Lesbian Mental Health, 19* (3), 244-260. doi: 10.1080/19359705.2014.999181

Pallikadavath, S., Garda, L., Apte, H., Freedman, J., & Stones, R. W. (2005). HIV/AIDS in rural India: Context and health care needs. *Journal of Biosocial Science, 37*, 641-655.

Paradies, Y. (2006). A systematic review of empirical research on self-reported racism and health. *International Journal of Epidemiology, 35*, 888-901. doi: 10.1093/ije/dy1056

Paradies, Y., Ben, J., Denson, N., Elias, A., Priest, N., Pieterse, A., …, & Gee, G. (2015). Racism as a determinant of health: A systematic review and meta-analysis. *PLOS ONE, 10*(9), e0139511.

Parker, R. (2002). The global HIV/AIDS pandemic, structural inequalities, and the politics of international health. *American Journal of Public Health, 92*(3), 343-347.

Parker, R., & Aggleton, P. (2003). HIV and AIDS-related stigma and discrimination: A conceptual framework and implications for action. *Social Science & Medicine, 57*(1), 13-24. doi: 10.1016/S0277-9536(02)00304-0

Pascoe, E., & Richman, L. S. (2009). Perceived discrimination and health: A meta-analytic review. *Psychological Bulletin, 135*(4), 531-554. doi: 10.1037/a0016059

Patterson, S. E., Milloy, M-J., Ogilvie, G., Greene, S., Nicholson, V., Vonn, M., …, & Kaida, A. (2015). The impact of criminalization of HIV non-disclosure on the healthcare engagement of women living with HIV in Canada: A comprehensive review of the evidence. *Journal of the International AIDS Society, 18*(1): 20572. doi: 10.7448/IAS.18.1.20572

Pavalko, E. K., Mossakowski, K. N., & Hamilton, V. J. (2003). Does perceived discrimination affect health? Longitudinal relationships between work discrimination and women's physical and emotional health. *Journal of Health and Social Behavior, 43*, 18-33.

Porter, K., Babiker, A., Bhaskaran, K., Darbyshire, J., Pezzotti, P., & Walker, A. S. (2003). Determinants of survival following HIV-1 seroconversion after the introduction of HAART. *Lancet, 362*, 1267-1274.

Pulerwitz, Michaelis, Lippman, Chinaglia, & Díaz. (2008). HIV-related stigma, service utilization, and status disclosure among truck drivers crossing the Southern borders in Brazil. *AIDS & Care, 20*(7), 764-770. doi: 10.1080/09540120701506796

Reisner, S.L., White, J. M., Bradford, J. B., & Mimiaga, M. J. (2014). Transgender health disparities: Comparing full cohort and nested matched-pair study designs in a community health center. *LGBT Health, 1*(3), 177-184. doi: 10.1089/lgbt.2014.0009

Riggle, E. D. B., Rostosky, S. S., McCants, L. E., & Pascale-Hague, D. (2011). The positive aspects of a transgender self-identification. *Psychology and Sexuality, 2*, 147-158. doi: 10.1080/19419899.2010.534490

Rintamaki, L. S., Davis, T. C., Skripkauskas, S., Bennett, C. L., & Wolf, M. S. (2006). Social stigma concerns and HIV medication adherence. *AIDS Patient Care and STDs, 20*(5), 359-368. doi:10.1089/apc.2006.20.359.

Rispel, L. C., Metcalf, C. A., Cloete, A., Reddy, V., & Lombard, C. (2011). HIV prevalence and risk practices among men who have sex with men in two South African cities. *Journal of Acquired Immune Deficiency Syndrome, 57*(1), 69-76. doi: 10.1097/QAI.0b013e318211b40a.

Ronzani, T. M., Higgins-Biddle, J., & Furtado, E. F. (2009). Stigmatization of alcohol and other drug users by primary care providers in Southeast Brazil. *Social Science & Medicine*, *69*(7),1080-1084. doi: 10.1016/j.socscimed.2009.07.026

Sayles, J. N., Wong, M. D., Kinsler, J. J., Martins, D., & Cunningham, W. E. (2009). The association of stigma with self-reported access to medical care and antiretroviral therapy adherence in persons living with HIV/AIDS. *Journal of General Internal Medicine*, *24*(10), 1101-1108. doi: 10.1007/s11606-009-1068-8

Schmitt, M. T., Branscombe, N. R., Postmes, T., & Garcia, A. (2014). The consequences of perceived discrimination for psychological well-being: A meta-analytic review. *Psychological Bulletin*, *140*(4), 921-948. doi: 10.1037/a0035754.

Schneiderman, N., Ironson, G., & Siegel, S. D. (2005). Stress and health: Psychological, behavior, and biological determinants. *Annual Review of Clinical Psychology*, *1*, 607-628. doi: 10.1146/annurev.clinpsy.1.102803.144141.

Segerstrom, S. C., & Miller, G. E. (2004). Psychological stress and the human immune system: A meta-analytic study of 30 years of inquiry. *Psychological Bulletin*, *130*(4), 601-630. doi: 10.1037/0033-2909.130.4.601

Selye, H. (1956). *The stress of life*. New York, NY: McGraw-Hill.

Siegler, A. J., Sullivan, P. S., Voux, A., Phaswana-Mafuya, N., Bekker, L-G, Baral, S. D.,..., & Stephenson, R. (2015). Exploring repeat HIV testing among men who have sex with men in Cape Town and Port Elizabeth, South Africa. *AIDS Care*, *27*(2), 229-234. doi: 10.1080/09540121.2014.947914

Simbayi, L. C., Kalichman, S. C., Strebel, A., Cloete, A., Henda, N., & Mqeketo, A. (2007). Disclosure of HIV status to sex partners and sexual risk behaviors among HIV-positive men and women, Cape Town, South Africa. *Sexually Transmitted Infections*, *83*, 29-34. doi: 10.1136/sti.2006.019893

Smith, R., Rossetto, K., & Peterson, B. L. (2008). A meta-analysis of disclosure of one's HIV- positive status, stigma, and social support. *AIDS Care*, *20*(10), 1266-1275. doi: 10.1080/09540120801926977

Spaulding, A. C., Seals, R. M., Page, M. J., Brzozowski, A. K., Rhodes, W., & Hammett, T. M. (2006). HIV/AIDS among inmates of an releases from US correctional facilities, 2006: Declining share of epidemic but persistent public health opportunity. *PLOS ONE*, *4*(11), e7558. doi:10.1371/journal.pone.0007558

Stangl, A. L., & Grossman, C. I. (2013). Global Action to reduce HIV stigma and discrimination. *Journal of the International AIDS Society*, *16*(3Suppl 2), 18934. doi: 10.7448/IAS.16.3.18934

Steinbrook, R. (2007). HIV in India: A complex epidemic. *The New England Journal of Medicine*, *356*, 1089-1093. doi: 10.1056/NEJMp078009

Stock, M. L., Peterson, L. M., Gibbons, F. X., & Gerrard, M. (2013). The effects of racial discrimination on the HIV-risk cognitions and behaviors of black adolescents and young adults. *Health Psychology*, *32*(5), 543-550. doi: 10.1037/a0028815

Strachan, E. D., Bennett, W. R., Russo, J., Roy-Byrne, P. P. (2007). Disclosure of HIV status and sexual orientation independently predicts increased absolute CD4 cell counts over time for psychiatric patients. *Psychosocial Medicine*, *69*(1), 74-80. doi: 10.1097/01.psy.0000249900.34885.46

Stryker, S., & Serpe, R. T. (1982). Commitment, identity salience, and role behavior: A theory and research example. In *Personality, Role, and Social Behavior*, edited by William Ickes and Eric S. Knowles. New York: Springer-Verlag.

Sue, D. W., Capodilupo, C. M., Torino, G. C., Bucceri, J. M., Holder, A. M.,...& Esquilin, M. (2007). Racial microaggressions in everyday life: Implications for clinical practice. *American Psychologist*, *62*(4), 271-286.

Sullivan, M. (1986). In what sense is contemporary medicine dualistic? *Culture, Medicine, and Psychiatry*, *10*(4), 331-350.

Sullivan, P. S., Hamouda, O., Delpech, V., Geduld, J. E., Prejean, J., Semaille, C., ..., & Annecy MSM Epidemiology Study Group (2009). *Annals of Epidemiology*, *19*(6), 423-431. doi: 10.1016/j.annepidem.2009.03.004

Tajfel, H., & Turner, J. C. (1986). The social identity theory of intergroup behavior. In S. Worchel & W. G. Austin (Eds.), *Psychology of intergroup relations* (2nd ed., pp.7-24). Chicago: Nelson-Hall.

Tewksbury, R., & McGaughey, D. (1998). Identities and identity transformations among persons with HIV disease. *International Journal of Sexuality and Gender Studies*, *3*(3), 213-232. doi: 10.1023/A:1023243032307

The Migrants Working Group on behalf of COHERE in EuroCoord. (2015). Mortality in migrants living with HIV in western Europe (1997-2013): A collaborative cohort study. *The Lancet*, 2(2), e540-e549. doi: 10.1016/S2352-3018(15)00203-9

Thoits, P. A. (1985). Self-labeling processes in mental illness: The role of emotional deviance. *American Journal of Sociology*, *91*, 221-249.

Thoits, P. A. (2010). Stress and health: major findings and policy implications. *Journal of Health and Social Behavior*, *51*, s41-s53.

Ti, L., Hayashi, K., Kaplan, K., Suwannawong, P., Wood, E., Montaner, J., & Kerr, T. (2013). HIV test avoidance among people who inject drugs in Thailand. *AIDS & Behavior*, *17*(7), 2474-2478. doi: 10.1007/s10461-012-0347-2

Tucker, J., Ren, X., Sapio, F. (2010). Incarcerated sex workers and HIV prevention in China: Social suffering and social justice countermeasures. *Social Science and Medicine*, *70*(1), 121-129. doi: 10.1016/j.socscimed.2009.10.010

Turner, R. J., & Lloyd, D. A. (1999). The stress process and the social distribution of depression. *Journal of Health and Social Behavior*, *40*(4), 374-404.

UNAIDS (2015). Global AIDS response progress reporting. Retrieved from http://www.unaids.org/sites/default/files/media_asset/global-AIDS-update-2016_en.pdf

Van Griensven, F., Na Ayutthaya, P. P., & Wilson, E. (2013). HIV surveillance and prevention   in transgender women. *Lancet*, *13*(3), 185-186. doi: 10.1016/S1473-3099(12)70326-2

Watkins-Hays, C. (2014). Intersectionality and the sociology of HIV/AIDS: Past, resent, and future research directions. *The Annual Review of Sociology*, *40*, 431-457. doi: 10.1146/annurev-soc-071312-145621

Williams, D. R., & Neighbors, H. (2001). Racism, discrimination, and hypertension: evidence and needed research. *Ethnicity and Disease*, *11*(4), 800-816.

Williams, D. R., & Williams-Morris, R. (2000). Racism and mental health: The African American experience. *Ethnicity & Health*, *3-4*, 243-268.

World Health Organization. (2016). *HIV/AIDS: Data and statistics*. Retrieved from http://www.who.int/hiv/data/en/

Yi, H., Mantell, J. E., Wu, R., Lu, Z., Zeng, J., & Wan, Y. (2010). A profile of HIV risk factors in the context of sex work environments among migrant female sex workers in Beijing, China. *Psychology, Health, & Medicine*, *15*(2), 172-187. doi: 10.1080/13548501003623914

Yoshioka, M. R., & Schustack, A. (2001). Disclosure of HIV status: Cultural issues of Asian patients. *AIDS Patient Care & STDs*, *15*(2), 77-82.

CHAPTER 5

Perspectives on World Sleep Disturbances

Kathy Sexton-Radek and Alissa Rubinfeld

Sleep disturbances are a common presentation problem in the medical community. Disruption in the sleep cycle exacerbates medical conditions with recent evidence identifying diabetes, cardiovascular disease, and depression worsening with poor sleep quality. These findings accompany a growing awareness of the impact of sleep disturbance on general functioning (e.g., lower grades in school, absentees, and industrial errors). The World Health Organization (WHO) has identified non-communicable diseases (cardiovascular disease, diabetes, cancer, and chronic respiratory diseases), neuropsychiatric conditions, and road traffic accidents as being related to mortality. While the impact of sleep disturbance on these conditions is receiving focus in medical literature, worldwide perspectives are lacking. This chapter will address the extent of sleep disturbances globally and indicate representative treatments aimed at reducing the impact of poor sleep quality on general functioning. Specific focus will be given to the prevalence of sleep disturbances by country. Representative medical and psychological interventions to treat the sleep disturbances will be presented, followed by a summarization of future directions.

Perspectives on World Sleep Disturbances

Humans spend a third of their lives in sleep. For many, sleep is a delightful repose resulting in rejuvenation and pleasant recollections of dreams; however, for others, sleep is disturbed. Restless legs, anxiety, and breathing disorders may disrupt sleep (World Health Organization [WHO],

131

1995; Sexton-Radek, Pendle & Marvi, 2015; Shankar, Charumathi, Kalidindi, 2008).

Sleep is determined by two factors: sleep drive and timing of sleep. As we wake in the morning, our sleep propensity begins its assent. At our typical bedtime, the degree of sleep need combined with a relaxed state allow sleep to follow. The typical bedtime is determined in young adulthood with the maturation of brain-regulating mechanisms in the hypothalamus. Thus, our typical bedtimes mark the start of our personal sleep pattern (i.e., our circadian rhythm). Global travelers outside of their typical time zone can attest to their bodily response when forced to be awake when they are typically sleeping. In addition to the biological factors that drive the need for sleep, there exists a second aspect of sleep – the timing of the sleep interval. This timing of sleep is based on a twenty-four hour schedule and is referred to as a circadian rhythm. It is the circadian rhythm that keeps a person asleep. Additionally, behavioral factors such as excessive worry or stress influence the biological determinants of sleep (Friborg, Bjorvatin, Amponsah & Pallesen, 2012).

There are two types of sleep that alternate throughout a restful night: Rapid Eye Movement sleep (REM) and non-Rapid Eye Movement sleep (nREM). An epoch of sleep is the gradual stage, shifting from wake to nREM light sleep (stage 1), to nREM sleep (stage2), and then to deep sleep (stage 3/4). This staging from wake to nREM is approximately ninety minutes and is followed by a stage of REM. Thus, Stage 1 through REM is considered an epoch; a night of sleep is three to four of these epochs (all of which are similar in composition). Sleep Medicine research has identified the importance of sleep, the substantive nature of each type of sleep, and the essential condition of well-ordered sleep, which is called sleep architecture. In general, sleep is an altered state of consciousness of varying levels of increasingly complex physiological processing. For more information on the physiological basis of sleep, see works in the reference list provided (Appendix A*).

Besides the astronomical beauty of the night sky, it has been found that darkness is conducive to sleep as visible light stimulates the brain structures related to sleep to move to wakefulness. To the majority, light is a time-giver or zeitgeber that wakes us or prevents sleep; however, for part of the world population, going to sleep at "night time" happens despite the sky's brightness (Friborg et al., 2012; (World Health Organization [WHO], 1995). An investigation of this natural light at "night time" found moderate seasonal differences in insomnia and fatigue as well as weak differences in mood level on studies of Ghana (5o) and Norway (69o) (Friborg et al.,

---

* Appendices for this chapter can be found at: http://tinyurl.com/wghm-attachments

2012). Light will impose upon sleep, and to those unaccustomed to a bright sky at night, sleep will be difficult (Friborg et al., 2012). Those in darkened or light sky extremes have acclimated to a sleep schedule. Light exposure does not necessarily affect sleep duration, but does influence the timing of bedtimes and rise-times. For example, increased sunlight in countries in the southern hemisphere causes a delayed onset of bedtime (i.e., Ghana compared to Norway) (Friborg et al., 2012). Temperature extremes can also disrupt sleep; it has been found that those unaccustomed to extreme climates experience sleep disturbance as a result (Friborg et al., 2012).

Sleep Disorders Worldwide

Poor sleep quality has been reported to be a worldwide problem with higher incidence in developing nations (Stranges, Tigbe, Gomez-Olivé, Thorogood, & Kandala, 2012). The WHO reports that non-communicable diseases are the leading cause of death in the world's low- and middle-income population. In fact, cardiovascular disease, diabetes, cancer, and chronic respiratory disease are responsible for 63% of deaths globally (WHO, 2011, p. 1). Cumulative, long-term effects of sleep loss and sleep disorders are associated with non-communicable diseases, particularly cardiovascular disease, diabetes mellitus, depression, and obesity. Shorter sleep times are associated with obesity and impaired glucose tolerance.

Sleep inefficiency is associated with motor vehicle accidents, industrial disasters, and other human errors. Using an American sample, the CDC (2016) reported poor attention as the most prevalent, self-reported result of sleep disturbance. Statistics from the National Department of Transportation (2015) show that drowsy driving is linked to 1,550 fatalities and 40,000 non-fatal injuries in the United States (Centers for Disease Control & Prevention, 2011, p. 1).

Sleep Epidemiology

The epidemiological study of sleep examines groups of people and sleep quality/disturbance variables (Ferrie, Kumari, Salo, Singh-Manoux & Kivimaki, 2011). Hafner, Stepanek, Taylor, Troxel, and VanStolk (2016) reported sleep loss in industrialized countries as reduced overall. Reports of sleep percent per day resulted in the following rank (in descending order): Japan, the United States, Germany, Canada, and the United Kingdom (Hafner et al., 2014, p. xi). Similar research in sleep epidemiology examines sleep in large groupings using four major factors (Ferrie, et al., 2011). First, estimates of worldwide motor-vehicle crashes attributed to poor sleep have increased (Ferrie, et al., 2011). Second, an increased number of adults complain of sleep disturbance. Third, according to Ferrie, et al. (2011), the common condition of sleep disturbance is at a chronic level. 10% of individuals complain of chronic sleep disturbance (p. 1432). A decline in sleep length per night has occurred in the recent past (Ferrie, et al., 2011). Shortened sleep length has been associated with mortality and chronic health conditions. It seems that extremes of sleep (too short or too long) outside developmental expectations are associated with mortality, cardiovascular conditions (due to increased inflammation), diabetes mellitus, obesity, and depression (Rajaratnam & Arendt, 2001; Sexton-Radek & Graci, 2009; Sexton-Radek, 2015). Furthermore, anxiety has been found to be related to insomnia, a form of sleep disturbance. The fourth variable relates to the need to carry out more large-scale epidemiological studies to better understand the patterns and quality of individual sleep.

Sleep epidemiologists have advanced the empiricism of the sleep medicine field by designing psychometrically valid assessment measures (e.g., Pittsburgh Sleep Quality Index [PSQI]) (Ferrie et al., 2011). In terms of methodology, it is recommended that the change in sleep disturbances be measured by daily sleep loggings, not just a single measurement. For example, in a report of a cohort of 25,000 Finnish employees, repeated measurements of sleep disturbance compared to single measurement improved prediction of future work disability by over 10% (Ferrie, et al., 2011, p.1433). Furthermore, recent findings from brain imaging studies have identified changes in brain and cognitive functioning across the lifespan. These age-related brain and cognitive changes are thought to be similar to chronic insomnia sleep-disturbed states. Further study in this area of neuroscience reveals investigation of the associations between brain, sleep quality, and health outcomes (Ferrie, et al., 2011, p. 1433).

Specific to insomnia, Lichstein, Durrence, Riedel, Taylor, and Bush (2004) conducted a stratified sampling of adults in the Memphis, Tennessee area. This research provides a normative standard for common sleep variables such as sleep length, minutes to fall asleep, napping/nap length, and ratings of sleep quality by age and gender. This prospective, stratified, randomized epidemiological study was across the adult lifespan and included racially diverse samplings (Lichstein, et al., 2004). These studies identified the prevalence of worry about work and finances, which was believed to lead to an increased number of minutes required to fall asleep (Lichstein, et al., 2004).

According to Sexton-Radek et al. (2015), a global sample of respondents reported insomnia symptoms lasting ten years or more. Furthermore, in another global study, the majority of respondents indicated that their sleep quality influenced their overall health and well-being, but they were not engaging in any actions to remedy this (Ng, Kowal, Kakn, et al., 2010).

Life and Sleep Issues

The literature representing international studies/populations has identified the disruptive nature of poor sleep. Sleep-related accidents as a result of increased impulsivity and cognitive impairment of police officers in Italy were reported to be related to sleep deprivation (Mucci, Montalti, Bini, Cupelli, Arcangeli, 2012). In Japan, shift workers (as compared to non-shift workers) reported more daytime sleepiness (Grunstein, 2012). In an investigation of sleep quality in Singapore, shift workers with naps had better health care outcomes than those without naps (Grunstein, 2012; Kronholm, Harme, Hublin, Aro, & Partonen, 2006). In a comparison investigation of occupation and sleep quality between non-Hispanic/Caribbean employees and white workers, it was found that non-Hispanic/Caribbean experienced more night shift work and job strain. It has been estimated that the number of workers working a nightshift has increased (Lombardi, Folkard, Willetts, & Smith, 2010). Onsite health care programs to prevent symptoms and disease have been reported as an essential element to address potential sleep/health disturbances (Bliwise, 2008; Mathers, & Loncar, 2006; Nakata, 2011; Ng, et al., 2010). Resources about programs and practitioners addressing sleep disturbances are listed in Appendices A and B.

Sleep apnea in infants and children is another sleep issue that has reached worldwide concern. A comprehensive review of the literature with data from sources worldwide had been collected for a database for pediatrician review (Mathers & Loncar, 2006). Detecting obstructive sleep apnea in infants and children is essential to their health and maturation (Mathers & Loncar, 2006). In Taipei, researchers have identified prevalence of asthma among children using the International Study of Asthma and Allergies in Childhood core written questionnaires (WHO, 2011). The findings from this study indicated an increase in both prevalence and severity of allergic rhinitis and atopic eczema (Grunstein, 2012). Nocturnal asthma (NA) is a global problem (Stranges, et al., 2012). As a result of these conditions, sleep is fragmented, and the child suffers from excessive daytime sleepiness. To date, pediatricians typically suggest interventions such as parent detection training and prescribed medicine. Some researchers are evaluating an automated wheeze detection device (Brouillette, Horwood, Constantin, Brown & Ross, 2011).

In Switzerland, regions of high migrations have been a source of study. In these regions, as a response to divergent childhood weight and eating patterns, an intervention focused on educating and providing physical fitness and course work in good sleep and nutrition behaviors. The outcome measures of the physical fitness evaluation revealed moderate success from the intervention that resulted in better sleep quality (Jaung, Yu, Stallones & Ziang, 2009).

Additionally, traffic accidents resulting from poor sleep quality are a global concern (Sexton-Radek, 2013). In rural China, sleepy drivers have increased the rates of road traffic injuries (Dinges, 1995). Naturally, this has increased both the risk posed to children who walk to school as well as their school-related stress (Jaung, Yu, Stallones & Xiang, 2009). Another trend that poses issues for children is co-sleeping. Co-sleeping results in interrupted sleep, which causes excessive daytime sleepiness.

Assessment

Insomnia is a global sleep problem (Kronholm, et al., 2008; Ohayon, Carskadon, Guillemenault, & Vitiello, 2004; Ohayon, Roberts, Zulley, Smirne, & Priest, 2000). Though behavioral interventions have been shown to be effective (and even advantageous) over medication, their use worldwide in unknown (Sexton-Radek, 2013). Core outcome measures of behavioral interventions for insomnia such as the PSQI have strong psychometric properties and have been translated into several languages. Other traditionally-used outcome measures include sleep quality (e.g., sleep time, number of awakenings, and amount of time awake) and sleep duration as computed from sleep logs.

Treatment

In addition to cognitive behavioral therapy (the first line of treatment for insomnia), a myriad of approaches with varying levels of effectiveness exist (Baglioni, et al., 2011). Sleep hygiene instructions are common; in this approach, the patient is advised to change sleep environment and lifestyle factors (e.g., noise level, irregular bedtimes etc.) that may perturb their sleep. The appendices contain references and resources for examples of these factors and treatments of sleep disturbances. For night workers, interventions need to be conducted both individually and at the patient's worksite. Poor sleep in workers often results in reduced productivity (Baglioni et al., 2011).

Sleep specialists are highly trained professionals in the area of sleep medicine. There are board certifications at the medical doctor level and at the psychologist level. A list of sleep associations representing the sources of credentialing and training can be found in Appendix B. Specialists are trained in diagnosis, assessment, sleep study conduction and interpretation, and pharmacological and behavioral sleep treatments. With the increase in sleep disturbances, additional sleep specialists are needed to address sleep disturbance problems (Sexton-Radek, 2013.)

Investigations of the prevalence of cross-national sleep problems reflect considerable variability (Van de Staat & Bracke, 2015). A higher likelihood of sleep problems in older women was identified by Van de Staat & Bracke (2015) in a study of nineteen European countries. They also identified availability of health care as cofactors to the poor sleep outcome. Horzum et al. (2015) identified a higher level of "morningness" (peak energy level and readiness for the day in the early morning) in Turkish adolescents than in their German counterparts. The timing of a signal called "daum" (i.e., phase shift hypothesis) synchronizes the circadian rhythm and consequent day length. Interestingly, using the measurement of Twitter feeds, Gulder and Macy (2011) found seasonal circadian changes across countries despite mood variations.

Cultural Legends

Stories inform us of our legacy and our potential, and stories about sleep are no different. The American tales of Rip Van Winkle sleeping for twenty years and awakening to find his children grown address both hypersomnia as much as the meta message of paying attention to our children. Grimm's fairy tales provide a European view of sleep through the depiction of Sleeping Beauty. The culturally-based story of the sandman can be found in Asian, South American, and North American heritage – a mythical creature that induces sleep. The sandman is a popular focus of a graphic novel series as well. Hindu mythology identifies the god Vishnu on his cosmic journey, bringing forth the world as he lies on the ocean while sleeping. This implies that sleep is an opportunity for creatively examining one's existence. The Hindu text *Vedanta* presents four states of mind, three of which we experience in everyday life including Jagrat (waking), Svapna (dreaming), and Susupti (deep sleep but no dreams). The fourth is Turlya (pure consciousness). In ancient Greek mythology, Hypnos is the god of sleep and Nyx is the goddess of the night. Hypnos's mother, Morpheus, and brothers, Phobetor and Phantasos, bring dreams to people, animals, and inanimate objects. Hypnos lives in a cave on the island of Lemnos through which the river Lethe (river of forgetfulness) flows. Greek philosophers such as Democritus of Abdera and Plato both wrote about divine dreams in works that allowed for hypotheses and theory in the day.

This collection of cultural legends share a common message about the value of sleep. Sleep is an opportunity to explore one's existence, to increase one's health with a sleep interval that includes light sleep, deep sleep, and dream sleep, and to prepare oneself for the next day. In summation, the messages from the cultural legends reflect a need to attend to one's sleep.

Conclusions – What is Needed to Address Sleep Issues Worldwide

The medical literature has identified the scope of sleep disturbances globally. To date, such literature accounts for descriptions with some clinical utility. The WHO and the International Classification Diagnostic System-10 provide a reliable means by which to identify sleep disturbances; however, applications to epidemiological studies are necessary. While there are some sleep disturbance interventions at the individual level, uniform applications of empirically supported treatments (such as Cognitive Behavior Therapy) appear to be undocumented.

Furthermore, sleep problems are thought to represent unrecognized public health issues worldwide (Czeisler, 2011; Danner & Phillips, 2008; Abdel-Khalek, 2004). In low-income countries struggling with infectious diseases and poor nutrition, non-communicable diseases (to which sleep problems contribute directly), are emerging (Stranges, et al., 2012). In some countries, such as the United States, a gender difference exists – females report sleep disturbance more than males (Arber, Bote, & Meadows, 2009; Lichstein, et al., 2004).

Sleep disturbances by age group has been identified in the global sleep literature. Gradisar, Gardner, and Dohnt (2011) report the expected delay in sleepiness in Asian, North American, Australian, and European adolescents (Gibson, et al., 2012). The sleep pattern is delayed with this later onset of sleep causing difficulties for the adolescent, globally, to still wake in the morning and participate in a full day at school (Chung, Cheung, 2008). Adolescents' self-perceptions as students and workers were eroded secondary to the poor performance given the poor sleep quality (e.g., impact of Insomnia and Delayed Sleep Onset Disorder).

Additionally, there is a global trend of sleep disturbance occurring in the elderly (Byass, 2008; Foley, Ancoli-Israel, Britz & Walsh, 2003; Gureje, Oladeji, Abiona, Makanjuola & Esan, 2011). Cultural factors were identified in this systematic review of adolescent sleep patterns across the world. (Gradisar, et al., 2011).

In aggregate, studies of sleep health resources contained in this chapter have identified the need to attend to one's sleep health. Sleep health, when compromised, erodes one's overall health, and considering the rates of sleep disturbances on the global scale, global health is at risk as well.

References

Abdel-Khalek, A.M. (2004). Prevalence of reported insomnia and its consequences in a survey of 5044 adolescents in Kuwait. *Sleep, 27*, 726-731.

Arber, S., Bote, M., Meadows, R. (2009). Gender and socio-economic patterning of self-reported sleep problems in Britain. *Social Science Medicine, 68*(2), 281-289.

Baglioni, C., Battagliese, G., Feige, B., Speigelhalder, K., Nissen, C., Vonderholzer, U., Lombardo, C., Riemann, D., (2011). Insomnia as a predictor of depression: A meta-analytic evaluation of longitudinal epidemiological studies. *Journal of Affective Disorders, 135*, 10-19.

Bliwise, D.L. (2008). Invited commentary: Cross-cultural influences on sleep—broadening the environmental landscape. *American Journal of Epidemiology, 168*, 1365-1366.

Brouillette,R.T., Horwood, L., Constantin, E., Brown, K., Ross, N.A. (2011). Childhood sleep apnea and neighborhood disadvantage. *Journal of Pediatrics, 158*(5), 789-795.

Byass, P. (2008). Towards a global agenda on aging. *Global Health Action, 1*, 10.3402/gha.v1i0.1908. http://doi.org/10.3402/gha.v1i0.1908

Centers for Disease Control and Prevention (2011). Insufficient sleep is a public health problem. Retrieved from https://www.cdc.gov/features/dssleep/

Chung, K., Cheung, M. (2008). Sleep-wake patterns and sleep disturbance among Hong Kong Chinese adolescents. *Sleep, 31*, 185-194.

Czeisler, C.A. (2011). Impact of sleepiness and sleep deficiency on public health-utility of biomarkers. *Journal of Clinical Sleep Medicine, 7*, S6-8.

Danner, F., & Phillips, B. (2008). Adolescent sleep, school start times, and teen motor vehicle crashes. *Journal of Clinical Sleep Medicine, 4*, 533-535.

Dinges, D.F. (1995). An overview of sleepiness and accidents. *Journal of Sleep Research, 4*(S2), 4-14.

Ferrie, J.E., Kumari, M., Salo, P., Singh-Manoux, A. & Kivimaki, M. (2011). Sleep epidemiology – a rapidly growing field. *International Journal of Epidemiology, 40*, 1431-1437. doi:10:1093/ijehdyr203

Foley, D., Ancoli-Isreal, S., Britz, P., Walsh, J. (2003). Sleep disturbances and chronic disease in older adults: results of the 2003 National Sleep Foundation Sleep in America Survey. *Journal of Psychosomatic Research, 56*, 497-502.

Friborg, O., Bjorvath, B., Amponsah, B., & Palleson, S. (2012). Associations between variation in day length (photo period), sleep timing, sleep quality and mood: Comparison between Ghana (5o) and Norway (69o). *Journal of Sleep Research, 21*, 176-184. doi: 10.1111/j. t 365-2819.2011.00 982x.

Gibson, E.S., Powles, A.C.P., Thhabane, L. O'Brien, S., Molnar, D.S., Trajanovic, N., et al. (2006). "Sleepiness" is serious in adolescence: Two surveys of 3235 Canadian students. *Biomedical Public Health, 6*, 116-125.

Gradisar, M., Gardner, G., & Dohnt, H. (2012). Recent worldwide sleep patterns and problems during adolescence: A review and meta-analysis of age, region and sleep. *Sleep Medicine, 12*(2), 110-118.

Grunstein, R.R. (2012). Global perspectives on sleep and health issues. *Journal of National Institute of Public Health, 61*(1), 35-42.

Gulder, S.R. & Marcy, M.W. (2011). Diurnal and seasonal mood vary with work, sleep and day length across diverse cultures. *Science, 333*, 1878-1881.

Gureje, O., Oladeji, B.D., Abiona, T., Makanjuola, V., Esan, O. (2011). The natural history of insomnia in the Ibadan study of aging. *Sleep, 34*, 965-973.

Hafner, M., Stepanek, M., Taylor, J., Troxel, W.M., & Van Stolk, C. (2016). Why sleep matters—the economic costs of insufficient sleep: A cross-country comparative analysis. Retrieved from http://www.rand.org/pubs/research_reports/RR1791.html

Horzum, M.B., Randler, C., Masal,E., Besolck, S., Onder, I. & Voltner, C. (2015). Morningness – eveningness and the environment hypothesis – A cross-cultural comparison of Turkish and German adolescents. *Chronobiology International, 32*(6), 814-821.

Jaung, M.S., Yu, S. Stallones, L., Xiang, H (2009). Road traffic injuries among middle school students in a rural area of China. *Traffic Injuries Prevalence, 10*, 243-251.

Kronholm, E., Harma, M., Hublin, C., Aro, A.R., Partonen, T. (2006). Self-reported sleep duration in Finnish general population. *Journal of Sleep Research, 15*, 276-290.

Kronholm, E., Partonen, T., Laatikainen, T., et al. (2008). Trends in self-reported sleep duration and insomnia-related symptoms in Finland from 1972 to 2005: A comparative review and re-analysis of Finnish population samples. *Journal of Sleep Research, 17*, 54-62.

Lichstein, K.L., Durrrence, H.H., Riedel, B.W., Taylor D.T., & Bush, A.J. (2004). *Epidemiology of sleep: Age, gender, and ethnicity.* Mahwah, NJ: Lawrence Erlbaum Publishers.

Lombardi, D.A., Folkard, S., Willetts, J.S., Smith, G.S. (2010). Daily sleep, weekly working hours and risk of work-related injury: US national health interview survey (2004-2008). *Chronobiology International, 27*, 1013-1030.

Mathers, C., Loncar, D. (2006). Projections of global mortality and burden of disease from 2002 to 2030. *PLoS Medicine, 3*, 2011-2030.

Mucci, N., Montalti, M., Bini, C., Cupelli, V., Arcangeli, G. (2012). Evaluation of the impact of night-work on health in a population of workers in Tuscany. *Giornale Italiano di Medicina de Lavoro ed Ergonomia, 34*, 381-384.

Nakata, A. (2011). Work hours, sleep sufficiency, and prevalence of depression among full-time employees: A community-based cross-sectional study. *Journal of Clinical Psychiatry, 72*, 605-614.

Ng, N., Kowal, P., Kahn, D., et al. (2010). Health inequalities among older men and women in Africa and Asia: Evidence from eight health and demographic surveillance system sites in the INDEPTH WHO-SAGE study, *Global Health Action, 3*(10), 3402.

Ohayon, M.M., Carskadon, M.A., Guillemenault, C., Vitiello, M.V. (2004). Meta-analysis of quantitative sleep parameters from childhood to old age in healthy individuals developing normative sleep values across the human lifespan. *Sleep, 27*, 1255-1273.

Ohayon, M.M., Roberts, R.E., Zulley, J., Smirne, S., Priest, R.G. (2000). Prevalence and patterns of problematic sleep among older adolescents. *Journal of American Academy of Child and Adolescent Psychiatry*, 1549-1556.

Rajaratnam, S.M., Arendt, J. (2001). Health in a 24-h society. *Lancet, 358*, 999-1005.

Sexton-Radek, K. (2013). A look at worldwide sleep disorders. *Journal of Sleep Disorders & Therapy, 2*(3), http://dx.doi.org/10.4172/2167-0277.1000115.

Sexton-Radek, K. & Graci. G. (2009). *Combating sleep disorders.* Westport, CT: Greenwood Publishers.

Sexton-Radek, K. Pendle, R.P. Marvi, F. (2015). A global perspective of falling asleep. Poster presentation of Special Interest Group: Behavioral Sleep Medicine at Association for Behavioral and Cognitive Therapies conference, Chicago, Illinois.

Shankar, A., Charumathi, S., Kalidindi, S. (2008). Sleep duration and self-rated health: The national health interview survey. *Sleep, 34*, 1173-1177.

Stranges, S. Tigbe, W., Gomez-Olivé, F., Thorogood, M., & Kandala, N. (2012). Sleep problems: An emerging global epidemic? Findings from the INDEPTH WHO-SAGE study among more than 40,000 older adults from 8 countries across Africa and Asia. *Sleep, 35*(8), 1173-1181.

Van de Straat, V. & Bracki, P. (2015). How well does Europe sleep? A cross-national study of sleep problems in European older adults. *International Journal of Public Health, 60*, 643-650.

World Health Organization. (2011). Global status report on non-communicable disease 2010. Retrieved from www.worldcat.org

CHAPTER 6

The Role of Neuropsychological Assessment in the Global Action against Dementia

Octavio A. Santos and Caroline D. Bergeron

In 2012, dementia was identified by the World Health Organization as a threat to global health (World Health Organization, 2012). Approximately 47.5 million people worldwide suffer from dementia, with these numbers expected to triple in the next few decades (Klimova & Kuca, 2015, p. 2). While the 2015 World Alzheimer Report discusses the global impact of dementia in terms of prevalence, incidence, and costs (Alzheimer's Disease International, 2015a), it neglects the important role of formal neuropsychological assessment (NPA) in patients with suspected or known cognitive deficits for early detection, diagnosis, and treatment of mild cognitive impairment or dementia. NPAs are increasingly viewed as an integral part of the work-up of these patients. The purpose of this chapter is to summarize (1) appropriate referral situations for NPA, (2) the cognitive domains frequently examined in the NPA of neurocognitive disorders (NCDs), (3) common barriers faced by patients, caregivers, and health professionals in the utilization of NPA in NCDs, and (4) next steps needed at the individual and societal level to decrease the risks of developing dementia and take action for global health.

The Role of Neuropsychological Assessment in the Global Action against Dementia

Mild cognitive impairment (MCI) is an intermediate stage between the expected cognitive decline of normal aging and the neurodegenerative decline of dementia (Albert et al., 2011). MCI is associated with greater-than-normal, age-related changes (Albert et al., 2011). Dementia is a term grouping together a set of symptoms associated with a decline in memory or other thinking skills severe enough to reduce one's ability to perform everyday activities (Alzheimer's Association, 2016a). Neurocognitive disorders (NCDs) describe a group of clinical syndromes characterized by a loss of cognitive functions that have an impact on social, occupational, interpersonal, and/or personal functioning (American Psychiatric Association, 2013).

Dementia was identified in 2012 by the World Health Organization (2012) as a threat to global health. The risk of dementia increases with age – the prevalence of dementia doubles with every 6.3 years (Alzheimer's Disease International, 2015a, p. 32). Approximately 47.5 million people worldwide suffer from dementia, with these numbers expected to triple in the next few decades (Klimova & Kuca, 2015, p. 2). Every 3.2 seconds, someone in the world develops dementia (Alzheimer's Disease International, 2015a, p. 33). Older women suffer the greater burden of dementia because they typically live longer than men (National Institute on Aging, 2012). In certain regions of the world, including East and South Asia, Western Europe, Latin America and the Caribbean, the prevalence of dementia for men is close to 30% lower than for women (Alzheimer's Disease International, 2015a, p. 18). It is estimated that 58% of people with dementia currently live in low or middle income countries, which are also expected to have the largest increase in incidence and prevalence of dementia by 2050 (Alzheimer's Disease International, 2015a, p. 22). Despite these numbers, low- to middle-income countries also have limited resources for dementia diagnosis and treatment (Maestre, 2012), such as a shortage of primary care physicians with dementia training and of neuropsychological services (Mathew & Mathuranath, 2008; Patel & Prince, 2001).

This shortage of trained professionals in the global action against dementia may explain why the 2015 World Alzheimer Report (2015a) neglected to mention the important role of neuropsychological assessment (NPA) in detecting, diagnosing, and treating MCI or dementia. However, NPA is uniquely able to discriminate normal aging from the presence of NCDs. NPA is also increasingly viewed as an integral and valuable part of the work-up of patients with suspected cognitive decline. Specifically, NPA can help to determine whether there is a functional or organic cause to the symptoms that may potentially be reversible, localize brain lesions, define patients' cognitive strengths and weaknesses, identify targets for rehabilitation, and monitor treatment response (Elamin, Bak, Doherty, Pender, & Abrahams, 2016; Scott, Ostermeyer, & Shah, 2016). Early dementia detection and diagnosis via NPA can allow patients and their caregivers to access earlier treatments, build a care team, and participate in support services. This can result in significant improvements in patients' quality of care and quality of life (Alzheimer's Association, 2015).

The purpose of this chapter is to raise awareness of NPA and to encourage its increased use in the global, long-term fight against dementia. Specifically, this chapter aims to (1) summarize appropriate referral situations, (2) describe accepted cognitive domains frequently examined in the NPA of NCDs, (3) list common barriers faced by patients, caregivers, and health professionals in the utilization of NPA in NCDs, and (4) discuss next steps needed at the individual and societal level to decrease the risks of developing dementia and take action for global health.

Referring a Patient for Neuropsychological Assessment

Referring patients in the early stages of an NCD is more likely to yield disease-specific cognitive profiles and earlier interventions. Common reasons for referral for NPA include difficulties with memory, expressive/receptive language, visuospatial awareness, decision-making, and attention/concentration as well as changes in behavior/personality and deterioration in functioning (e.g., performing at work, managing finances/medications, driving, etc.) (Attix & Welsh-Bohmer, 2013; Elamin et al., 2016). Referral eligibility can also be determined from a cognitive standpoint for certain medical procedures and postsurgical outcomes, such as transplant candidacy (Mooney et al., 2007), epilepsy and brain tumor surgery (Duffau, 2011), and deep brain stimulation (Witt et al., 2008) among others.

Temple, Carvalho, and Tremont (2006) found that North American physicians most frequently referred for NPA to establish or confirm a diagnosis. Patients are referred for diagnostic clarification to elucidate whether cognitive symptoms and functional impairment are associated with pseudodementia (i.e., depression), Alzheimer's disease (AD), or a less common form of dementia (e.g., frontotemporal dementia [FTD], Huntington's disease [HD], etc.) and to establish a baseline of cognitive/emotional functioning. In other words, NPA can assist in discriminating the contributions of neurologic and emotional factors in the patient's presenting complaints. Referral sources may also want to document whether cognitive deficits are present, particularly in conditions where deficits are relatively common (e.g., Parkinson's disease [PD]), and/or to document disease progression or treatment response in patients with a known cognitive impairment (Attix & Welsh-Bohmer, 2013; Elamin et al., 2016; Scott et al., 2016).

Referrals for NPA may also be made based on lower-than-expected scores on cognitive screenings, such as the Mini-Mental State Examination (MMSE) (Folstein, Folstein, & McHugh, 1975) and the Montreal Cognitive Assessment (MoCA) (Nasreddine et al., 2005). Compared to the MMSE, the MoCA has a higher sensitivity in distinguishing cognitively normal individuals from patients with AD, MCI, PD with dementia, HD, and FTD, but also variable specificity in distinguishing dementia patients from controls (Damian et al., 2011; Freitas, Simões, Alves, Duro, & Santana, 2012; Hoops et al., 2009; Nasreddine et al., 2005; Videnovic et al., 2010). The MoCA is also freely accessible online at www.mocatest.org. Both the MMSE and the MoCA have been translated into several languages and have age- and education-corrected norms (e.g., Crum, Anthony, Bassett, & Folstein, 1993; Malek-Ahmadi et al., 2015; Rossetti, Lacritz, Cullum, & Weiner, 2011) that clinicians are encouraged to use to better determine the presence of cognitive impairment that may warrant NPA.

Neuropsychological Assessment (NPA)

NPA employs both quantitative and qualitative methods to evaluate premorbid, cognitive, behavioral, and emotional functioning in order to identify subtle deficits early in the course of NCDs. NPA has been used for assisting with differential diagnosis, determining functional capacity, assessing pre- or post-treatment change, and providing recommendations. NPA enables documenting the presence and degree of cognitive deficits based on standardized tests with normative data (i.e., a method of test administration, scoring, and interpretation resulting in reproducible, valid, and reliable results). NPA also contributes to determine the expected course of the disease and extrapolation to patient management needs, while providing recommendations to assist with maximizing care and functioning (Attix & Welsh-Bohmer, 2013; Elamin et al., 2016; Schoenberg & Scott, 2011; Scott et al., 2016).

NPA has become increasingly complex and generally requires specialized training in clinical neuropsychology (CNP) (Scott et al., 2016). For example, in the United States (U.S.), neuropsychologists are required to obtain doctoral, internship, and postdoctoral training in CNP according to the Houston Conference Guidelines (Bodin, Butts, & Grote, 2016; Hannay et al., 1998). Neuropsychologists are also required to become licensed to practice psychology in their state and are increasingly expected to become board certified in CNP (Grote, Butts, & Bodin, 2016). However, CNP is less regulated in other countries as evidenced by the variability in required training among other professional challenges (e.g., Chan, Sze, Cheung, & Han, 2016; Chan, Wang, Wang, & Cheung, 2016; Egeland et al., 2016; Fernandez, Ferreres, Morlett-Paredes, Rivera, & Arango-Lasprilla, 2016; Hokkanen, Nybo, & Poutiainen, 2016; Janzen & Guger, 2016; Kim & Chey, 2016; Kumar, 2010; Olabarrieta-Landa et al., 2016; Ostrosky Shejet, & Velez Garcia, 2016; Ponsford, 2016; Sakamoto, 2016; Vakil & Hoofien, 2016; Watts & Shuttleworth-Edwards, 2016).

NPA is usually composed of a clinical interview, behavioral observations, neurobehavioral exam, and standardized neuropsychological testing. The initial interview serves to gather patients' background information and insight into their cognitive problems. Specifically, information on the patient's demographics, acculturation and language preference (if applicable), and educational, occupational, medical, neurological, and psychiatric histories is collected to answer the referral question and tailor the evaluation accordingly (e.g., accommodation to physical disabilities, use of certified interpreters, etc.). Given that patients can have limited insight into their deficits, it is recommended, whenever possible, to interview an informant (e.g., a family member) after obtaining the patient's consent to corroborate or gather more information on the course of the presenting cognitive/behavioral complaints (i.e., duration, scope, and severity of problems), as well as on basic and instrumental activities of daily living (e.g., bathing, grooming, cooking, managing medications). Behavioral observations and qualitative assessment provide valuable information about the patient's expressive/receptive speech, sensory/motor functioning (e.g., arousal, visual acuity and fields integrity, cranial nerve functioning, gait, balance, reflexes, etc.), self-care/hygiene, and mood/affect. It also informs about the presence of attentional difficulties, perseveration, disinhibition, or impulsivity. Certain conditions that may affect the patient's ability to cooperate may include secondary gain, severe physical illness, and active psychiatric difficulties (e.g., psychosis or delirium) (Attix & Welsh-Bohmer, 2013; Elamin et al., 2016; Fujii, 2017; Lezak et al., 2012; Parsons & Hammeke, 2014; Schoenberg & Scott, 2011; Scott et al., 2016).

NPA often includes tests that rely on one's knowledge base and are resilient to neurological insult (i.e., "hold measures") to quantitatively estimate a decline from previous level of premorbid functioning. Common hold measures include the Test of Premorbid Functioning (TOFP) (Psychological Corporation, 2009) as well as Vocabulary and Information from the Wechsler Adult Intelligence Scale-Fourth Edition (WAIS-IV) (Wechsler, 2014), with the caveat that these tests are highly sensitive to English language level, cultural background, and education. In addition to premorbid functioning measures, NPA includes psychopathology, personality, and embedded and stand-alone symptom/performance validity measures (S/PVTs). These measures are routinely administered and considered when interpreting a patient's overall cognitive performance and ruling out psychiatric conditions or poor task engagement. Regarding the latter, most PVTs are based on the assumption that patients with significant deficits can successfully pass these tests, and that scores below or above established cut-offs indicate invalid performance. Commonly used self-report measures include the Geriatric Depression Scale (GDS) (Yesavage et al., 1983) and the Geriatric Anxiety Scale (GAS) (Segal et al., 2010). Frequently used SPVTs include the Minnesota Multiphasic Personality

Inventory–2 Restructured Form (MMPI-2-RF) (Ben-Porath & Tellegen, 2008/2011), the WAIS-IV Reliable Digit Span (Schroeder, Twumasi-Ankrah, Baade, & Marshall, 2012), the Test of Memory and Malingering (TOMM) (Tombaugh, 1996), and the Word Memory Test (WMT) (Green, Allen, & Astner, 1997).

NPA also involves a brief or comprehensive evaluation of multiple cognitive domains, including sensory-motor, perceptual/visuospatial, processing speed, attention/concentration, language, memory, executive, emotional and behavioral functioning (Attix & Welsh-Bohmer, 2013; Elamin et al., 2016; Lezak et al., 2012; Parsons & Hammeke, 2014; Schoenberg & Scott, 2011; Scott et al., 2016; Siri, Benaglio, Frigerio, Binetti, & Cappa, 2001). The patient's performance on neuropsychological measures is compared against both estimated premorbid functioning and group normative data. The latter is based on cognitively normal individuals or samples with specific neurologic/psychiatric conditions. Given that test performance is affected by many factors (e.g., age, quantity/quality of education, language proficiency, acculturation, etc.), validated tests with appropriate norms are fundamental for accurate test interpretation, diagnosis, and treatment recommendations; otherwise, limited or erroneous conclusions can be drawn (Elamin et al., 2016; Fujii, 2017; Lezak et al., 2012; Mitrushina et al., 2005; Parsons & Hammeke, 2014; Schoenberg & Scott, 2011; Scott et al., 2016; Strauss et al., 2006). Age- and/or education-corrected norms for common neuropsychological tests are available in the U.S., Western European, and some Latin American countries (Fujii, 2017). The following are important considerations when determining the psychometric properties of tests and the strength of evidence for cross-cultural validity: study design, sampling selection, size and demographics, and adequacy of outcome measures and statistical analysis (Fujii, 2017).

In addition to statistical comparison of the patient's test performance, data interpretation is conducted in an integrated way by examining a hierarchy of functions and localization/lateralization of cognitive/sensory-motor functioning. That is, failure at basic cognitive/sensory-motor skills makes the interpretation of higher cognitive order skills less definite. Also, localizing/lateralizing prediction decreases as skills get more complex. For example, language comprehension is a prerequisite for accurate interpretation of attention/memory tests and is also highly lateralized in the left hemisphere for most right-handers, while abstraction/problem solving do not localize/lateralize well. Data are also interpreted in reference to a pathognomonic symptom (i.e., loss of a previously acquired skill or the failure to normally develop a universal skill within a given time), and to statistically expected performance between skills within a person and relative to a normative group for patterns consistent with varying NCDs (Lezak et al., 2012; Parsons & Hammeke, 2014; Schoenberg & Scott, 2011;

Scott et al., 2016; Strauss et al., 2006).

Cognitive Domains Examined in Neuropsychological Assessment

The major cognitive domains frequently evaluated during NPA for the most common forms of NCDs are briefly discussed next along with their main components, neural substrates, tests frequently used, and examples illustrating the clinical relevance of testing that domain. Although the domains and measures are categorized for illustrational and organizational purposes, there is significant overlap between them.

Sensorimotor and Perceptual/Visuospatial Functioning

Sensorimotor testing evaluates basic sensory (visual, auditory, and tactile) thresholds and integrity (Lezak et al., 2012; Parsons & Hammeke, 2014; Schoenberg & Scott, 2011; Scott et al., 2016; Strauss et al., 2006). It also assesses manual strength, fine motor speed, and manual dexterity to determine the presence of lateralized hand discrepancy. Commonly used measures to assess motor skills include the Hand Dynamometer (Dodrill, 1978), the Finger Tapping Test (Reitan & Wolfson, 1989), and the Grooved Pegboard Test (Roy & Square, 1994). Tactual functioning is generally assessed by asking the patient to identify numbers/letters drawn on the palm of each hand or on the tip of each finger with closed eyes, or to identify drawn shapes/objects using the Tactile Form Recognition Test (Benton, 1994). Auditory discrimination is assessed by producing highly similar rhythmic patterns or speech sounds played on a recording (Reitan & Wolfson, 1985, 1989). Overall, sensory and motor functions are evaluated qualitatively for pathognomonic signs (Scott et al., 2016).

Regarding perceptual and visuospatial functioning, interpretation of deficits is generally based on the two (ventral and dorsal) stream hypothesis. The ventral stream (i.e., the "what pathway") ends in the temporal lobe and is involved in object recognition. Damage to the ventral stream is usually due to bilateral temporal or fusiform lesions, leading to the inability to visually recognize objects (agnosia), colors (acromatosia), and/or faces (prosopagnosia). The dorsal stream (i.e., the "where pathway") projects to the parietal lobe and is involved in processing where an object is in space and guiding/perceiving actions. Damage to the dorsal stream is often due to bilateral superior parieto-occipital region, leading to difficulty perceiving moving objects (akinetopsia), lack of awareness of things or body parts in one hemifield (hemispatial neglect), and Balint's syndrome. The latter is characterized by the inability to perceive more than one component of a scene or object simultaneously (simultanagnosia), guide movement visually (visual optic ataxia), direct one's gaze to a visual stimulus/target (ocular apraxia), and may also include other symptoms, such as searching for a target by moving one's head and functional blindness in severe cases

(Elamin et al., 2016; Lezak et al., 2012; Parsons & Hammeke, 2014; Schoenberg & Scott, 2011; Scott et al., 2016; Strauss et al., 2006).

Posterior cortical atrophy (PCA; also called posterior/visual variant of AD) involves significant visuospatial perception deficits and is associated with occipito-parietal compromise (Nestor, Caine, Fryer, Clarke, & Hodges, 2003). Common symptoms include problems with reading, driving or parking, and walking in the presence of uneven or patterned ground, stairs, sidewalk borders, or escalators due to impaired depth or form perception. However, classical AD and atypical Parkinsonian syndromes, particularly Dementia with Lewy Bodies (DLB) and Corticobasal Degeneration (CBD), also show decline in visuospatial skills. Tasks to test visuospatial skills often include replication of complex drawing, judgment of angles, and reading disintegrating letters. Commonly used tests of perceptual/visuospatial functioning include the Judgment of Line Orientation Test (Benton, Hamsher, Varney, & Spreen, 1983), the Rey Osterrieth Complex Figure (Meyers & Meyers, 1995), and the Hooper Visual Organization test (Hooper, 1983). However, drawing tests can be confounded by motor disability and by poor organizational skills due to dysexecutive deficits (Elamin et al., 2016).

Apart from intact motor and sensory systems, carrying out complex motor actions (praxis) requires at least two processes: (1) accessing semantic knowledge on how to perform a specific task and its required objects and (2) accessing a previously acquired "action plan." Praxis and egocentric/allocentric right-left orientation are generally assessed. Neuroanatomically, the left frontal premotor and fronto-parietal cortex is associated with the storage of action plans, while the primary motor cortex along with the cerebellum and basal ganglia are associated with their execution. Apraxia is a difficulty with motor planning to perform a task or execute movements upon command despite intact language comprehension and sensorimotor skills. Apraxia is frequently seen in NCDs, particularly CBD as well as mid to late stages of AD and primary progressive aphasia (PPA) (Attix & Welsh-Bohmer, 2013; Elamin et al., 2016; Parsons & Hammeke, 2014; Schoenberg & Scott, 2011; Scott et al., 2016). The two most common types of apraxia are ideational apraxia and ideomotor apraxia.

Ideational apraxia is the inability to access the semantic knowledge related to the action and can be subdivided into conceptual and sequencing apraxia. Conceptual apraxia is commonly observed in AD and may involve difficulty producing an action upon command, imitating the examiner, identifying an action when presented with multiple choices or a situation that needs intervention, and selecting the appropriate tool for a specific action (e.g. using a hammer to cut paper) despite intact naming skills. Sequencing apraxia involves difficulty conducting an action in the appropriate sequence. It is associated with left occipito-parietal cortex and tested by asking the patient to perform a multi-step action (e.g., making a sandwich) (Attix & Welsh-Bohmer, 2013; Elamin et al., 2016; Schoenberg & Scott, 2011).

Ideomotor apraxia refers to impaired activation of an action plan and is often associated with lesions in the left frontal premotor and parietal cortex. These patients are unable to perform the action either on command or imitation, but can identify a situation requiring an action or performed by the examiner and choose the appropriate tool. Specific motor errors may include inaccurate timing/tempo of an action, using the wrong part of the body or a body part as a tool (e.g. using a finger as a toothbrush), and incorrectly aligning the limbs in space or moving the limbs or tool inappropriately in the spatial plane. Both ideational and ideomotor apraxia are commonly observed in corticobasal degeneration (CBD), with initial deficits usually confined to one hand (Attix & Welsh-Bohmer, 2013; Elamin et al., 2016; Schoenberg & Scott, 2011), but are also seen in other NCDs.

Processing Speed and Attention/Concentration

Processing speed (PS) is a measure of cognitive efficiency in processing information and is closely associated with attention and working memory. PS is typically assessed directly using reaction time (RT) or timed tasks (e.g., Continuous Performance Test [CPT], which requires pressing the space bar when an "X" is shown on the screen or not pressing it if any other letters are presented; Conners et al., 2000) or indirectly using speeded attentional and verbal fluency tasks described below. PS has limited lateralizing/localizing value and can be negatively impacted by lesions or degenerative conditions throughout the brain. Despite that, impaired PS is commonly seen in PD and HD, but can also be confounded by motor deficits (Elamin et al., Scott et al., 2016).

Attentional processes are assessed on a continuum from simple attention to rapid alternation and sustained attention. Simple attention is frequently evaluated using the WAIS-IV Digit Span Forward subtest in which the patient is asked to repeat a string of numbers in order. Sustained attention, or vigilant readiness to respond, is also commonly assessed with the CPT's omission errors (i.e., failure to press the spacebar when the "X" appears) and associated with right noradrenergic connections of the locus coeruleus, right prefrontal cortex, and right parietal lobe (Parasuraman, Warm, & See, 1998). Rapid alternation and redirection of attentional focus are typically assessed with coding transposition or symbol substitution tasks, such as the Symbol Digits Modalities Test (Smith, 1982) and the WAIS-IV Symbol Digit subtest (Elamin et al., Scott et al., 2016).

Language Skills

Language is a complex domain with identified networks, including Broca's and Wernicke's area as well as the supramarginal and angular gyri. Language difficulties are the most salient symptoms in patients with PPA, but can also occur in other NCDs, including AD, CBD, and progressive supranuclear palsy (PSP). The most commonly observed language problems include inability to: name objects while knowing what they are (anomia) that usually extends to both speech and writing; express, repeat, and/or comprehend language (aphasia); and read (alexia) or write (agraphia) (Attix & Welsh-Bohmer, 2013; Elamin et al., 2016; Parsons & Hammeke, 2014; Schoenberg & Scott, 2011; Scott et al., 2016).

In contrast with aphasia observed after stroke, the impairment in the language network associated with NCDs is gradual and progressive (Mesulam et al., 2014), involving a selective loss of cortical neurons that leads to more complex and subtle dissociations. For example, the term "discourse" refers to the process of conveying meaning concisely and accurately, including speech content and non-verbal cues (e.g., prosody, facial expressions, and gestures). Effective discourse is primarily dependent on the right hemisphere, damage to which can cause vague speech and poor expression/comprehension of non-verbal clues (Elamin et al., 2016). Dysfunctional discourse is commonly seen in the behavioral variant frontotemporal dementia (bvFTD) due to widespread right hemispheric involvement (Pakhomov et al., 2010).

Naming is a commonly assessed language component within NPA, given that difficulties in naming and word retrieval are pervasive across several NCDs. Specifically, anomia is often the presenting feature of PPA, but it can also be observed in AD and other NCDs affecting the posterior temporal areas. PPA is often classified under the umbrella of FTD and has three clinical variants: Agrammatic/non-fluent (nfvPPA), logopenic (lvPPA), and semantic (svPPA). Similar to Broca's aphasia, impaired speech fluency and grammar are the hallmarks of nfvPPA. Specifically, nfvPPA usually involves effortful, halting speech, speech apraxia (i.e., inability to translate conscious speech plans into motor plans), distorted word order, omissions of articles and propositions, poor use of pronouns, impaired repetition and comprehension of grammatically/syntactically complex sentences, and loss of normal prosody. It is associated with changes in left posterior fronto-insular region, including inferior frontal gyrus, insula, premotor and supplementary motor areas. Anomia is often the most salient and disabling feature of lvPPA, but it also includes poor repetition and speech fluency (due to impaired word retrieval) as well as comprehension and repetition of long unfamiliar sentences (likely due to phonological working memory impairment); however, grammar is usually intact. LvPPA is associated with changes in the left posterior perisylvian tempero-parietal regions, including posterior temporal, supramarginal, and angular gyri. Finally, patients with svPPA have naming difficulties due to impaired access to semantic knowledge, replacing low-frequency nouns with high-frequency nouns (e.g. "dog" for "boar") and using supra-ordinate categories (e.g. "animal" for "cow"). These patients often suffer from surface alexia (i.e., difficulty reading irregular words) and, although they may understand complex abstract concepts (e.g., is justice more important than mercy?), they have difficulty understanding simpler questions that depend on semantic knowledge of common objects (e.g., do people ride pineapples to get to work?). In svPPA, neuroimaging shows abnormalities in both anterio-lateral temporal lobes, generally left greater than right (Elamin et al., 2016; Gorno-Tempini, 2011; Mesulam, 2001; Scott et al., 2016). Commonly used test to measure language skills are the Boston Diagnostic Aphasia Examination (Kaplan, 1983), the Token Test (De Renzi & Vignolo, 1962), and the Boston Naming Test (Kaplan, Goodglass, & Weintraub, 2001).

Memory Skills

Although decline in memory is the hallmark of AD, memory deficits may also be observed in other NCDs (e.g., bvFTD, PD, and HD), and their cognitive underpinnings may differ. First, it is important to know that multiple memory systems are used to carry out daily activities. Such systems can be broadly classified as short-term memory (STM) and long-term memory (LTM). STM, also called working memory, is responsible for temporary storage and manipulation of information for seconds, and is closely linked to attention and executive functions described below. Contrarily, information can be stored for long periods of time in LTM, which can be divided into non-declarative memory and declarative memory (Attix & Welsh-Bohmer, 2013; Beaumont, 2008; Elamin et al., 2016; Schoenberg & Scott, 2011; Scott et al., 2016).

Non-declarative or procedural memory involves implicit and unconscious learning/recall (e.g., riding a bicycle) and is closely linked to the supplementary motor cortex, cerebellum, and basal ganglia. Patients with PD or HD generally have damage to these structures, leading to impaired acquisition of new procedural learning. Contrarily, declarative memory involves conscious recollection of facts/events and can be further subdivided into semantic and episodic memory. Semantic memory is involved in retaining facts about the world and is closely related to language processing, such that deficits in semantic memory usually present as language difficulties. Both anterior-lateral temporal lobes play a key role in semantic memory (Attix & Welsh-Bohmer, 2013; Elamin et al., 2016; Scott et al., 2016).

Episodic memory stores personally experienced events within a specific time and place. It involves registration, encoding, consolidating, and retrieval of that information. Episodic memory is assessed by having the patient recall previously presented lists of words, stories, or figures. Commonly used memory tests include the Wechsler Memory Scale (WMS-IV; Wechsler, 2014), the California Verbal Learning Test (Delis, Kramer, Kaplan, & Ober, 2000), the Rey Auditory Verbal Learning (Rey, 1964), and the Rey Osterrieth Complex Figure (Meyers & Meyers, 1995). Neuroanatomically, episodic memory involves the medial temporal lobe, particularly the hippocampus and the extra hippocampal regions (perirhinal, entorhinal, parahippocampal cortices), frontostriatal regions (including the basal ganglia and frontal lobes), and the Papez circuit (Papez, 1937), which starts and ends in the hippocampus and includes the fornix, mammillary bodies, mammillothalamic tract, anterior thalamic nucleus, cingulum, and entorhinal cortex. Thus, damage to the temporal lobes or structures of the Papez circuit impairs the ability to retain new memories, as evidenced by patients with amnesia after bilateral medial temporal lobotomy (e.g., famous case of HM; Scoville & Milner, 1957), Korsakoff's syndrome involving mammillary body damage, and thalamic stroke (Elamin et al., 2016; Schoenberg & Scott, 2011; Scott et al., 2016).

Distinctions between the types of information to be remembered, the mode of recollection, and when the information was acquired may also provide clues on lesion location. For instance, left and right temporal lobe damage are typically associated with verbal and non-verbal/visuospatial memory impairments, respectively. Also, recollection of specific contextual information is dependent on retrieval processes and strategic search associated with the parahippocampal cortex. However, recognition memory can also depend on familiarity judgement associated with the perirhinal cortex – that is, information recognized without retrieval of specific contextual details (e.g. "I think I've seen that woman before, but don't remember where") (Daselaar, Fleck, & Cabeza, 2006; Haskins, Yonelinas, Quamme, & Ranganath, 2008).

To assess associative memory, patients are often asked to recall lists of semantically unrelated word pairs (e.g., whale and corn). Impairment on these tasks, with relative sparing of item memory and familiarity, is typically seen after focal hippocampal pathology and may be found early in AD when older memories show less degradation than recent memories. Contrarily, PD and HD often present with a flat temporal gradient. Additionally, patients with frontal lobe lesions may have significant episodic memory difficulties, particularly in retrieval, that often improve with category (e.g., a type of color) or context clues or multiple choice cueing during recognition tasks. This distinction is often helpful when differentiating bvFTD and AD, given that bvFTD patients generally perform better in cued and recognition memory tasks. Of note, this improvement in performance following cueing can also be seen in pseudodementia (Kang et al., 2014) and NCDs, including subcortical vascular dementia (Grober, Hall, Sanders, & Lipton, 2008) and PD (Emre, 2003), which implies that the new information was stored, but not readily accessed. Also, better performance with cueing can be adversely influenced by repeating a response in the absence/cessation of a stimulus (perseverations) and a tendency towards "yes" responses (response biases) (Attix & Welsh-Bohmer, 2013; Beaumont, 2008; Elamin et al., 2016; Schoenberg & Scott, 2011; Scott et al., 2016).

Executive Functions

Executive functions (EFs) are a heterogeneous group of higher order cognitive processes that represent functional capacities with real-world implications, including problem-solving, planning, goal-directed behavior, abstract thinking, concept formation, error monitoring, sustain/selective attention, inhibition of unwanted responses/impulses, sequencing, mental flexibility, and set-shifting. For instance, anticipating medication refills during a future trip requires planning, deductively reasoning the impending shortage of medication, and considering options when faced with potential problems (e.g., losing medications, staying longer than expected, etc.). EFs rely on both frontal and non-frontal lobe structures. A brain network that play a critical role in multiple cognitive EFs is the dorsolateral frontal sub-cortical circuit, which projects to and from the dorsolateral prefrontal cortex (DLPFC) and includes the dorsolateral head of the caudate nucleus, globus pallidus, and ventro-anterior and medio-dorsal thalamic nuclei. Dysexecutive deficits can display significant difficulties in instrumental activities of daily living and are typical features of both bvFTD and amyotrophic lateral sclerosis (ALS) (Attix & Welsh-Bohmer, 2013; Beaumont, 2008; Elamin et al., 2016; Goldstein & McNeil, 2013; Horton & Wedding, 2008; Lezak et al., 2012; Parsons & Hammeke, 2014; Strauss et al., 2006; Schoenberg & Scott, 2011; Scott et al., 2016).

The inability to inhibit unwanted responses/impulses can lead to impulsivity, perseveration, imitating other people's speech (echolalia) or action (echopraxia), and spontaneously picking up objects and using them (utilization behavior). The Stroop Color Word Test (Stroop, 1935) is a commonly used task to assess inhibitory control in which the patient has to name a colored word instead of reading it, and is associated with anterior cingulate, insula, premotor and inferior frontal regions (Leung, Skudlarski, Gatenby, Peterson, & Gore, 2000). The ability to rapidly generate responses (energization) is typically tested using verbal fluency tasks in which the patient is asked to rapidly generate words using either phonemic cues (e.g. words starting with the letter "S") or semantic cues (e.g., animal names) (Stuss, 2011). Overall, patients with frontal lobe lesions produce fewer correct words and make more errors. Phonemic fluency is associated with the left DLPFC and anterior cingulate, whereas semantic fluency is more associated with temporal lobe functions (Elamin et al., 2016).

Monitoring and updating are also heavily reliant on attention and working memory (WM). WM is essential for understanding and tracking information over time (e.g., doing simple mental calculations). A widely accepted model of WM proposes a "central executive" that supervises two slave systems whose function is to store and manipulate information for brief periods of time: the phonological loop and the visuospatial sketchpad (Baddley, 1986). The former stores and rehearses verbal material and is associated with the left perisylvian region, whereas the latter serves to store and manipulate images and is associated with the right inferior prefrontal and parietal cortex. Tasks used to assess these functions include the WAIS-IV Digit Span Backward and Arithmetic subtests (Elamin et al., 2016; Scott et al., 2016).

Planning involves identifying and organizing the steps required to successfully achieve a goal (i.e., strategy formation). Cognitive flexibility (CF) allows to change a strategy to accommodate new demands to changing environments or because of an unwanted outcome. CF is a critical requirement for problem-solving and is closely linked to creativity and to the ability to shift sets/tasks; thus, impairments in CF leads to mental rigidity. Planning, CF, and set-shifting are associated with the DLPFC and are generally assessed using sorting and sequencing tasks, such as the Wisconsin Card Sorting Test (Heaton, Chelune, Talley, Kay, & Curtiss, 1993), the Tower of London (Shallice, 1982), and the Trail Making Test (Reitan, 1992).

Verbal and nonverbal abstraction and reasoning are typically assessed with novel tasks that require convergent/divergent abstract reasoning, hypothesis testing, and sequencing skills. Deductive reasoning tests assess the ability to reason logically, often involve a transitive inference task, and may include meaningful/familiar or non-specific/unfamiliar situations (Goel, 2007). Reasoning about meaningful and familiar situations is thought to rely on background knowledge/beliefs (i.e., semantic knowledge) and is linked to the frontal-temporal lobes, particularly the left temporal lobe. Reasoning about non-specific, unfamiliar situations where semantic knowledge is not useful is associated with a parietal system and involves visuospatial imagery. Both types of reasoning share links to the basal ganglia, cerebellum, fusiform gyri, and frontal lobes. Tasks of abstract conceptualization also evaluate the ability to work out new concepts and abstract ideas and usually involve the recognition of patterns/similarities between shapes and figures. Metaphorical thinking is often tested using proverb comprehension. Overall, impaired deductive reasoning, abstract conceptualization, and literal interpretation of metaphors are typically observed in patients with bvFTD, particularly using deductive reasoning tasks involving familiar situations compared to similar tasks involving unfamiliar environments (Elamin et al., 2016).

Emotional and Behavioral Functioning

NCDs are generally accompanied by behavioral/personality changes. Frequently reported changes include apathy, impulsivity, risk-taking and/or obsessive-compulsive behavior, lack of empathy and insight, mental rigidity, irritability, disinhibition, social misconduct, and emotional dysregulation. These changes have been linked to frontal lobe and right hemispheric involvement, and their severity and pattern relative to any co-existing cognitive abnormalities offer clues to the potential underlying NCD. Although changes in behavior/personality are the defining feature of bvFTD, which may occur despite intact or slightly lower than expected cognitive performance on neuropsychological tests, these changes may also be present in PPA, ALS without co-morbid dementia, AD, and HD. Bilateral lesions along the cortico-bulbar tract can produce spontaneous episodes of crying or laughing (i.e., pseudo-bulbar affect). Patients may also have emotional reactions to having a neurologic condition and develop reactive emotional disorders or have exacerbations of prior psychopathology (Attix & Welsh-Bohmer, 2013; Beaumont, 2008; Elamin et al., 2016; Goldstein & McNeil, 2013; Horton & Wedding, 2008; Lezak et al., 2012; Parsons & Hammeke, 2014; Schoenberg & Scott, 2011; Scott et al., 2016; Strauss et al., 2006).

Behavioral/personality changes often cause significant strain on family and caregivers, and are a more reliable predictor of caregiver burden than physical disability or cognitive impairment (van der Lee, Bakker, Duivenvoorden, & Dröes, 2014). Although standard neuropsychological tests do not tap into these behavioral/personality changes, the latter are typically assessed though direct observation of the patient, interviews with an informant, collateral report and, to a lesser extent, neurobehaviorally. Information on emotional functioning and behavioral/personality change can also be obtained using self-reported measures, such as the GDS, GAI, MMPI-2-RF, and the Frontal Systems Behavior Scale (Grace & Molloy, 2001). Of note, accurate documentation of behavioral/personality changes may be confounded by the patient's premorbid personality, level of insight, and cultural background as well as by informant characteristics.

As discussed, NPA is a complex process that involves a good understanding of NCDs, various cognitive domains, and a broad range of neuropsychological tests administered to assess cognitive deficits. NPA is also crucial in the early identification and intervention of dementia. However, several barriers prevent the full use of NPA around the world. Some of these barriers are discussed next.

Common Barriers in Using Neuropsychological Services
for Dementia Assessment

Detecting and diagnosing dementia can significantly outweigh the costs of the diagnosis and may also result in long-term savings. In fact, in high-income countries, the estimated cost for one person with dementia is $36,669 USD (Alzheimer's Disease International, 2015a, p. 63), while the estimated cost for a dementia diagnosis is approximately $5,000 USD (Alzheimer's Disease International, 2011, p. 5). Investments in early diagnosis can ultimately lead to savings of approximately $10,000 USD per person with dementia, for example, by delaying institutionalization (Alzheimer's Disease International, 2011, p. 5). While these costs are significant and important to consider, other barriers prevent patients with suspected NCDs, caregivers, and health professionals from using NPA.

Barriers Faced by Patients

Both cognitive and structural barriers may impact patients' use of NPA. Regarding cognitive barriers, patients may have limited knowledge of dementia and may believe that memory loss is a normal part of aging (Alzheimer's Association, 2014). Patients may have little knowledge about the role of NPA in the diagnosis and treatment of dementia (Shaaf, Stevens, Holcomb, Smith, Artman, & Kreutzer, n.d.). Patients may also think that they do not need NPA or may be afraid of the results or stigma associated with being diagnosed with an NCD (Bamford, Lamont, Eccles, Robinson, May, & Bond, 2004; Bunn et al., 2012). Indeed, the diagnosis of dementia can have a major impact on the patient's identity, roles, and relationships in addition to leading to feelings of denial, loss, anger, fear, or frustration. These reasons may likely account for why patients would delay or refuse to undergo NPA if available (Aminzadeh, Byszewski, Molnar, Eisner, 2007; Bunn et al., 2012; Vernooij-Dassen et al., 2005). Among key structural barriers, lack of awareness, accessibility, and health insurance may prevent patients from using NPA. For example, patients may be unaware of existing neuropsychological services in their community and, therefore, may not reach out for help when experiencing memory loss or other cognitive deficits. It is also possible that such services may simply not be available in the patients' area, may involve waiting for several months to consult a specialist, and require health insurance or cover co-pays, which can significantly limit access.

Barriers Faced by Caregivers

Most caregivers, including family members and friends, agree that obtaining a diagnosis helps to finally know what is "wrong" with the patient (Alzheimer's Association, 2012). While caregivers may play a key role in the diagnosis and management of dementia, they may face several barriers to using neuropsychological services for diagnosis and treatment of NCDs. Similar to patients, caregivers may lack an understanding of the role of NPA in diagnosing and helping to better manage the disease and prepare for future cognitive decline. They may also lack time or resources to bring the patient for NPA. If interviewing during NPA, caregivers may not report relevant information on the patient's symptoms due, among other reasons, to being in denial or lack of frequent contact with the patient. A diagnosis of dementia has important implications for caregivers and may bring about a change in identity and relationship with the patient (e.g., transitioning from a spouse's role to a caretaker's role), which may prevent caregivers from reaching out for help (Aminzadeh, Byszewski, Molnar, Eisner, 2007; Bunn et al., 2012; Vernooij-Dassen et al., 2005). Caregivers may also face the same structural barriers as patients, including lack of awareness of available services, access to NPA in the community, and health insurance, and/or financial resources to cover the costs of services.

Barriers Faced by Professionals

The main barriers that health professionals may face in using NPA of dementia include lack of training, trained professionals, and/or valid measures and norms for diverse populations. Healthcare providers may not have received training in dementia care and may not easily be able to recognize signs of cognitive impairment (Bradford, Kunik, Schulz, Williams, & Singh, 2009; Chodosh et al., 2004). They may also have limited time with their patients and/or may doubt the value of detecting dementia early if there are limited treatment options available (Bradford et al., 2009). Additionally, there are few clinical neuropsychologists around the world. For example, according to U.S. Bureau of Labor Statistics data, there are approximately 17,000 neuropsychologists in the U.S. or approximately one for every 19,000 patients (O-Net Online, 2014, para. 1). Data in other countries are similarly inadequate, which help portray the important need to invest in developing this workforce (Maestre, 2012).

Neuropsychological measures are also an important barrier because there is a shortage of valid tests for culturally and linguistically diverse populations. This is due in part to the fact that clinical neuropsychology was created in developed countries and, although some measures have been translated in languages other than English, they may not "embody the challenges that a particular culture poses on cognition" (Parra, 2014, p. 95). For example, a study found that performance on verbal fluency across four different Spanish-speaking subgroups from Chile, Dominican Republic, Puerto Rico, and Spain varied greatly, although the tests were all administered by native speakers from their respective countries (Buré-Reyes et al., 2013). Therefore, there are several cultural variables that pose a challenge when working with diverse clients that require extra training/knowledge and resources to provide adequate neuropsychological services.

Next Steps

As the burden of dementia increases, several steps can be taken, both at the individual level and the societal level, to decrease the risks of developing dementia and address this global health issue. At the individual level, having a healthy lifestyle (e.g., being tobacco-free), maintaining a normal blood pressure around 120/80 mm Hg, engaging in regular physical activity, and being socially active may help lower the individual risk of dementia or delay its onset (Alzheimer's Disease International, 2015a; Fratiglioni, Paillard-Borg, & Winblad, 2004; Paillard-Borg, Fratiglioni, Xu, Winblad, & Wang, 2012). Having a Mediterranean diet has also been associated with reduced risks of dementia (Lourida et al., 2013). This diet typically involves high consumption of plant foods, olive oil, and fish, which have important nutrients, such as monounsaturated fatty acids, vitamins B12, folate, and antioxidants, and are considered protective against cognitive dysfunction (Féart et al., 2009).

Important efforts can be made at the societal level in the global action against dementia. The development and implementation of government dementia policies, such as The Netherlands' *National Dementia Programme* or South Korea's *War on Dementia*, have been strongly recommended by international organizations (Bupa & Alzheimer's Disease International, 2013). Such programs involve concrete strategies and accountability to raise awareness of dementia to combat stigma, as well as to assess and improve availability and access of NPA to improve dementia care worldwide (Alzheimer's Disease International, 2016; Bupa & Alzheimer's Disease International, 2013). To decrease dementia-related stigma, all organizations, including businesses and public services, can follow recommendations and best practices from dementia-friendly communities and encourage respect and empowerment of people living with dementia (Alzheimer's Disease International, 2015b).

In addition, the field of clinical neuropsychology should be promoted and encouraged so that a larger, more diversified workforce is available to meet the current and upcoming needs of patients with dementia and their caregivers. The curricula for medicine, nursing, and other health professions should include training in dementia and NCDs in case of limited access to neuropsychologists in the region. Finally, NPA should be strongly encouraged and used to increase and improve the early detection and treatment of dementia. Early detection can help families receive key information and advice, allow individuals to make financial, legal, and health care plans while they are still capable of doing so, and take some control over the condition by accessing medical care, treatment, and support services (Alzheimer's Association, 2016b; National Health Service, 2015).

Conclusions

Dementia is and will continue to be an important threat to global health. NPA is critical in the evaluation of NCDs to detect, diagnose, and treat people with suspected or known cognitive impairment in the aging population. A strong global action is needed to encourage the use of NPA in more countries and regions around the world, so that a greater proportion of individuals has an equal opportunity to achieve the quality of care and quality of life that they deserve. Achieving this goal is certainly challenging given the many barriers faced by patients, caregivers, and healthcare professionals. However, focusing on prevention by promoting healthy lifestyles as well as building a well-trained and diverse workforce in neuropsychology are essential to better address the growing dementia epidemic.

Acknowledgments

We would like to acknowledge Jason R. Soble, Ph.D., ABPP for his review of earlier drafts of this manuscript.

References

Albert, M. S., DeKosky, S. T., Dickson, D., Dubois, B., Feldman, H. H., Fox, N. C., ... & Snyder, P. J. (2011). The diagnosis of mild cognitive impairment due to Alzheimer's disease: Recommendations from the National Institute on Aging-Alzheimer's Association workgroups on diagnostic guidelines for Alzheimer's disease. Alzheimer's & Dementia, 7(3), 270-279.

Alzheimer's Association. (2012). Increasing disclosure of dementia diagnosis. Retrieved from http://www.alz.org/documents_custom/inbrief_disclosure.pdf

Alzheimer's Association. (2014). Press release on the Alzheimer's & brain awareness month international survey. Retrieved from http://www.alz.org/documents_custom/abam_intl_survey_release.pdf

Alzheimer's Association. (2015). Early detection and diagnosis of Alzheimer's Disease. Retrieved from https://www.alz.org/publichealth/downloads/policy-brief.pdf

Alzheimer's Association. (2016a). What is dementia? Retrieved from http://www.alz.org/what-is-dementia.asp

Alzheimer's Association. (2016b). Early detection. Retrieved from http://www.alz.org/publichealth/early-detection.asp

Alzheimer's Disease International. (2011). World Alzheimer Report 2011: The benefits of early diagnosis and intervention. Retrieved from https://www.alz.co.uk/research/WorldAlzheimerReport2011.pdf

Alzheimer's Disease International. (2015a). World Alzheimer Report 2015: The global impact of dementia. Retrieved from https://www.alz.co.uk/research/WorldAlzheimerReport2015.pdf

Alzheimer's Disease International. (2015b). Dementia friendly communities: Key principles. Retrieved from https://www.alz.co.uk/adi/pdf/dfc-principles.pdf

Alzheimer's Disease International. (2016). Alzheimer's and dementia plans. Retrieved from https://www.alz.co.uk/alzheimer-plans

American Psychiatric Association. (2013). Diagnostic and statistical manual of mental disorders: DSM-5. Washington, D.C: American Psychiatric Association.

Aminzadeh, F., Byszewski, A., Molnar, F. J., & Eisner, M. (2007). Emotional impact of dementia diagnosis: Exploring persons with dementia and caregivers' perspectives. *Journal of Aging and Mental Health, 11*(3), 281-290. doi: 10.1080/136070600963695

Attix, D. K., & Welsh-Bohmer, K. A. (Eds.). (2013). *Geriatric neuropsychology: Assessment and intervention.* New York, NY: Guilford Publications.

Baddeley, A. D. (1986). *Working Memory.* Oxford, UK: Oxford University Press.

Bamford, C., Lamont, S., Eccles, M., Robinson, L., May, C., & Bond, J. (2004). Disclosing a diagnosis of dementia: a systematic review. *International Journal of Geriatric Psychiatry, 19*(2), 151-169.

Beaumont, J. G. (2008). *Introduction to Neuropsychology: Second Edition.* New York, NY: Guilford Press.

Ben-Porath, Y. S., & Tellegen, A. (2011). *MMPI-2-RF: Manual for administration, scoring and interpretation.* Minneapolis, MN: University of Minnesota Press.

Benton, A. L. (1994). *Contributions to neuropsychological assessment: A Clinical Manual.* New York, NY: Oxford University Press.

Benton, A. L., Hamsher, K. D., Varney, N. R., & Spreen, O. (1983). *Judgment of line Orientation.* New York, NY: Oxford University Press.

Bodin, D., Butts, A. M., & Grote, C. L. (2016). Postdoctoral training in clinical neuropsychology in America: how did we get here and where do recent applicants suggest we go next? *The Clinical Neuropsychologist, 30*(8), 1371-1379.

Bradford, A., Kunik, M. E., Schulz, P., Williams, S. P., & Singh, H. (2009). Missed and delayed diagnosis of dementia in primary care: Prevalence and contributing factors. *Alzheimer Disease & Associated Disorders, 23*(4), 306-314.

Bunn, F., Goodman, C., Sworn, K., Rait, G., Brayne, C., Robinson, L., … & Iliffe, S. (2012). Psychosocial factors that shape patient and carer experiences of dementia diagnosis and treatment: A systematic review of qualitative studies. *PLOS Medicine, 9*(10), e1001331. doi: 10.1371/journal.pmed.1001331

Bupa, & Alzheimer's Disease International. (2013). Ideas and advice on developing and implementing a National Dementia Plan. Retrieved from http://www.alz.co.uk/sites/default/files/pdfs/global-dementia-plan-report-ENGLISH.pdf

Buré-Reyes, A., Hidalgo-Ruzzante, N., Vilar-López, R., Gontier, J., Sánchez, L., Pérez-García, M., & Puente, A. E. (2013). Neuropsychological test performance of Spanish speakers: Is performance different across different Spanish-speaking subgroups? *Journal of Clinical and Experimental Neuropsychology, 35*(4), 404-412.

Chan, A. S., Sze, S. L., Cheung, M. C., & Han, Y. M. (2016). Development and application of neuropsychology in Hong Kong: implications of its value and future advancement. *The Clinical Neuropsychologist, 30*(8), 1236-1251.

Chan, R. C., Wang, Y., Wang, Y., & Cheung, E. F. (2016). Practice, training, and research in neuropsychology in mainland China: challenges and opportunities. *The Clinical Neuropsychologist, 30*(8), 1207-1213.

Chodosh, J., Petitti, D. B., Elliott, M., Hays, R. D., Crooks, V. C., Reuben, D. B., … & Wenger, N. (2004). Physician recognition of cognitive impairment: Evaluating the need for improvement. *Journal of the American Geriatrics Society, 52*(7), 1051-1059.

Conners, C. K., Staff, M. H. S., Connelly, V., Campbell, S., MacLean, M., & Barnes, J. (2000). Conners' continuous performance Test II (CPT II v. 5). *Multi-Health Systems Inc., 29*, 175-96.

Crum, R. M., Anthony, J. C., Bassett, S. S., & Folstein, M. F. (1993). Population-based norms for the Mini-Mental State Examination by age and educational level. *Journal of the American Medical Association, 269*(18), 2386-2391.

Damian, A. M., Jacobson, S. A., Hentz, J. G., Belden, C. M., Shill, H. A., Sabbagh, M. N., ... & Adler, C. H. (2011). The Montreal Cognitive Assessment and the Mini-Mental State Examination as screening instruments for cognitive impairment: item analyses and threshold scores. *Dementia and Geriatric Cognitive Disorders*, *31*(2), 126-131.

De Renzi, A., & Vignolo, L. A. (1962). Token test: A sensitive test to detect receptive disturbances in aphasics. *Brain: A Journal of Neurology*, *85*, 665-678.

Delis, D. C., Kramer, J. H., Kaplan, E., & Ober, B. A. (2000). *CVLT-II: California Verbal Learning Test: Adult Version*. San Antonio, TX: Psychological Corporation.

Daselaar, S. M., Fleck, M. S., & Cabeza, R. (2006). Triple dissociation in the medial temporal lobes: recollection, familiarity, and novelty. *Journal of Neurophysiology*, *96*(4), 1902-1911.

Dodrill, C. B. (1978). The hand dynamometer as a neuropsychological measure. *Journal of Consulting and Clinical Psychology*, *46*(6), 1432-1435.

Duffau, H. (Ed.). (2011). *Brain Mapping: From Neural Basis of Cognition to Surgical Applications*. Vienna, Austria: Springer Science & Business Media.

Egeland, J., Løvstad, M., Norup, A., Nybo, T., Persson, B. A., Rivera, D. F., ... & Arango-Lasprilla, J. C. (2016). Following international trends while subject to past traditions: neuropsychological test use in the Nordic countries. *The Clinical Neuropsychologist*, 1-22.

Elamin, M., Bak, T. H., Doherty, C. P., Pender, N., & Abrahams, S. (2016). Role of neuropsychology in neurodegeneration. Hardiman O., Doherty, C. P., Elamin, M., & Bede, P. (Eds.) *Neurodegenerative Disorders* (pp. 29-55). Dublin, Ireland: Springer International Publishing.

Emre, M. (2003). Dementia associated with Parkinson's disease. *The Lancet Neurology*, *2*(4), 229-237.

Féart, C., Samieri, C., Rondeau, V., Amieva, H., Portet, F., Dartigues, J. F., ... & Barberger-Gateau, P. (2009). Adherence to a Mediterranean diet, cognitive decline, and risk of dementia. *Journal of the American Medical Association 302*(6), 638-648.

Fernandez, A. L., Ferreres, A., Morlett-Paredes, A., Rivera, D., & Arango-Lasprilla, J. C. (2016). Past, present, and future of neuropsychology in Argentina. *The Clinical Neuropsychologist*, *30*(8), 1154-1178.

Folstein, M. F., Folstein, S. E., & McHugh, P. R. (1975). "Mini-mental state": A practical method for grading the cognitive state of patients for the clinician. *Journal of Psychiatric Research*, *12*(3), 189-198.

Fratiglioni, L., Paillard-Borg, S., & Winblad, B. (2004). An active and socially integrated lifestyle in late life might protect against dementia. *The Lancet Neurology*, *3*(6), 343-353.

Freitas, S., Simões, M. R., Alves, L., Duro, D., & Santana, I. (2012). Montreal Cognitive Assessment (MoCA): validation study for frontotemporal dementia. *Journal of Geriatric Psychiatry and Neurology*, *25*(3), 146-154.

Fujii, D. (2017). *Conducting a Culturally Informed Neuropsychological Evaluation*. Washington, DC: American Psychological Association

Goel, V. (2007). Anatomy of deductive reasoning. *Trends in Cognitive Sciences*, *11*(10), 435-441.

Gorno-Tempini, M. L., Hillis, A. E., Weintraub, S., Kertesz, A., Mendez, M., Cappa, S. E. E. A., ... & Manes, F. (2011). Classification of primary progressive aphasia and its variants. *Neurology*, *76*(11), 1006-1014.

Grace, J., & Malloy, P. F. (2001). *Frontal Systems Behavior Scale Professional Manual*. Lutz, FL: Psychological Assessment Resources.

Green, P., Allen, L., & Astner, K. (1997). *The Word Memory Test: A Manual for the Oral and Computerized Forms*. Durham, NC: CogniSyst, Inc.

Grober, E., Hall, C., Sanders, A. E., & Lipton, R. B. (2008). Free and cued selective reminding distinguishes Alzheimer's disease from vascular dementia. *Journal of the American Geriatrics Society*, *56*(5), 944-946.

Grote, C. L., Butts, A. M., & Bodin, D. (2016). Education, training and practice of clinical neuropsychologists in the United States of America. *The Clinical Neuropsychologist*, *30*(8), 1356-1370.

Hannay, J., Bieliauskas, L., Crosson, B. A., Hammeke, T. A., Hamsher, K., & Koffler, S. (1998). Proceedings of The Houston Conference on specialty education and training in clinical neuropsychology [Special issue]. *Archives of Clinical Neuropsychology, 13*, 157–250.

Haskins, A. L., Yonelinas, A. P., Quamme, J. R., & Ranganath, C. (2008). Perirhinal cortex supports encoding and familiarity-based recognition of novel associations. *Neuron, 59*(4), 554-560.

Heaton, R. K., Chelune, G. J., Talley, J. L., Kay, G. G., & Curtiss, G. (1993). Wisconsin card sort test manual: Revised and expanded. Odessa, FL: Psychological Assessment Resources.

Hokkanen, L., Nybo, T., & Poutiainen, E. (2016). Neuropsychology in Finland–over 30 years of systematically trained clinical practice. *The Clinical Neuropsychologist*, 30(8), 1214-1235.

Hooper HE. (1983). *Hooper Visual Organization Test Manual.* Los Angeles, CA: Western Psychological Services.

Hoops, S., Nazem, S., Siderowf, A. D., Duda, J. E., Xie, S. X., Stern, M. B., & Weintraub, D. (2009). Validity of the MoCA and MMSE in the detection of MCI and dementia in Parkinson disease. *Neurology, 73*(21), 1738-1745.

Horton, A. M., & Wedding, D. (2008). *The Neuropsychology Handbook, 3rd edition.* New York, NY: Springer Publishing Company.

Janzen, L. A., & Guger, S. (2016). Clinical neuropsychology practice and training in Canada. *The Clinical Neuropsychologist*, 30(8), 1193-1206.

Kang, H., Zhao, F., You, L., Giorgetta, C., Venkatesh, D., Sarkhel, S., & Prakash, R. (2014). Pseudo-dementia: A neuropsychological review. *Annals of Indian Academy of Neurology, 17*(2), 147-154.

Kaplan, E. (1983). *Boston diagnostic aphasia examination booklet.* Philadelphia, PA: Lea & Febiger.

Kaplan, E., Goodglass, H., & Weintraub, S. (2001). *The Boston Naming Test.* Philadelphia, PA: Lea & Febiger.

Kim, M. S., & Chey, J. (2016). Clinical neuropsychology in South Korea. *The Clinical Neuropsychologist, 30*(8), 1325-1334.

Klimova, B., & Kuca, K. (2015). Alzheimer's disease: Potential preventive, non-invasive, intervention strategies in lowering the risk of cognitive decline – A review study. *Journal of Applied Biomedicine, 13*(4), 257-261.

Kolb, B., & Whishaw, I. Q. (2009). *Fundamentals of Human Neuropsychology.* New York, NY: Worth Publishers.

Kumar, J. K. (2010). Neuropsychology in India. In *The Neuropsychology of Asian Americans*, 219-236. Fujii, D. E. (Ed). New York, NY: Psychology Press.

Leung, H. C., Skudlarski, P., Gatenby, J. C., Peterson, B. S., & Gore, J. C. (2000). An event-related functional MRI study of the Stroop color word interference task. *Cerebral Cortex, 10*(6), 552-560.

Lezak, M. D., Howieson, D. B., Bigler, E. D., & Tranel, D. (2012). *Neuropsychological Assessment* (5th edition). New York, NY: Oxford University Press.

Lourida, I., Soni, M., Thompson-Coon, J., Purandare, N., Lang, I. A., Ukoumunne, O. C., & Llewellyn, D. J. (2013). Mediterranean diet, cognitive function, and dementia: a systematic review. *Epidemiology, 24*(4), 479-489.

Maestre, G. E. (2012). Assessing dementia in resource-poor regions. *Current Neurology and Neuroscience Reports.* 12(5), 511-519.

Malek-Ahmadi, M., Powell, J. J., Belden, C. M., O'Connor, K., Evans, L., Coon, D. W., & Nieri, W. (2015). Age-and education-adjusted normative data for the Montreal Cognitive Assessment (MoCA) in older adults age 70–99. *Aging, Neuropsychology, and Cognition, 22*(6), 755-761.

Mathew, R., & Mathuranath, P. S. (2008). Issues in evaluation of cognition in the elderly in developing countries. *Annals of Indian Academy of Neurology, 11*(2), 82-88.

Mesulam, M. (2001). Primary progressive aphasia. *Annals of Neurology, 49*(4), 425-432.

Mesulam, M. M., Rogalski, E. J., Wieneke, C., Hurley, R. S., Geula, C., Bigio, E. H., ... & Weintraub, S. (2014). Primary progressive aphasia and the evolving neurology of the language network. *Nature Reviews Neurology, 10*(10), 554-569.

Meyers, J. E., & Meyers, K. R. (1995). *Rey Complex Figure Test and Recognition Trial Professional Manual.* Lutz, FL: Psychological Assessment Resources.

Mitrushina, M., Boone, K. B., Razani, J., & D'Elia, L. F. (2005). *Handbook of Normative Data for Neuropsychological Assessment.* Oxford, UK: Oxford University Press.

Mooney, S., Hasssanein, T. I., Hilsabeck, R. C., Ziegler, E. A., Carlson, M., Maron, L. M., ... & Program, T. U. H. N. R. (2007). Utility of the Repeatable Battery for the Assessment of Neuropsychological Status (RBANS) in patients with end-stage liver disease awaiting liver transplant. *Archives of Clinical Neuropsychology, 22*(2), 175-186.

Nasreddine, Z. S., Phillips, N. A., Bédirian, V., Charbonneau, S., Whitehead, V., Collin, I., ... & Chertkow, H. (2005). The Montreal Cognitive Assessment, MoCA: a brief screening tool for mild cognitive impairment. *Journal of the American Geriatrics Society, 53*(4), 695-699.

Nasreddine, Z. S., Phillips, N. A., Bédirian, V., Charbonneau, S., Whitehead, V., Collin, I., ... & Chertkow, H. (2005). The Montreal cognitive assessment, MoCA: A brief screening tool for mild cognitive impairment. *Journal of the American Geriatrics Society, 53*(4):695-699.

National Health Service. (2015). Benefits of early dementia diagnosis. Retrieved from http://www.nhs.uk/Conditions/dementia-guide/Pages/dementia-early-diagnosis-benefits.aspx

National Institute on Aging. (2012). Health disparities and Alzheimer's disease. Retrieved from https://www.nia.nih.gov/alzheimers/publication/2011-2012-alzheimers-disease-progress-report/health-disparities-and

Nestor, P. J., Caine, D., Fryer, T. D., Clarke, J., & Hodges, J. R. (2003). The topography of metabolic deficits in posterior cortical atrophy (the visual variant of Alzheimer's disease) with FDG-PET. *Journal of Neurology, Neurosurgery & Psychiatry, 74*(11), 1521-1529.

Olabarrieta-Landa, L., Caracuel, A., Pérez-García, M., Panyavin, I., Morlett-Paredes, A., & Arango-Lasprilla, J. C. (2016). The profession of neuropsychology in Spain: results of a national survey. *The Clinical Neuropsychologist, 30*(8), 1335-1355.

O-Net Online. (2014). Summary report for 19-3039.01 - Neuropsychologists and clinical neuropsychologists. Retrieved from http://www.onetonline.org/link/summary/19-3039.01#WagesEmployment

Ostrosky Shejet, F., & Velez Garcia, A. (2016). Neuropsychology in Mexico. *The Clinical Neuropsychologist, 30*(8), 1296-1304.

Paillard-Borg, S., Fratiglioni, L., Xu, W., Winblad, B., & Wang, H. X. (2012). An active lifestyle postpones dementia onset by more than one year in very old adults. *Journal of Alzheimer's Disease, 31*(4), 835-842.

Pakhomov, S. V., Smith, G. E., Chacon, D., Feliciano, Y., Graff-Radford, N., Caselli, R., & Knopman, D. S. (2010). Computerized analysis of speech and language to identify psycholinguistic correlates of frontotemporal lobar degeneration. *Cognitive and Behavioral Neurology, 23*(3), 165.

Parasuraman, R., Warm, J. S., & See, J. E. (1998). Brain systems of vigilance. Parasuraman R. (Ed.) *The Attentive Brain* (pp. 221-256). Cambridge, MA: The MIT Press.

Parra, M. A. (2014). Overcoming barriers in cognitive assessment of Alzheimer's disease. *Dementia & Neuropsychologia, 8*(2), 95-98.

Parsons, M. W., & Hammeke, T. A. (2014). *Clinical Neuropsychology: A Pocket Handbook for Assessment.* P. J. Snyder (Ed.). Washington, DC: American Psychological Association.

Patel, V., & Prince, M. (2001). Ageing and mental health in a developing country: Who cares? Qualitative studies from Goa, India. *Psychological Medicine, 31*(1), 29-38.

Ponsford, J. (2016). The practice of clinical neuropsychology in Australia. *The Clinical Neuropsychologist*, 30(8), 1179-1192.Psychological Corporation. (2009). *Advanced Clinical Solutions: Clinical and Interpretive Manual*. San Antonio, TX: Pearson.

Putzke, J. D., Williams, M. A., Millsaps, C. L., Azrin, R. L., LaMarche, J. A., Bourge, R. C., ... & Boll, T. J. (1997). Heart transplant candidates: A neuropsychological descriptive database. *Journal of Clinical Psychology in Medical Settings*, 4(3), 343-355.

Reitan, R. M. (1992). *Trail Making Test: Manual for Administration and Scoring*. Tucson, AZ: Reitan Neuropsychology Laboratory.

Reitan, R. M., & Wolfson, D. (1985). *The Halstead-Reitan Neuropsychological Test Battery: Theory and Clinical Interpretation* (Vol. 4). Tucson, AZ: Neuropsychology Press.

Reitan, R. M., & Wolfson, D. (1989). The Seashore Rhythm test and brain functions. *The Clinical Neuropsychologist*, 3(1), 70-78.

Rossetti, H. C., Lacritz, L. H., Cullum, C. M., & Weiner, M. F. (2011). Normative data for the Montreal Cognitive Assessment (MoCA) in a population-based sample. *Neurology*, 77(13), 1272-1275.

Roy, E. A., & Square, P. A. (1994). Neuropsychology of movement sequencing disorders and apraxia. Zeidel, D. W. (Ed.) *Neuropsychology* (pp. 183-218). London, UK: Academic Press.

Sakamoto, M. (2016). Neuropsychology in Japan: history, current challenges, and future prospects. *The Clinical Neuropsychologist*, 30(8), 1278-1295.

Schoenberg, M. R., & Scott, J. G. (Eds.). (2011). *The Little Black Book of Neuropsychology: a Syndrome-based Approach*. New York, NY: Springer Science & Business Media.

Schroeder, R. W., Twumasi-Ankrah, P., Baade, L. E., & Marshall, P. S. (2012). Reliable digit span: A systematic review and cross-validation study. *Assessment*, 19(1), 21-30.

Scoville, W. B., & Milner, B. (1957). Loss of recent memory after bilateral hippocampal lesions. *Journal of Neurology, Neurosurgery & Psychiatry*, 20(1), 11-21.

Scott, J. G., Ostermeyer, B., & Shah, A. A. (2016). Neuropsychological assessment in neurocognitive disorders. *Psychiatric Annals*, 46(2), 118-126.

Segal, D. L., June, A., Payne, M., Coolidge, F. L., & Yochim, B. (2010). Development and initial validation of a self-report assessment tool for anxiety among older adults: the Geriatric Anxiety Scale. *Journal of Anxiety Disorders*, 24(7), 709-714.

Shaaf, K. W., Stevens, L. F., Holcomb, M., Smith, S., Artman, L., & Kreutzer, J. S. (n.d.). Frequently asked questions about neuropsychological evaluation. Retrieved from http://www.tbinrc.com/Websites/tbinrcnew/images/Neuropsych_FAQ.pdf

Shallice, T. (1982). Specific impairments of planning. *Philosophical Transactions of the Royal Society of London B: Biological Sciences*, 298(1089), 199-209.

Siri, S., Benaglio, I., Frigerio, A., Binetti, G., & Cappa, S. F. (2001). A brief neuropsychological assessment for the differential diagnosis between frontotemporal dementia and Alzheimer's disease. *European Journal of Neurology*, 8(2), 125-132.

Smith A. (1982) *Symbol Digits Modalities Test*. Los Angeles, CA: Western Psychological Services.

Strauss, E., Sherman, E. M., & Spreen, O. (2006). *A Compendium of Neuropsychological Tests: Administration, Norms, and Commentary*. Oxford, UK: Oxford University Press..

Stroop, J. R. (1992). Studies of interference in serial verbal reactions. *Journal of Experimental Psychology*, 121(1), 15-23.

Stuss, D. T. (2011). Functions of the frontal lobes: Relation to executive functions. *Journal of the International Neuropsychological Society*, 17(5), 759-765.

Temple, R. O., Carvalho, J., & Tremont, G. (2006). A national survey of physicians' use of and satisfaction with neuropsychological services. *Archives of Clinical Neuropsychology*, 21(5), 371-382.

Vakil, E., & Hoofien, D. (2016). Clinical neuropsychology in Israel: history, training, practice and future challenges. *The Clinical Neuropsychologist*, 30(8), 1267-1277.

van der Lee, J., Bakker, T. J., Duivenvoorden, H. J., & Dröes, R. M. (2014). Multivariate models of subjective caregiver burden in dementia: a systematic review. *Ageing Research Reviews, 15*, 76-93.

Vernooij-Dassen, M. J. F. J., Moniz-Cook, E. D., Woods, R. T., Lepeleire, J. D., Leuschner, A., Zanetti, O., ... & Iliffe, S. (2005). Factors affecting timely recognition and diagnosis of dementia across Europe: From awareness to stigma. *International Journal of Geriatric Psychiatry, 20*(4), 377-386.

Videnovic, A., Bernard, B., Fan, W., Jaglin, J., Leurgans, S., & Shannon, K. M. (2010). The Montreal Cognitive Assessment as a screening tool for cognitive dysfunction in Huntington's disease. *Movement Disorders, 25*(3), 401-404.

Watts, A. D., & Shuttleworth-Edwards, A. B. (2016). Neuropsychology in South Africa: confronting the challenges of specialist practice in a culturally diverse developing country. *The Clinical Neuropsychologist, 30*(8), 1305-1324.

Wechsler, D. (2014). Wechsler Adult Intelligence Scale–Fourth Edition (WAIS–IV). London, UK: Pearson.

Witt, K., Daniels, C., Reiff, J., Krack, P., Volkmann, J., Pinsker, M. O., ... & Wojtecki, L. (2008). Neuropsychological and psychiatric changes after deep brain stimulation for Parkinson's disease: a randomised, multicentre study. *The Lancet Neurology, 7*(7), 605-614.

World Health Organization. (2012). Dementia: a public health priority. Retrieved from http://www.who.int/mental_health/publications/dementia_report_2012/en/

Yesavage, J. A., Brink, T. L., Rose, T. L., Lum, O., Huang, V., Adey, M., & Leirer, V. O. (1983). Development and validation of a geriatric depression screening scale: A preliminary report. *Journal of Psychiatric Research, 17*(1), 37-49.

CHAPTER 7

A Recurring Global Syndrome:
Challenges in Treating an Epidemic of Communal Trauma

Steve Olweean and Myron Eshowsky

Five years into the Syrian crisis, the damage, according to the 2015 Office of the United Nations High Commissioner for Refugees (UNHCR) report, has been catastrophic, with over half a million people seriously injured, approaching that number killed, and countless numbers traumatized (p. 1). The report further shares that at least half of homes are damaged, and nearly half of all Syrians are displaced, the majority of whom are children and women (p. 1). The refugees are crammed into insecure camps, dilapidated buildings, or the streets; however, psychological damage is even more severe, harder to repair, and sorely neglected. Without adequate healing, it is difficult to imagine how Syrian society can be put back together after years of hatred, violence, and profound loss and trauma at all levels.

Olweean (2001) points out that when humanitarian disaster occurs, aid efforts historically tend to focus on food, clothing, shelter, medical attention, physical security, and economic need. Despite widespread acknowledgement of high levels of traumatization within displaced populations in the past and present, including within the Syrian society, there is a lack of awareness and understanding of large-scale wounds that profoundly impact on the psycho-social-biological-spiritualdimensions as a major global health issue.

In the face of old, ineffective models of intervention, new models are needed for addressing communal trauma, building communal resiliency, adapting culturally-specific methods for healing, local capacity-building skills training at the grassroots and professional levels for treating mass traumatization, and strategic collaboration among humanitarian response groups (p. 271).

Through the work of the Social Health Care (SHC) model (a program of Common Bond Institute [CBI] and International Humanistic Psychology Association), this chapter describes massive communal trauma permeating the entire Syrian population as one example of a central and chronic global health risk historically afflicting the world population. It underscores the necessity of understanding communal and transgenerational trauma and developing new, culturally-sensitive healing responses to effectively promote recovery and to prevent unresolved, trans-generational trauma from becoming embedded in the consciousness of a society.

Syrian Refugee Crisis in the Middle East

According to Mercy Corps's (2016) report on the Syrian refugee crisis, every minute, 24 more people in the world are forced into migration by war, poverty, violence, or environmental issues, amounting to a total of over 65 million at the end of 2016 (para. 1). Mercy Corps (2016) states the Syrian refugee crisis is truly a global one as it accounts for the largest and fastest-growing displacement of people in the world (para. 2). This far-reaching displacement sits on a backdrop of the Syrian civil war, which exacerbates the splintering of social structures down to the family level. Many men have died in the war, so the majority of the refugee population is women and children. This adds to the criticality of increasing access to resources for an already vulnerable population (UNHCR, 2015, p. 1).

The UNHCR (2015) estimates that since the beginning of the conflict in 2011, over 400,000 people have been killed, and well over half of the Syrian population has been displaced either internally or externally (p. 1). Although the UNHCR (2016) estimates that 6.5 million are externally displaced, this approximation does not reflect undocumented refugees that significantly increase the actual figures (p. 1). Of these, the vast majority have settled into the four closest neighboring countries of Jordan, Lebanon, Turkey, and Iraq.

Resources in these host countries are limited and severely stretched. The massive influx of refugees is adding stress to the political and economic situations in each of these countries. The situation is especially dire for women and children languishing in these new lands. The UNHCR (2015) reports that four out of five refugee households are led by women, and most are struggling for basic resources to survive (p. 3). In general, refugees are not allowed to work in host countries that are already burdened by large-scale unemployment. According to the UNHCR (2015), over half of refugees are children under the age of 18 (p. 3). Many girls under 18 must confront the burden of being married off, as parents often believe doing so reduces their daughters' chances of being victimized by exploitation and rape. In fact, the UNHCR (2016) reports that girls as young as 11 or 12 are being married for these reasons (p. 14). Financial stresses have led to child labor, prostitution, and black market economic activity that undermines both the host and refugee communities.

While the priorities that humanitarian aid services typically concentrate on are the most concrete and immediately visible needs, increasingly, organizations that are addressing refugee health issues are identifying widespread trauma and expressing the critical need for psychosocial services. The World Health Organization (WHO), Doctors without Borders, International Medical Corps, and others have released reports on the degree of distress found amongst the refugees. The Migration Policy Institute's (2015) research of Syrian refugees in Turkey found that among female led families: one-third report being distressed and disturbed to the point of being unable to carry out activities of daily living in the last two weeks, one-third report this being an all-the-time occurrence, and two-thirds felt unable to care for their children. It is estimated that less than 13 percent of these families receive any form of even limited psychosocial support services (İçduygu, 2015, p. 11).

Children are the most vulnerable to the immediate effects of war and atrocities. They have witnessed bombardments, destruction, killings, torture, and loss of family members. They have experienced displacement and the loss of the familiarity of family, home, school, and community. In many cases, they have been tortured themselves. Machel (2000) argues, "One of the most significant of war traumas of all, particularly for younger children, is separation from parents – often more distressing than the war activities themselves" (p.10).

In attempting to assess the psychosocial impact of mass exposure to displacement and trauma that the Syrian refugee population has experienced, it is important to understand the role of cultural influences in shaping the collective experience of extreme stress. Wilson (2005) argues that culture shapes the way individuals form trauma complexes after a traumatic experience. He argues that emotional experience (such as hyper-arousal, startle response, irritability, and depression) may have different effects based on cultural overrides. Smith, Lin, and Mendoza (1993) state:

> Humans in general have an inherent need to make sense out of and explain their experiences. This is especially true when they are experiencing suffering and illness. In the process of this quest for meaning, culturally shaped beliefs play a vital role in determining whether a particular explanation and associated treatment plan will make sense to the patient. (p. 38)

Husain, Nashwan, and Howard (2016) point out that the influence of cultural traditions in the Middle East discourages verbal displays of emotion, and traumatic stress manifests as somatic complaints. Complaints such as chest constriction, heartache, bedwetting (children), attention deficit disorder, sleep disturbances, and eating difficulties may be somatic indicators of how refugees experience their traumatization. Husain, Nashwan, and Howard go on further to explain the critical role of gender dynamics while providing care. Examples of this were male professionals maintaining appropriate physical distance from a female Arab client, and, for female professionals working with an Arab male, taking the time to develop rapport and establish themselves as an expert in the field.

According to the UNHCR (2015), regarding refugee psychosocial needs, various psychological responses have been observed in refugee children, including attachment difficulties, increased clinginess, sleep disturbances, bedwetting, easily startled by loud noises, anxiety, chronic stomach aches or headaches, mutism, and eating difficulties (p. 20). According to our own experiences in SHC psychosocial clinics, parents most commonly bring their children in with complaints of bedwetting, nightmares, stomach aches, inability to stay still, or difficulty getting them to eat. Additionally, signs of unhealed traumatization witnessed in our clinics include: numerous reports of refugee children being bullied at school by host-country children, reports of intrusive negative and hostile thoughts, panic responses to jets flying over the area, aggressive behaviors by young and adolescent boys, and self-mutilation/cutting.

Increasingly, Syrian refugees are referred to as a "lost generation." Education Cluster (2015) reports that prior to the civil war in Syria, school attendance was universal and the country as a whole had an upper 90% literacy rate, ranking amongst the highest in the world (p. 2). Research by The Migration Policy Institute (2016) found that while there has been some improvement in school attendance since the beginning of the mass forced migration, in general, attendance rates are sporadic and overall quality of education is inadequate (p. 11). As a result, Education Cluster (2015) found Syria to be currently ranked second-lowest in education globally (p.3). Furthermore, all the countries where the refugees have migrated report overwhelming psychological/mental health needs amongst the refugees.

Only a small percentage of refugees receive any form of psychosocial services to address the severe and pervasive depression, anxiety, post-traumatic stress disorder (PTSD), and other mental health disorders that service providers are witnessing throughout the population. An exact figure of how many refugees are receiving psychosocial services is difficult to assess. In many cases, due to reporting criteria among various humanitarian aid organizations, a service that is reported as "psychosocial" may simply be documenting an assessment of needs, with no capacity to actually offer direct treatment services. Additionally, there are cultural stigmas which restrict refugee participation in accessing these extremely scarce psychological and psychiatric services. A typical response at SHC field clinics is, "I'm not crazy. Why were we sent here?" In summary, the loss of family and community, education and employment possibilities, and cultural self-identity in addition to festering, unhealed psychological wounds raise serious concerns about the transmission of these unresolved traumas into future generations – a phenomena known as transgenerational trauma.

The Challenge of Communal and Transgenerational Trauma

Psychological trauma due to war and violence is historically an oft-ignored problem, allowing devastating, unhealed, communal wounds to be inherited by future generations. This transgenerational trauma is a complex global syndrome that weakens internal resilience, damages the capacity to form healthy relationships, divides, polarizes, and perpetuates enemy images. It has been a central basis for past conflict and wars and is an underlying, potent fuel for the eruption of violence and victimization in the present and the future.

Contemporary models of healing individual trauma, while useful tools, are inadequate in addressing larger, shared, communal trauma and its implications for the future. While a large range of literature has been developed to address the issues traumatized individuals face in their healing journey, there is a dearth of understanding the dynamics and implications of communal trauma and its evolution into transgenerational trauma when this trauma goes unhealed. New, innovative, and practical models and methodologies at the large-scale societal level are needed to effectively treat trauma wounds at this level and prevent their transfer into future generations. This task is essential to bring healing and reconciliation within and between communities, establishing compassionate local and global relations, and achieving sustainable peace.

There are a number of mechanisms cited to explain the transmission of the effects of trauma across generations. Milroy (2005) states:

The trans-generational effects of trauma occur via a variety of mechanisms including the impact on the attachment relationship with caregivers; the impact on parenting and family functioning; the association with parental physical and mental illness; disconnection and alienation from extended family, culture and society. These effects are exacerbated by exposure to continuing levels of stress and trauma including multiple bereavements and other losses, the process of vicarious traumatization where children witness the on-going effect of the original trauma which a parent or other family member has experienced. Even where children are protected from the traumatic stories of their ancestors, the effects of past traumas still impact on children in the form of ill health, family dysfunction, community violence, psychological morbidity, and early mortality. (p. 3)

Danieli (1998) presents a model for understanding psychological mechanisms of transmission in transgenerational trauma. Paraphrasing her model, these mechanisms include: a conspiracy of silence, over-disclosure, identification with family members, and reenactments.

- A conspiracy of silence (society, individuals) helps maintain and exacerbate the effects of trauma. It might have been an empathic response to not stir up the painful issues, as a parent may react with anxiety, extreme rage, or flashbacks.
- Over-disclosure, especially with children, makes them bear witness to traumatic experiences that can challenge even the most firmly held beliefs that the world is a safe place.
- Identification with parents/other family members leaves children tending to feel responsible for parents' or other family members' distress, and if they were only good enough, parents would not be so angry or sad. Children may experience a type of survivor guilt.
- Trauma survivors tend to reenact their traumatic events with family and significant others. (p. 4)

Research in epigenetics indicates that trauma can and does pass from one generation to the next. Rachel Yehuda (2009), a professor in psychiatry and neuroscience at Mount Sinai School of Medicine, examined the neurobiology of PTSD in Holocaust survivors and their children. Her research on cortisol levels (the stress hormone that helps our body return to normal after we experience a trauma) and its effect on brain function has revolutionized thinking about PTSD. People with PTSD relive feelings and sensations associated with a trauma despite the trauma having occurred in the past.

Yehuda and her team found that children of Holocaust survivors with PTSD were born with low cortisol levels (similar to their parents), predisposing them to relive the PTSD symptoms of the previous generation. Her discovery of low cortisol levels in people who experience an acute traumatic event was considered controversial for previous theory held that stress is associated with high cortisol levels. Yehuda also discovered low cortisol levels in war veterans and pregnant mothers (and later in their children) who developed PTSD after being exposed to the World Trade Center attacks on September 11, 2001. In her research, a person is three times more likely to experience symptoms of PTSD if one of their parents had PTSD (p. 131).

Eduardo Duran (2006) expresses the view that we have all internalized much of the personal and collective wounding of our cultures. In his view, the wounding expressed in the opposition of war creates an identity that predisposes us to future trauma. In his research with American Indians, he found that many identified with tribal historical losses, which brought on symptoms of emotional distress including anger, anxiety, and depression. This process of identity formation is what leads to what Vamik Volkan

(1997) calls "victim identities." As he states, "People kill for the sake of protecting and maintaining their large group identities. Why are they compelled to take revenge for the wrongs inflicted on their ancestors and others belonging to their bloodlines?" (p.17). Even if the civil war in Syria were to come to a point of cessation, we would argue there will be a strong need for healing processes to address the collective wounding across "bloodlines."

Diagnoses such as PTSD are unable to capture the levels of chronic, ongoing stress that many refugees experience in their everyday lives. The sources of this stress are multiple, repeated, and of great severity. The sources of their stress are unacceptably high and compounded by:

· The inability to identify and overcome a single source of stress, due to stressors on multiple levels, that feeds a sense of helplessness
· The presence of cumulative stressors
· The realization that many of these stressors are inflicted by people well-known to the victims.

Not only does this speak to the inadequacy of diagnosis, but also to the larger problems of how to build levels of capacity to address the individual and communal traumas in the present and future. An effect of these complex stressors on the refugee population is reflected in a collective sense of hopelessness and desperation. Current examples of how this effect is exhibited within the Syrian refugee population include: an inability to acquire adequate life skills due to high rates of youth receiving no education or vocational training; increasingly disaffected youth being lured to radical groups by promises of money and revenge; a breakdown in the family structure, a growing trend of aggressive gangs being formed particularly amongst unaccompanied minors; early marriages of young girls to provide protection and security; and an unprecedented prevalence of substance abuse as a means to cope. If left unaddressed the impact of these stressors can be expected to result in a high probability of future problems within and between communities, including re-traumatization.

Peter Levine (2007) cites cultural anthropologist Merida Blanco, PhD's (2004) unpublished manuscript which develops a model of an intergenerational diagram spanning five lifetimes following violence perpetrated by one social group against another:

· First Generation: In the first generation to be conquered, the males are killed, imprisoned, enslaved, or in some other way deprived of the ability to provide for their families
· Second Generation: Many of the men turn to alcohol or drugs, as their cultural identity has been destroyed with a predictable, accompanying loss of self-worth

- Third Generation: Spousal abuse and other forms of domestic violence are spawned. By this generation, the connection to its antecedent from societal trauma only two generations before has been weakened or lost.
- Fourth Generation: At this stage, abuse moves from spousal abuse to child abuse or both.
- Fifth Generation: This cycle repeats itself over and over as trauma begets violence and more trauma and violence, with increasing societal degradation, including abuse of our Earth and her natural resources as sustainability is disregarded. (p. 438)

Duran and Duran (1995) suggested that historical (communal) trauma becomes embedded in the cultural memory of a people, is passed on by the same mechanisms by which culture is generally transmitted, and therefore becomes "normalized" within that culture. They argue that this communal trauma provides a link between the transmission of generational trauma and what they call "dysfunctional community syndrome" (DCS):

[DCS is] A situation whereby multiple violence types are occurring and appear to be increasing over generations, both quantitatively (numbers of incidents) and in terms of the intensity of violence experiences, for example, victims of sexual abuse include very small children; pack rape is being committed by boys as young as 10 years old. (p.51)

Memmot et al. (2001) looked at typical clusters of violence in a dysfunctional community. The clusters include: male on male violence, female on female violence, child abuse, substance abuse and related violence, male suicide, gang rape, infant rape, rape of grandmothers, self-mutilation, domestic violence, and homicide. They argue that when a community deteriorates to the level of DCS, it has immediate and generational effects on community members, particularly on children.

On the individual level, certain factors have shown themselves in our work at SHC to be helpful for personal recovery:

- Actively learning about trauma and its effects to help people make appropriate decisions about healthcare
- Developing new community where possible to help give a feeling of belonging as anecdote to isolation
- Establishing some sort of daily and weekly routine such as exercise, attending religious services, or participation in community support programs
- Learning skills of active listening so family and friends can vent their feelings as well as being able to express one's own needs
- Learning stress management skills and cognitive behavioral strategies for addressing helplessness and negative thinking.

· Offering support services where on the grassroots level, refugees can restore self and the community through being able to be of help to others

The task of reparation for survivors of communal trauma according to Volkan (2004) asks how to:

...reverse shame and humiliation, to turn passivity into activity, to tame the sense of aggression, and to mourn the losses associated with the trauma (the actual deaths of relatives and friends in the original tragedy, the loss of self-esteem and prestige, and the loss of land and other valuable things). (p. 15)

Among examples of approaches that can help contribute to community cohesiveness and healing of collective trauma are:

· Community rituals such as: grief rituals to help release shared trauma and loss and rituals for promoting acknowledgement, forgiveness, and healing
· Use of memorialization with emphasis on social reconciliation
· Truth and Reconciliation commissions and public apologies
· Communal food sharing to restore sense of community
· Community use of music, the arts, and dance as a way of restoring community relations

For refugees from the Syrian culture, where communal identity is central to individual identity, the sense of home and neighborhood has been lost and along with it, communal life as they knew it. In the early days of the conflict, most refugees reported that they wanted to return to their homes in Syria as soon as the conflicts ended. Although still prevalent, this sentiment is gradually diminishing as the fighting drags on and the reality of the level of destruction sets in. Renos Papadapolous (2002) makes the argument that clinicians often mistake the loss of place (what he calls "nostalgia disorientation") for individual symptoms of personal traumatization. It is a pain associated with the desire to return home.

Unlike PTSD, which is a widely accepted syndrome describing the behavior of affected individuals, there is no similar agreement on the existence of a syndrome describing the behavior of societies affected by large-scale violence. Volkan (2004) holds with respect to shared communal trauma that "...the collective mental representation of an event has caused a large group to face common losses, to feel helpless and victimized by another group, and to share a humiliating injury" (p.14).

Collective trauma, according to Judy Atkinson (2011), seeps slowly and insidiously into the fabric and soul of relations and beliefs of people as community. People feel an overwhelming sense of grief with the loss of their cultural surroundings, family, and friends.

Survivors of violent events (in this case Syrians) not only experience a sense of loss but can also be singled out by the Assad regime for victimization and punishment. The resulting trauma for the community generates feelings of humiliation, helplessness, and loss of human dignity. Deep desires for revenge and glory to overcome the undercurrents of communal pain becomes fuel for future conflicts and further communal traumatization.

One the unfortunate consequences of the Syrian crisis has been the massive loss of fathers and other adult male role models in a society where the male head of household plays a pivotal role. SHC has witnessed several instances in which packs of young boys aggressively act out in our triage medical clinics. Generally, these situations are handled with staff interventions to engage them directly, such as holding, soothing, and engaging them in constructive physical activities that reduce stress and increase a sense of internal control. Many of these boys have little to no adult supervision or adult male role models and are becoming under-socialized. In certain cases, acting out reflects deep desires for revenge and glory. Increasingly, we are witnessing a growth in gangs (which promote the reenactment of past traumatic violence) amongst the refugee population.

Collective trauma is further compounded as bureaucratic responses dismantle basic, essential, social-cultural support structures, traditions, and networks within the traumatized community during times of crisis when these supports are most needed. Examples of this include: temporary refugee camps not allowing family/community cooking or social activities; unclear policies on how to transfer out of the camps and reestablish independent life; forced housing of historically-incompatible groups from within and outside countries of origin; housing refugees together in close quarters with different cultures, languages, races, and religions; housing structures that create significant lack of basic privacy; and integration policies forcing immediate adaptation to the dominant host culture at the expense of their own culture. In addition, these residential centers are seriously understaffed and under great stress

A Model for Addressing These Challenges:
The Social Health Care (SHC) Training and Treatment Program

CBI's SHC program addresses these needs as it invests in the local human service system of Jordan, Lebanon, Turkey, and eventually Syria, in four ways.

Local Capacity Building Skills Training

A holistic, interdisciplinary, and culturally adapted psychosocial skills training, equips a growing pool of local, skilled psychosocial service providers with the ability to deliver essential services to large numbers of people from both the refugee and host communities. The SHC program follows a psycho-social, somatic, spiritual/transpersonal/philosophical approach and includes identifying and integrating traditional healing and recovery rituals, ceremonies, and approaches that promote resilience within the community itself.

Trainees are members of both the displaced and traumatized population and the host community and include humanitarian aid staff, health care professionals, students, relief workers, and community volunteers. Training is a progressive curriculum that prepares professionals, para-professionals, and lay helpers to deliver a range of direct support and treatment services, from emotional support, immediate care, and crisis stabilization, to more in-depth and longer-term mental health therapy.

Based on the Catastrophic Trauma Recovery (CTR) model developed by CBI at the end of the Balkan Wars, the SHC program operates on the central premise of promoting self-healing communities that build communal resilience, cohesion, confidence, and empowerment, and promote individual and communal narratives of resilient survivors rather than victims. Employing the human resources of the community itself to become the primary provider of healing is a central characteristic of the SHC program and is fundamental to communal healing.

In addition to programs conducted in the Middle East, CBI is now extending the SHC program to collaborating with non-governmental organizations (NGOs) in Europe by launching a bi-regional, cross-training initiative between psychosocial treatment professionals in Germany, Jordan, and Lebanon. This joint project will increase the capacity to provide effective, culturally adapted treatment services to the refugee populations in each country. CBI will offer orientation and recommendations to German humanitarian services in designing, implementing, and evaluating culturally and linguistically competent service delivery systems addressing multiple needs of large Middle Eastern populations in crisis, as well as offering training for working with large groups and communal trauma.

The intent is to build mutual support and shared purposes in assisting refugees and asylum seekers to successfully integrate into a new, fruitful, and productive life in Germany, while also helping them to heal emotionally, recover within their home culture, and reduce the need for them to flee the Middle East. CBI is also working with cooperating organizations in developing an international professional mentor network to support local service providers in each region and newly emerging psychosocial services in the Middle East.

Direct Services and Modeling Community-Based, Multi-Modal Service Systems

CBI's SHC program also conducts Disaster Health Care field clinics and establishes pilot, community-based service programs to:

- Provide direct treatment services to the refugee community
- Demonstrate treatment methods and skills to trainees
- Provide supervised field work opportunities for trainees to apply skills learned
- Demonstrate models for developing, operating, and sustaining community-based, psychosocial services in situations where there is high need, the local human service system is largely underdeveloped, and skill and financial resources are scarce. In line with CBI's commitment to local capacity building, models used rely on collaboration and shared programming between local humanitarian NGOs, as well as a strong orientation towards equipping members of the client population with self-help skills in order to create a larger, more comprehensive service network and more effective continuity of care.

Investing in the Local Academic System

There is a lack of practical, mental health-related, academic or professional training programs that offer a practical internship component in Syria and surrounding countries hosting Syrian refugees. This deficit has historically prevented the development of an adequate, local, mental health service system within the region as a whole. With the current crisis of massive trauma and psychological stressors due to displacement and loss throughout the region, this lack of a mechanism for training skilled professionals is all the more glaring.

In response, CBI is establishing certified and accredited professional training programs at local universities and institutes that include the missing locally-based professional, practical internships in the mental health disciplines. Current examples include:

- A Certified Diploma in Clinical Social Work at Yarmouk University in Jordan. This is a partnership between CBI, Yarmouk University, the Queen Rania Center, Michigan State University, and the International Humanistic Psychology Association that prepares local students with practical skills training and field experience in practical, psychosocial treatment services that enable them to provide critical services to under-served and at-risk communities
- Development of a practical master's degree in Community Mental Health with a local internship in Jordan, in partnership with CBI, Yarmouk University, and Michigan State University

Consultation to Public Policy Makers and Public Education

Through a series of bi-regional working conferences organized by CBI in Germany and Jordan, organizational representatives, government representatives, and professionals directly involved in working with refugees are developing a formal body of fact-based recommendations and guidelines. Recommendations have been made for developing proven operational structures and systems for effectively responding to the multiple and interrelated needs of refugees. The goal is successfully resettling and integrating refugees into the local society, and supporting the unique needs of communities and societies receiving refugees. The purpose is to make the information and consultation available to national and community public policy makers responsible for developing official logistical structures, policies, and procedures affecting refugees. These formal recommendations and guidelines are supported and endorsed by a growing international list of universities, professional associations, training institutes, and NGOs with expertise in the field. An active public education process is also being jointly developed to increase intercultural understanding and sensitivity, and to reduce and prevent polarization in the host society.

Conclusion

According to Olweean (2001), regardless of place, time, or original motivation of the conflict, unresolved, inherited, communal psychological wounds are one of the most powerful fuels of violence. The pervasive presence of such a substantial segment of traumatized members in a society poses perhaps the most formidable barrier to recovery and future peace.

While communal trauma is not a new phenomenon historically, it is typically ignored by the healing professions out of a sense of futility due to its size and span. Treating large civilian populations that are experiencing catastrophic psychological trauma due to war and violence poses unique challenges that are typically not focused on in the therapeutic literature or conventional clinical practice, where historical applications are with individuals or small groups. When the society is one in which human services are seriously underdeveloped or absent, and when the integrity of the existing social support system itself is critically compromised by a disastrous situation, this challenge can be overwhelming (p. 271-272).

Although needs assessments conducted in the region over the years by various international aid organizations have consistently identified this critical and predominantly unmet need, and although NGO coordinating agencies and relief organizations confirm this as a present and growing condition, there has been far too little provided in the way of adequate direct treatment services or local training in trauma treatment. This lack of action has been primarily due to a lack of workable models and methodologies in the field of mental health for undertaking such an immense, long-term task of treating on the societal level, particularly where the local human service infrastructure is significantly lacking.

Olweean (2001) further states that concerted efforts to develop new models and methods oriented toward treating large populations are required (p. 272), particularly in societies where trauma has become systemic and the needed skills, services, infrastructure, and financial resources are scarce. These approaches must incorporate an integrated and multi-level flow of services and supports designed to respond to both immediate and long-term effects of trauma in order to prevent the transfer of trauma into future generations. A key feature is that the capacity to provide and quickly expand these services on an ongoing basis is designed to be instilled within the local community itself by tapping into its own skills and human resources. The deep symbolism of a community healing itself is vital to regaining a sense of empowerment, value, and dignity that is threatened and undermined by the trauma experience. It is noteworthy that these qualities within a community also support compassion and tolerance toward others that can help defuse defensiveness and impulses toward revenge and retribution.

It is imperative that any model also be sensitive and appropriate to the cultural context of both the trauma experience and treatment. Thus, in addition to adaptations of highly effective mental health treatment methods, it is important to enlist traditional healing aspects of the society, including its cultural and spiritual resources.

Through the SHC model, CBI has worked to be an example of what is called for in effectively addressing large-scale collective trauma and to promote the creative development of more expanded approaches to healing that move beyond the limits of traditional mental health practices in order to meet the historical, global health challenge of communal trauma.

References

Atkinson, J., Nelson, J., & Atkinson, C. (2010). Trauma, transgenerational trauma and effects on community wellbeing. In Purdie, N., Dudgeon, P., & Walker, R. (Eds.), *Working together: Aboriginal and Torres Strait Islander mental health and wellbeing* (pp. 135-144). Canberra, Australian Health and Welfare.

Danieli, Y. (1998). *International handbook of multigenerational legacies of trauma.* NY: Plenum Press.

Duran, E. (2006). *Healing the soul wound: Counseling with American Indians and other native peoples.* NY: Teachers College Press.

Duran, E. & Duran, B. (1995). *Native American post-colonial psychology.* Albany, New York: State University of New York.

Husain, A., Nashwan, A., & Howard, S. (2016). Middle Eastern immigrant and refugee Families. In Dettlaff, A. & Fong, R. (Eds.), *Immigrant and refugee children and families: Culturally responsive practice.* NY: Columbia University Press.

İçduygu, A. (April 2015). Syrian refugees in Turkey: Long road ahead. *Migration Policy Institute.* Retrieved from http://www.migrationpolicy.org/research/syrian-refugees-turkey-long-road-ahead

Levine, P. & Kline, M. (2007). *Trauma through a child's eyes: Awakening the ordinary miracle of healing, infancy through adolescence.* Berkeley, CA: North Atlantic Books.

Machel, G. (2000). *The impact of armed conflict on children: A critical review of progress made and obstacles encountered in increasing protection for war affected children.* NY,UNICEF.

Memmot, P., Stacy, P., Chambers, C. and Keys, C. (2001). *Violence in indigenous communities.* Canberra: Commonwealth Attorney General's Department.

Milroy, H. and S.R.Zubrick, *The Western Australian Aboriginal Child Health Survey: The social and emotional wellbeing of Aboriginal children and young people,* Perth, Curtin University, 2005

Mercy Corps (2016). It's not just Syria: Refugee crisis is 60 million and growing. retrieved from https://www.mercycorps.org/articles/its-not-just-syria-refugee-crisis-60-million-and-growing

Olweean,S. (2001) "When society is the victim:The catastrophic trauma recovery project", *The psychological impact of war trauma on civilians:An international perspective.* Westport,CT:Praeger Press

Papademetriou, D., & Fratzke, S. (November 2016). Beyond care and maintenance: Rebuilding hope and opportunity for refugees. *Migration Policy Institute.* Retrieved from http://www.migrationpolicy.org/research/beyond-care-and-maintenance-rebuilding-hope-and-opportunity-refugees-transatlantic-council

Papadopoulos, R. K. (Ed.). (2002). *Therapeutic care for refugees: No place like home.* London: Karnac Press.

Smith, M., Lin, M. K., & Mendoza, R. (1993). Non-biological issues affecting psychopharmacology: Cultural considerations. In Lin, K.M., et al. (Eds.), *Psychopharmocology and psychobiology of ethnicity.* Washington, D.C.: American Psychiatric Press.

UNHCR. (June 2015). Regional refugee and resilience plan 2015-2016 in response to the Syria crisis. Retrieved from data.unhcr.org/syrianrefugees/regional.php

UNHCR. (June 2016). Regional refugee and resilience plan 2015-2016 in response to the Syria crisis. Retrieved from http://www.3rpsyriacrisis.org/the-3rp/strategic-overview/

UNICEF. (March 2015). Syria: Education caught in the crossfire. *Education Cluster.* Retrieved from http://educationcluster.net/syria-education-caught-crossfire-conflict/

Volkan, V. (2004). *Blind trust: Large groups and their leaders in times of crisis and terror.* Charlottesville, Virginia: Pitchstone Publishing.

Volkan, V. (1998). *Bloodlines: From ethnic pride to ethnic terrorism.* Boulder, CO: Westview Press.

WHO. (2016). Syria regional refugee and resilience plan. Retrieved from http://www.who.int/hac/crises/syr/appeals/syria3RP2016/en/

Wilson, J. P. & So-kum Tang, C. (Eds.). (2010). *Cross-cultural assessment of psychological trauma and PTSD.* NY: Springer Science.

Yehuda, R. & Bierer, L. (2009). Relevance of epigenetics to PTSD: Implications for DSMV. *Journal of Traumatic Stress, 22*(5), 427-434.

Yehuda, R. & Bierer, L. (2007). Transgenerational transmission of cortisol and PTSD risk. *Progress in Brain Research Journal, 167,* 121-135.

CHAPTER 8

Activating Compassion into Meaningful Impact

Neena S. Jain and A. Maya Casagrande

Introduction

> *"Haiti was littered with the skeletons of 'successful' aid projects."*
> *- Dr. Nigel Fisher, former U.N. Humanitarian Coordinator for Haiti*
> *(personal communication, 2015)*

If we truly believe in compassion as a renewable resource and driver of change, how can we optimally focus and direct its power in meaningful ways? How can we harness compassion to lead personal, organizational, and global positive impact? What examples of critical ingredients in this process exist from work with communities around the world in humanitarian emergencies and international development contexts? What case studies from pre-departure or pre-engagement preparations can serve as best practices for individual and collective change?

We know from past efforts, scores of examples, and much research and writing that good intentions are not enough in this endeavor. Accepting that, perhaps one of the most fundamental and profoundly important foundations to forge new paths toward meaningful progress is to first critically examine failure.

Accept Failure – and Dissect It

We have all read articles about "failure," "intelligent failure," or the "5 simple tools" to accepting and reporting failure, moving on, etc. Such articles are prolific in the non-governmental organization (NGO) space and testify to the need for, and the complex difficulties of, sharing failures publicly (Barrington & Tufa, 2014). However, far less has been written on the definition of the word "failure" and who decides its meaning.

This conversation is long overdue. While it is clear that the nonprofit, international aid, and development communities should embrace sharing both successes and failures across the entire NGO stakeholder chain, we cannot afford to stop there. We must also embrace updated, inclusive definitions of success and failure that go far beyond traditional measures to more fully reflect the reality of our programs as well as the communities with whom we work.

> *"What impact are you talking about? The impact is just spending money. Goods are delivered with no sense of social development. There is no interest to develop people; it's all reduced to practicality. Just know how to write a report. The focus is on skills put in the framework of outputs with no reflection included."*
> *- Director of a local NGO in Lebanon*
> *(Anderson, Brown, & Jean, 2012, p. 41).*

It can be difficult to disclose and discuss failures in a world where nonprofits, international aid, and development are all deeply analyzed and frequently criticized. We are working during a time when some donors give based on interests and compassion – trusting that donation dollars will be well spent – while others are more restricted or skeptical. An increased scrutiny of international aid and development is an opportunity to rethink our operating models. Are we truly working in the most meaningful and impactful ways possible?

Learning from our failures can be the strongest catalyst to change in order to do better (Giang, 2015). When we choose to ignore our failures, we diminish our effectiveness and undermine our work. And it happens all too often. Indeed, hiding failure in the NGO world is, "an ugly dishonesty that runs through almost all aid work, a painful underbelly to the very obvious idealism and good intentions" (Bunting, 2011, para. 5).

However, many NGOs find themselves stuck between competing demands for time and resources as well as between measures of perfunctory versus constructive evaluation. Externally, NGOs are often simplistically rated on the breakdown of their work, or what percentage of their time or money is spent on major expenditure categories like administration, fundraising, and programming. Internally, the definitions by which they frequently define success or failure have stayed static and unyielding to community-specific perspectives and changing landscapes. NGOs often both complain about and yield to simply having to "check the boxes" in order to fulfill stakeholder needs. This status quo, perpetuated by a variety of factors and players in the nonprofit sector, has played a large part in the stagnation of much of the development and aid sectors as well as in the growing frustration of many communities, nonprofit members/staff, and philanthropists.

In evaluating programs and impact, distinctions between success and failure are only important if they can be accurately and directly utilized toward tangible improvement. Often, the way an organization defines success or failure is more a reflection of the NGO or donor priorities rather than those of the community. As just one example, in an effort to collect stories from program participants (to meet the never-ending, relentless demands to be "storytellers"), NGOs tend to gear questions (and thus, listening) toward what they would like or need to hear instead of toward being truly investigatory. The practice of consistently asking questions based on the premise that programs are strong and effective may result in never realizing that that same premise, intended as building blocks for a house, could, in actuality, be built on sand. Current research and our collective track record amongst NGOs demand a paradigm shift in how we view and share our definitions of success and failure throughout the entire NGO stakeholder network – we must put communities first and foremost.

At the recent American Anthropological Association Annual Meeting, emBOLDen Alliances had the opportunity to lead a session titled "Redefining Successes and Failures" for a group of NGO leaders, anthropologists, and ethnographers. The session sought to reflect on definitions of success and failure as well as to highlight how a paradigm shift is needed across the NGO spectrum in order to meaningfully increase the impact of service. During the presentation, we cited Dr. Nigel Fisher, former U.N. Humanitarian Coordinator for Haiti, who said: "Haiti [for example] was littered with the skeletons of 'successful' aid projects" (personal communication, 2015). We use this reference with peers and partners, as well as within emBOLDen Alliances, to prompt each of us to think deeply about this truth and ask the following questions:

· What have our past lessons taught us?
· How do we define "success"? Who is defining it?
· What are our barriers to fundamental change?

In the book *Time to Listen: Hearing People on the Receiving End of International Aid*, an international NGO project manager explains:

The phrase "paradigm shift" is scary for many people. It calls into question everything they are doing and they think they have to start from scratch, relearn everything...[when], in fact, it is precisely the hard-won experience that prompts the shift. (Anderson et al., 2012, p. 136)

The book – an excellent resource that is based on conversations in 20 countries with over 6,000 individuals, 125 organizations, and 150 donors (Anderson et al., 2012, p. ii) – summarizes that:

1) international aid is positive and appreciated;

2) assistance as it is currently provided is falling short of its intent;
3) the way that aid is provided must change significantly if it is to become an effective tool in support of positive economic, social, and political change; and
4) these changes are possible (Anderson et al., 2012).

These findings offer us a wonderful opportunity to reflect on and change both our individual and our organizational or institutional practices, and thus, the paradigm itself. For nonprofits and international aid to deliver on the promise of supporting "positive economic, social, and political change" (Anderson et al., 2012, p. 2), we must:

· Identify the basic terms we are using to define this support
· Ask from whose perspective are these terms currently being defined
· Reevaluate from whose perspective should they be
· Re-identify how each of us can lead that change

Utilizing a combination of common sense, history, and in-depth working experience with locally-based organizations, emBOLDen Alliances defines success and failure in collaboration with community partners. We know that a deep and continuing conversation, starting at the beginning stages of any intervention, is necessary to ensure that the definitions of success and failure are adequately aligned with local priorities. Not only do we employ intentional listening with every partner organization in order to build for success or recognize failure, but we also advocate for the universal adoption of this critical process.

Can a measure of listening and collaborative definitions of success and failure with communities drive the paradigm shift that international aid so clearly requires? Consider the following: What if each of us rated the organization we choose to support (and the projects we're involved in) on *the percentage of time spent listening* as a component of the criteria we use to guide our support and donations? What if NGOs included metrics on *listening* as a part of their evaluation of success?

Compassion alone is not enough. We must strive to constructively and collaboratively define success and failure, and we must integrate a deep and ongoing process of listening to the communities with whom we work. This is how we collectively drive a paradigm shift in international aid toward real impact. We must let go of stagnant and skewed premises that dictate our measures of success and failure. Through this, we can actually realize the true betterment of communities as they define betterment for themselves and achieve more meaningful, durable impact.

How Can I Help?

Having examined the current status of international aid and having determined a new path forward to shift the paradigm overall, we now turn our attention to how an individual can identify and direct change on a personal level.

How many times have you read the words, "Lather, rinse, repeat," on the back of a shampoo bottle? How many times have you skipped that last step, either because you know it's a waste of shampoo and water or for myriad other valid reasons? According to the Urban Dictionary, those three words are defined and used in everyday parlance to signify "mindlessly repeating past patterns or behaviors without critical thought" (Urban Dictionary, 2013).

However, what if we looked at those simple words differently – as an opportunity for thoughtful, critical analyses? What does that look like? How can this simple examination help us to find our way in this shared global humanity? How can it help each of us to define where to best direct our compassion? Try: *Listen. Act. Repeat.*

You may have awakened one morning to the horrible news of the 7.8 magnitude earthquake in Nepal on April 25, 2016 (Shrestha, 2016, para. 2), or to the news of a community in your own state broken down by senseless violence, or to the news of the devastating tsunami on December 26, 2004 (UNHCR, 2004, para. 1). As you heard about the devastation, perhaps you were touched in your core. Perhaps you hurt for other humans who suffered. If so, you likely began to listen attentively and started to think: "What can I do to help?"

These moments of human compassion can be of the utmost authenticity and a true indication that we are all unified on this planet. These moments remind us that we all breathe air, that we all bleed red, and that we all have the capacity to love. In addition, in that moment of wanting to help, we are reminded that human instinct is to reach out and help one another. So, now what? What do you actually do? Where do you turn? This is where the listening becomes even more important – no, critical.

Listen to yourself. No one else can decide what you should do or how you can best help another person. Take an honest inventory of your resources and your skills. Do you have money to donate to aid organizations or to support the effort? If so, thoroughly research those organizations to find those that most align with your values and that have the solid experience and programming to deserve your investment.

Do you have time or necessary skills? How much time can you give, and in what capacity are you willing to serve? What if you arrive in the target community as a skilled physician, but what is really needed is someone to help offload shipments of supplies? Are you able to roll up your sleeves and dive in?

Listen to those immediately around you. Chances are, you have friends and family who also want to help in whatever ways they can. Can you build a project, large or small, to help the affected community from where you are? Can you build awareness on social media or in other ways to inspire others?

In other words, are there ways in which you can bring compassion together constructively so that we are united in strength, rather than paralyzed in despair? What is your own community saying and why? How will your actions influence and affect those immediately around you? For example, deciding to work in West Africa for the Ebola crisis requires careful consideration of how to manage a 21-day return quarantine, especially in the context of family or work responsibilities.

Listen to those outside your circle. Where will you be most helpful, or where might you become a liability? After Typhoon Haiyan, the Government of the Philippines requested that all assistance teams arriving carry their own supplies, food, and water so as to reserve the limited resources in communities for their own community members (Hall, 2015).

Would you help most effectively by jumping on a plane and traveling to the target community because you have the best experience, skills, and resources and are completely physically and mentally prepared? Or, might you best assist in your own city by helping immigrant families from the affected country who may have lost loved ones in the event?

Act with these thoughts in mind. Then, Repeat. Go back to Listening and never be far from it. Only through iterating, listening, trying, failing, succeeding, and iterating again can we hope to find the "right" ways forward.

Remember, all of our ripples, both positive and negative, travel far. We all strive to make them as positive as we can. In the spirit of our mission at emBOLDen Alliances, the positive translation of compassion (which is an ever-renewable resource) into maximum positive impact creates durable change for communities globally.

> *One of the sayings in our country is Ubuntu – the essence of being human. Ubuntu speaks particularly about the fact that you can't exist as a human being in isolation. It speaks about our interconnectedness. You can't be human all by yourself, and when you have this quality – Ubuntu – you are known for your generosity. We think of ourselves far too frequently as just individuals, separated from one another, whereas you are connected and what you do affects the whole world. When you do well, it spreads out; it is for the whole of humanity. (Harees, 2012)*
> *– Archbishop Desmond Tutu (The South African Ubuntu Foundation, 2011)*

It turns out you can learn life lessons about turning compassion into action from everyday objects. Even a shampoo bottle.

Teamwork

> *"It is better to lead from behind and to put others in front, especially when you celebrate victory when nice things occur. You take the front line when there is danger. Then people will appreciate your leadership." (Hung, 2013)*
> -Nelson Mandela

By using the power of individual compassion and action as building blocks for larger, consolidated efforts, we can effect widespread, meaningful, and durable impact, particularly when efforts are not only well-intentioned, but also well-led and thoughtfully designed and implemented. In business management, much has been written about the concept of leading from behind. As expected, there is a lot of debate and discussion surrounding the usage (and misusage) of the concept. But why do we talk about this so much more in the world of for-profit business than in the world of international nonprofits and humanitarian response?

Sophie Johnson (n.d.) states in her piece, *The Theory of Leading from Behind*, "…since leading from behind promotes cooperative initiatives from within teams, this style of leadership can be a good fit for businesses dedicated to working for the common good" (para. 5). Isn't it desirable and critical to fully integrate this methodology into the world of humanitarian assistance, specifically in terms of engaging donors, delivering programs, reporting on successes and failures, and evaluating actions?

emBOLDen Alliances' executive director witnessed an event when working on earthquake response in Nepal that simultaneously bothered and inspired her. This event gave her pause about the structure and expectations of donors, international aid, NGOs, and emBOLDen itself.

Amid the aftermath of the April 2015 Nepal Earthquake, a young Nepalese man worked tirelessly to source, collect, and deliver food, flashlights, blankets, and shelter supplies to his community and its surrounding villages. He arranged multiple deliveries to these villages for many days, beginning within 48 hours post-earthquake. During one delivery, the young Nepalese man encountered an international NGO director. The NGO director heard the young man's story and immediately saw an opportunity for his own organization. Unbeknownst to the Nepalese man, the NGO director was quickly nearing the end of his time in Nepal and was feeling the pressures of not having delivered sufficient work to satisfy his donors.

The NGO director offered to pay for transportation of the Nepalese man's goods on the condition that someone of his choosing would wear his NGO's shirt and logo, accompany the items to the delivery point, shoot video, and take photos. The director was completely unaware that the person he chose did not speak Nepali or the local language of the village, had never been to those villages before, and had not been involved in any of the collections or prior deliveries of items. This individual was now going to be the "poster" person for this aid effort. What the director cared about most, it would seem, was logo placement and marketing.

Unfortunately, this type of situation is all too frequently the image of international, nonprofit work. While the upside of this situation is undeniable (the goods were delivered), it is inappropriate that the emphasis is on the organization's general "need" to "plant its flag" through photographs littered with logos for the sake of accountability in the name of doing good.

The book *Time to Listen: Hearing People on the Receiving End of International Aid* involved over 6,000 conversations globally in order to understand the long-term effects of international aid efforts on communities (Anderson et al., 2012, p. 1). Many respondents "believe aid providers depend on the recipients' 'needs' because responding to these needs justifies the providers' existence and work" (Anderson et al., 2012, p.2).

In response to this, we should instead prioritized the characteristics of those who lead from the middle and from behind to guide principled action, team building, and innovation. *Lead from the Middle: The 9 New, New Leadership Principles* (Mertz, 2011) discusses the following approaches:

· Facilitate open and honest debates
· Listen mindfully
· Set clear goals but be flexible
· Be measurably accountable
· Fail valuably
· Learn relentlessly
· Give 100% real action
· Lead from within—with soul

Aren't these principles what we ultimately value the most in an NGO that delivers assistance to those in need? *Lead from the Middle* also states, "[i]t is about being in the middle of it, not directing, not dictating, and not doing it all" (Mertz, 2011, para. 12). International NGOs cannot do it all, nor should we expect to, particularly when community partners are already doing so much and can use support that is given without the risk of being overrun.

So, at every instant in humanitarian assistance and international development, can we fundamentally shift our paradigm to one that values and promotes an organization's ability to support local efforts, local networks, and local organizations rather than its temptation to stamp a logo, take photos, and wave goodbye? Perhaps we would all better serve communities by taking a few steps back and lead from the middle and/or behind.

These findings offer us the opportunity to reflect on and change our practice, and thus, the paradigm. For international aid to deliver on the promise of supporting "positive economic, social, and political change" (Anderson et al., 2012, p. 2), we must reevaluate the basic terms we use to define success and failure as well as our roles and responsibilities as students, donors, community members, emergency responders, and global citizens.

Compassion alone is not enough. However, compassion can be exponentially transformative when coupled with the power and practice of understanding and redefining failure, knowing ourselves and listening, translating compassion into meaningful impact, and cultivating thoughtful, mindful leaders.

References

Anderson, M.B., Brown, D. and Jean, I. (2012). *Time to listen: Hearing people on the receiving end of international aid.* Cambridge, Massachusetts: CDA Collaborative Learning Projects.

Barrington, D., and Tufa, T. (2014, April). *Why NGOs need to admit failure.* Retrieved from http://www.whydev.org/why-ngos-need-to-admit-failure/.

Bunting, M. (2011, January). NGO hopes to benefit from failure. *The Guardian.* Retrieved from https://www.theguardian.com/global-development/poverty-matters/2011/jan/17/ngos-failure-mistakes-learn-encourage.

Giang, V. (2015, January). The skills you need to make failure productive. *Fast Company.* Retrieved from https://www.fastcompany.com/3040357/hit-the-ground-running/the-skills-you-need-to-make-failure-productive.

Hall, J. (2015). Typhoon Haiyan: Lessons from the Response and How to Prepare for the Future. In *Humanitarian exchange, special feature: the typhoon haiyan response.* Retrieved from http://odihpn.org/wp-content/uploads/2015/01/HE_63_new_web2_.pdf.

Harees, L. (2012). The Mirage of dignity on the highways of human 'progress': The bystander's perspective. Bloomington, IN: AuthorHouse.

Hung, W. (2013 December 10). *The Words Of Nelson Mandela (1918 – 2013) That Forever Inspire Our World.* Retrieved from http://jetsettimes.com/2013/12/10/nelson-mandela/

Johnson, S. (n.d.). The theory of leading from behind. *Small Business.* Retrieved from http://smallbusiness.chron.com/theory-leading-behind-76457.html.

Mertz, J. (2011, December). Lead from the middle. The 9 new, new leadership principles. *Thin Difference.* Retrieved from https://www.thindifference.com/2011/12/lead-from-the-middle-the-9-new-new-leadership-principles.

Shinagel, M. (n.d.). The paradox of leadership. Retrieved from http://www.dce.harvard.edu/professional/blog/paradox-leadership.

Shrestha, D. (2016, April). A year after Nepal quake, villagers rebuild from the ruins. *UNHCR.* Retrieved from http://www.unhcr.org/news/latest/2016/4/571dc9f86/year-nepal-quake-villagers-rebuild-ruins.html

UNHCR. (2004, December). UNHCR steps up response to Asian tsunami catastrophe. *UNHCR.* Retrieved from http://www.unhcr.org/news/press/2004/12/41d2c9374/unhcr-steps-response-asian-tsunami-catastrophe.html.

Urban Dictionary. (2013, September). Retrieved from http://www.urbandictionary.com/define.php?term=lather%20rinse%20repeat&utm_source=search-action.

van der Zee, B. (2015, October). Less than 2% of humanitarian funds 'go directly to local NGOs'. *The Guardian*. Retrieved from https://www.theguardian.com/global-development-professionals-network/2015/oct/16/less-than-2-of-humanitarian-funds-go-directly-to-local-ngos?CMP=ema-1702&CMP

PART 2

APPROACHES AND CLINICAL SOLUTIONS

CHAPTER 9

Meaningfulworld's Response to a Crisis in Global Trauma and Health

Daria Diakonova-Curtis, Ani Kalayjian, and Loren Toussaint

> *"When one helps another both become stronger."*
> *- Meaningfulworld's Motto*

Introduction

Traumatic events occur throughout the world and can adversely affect the communities that experience these events. Incidents deemed as traumatic can take several forms but are generally considered life-threatening and include natural as well as human-made disasters, such as earthquakes, war, military occupation, and forced relocation. It is well-documented that exposure to traumatic events negatively impacts one's psychological well-being (Kendall-Tackett, 2009; Perry, 2008; Wu, Schairer, Dellor, & Grella, 2010). After experiencing a traumatic event, individuals suffering from post-traumatic stress present with disruptions in sense-making systems, loss of faith, and feelings of anger (Carver, 1998; Frankl, 1962; Park & Ali, 2006). These can develop into syndromes such as depression, anxiety, acute stress disorder, and post-traumatic stress disorder (PTSD) (Deschenie, 2006; Kalayjian & Eugene, 2010a, b; Kessler, Sonnega, Bromet, & Hughes, 1995). Some level of post-traumatic stress is common following a traumatic event; PTSD is one of the most prevalent psychiatric diagnoses given to those who have experienced trauma (Kalayjian, 2010; Lantz & Buchalter, 2005). While both post-traumatic stress and PTSD are associated with decreased psychological well-being, PTSD is characterized as the more severe disorder with long-term outcomes. According to the

Diagnostic and Statistical Manual of Mental Disorders-5th Edition (DSM-5) (American Psychiatric Association, 2013), diagnostic criteria for PTSD include exposure to a traumatic event, after which at least two symptoms from each of three symptom clusters are present: (1) intrusive recollections, (2) avoidant/numbing behavior, and (3) physiological hyperarousal lasting more than one month and causing distress or impairment. (American Psychiatric Association, 2013). When left untreated, PTSD symptoms can become chronic and interfere with one's ability to function adaptively in society (Yehuda, 2002).

Because of their knowledge of the mental processes involved in responding to trauma, psychologists and mental health professionals are in a unique position to take on humanitarian roles. Humanitarian psychology work is an emerging field that makes use of psychologists' skills with the goal of healing communities either through direct services or by training health care workers to perform specific jobs, subsequently increasing access to health care in affected countries (American Psychological Association, 2016). This work is inherently connected to the sustainable development goals outlined by the United Nations (2015) which seek to increase global access to education and health and to establish peace, justice, and strong institutions throughout the world.

The work of one non-profit organization, the Association for Trauma Outreach & Prevention (ATOP) Meaningfulworld, provides an example of humanitarian action applied to global communities affected by trauma. It was founded in 1990 and is affiliated with the United Nations Department of Public Information. Meaningfulworld has been committed to service of humanity, fostering, healing, instilling peace and justice, and transforming generational pain and suffering. The organization utilizes state-of-the-art scientific theory and peace and consciousness research to promote education and the development of technical skills of mental health professionals, teachers, psychologists, art therapists, nutritionists, alternative medicine practitioners, clergy, nurses, mediators, interfaith ministers, and lay persons working in communities affected by trauma. Meaningfulworld's humanitarian outreach programs have transformed the lives of over a million people in over 46 countries in seven regions: Africa, Asia, North and South America, the Caribbean, Europe, the Middle East, and the Caucuses. This chapter will describe Meaningfulworld's approach to promoting health in communities affected by trauma and examine humanitarian outreach teams' work in Armenia, a country that has suffered from both a sizeable natural disaster and continuous human-made conflict with neighboring countries.

Approach to Humanitarian Action

The primary focus of Meaningfulworld is to transform trauma globally and promote healing through increased empowerment, emotional intelligence, inner peace, well-being, and harmony. Meaningfulworld's mission is to help to develop a meaningful, peaceful, and just world where everyone can enjoy good health on mind-body-eco-spirit levels. Meaning, peace, and justice are nurtured through a process of learning, reflection, mindfulness, and transforming old habits through new and integrated experiences with a sense of responsibility. This is facilitated by healthy relationships that foster honest and open communication, insight into forgiveness, love and spiritual connection, non-violent communication, compassion, empathy, and active collaborations. The ultimate goal is to promote a global society guided by love, peace, passion, and meaning (www.Meaningfulworld.com).

Meaningfulworld's view is that recovery following trauma is achieved primarily through two psychological processes: meaning-making and forgiveness. The ability to find meaning in the traumatic event and cultivate a sense of purpose in one's life has been described as one of the central components to healing from disasters (Frankl, 1962; Kalayjian & Eugene, 2010a,b). Meaning-making has been linked to better adjustment following stressful life events (Collie & Long, 2005; Skaggs & Baron, 2006) and lower severity of post-traumatic symptoms (Kalayjian, Shigemoto, & Patel, 2010). Those who are able to process and make personal sense of often incomprehensible and atrocious events have been shown to experience healing following a trauma.

Similarly, forgiveness has been identified as a way of coping with the effects of perpetrated, human-made trauma (Chapman, 2007; Kalayjian, 2010; Schaefer, Blazer, & Koenig, 2008; Staub, Pearlman, Gubin, & Hagengimana, 2005; Worthington, 2006), including events that occur in post-conflict societies (Swart, Turner, Hewstone, & Voci, 2011). Forgiveness is described as shifting from the automatic, ego reaction of hitting back (revenge, hurting back) to a conscious, empathic response that takes into account that the perpetrator is also human and is perhaps not acting mindfully (Kalayjian, 2010). This shift increases one's sense of peace and decreases incidents of anger, retaliation, and depression.

Furthermore, according to Frankl's theory (1962), forgiveness plays an important role in helping one achieve a sense of meaning regarding the traumatic event. Because forgiveness involves an internal shift from holding on to negative emotions (e.g., anger or shame) to experiencing positive states (e.g., a sense of calmness) (Berry, Worthington, O'Connor, Parrott, & Wade, 2005), it may be related to how one makes sense of the adverse event and how much one is affected by the post-traumatic symptoms afterwards. Forgiveness can decrease vengeful rumination, self-hate, and fearfulness following a transgression, which may in turn create the internal space needed to process the event and generate a sense of meaning about it. In other words, the more one has forgiven oneself and others for the event, the easier it may be to begin to make sense of it and thus find relief from post-traumatic stress (Toussaint, Kalayjian, & Diakonova-Curtis, in press).

Meaningfulworld provides outreach programs that consist of community building and data collection workshops that progress in nine phases: (1) pre-assessment, (2) assessment, (3) analysis, (4) community diagnosis, (5) planning, (6) implementation, (7) evaluation, (8) remodification, and (9) dissemination. This chapter will explain each of the nine phases and provide illustrations of Meaningfulworld's humanitarian work in Armenia as a case example.

Nine Phases of Global Humanitarian Work

Phase I: Pre-Assessment

This phase occurs immediately prior to journeying to the disaster community. Ideally, pre-assessment begins immediately after the disaster and continues through the onset of the assessment phase. Its primary goal is to familiarize humanitarians with the survivor community and to determine the extent of the damage. It is also important to determine what help is already offered, to consider how other professionals are diagnosing the community's needs, and to avoid duplicating other efforts.

The pre-assessment typically covers five critical areas. First, to understand the survivor community, helpers must learn about its characteristics, including geographic size of the region, history of both natural and human-made disasters in the region, ethnic background and nationalities of residents, and common religious or spiritual beliefs of the area. They must not only research by reading academic sources and recent media, but also by speaking with individuals who are familiar with and originally from the community.

Second, one must understand the characteristics of the disaster at hand. This includes the extent of the physical damage and casualties as well as the extent of infrastructure destruction – particularly its effect on housing, transportation, and communication systems, and also whether it calls for evacuation. Third, issues of disaster relief to that community are pre-assessed. These might include responses to the disaster on community, national, and international levels, the extent of assistance to the surviving community, and any political and economic issues affecting progress. Fourth, one should examine the pre-disaster sociopolitical and economic climates, as they directly influence the resources available to the survivor community. Finally, whenever facing unanticipated change, global mental health professionals need to consider the community's resistance to this change, to determine how to mobilize the community, and to utilize this resistance to benefit the affected community.

Phase II: Assessment

Assessment is the second phase in humanitarian outreach and provides a foundation for community diagnosis, planning, and implementation. This phase involves the collection, validation, and organization of data. Steps include comparing data for accuracy and clustering them into groups to identify patterns of health and illness. In this stage, information about the actual impact of the disaster is gathered firsthand and on-site. This phase may range from one day to one month in duration. A total assessment involves all areas of the surviving community: physical, psychological, sexual, economic, political, technological, cultural, and spiritual. Due to time limitations and the chaotic situation in disaster environments, it is essential to focus on the psychological assessment of survivors. It is also important to be familiar with likely responses during post-disaster community assessment. Emotional responses may include denial, sadness/weeping, anger/restlessness, or acceptance/hopefulness.

Phase III: Analysis

The analysis phase follows the pre-assessment and assessment sequentially. Data from the pre-assessment are used as a theoretical basis for clustering and organizing data regarding the surviving community and the overall environment. Data from the assessment are examined to identify the specific community strengths and needs, available and desirable resources, and the community's overall readiness and motivation for change.

Phase IV: Community Diagnosis

A "community diagnosis" is a statement describing the community's response to the disaster. Diagnoses are utilized as classifications to express conclusions based on the data gathered in the pre-assessment, assessment and analysis phases. Diagnoses are generally broad labels used by health professionals to help communities change and improve. They are also utilized to assist professionals in their planning and implementations of care.

Phase V: Planning

Planning is the prioritization of needs and organization of resources for individuals and their community. Planning results in the implementation process and is comprised of two components: short-term and long-term. Short-terms goals are developed to address the acute needs of the community. Long-term goals address the rehabilitation, education, and training needs of the community. These begin after the completion of the short-term goals and continue as long as necessary.

Phase IV: Implementation

Implementation is the stage in which the plan is put into effect. It is based on the specific and unique needs of individuals and their community. Ideally, the sooner the therapeutic implementation, the sooner the community will return to its pre-disaster state of equilibrium.

One of the ways that Meaningfulworld accomplishes its implementation goals is by utilizing the 7-step Integrative Healing Model through which traumatic experiences are assessed, identified, explored, described, released, processed, and eventually reintegrated. The model provides the basis of all humanitarian outreach programs (Kalayjian, 2002; Kalayjian & Sofletea, 2012). The model builds from the integration of multiple theories including: psychodynamic (Freud, 1910), interpersonal (Sullivan, 1953), existential and humanistic (Frankl, 1962), electromagnetic field balancing (Dubro & Lapierre, 2002), forgiveness and reconciliation (Kalayjian & Paloutzian, 2010), learning theory, flower essences, essential oils, physical release (van der Kolk, 1993), and Soul-Surfing (Kalayjian, 2015), prayers, and meditation. The seven steps of the model include: 1) assessing levels of distress, disagreement, or conflict, 2) encouraging expression of feelings, 3) providing empathy and validation, 4) encouraging discovery and expression of meaning, 5) providing information, 6) instilling eco-centered healing, and 7) learning breathing, movement-centered healing, and meditation. Each step of the model is expanded below.

The 7-Step Integrative Healing Model (The BioPsychosocial and Eco-Spiritual Model)
1) Assess Levels of Post-Traumatic Stress: Community residents are given the Harvard Trauma Questionnaire to determine severity of trauma, followed by questionnaires on forgiveness and meaning-making to indicate how these practices impact levels of traumatic stress. When completing questionnaires, community residents are asked to identify their feelings, measured on a scale of 0-10, with 10 indicating severe distress.
2) Encourage Expression of Feelings: When working with community survivors in group settings, participants are encouraged to express their feelings in the "here and now" in relation to the disaster they have experienced. Release of feelings is seen as therapeutic, and participants are told that sharing them may "help get distress off our chest, release the grip that the trauma has on us, and let it go."
3) Provide Empathy and Validation: Survivors' feelings are validated by group leaders using statements such as, "It makes sense that you are feeling this way." Leaders also share information about how

other survivors from around the world have coped during disasters. Intentional therapeutic touch, such as holding a survivor's hand, is also used, and the fact that the survivor may be feeling grief, fear, frustration, or anger is recognized. Participants are also encouraged to express positive feelings, such as joy due to their survival. When this model is practiced individually (not in a group setting), the survivor is encouraged to find an empathic and non-judgmental person with whom to share their trauma and from whom to receive support.

4) Encourage Discovery and Expression of Meaning: Survivors are asked, "What lessons, meaning, or positive associations might have you discovered as a result of this disaster?" This question is based on Viktor Frankl's logotherapeutic principle that there could be a positive meaning discovered in the worst catastrophe.

5) Provide and Gather Information: Practical tools and information are given on how to use the systematic desensitization process. The importance of preparation for natural disasters and mindfulness for human-made traumas is also reinforced. Information regarding forgiveness and self-healing is shared.

6) Eco-Centered Processing: Practical tools are shared to connect with Mother Earth. Group leaders guide discussions and exercises regarding environmental/global connections. The group considers ways to care for one's environment and ways to be mindful of our impact on the environment and of the environment's impact on humankind. At this point, Mother Earth is presented as a means to heal oneself and others through connecting with the sunrise and sunset, connecting with trees and flowers, and merging oneself in the ocean or sea for cleansing the body and soul. Flower remedies and flower essences are also used to minimize the negative impact of trauma and help regain a sense of self.

7) Breath Work, Movement Exercises, and Meditation: Breath is used as a natural medicine and healing tool. Since no one can control nature, others, or what happens outside of oneself, survivors are assisted in controlling how they respond to the disaster. Survivors are instructed on how to release fear, uncertainty, and resentments. They are also instructed on how to use breath towards self-empowerment and in order to engender gratitude, compassion, faith, strength, and forgiveness in response to disasters. Breath work is combined with a series of physical movements that focus on each energy center, its color vibration, and its use and benefit while balancing and energizing each center with affirmations specifically designed for each center. This combination of

movement, color identification, evaluation of the physical area, affirmation, and breath is called *Soul-Surfing*.

Phase VII: Evaluation

During the evaluation phase, the progress and effectiveness of the care provided are determined. In this phase, communication with several layers of the community is necessary to investigate the effectiveness of the plan. Examples of the people that may be involved in the evaluation phase include those directly affected by the disaster, their families, and providers of therapeutic care (including physicians, teachers, community leaders, and leaders of volunteer organizations, government officials, armed forces, and rescue workers).

Phase VIII: Remodification

Remodification is the process of tailoring the plan specifically to fit the needs of the survivor community. In this phase, the following steps may be taken: identifying areas of deficit in the original plan, prioritizing areas of community needs, and identifying new interventions. This is a circular process involving implementation and continuous remodification.

Phase IX: Dissemination and Education

Education and information are essential to providing support to survivors and the professionals working in the surviving community. Both survivors and caregivers value information as an important method by which to cope with disasters. Sharing information could occur on several levels, including formal and informal education, training, conferences, workshops, and networking. It is important to remember that training materials must be in the language of the community, and the reading level of the materials must be congruent to the levels reflected in the community. Finally, acknowledging and celebrating the work of caregivers and relief workers in the community is an essential step in the process of humanitarian outreach.

Case Example of Meaningfulworld's Humanitarian Outreach: Armenia

Cultural Context

Armenia is a small country situated in the mountainous Southern Caucasus region. In the last 25-30 years, Armenia has endured political conflicts from its larger neighbors, refugee migrations, and economic instability. From 1895-1923, the Armenia Nation was brought to the brink of annihilation – almost two million Armenians (more than half the Armenian population) were massacred by the Ottoman Turkish rulers

(Kupelian, Kalayjian, & Kassabian, 1998, p. 192). To this day, the genocide is denied by the current Turkish government. This denial causes tremendous feelings of anger and resentment with no reparation or resolution for many Armenians (Kalayjian, 1991a).

Until 1991, Armenia and several surrounding countries (e.g., Azerbaijan) were part of the Soviet Union, a regime that controlled the economies of its states and created territories according to its political plan, thus dividing land and instigating territorial conflicts (Kalayjian, 1995; Kalayjian, Shigemoto, & Patel, 2010). An example of such territorial conflict is the dispute over the region of Karapagh, which was an Armenian land given to the Azeris in 1923 as part of Stalin's "Divide and Conquer" campaign (Ware, 1998). After the collapse of the Soviet Union, the smaller countries were unable to form political and economic infrastructures quickly enough to deal effectively with the aftermath of such a major overhaul (World Bank Group, 2014). As the smaller countries gained independence, hundreds of thousands of Armenians were forced to flee from Azerbaijan and were displaced in Armenia's northern region. The conflict between Armenia and Azerbaijan over the Artsakh territory has led to more than 20,000 casualties, large numbers of refugees moving away from both Armenia and Azerbaijan, and expulsions of ethnic Armenians and Azeris from both sides (Geneva Academy of International Humanitarian Law and Human Rights, 2012, para. 1). People born during this decade were born into a country whose government was unable to deal with the economic burden of these events (World Bank Group, 2014).

During the 2000s, Armenia saw an increase in refugees due to wars occurring in nearby Syria and Iraq. The settling of refugees in this contested territory may have led to political clashes and an increase in violence between neighboring communities. The economic status of Armenia continues to be unstable, as both native and refugee communities compete for limited resources. When a country experiences an economic crisis, the population's psychological well-being oftentimes worsens because people are more likely to have feelings of anger, desperation, uncertainty, anxiety, depression, and suicidal ideation (Lee et al., 2010; Hong, Knapp, & McGuire, 2013). The traumatic events that Armenians have experienced include both a natural disaster (the earthquake) and human-made violence (conflict with neighboring countries, and the fighting for resources among several territories and factions).

Meaningfulworld has a long history of working in Armenia. It organized humanitarian outreach programs following the 1988 earthquake and also lead multiple follow-up missions and projects. On Wednesday, December 7, 1988, at 11:41 AM, a devastating earthquake shook the Republic of Armenia (Soviet Armenia) for roughly 20 seconds (Wood, Berrill, Gillon, & North, 1993, p. 256). This catastrophic destruction occurred in a zone where several plates of the earth's surface converge, a geological situation which occasionally results in devastating consequences when movement occurs (Wood et al., 1993, p. 253). Although the quake did not come as a total surprise to American and Soviet experts in the field, the community experienced the quake as traumatic due to gross unpreparedness and lack of emergency and evacuation plans (Fein, 1988a, para. 4-10). Measuring 6.8 on the Richter scale, the quake occurred in an area highly vulnerable to seismic activity (Cisternas et al., 1989, p. 675). It destroyed two-thirds of Leninakan, Armenia's second-largest city (now Gumri, population about 300,000), half of Kirovakan (now Vanatzor, population 150,000), and obliterated Spitak, the epicenter (a town of about 30,000) (Fein, 1988a, para. 3). It also destroyed 200 homes and heavily damaged 400 homes along the Turkish border (Fein, 1988a, para. 9). Although the Soviet authorities did not release official statistics (Fein, 1988b, para. 8), it is estimated that nearly half a million (one sixth of the Armenian population) were left homeless, many more were handicapped, and many children were orphaned (Fein, 1988b, para. 1; Wood et al., p. 281).

Most recently, humanitarian outreach has included continuous follow-up with the post-earthquake community, efforts with Armenians affected by the war in Iraq, the war in Syria, and the conflict with Azerbaijan, and work with those presenting with generational trauma from the 1915 Ottoman Turkish Genocide of Armenians. Next, we provide illustrations of the team's work in Armenia, which was originally organized to heal the community after the 1988 earthquake and which follows the nine phases as they pertain to providing outreach in mental health.

Pre-Assessment

The original pre-assessment of the community in Armenia after the earthquake revealed that, while most earthquakes are predicted, this event was largely unanticipated by the surviving community. It impacted a significant segment of the local population and caused tremendous property damage. All hospitals, schools, churches, and community centers were severely damaged or destroyed. Survivors were forced to head for the capital, Yerevan, to receive emergency medical care. This meant traveling four to six hours in extremely crowded conditions and on roads that were partially destroyed by the quake. In the earthquake region, survivors had intact community outlets through which to seek support. This made relocation a necessity and created additional stress and trauma. Assistance poured in from around the world, but Armenia's airport was not equipped to deal with such volume, and therefore many planes could not land. The planes that were able to land unloaded their goods directly onto the runway. Much of the assistance that went through Moscow did not make it to

Armenia in its entirety. This lasted until Armenian volunteer organizations took over the distribution and management of the funds and goods. Additionally, during the ten months preceding the quake, Armenia had been experiencing sociopolitical tension and was economically drained due to the conflict with neighboring Azerbaijan over Nagorno-Karabagh.

It became clear that the emphasis had been placed on the physical and material needs of the survivor community. Countries and organizations from around the world responded to the quake with offers of aid ranging from volunteer orthopedic surgeons to equipment designed to detect signs of life under rubble. All the material assistance notwithstanding, it was apparent that no one was addressing the mental health and emotional needs of the survivor community.

Assessment

Psychological and behavioral symptoms were first assessed systematically six to eight weeks after the earthquake. Over two hundred adults and two hundred adolescents and children constituted the assessment sample. Several layers of the community were observed in their natural environments. For example, school-aged children and adolescents were observed in their classrooms during recess, in hospitals, in shelters, or in their homes; adults were observed at their work places (if they were still employed), in hospitals, at government shelters, or at the homes of their relatives. Geographically, emphasis was placed on the quake zone: Leninakan, Kirovakan, Spitak, and several villages that were en route to the larger cities.

The most common psychological symptoms in children after the quake were separation anxiety (manifested as excessive clinging to parents or significant others, particularly at night, refusing to sleep or be left alone, or refusing to go to school) regressive behavior (such as thumb-sucking, enuresis or clinging behaviors, hyperactivity, withdrawal, inability to concentrate) somatic complaints (i.e., stomach ache, headache, joint aches, etc.), and sleep disturbances (i.e., bad dreams, frequent awakenings, or difficulty falling asleep). Adolescents manifested withdrawal, anger and increased aggression, regression, sleep disturbances and nightmares, increased daydreaming, inability to concentrate, irritability, and poor grades in the courses in which they excelled prior to the disaster. Adults most commonly presented with uncertainty and fear, anger, feelings of tension, feeling on-edge and jumpy, loss of appetite, sleep disturbances and nightmares, loss of interest or inability to engage in sexual activities, withdrawal, loss of concentration, inability to make decisions, and aggression turned inward or outward.

When survivors were asked an open-ended question eliciting the meaning they had attributed to the earthquake, 20% attributed a positive value and meaning to the disaster (Kalayjian, 1991b). This is congruent with Quarantelli's (1985) notion that disaster survivors are primarily attempting to cope with the meaning of the trauma and with Frankl's (1978) assertion that meaning is available under any condition, even the worst conceivable one. This is somewhat contrary to Figley's (1985) belief that one of the fundamental questions a victim needs to answer to become a survivor is "Why did it happen?" Findings from the outreach indicated that type of question forced the survivor to remain in the past, in the role of a victim, without a rational or satisfactory answer. It also left the survivor filled with feelings of self-induced guilt and often trapped in a cycle of destructive behavior. Viktor Frankl, the author of *Man's Search for Meaning*, labeled this type of "why" question as the "wrong question" (personal communication, June 28, 1991). Any question that begins with "why" presumes that there is a responsible party. In this case, it was the natural disaster. Survivors who were preoccupied with the "why" were dissatisfied with the scientific answer that the plates moved, pressure built up, and finally the tension was released. Findings at the one-year follow-up revealed that earthquake survivors exhibited increased anger and helplessness, consumption of alcohol, and reports of violence in the family (Kalayjian, 1994). This may have been partially due to the ongoing trauma from the conflict with Azerbaijan, the country's struggle for democracy and independence, or economic hardship.

Survivors who attributed a positive meaning focused instead on the present moment and the meaningful experiences they had gained by helping or receiving help from one another and from the world. As one survivor stated, "Look at how the world has come to help us, the closed Soviet system has opened its doors, there is more communication, caring, and sharing."

Community Diagnoses

After analyzing data from the assessment instruments following the quake, findings revealed that 86% of the children, 83% of adolescents, and 81% of adults met criteria for PTSD. Further, 80% of teachers and over 79% of leaders and government officials in Leninakan were survivors themselves. Eighty percent of the mental health professionals from the quake zone exhibited signs of burnout, and 98% of the survivors in the earthquake zone did not have a mental health professional available to provide care. There was only one community mental health outpatient clinic in Leninakan, and Spitak and some 56 affected villages had no mental health providers or centers.

Planning

Based on the assessment and community diagnoses, the following plan was formulated. The first short-term goal was coordinating humanitarian outreach teams of Armenian-speaking mental health professionals from the U.S., Canada, and Europe to provide direct care for individuals in the community. Fluency in the Armenian language, some knowledge of the culture, and emotional stability were key criteria in the selection of the volunteers. Though the surviving community was fluent in Armenian and Russian, only about 20% of university graduates had a working knowledge of the English language. The second goal was to include a psychiatrist, a psychologist, and a psychiatric nurse or psychiatric social worker in each outreach team. Psychologists in Armenia did not practice psychotherapy and were not permitted to care for individuals (as they held academic appointments and were supervised by the Ministry of Education and not the Ministry of Health). There were a handful of psychotherapists in Yerevan who were psychiatrists with a year of post-psychiatry training, which frequently took place in Moscow or Leningrad (now St. Petersburg), Russia. The third goal was to provide training, role-modeling, and workshops for the mental health professionals working in Armenia. This not only enhanced the sharing of a variety of theoretical perspectives and clinical interventions, but also informed and empowered the volunteers. Long-term goals included continuing to support the post-disaster community (primarily by providing training and workshops for mental health professionals in Armenia regarding trauma and interventions) and working with government officials to establish mental health resources in the community.

Implementation

The original humanitarian outreach was implemented in February 1989, with a six-month follow-up in August 1989. Utilized therapeutic techniques included art therapy, bio-feedback, the coloring storybook, drawings (structured and unstructured), family therapy, group therapy, instruction booklets, logotherapy, meditation, play therapy, pharmacotherapy, and short-term psychotherapy. Any therapeutic modality that could be done in a group format was desirable for the short-term component of the outreach program due to the large number of people affected by the disaster and the limited amount of time. Art therapy was utilized primarily with children and adolescents to facilitate the expressions of feelings. In accordance with primary trauma interventions in disasters, adults were able to tell their stories. This was done through a supportive, personalized, safe, interactive process between individuals in small groups, with a facilitator providing an opportunity to develop clarity and expression of the event and experience.

In addition to the expression of emotions through art or talking, therapeutic work in Armenia included a somatic component where survivors were encouraged to use movement to tell their stories with their bodies and thus notice any physical aspects of trauma. By utilizing movement-based expression, the trauma experiences do not go through the cognitive mind as words, but rather arise from sensations and perceptions. Somatic techniques also included meditation and breathing. Finally, attention was paid to rituals and community ceremonies. The act of making a ritual became healing in itself, as it allowed the community to assign meaning and find closure.

Evaluation

The surviving community was evaluated six months after the earthquake. Interviews with survivors (N = 180) revealed that those who received care by the humanitarian outreach's professional teams were coping more effectively, were less depressed, and scored lower on PTSD assessment instruments (Kalayjian, 1994). In comparison, those survivors who did not receive care from the professional teams continued to express feelings of hopelessness, helplessness, despair, and apathy. Those who did not receive any psychological support continued to exhibit signs of moderate to severe levels of PTSD, thoughts of suicide and homicide, aggressive outbursts, substance abuse, and spousal and child abuse. Meaningfulworld established mobile clinics in vans for the villages and towns, and permanent outpatient clinics were founded in Gumri, Vanatzor, and Spitak.

Overall, after six months, Armenia still struggled to provide adequate care for its surviving community: tents and makeshift sheds constituted basic shelter, air was still polluted with dust due to the rubble, there was no running water in many places for 15 hours a day, and there was no electricity for several hours a day. It was noted by humanitarian teams that only about 50% of the survivors had homes, 30% were in shelters and 20% had relocated to the U.S. or to other parts of what was then the Soviet Union. Less than 15% of the projected construction had been completed in the quake zone (these figures were obtained from personal communications with local officials during the humanitarian outreach follow-up, August 1989). Almost all aid from around the world had subsided, and the conflicts with neighboring countries continued. Therefore, Meaningfulworld has been committed to returning to Armenia in 2017 to maintain its humanitarian efforts, to continue the evaluation process, and to provide healing.

Remodification

In Armenia, according to the team's observations and evaluations, there was a need for at least a 20-year, continued, on-site, clinical intervention program with three groups: the earthquake survivors, refugees from Azerbaijan, and the former government's Communist Party leaders who were expressing feelings of shame, doubt, defeat, resentment, and uncertainty due to the collapse of Soviet Union. When addressing the educational arena in Armenia, it was recommended that a 20-year plan be established for schools in clinical psychology, social work, and nursing, with training programs in interpersonal and behavioral modalities. The American General Benevolent Union and the University of California have founded the American University of Armenia, which opened its doors in the fall of 1991. Future programs could be in the fields of clinical psychology with specialty programs in social work, counseling, and psychiatric nursing.

Continuous Follow-up

More recently, in 2014, the humanitarian outreach team travelled back to Armenia in accordance with its long-term plans to provide continuous care to the post-disaster community. The goals of the outreach were: 1) to train in the 7-Step Integrative Healing Model, 2) to train psychologist to work at Suicide Hotline, 3) to train psychology faculty and students in trauma healing, 4) to help transform Horizontal Violence, 5) to conduct research on the impact of trauma, forgiveness, and meaning-making, 6) to work with refugees from Syria, 7) to work with orphans in children's' centers, 8) to start a Suicide Hotline, and 9) to start Peace & Forgiveness Gardens.

During the outreach, team members provided workshops that targeted professors of psychology at Yerevan State University's Pedagogical Institute Psychological Department, with representatives from The Intra Mental Health Center, the Caucasus Institute of Gestalt and Family Therapy, the Armenia Round Table Foundation, and the State University. In one workshop, close to 30 psychology professors and master's degree students gathered at the Yerevan State Apovian Pedagogical University for a workshop on peace building, conflict transformation, and mindfulness. Participants were enthusiastic, involved, and curious. They asked many questions and shared their feelings and experiences (Steps 2 and 3 of the Healing Model). Five of the participants had read Frankl's Man's Search for Meaning; others participated in a discussion of meaning-making (Step 4 of the Healing Model). Forgiveness was a particularly complex concept to grasp, especially when participants referenced Armenian soldiers being killed daily at the Armenia-Azerbaijan border, and when they referenced conflict that continues regarding the Karapagh region. A few challenging questions arose: "How do we remember while forgiving? Why forgive, if the aggressor would repeat the violence? How do we send love to Turkey and Azerbaijan while they continue oppressing Armenia through blockade and ongoing gun fires?"

The team also conducted a workshop at the State University of Yerevan's Sociology Department. The theme of the workshop was Peace Building, Conflict Transformation, Forgiveness, and Mind-Body-Eco-Spirit Health. Forty third-level students participated with curiosity – they were eager to learn new and integrative healing models. Team members presented an interactive lecture and discussed coping with difficult feelings (i.e., anger) which interfere with peace-making. Participants were led to pledge to peace, and they enthusiastically participated. Also shared was the importance of developing Neighborhood Associations, Peace & Forgiveness Gardens, and Beautification Clubs in their neighbourhood and the university at first, and then in their city, Yerevan (Step 6 of the Healing Model). The majority responded positively to the Chakra Balancing Exercises (Step 7 of the Healing Model). Some students struggled with the body work and said they are not used to exercising. Recommendations to the community included beginning a campaign titled "Armenia is my home," developing an ecological club to bring greater aesthetic awareness, and adopting practices that enhance physical fitness. At the end of the workshop, the majority of participants expressed feelings of peacefulness, relaxation, lightness, awareness, and curiosity or excitement about the new skills and practices. The training ended with the Heart-to-Heart Circle of Gratitude, warm heart-centered hugs, and certificates distribution.

Furthermore, the team conducted a workshop on suicide assessment, intervention, and prevention. Twenty professional psychologists, social workers, teachers, and a few students of psychology gathered at the Armenian Center for Health and Education for this workshop. The workshop emphasized the importance of meaning-making, being open regarding cultural perspectives on suicide (particularly as they pertain to the concepts of shame and humiliation), and motivators like depression, addiction, loss of loved ones, financial status, health, and purpose in life. Appropriate and inappropriate interventions were outlined. In Armenia, the connection to meaning-making in suicide prevention was fairly unfamiliar. Shared recommendations included: starting a suicide hotline, training the police to handle suicidal emergencies, defining suicide as a health problem instead of a moral or religious one, and offering peer support groups for anyone working on a suicide hotline.

The team also travelled to the Civil Society Institute to meet with a group of mothers who had suffered the loss of their sons to snipers in the Azerbaijani conflict. Another training was provided through collaboration with the Minister of Health and the Armenian Red Cross that included close to 50 medical doctors, nurses, social workers, psychologists, and other health care professionals. They discussed the pain and suffering in Armenia following the genocide, the negative impact of the Soviet Regime, the devastating earthquake, the 25-year war with neighboring Azerbaijan, and leadership challenges after the nation's independence.

Finally, the team traveled to Gumri from Yerevan, to the Diramayr Armenian Orphanage (founded in 1991) to work with the orphans, staff, and teachers. Team members met with Sister Arousyag, who outlined the pressing issues that affect the children and staff of the orphanage, and then conducted a 2-hour workshop with close to 80 children, teachers, and staff on peace building, conflict resolution, self-love, forgiveness, healthy communication skills, and the signature Heart-to-Heart Circle of Love and Gratitude. The children also sang.

Meaningfulworld's team members have returned to Armenia for extended periods of time through Fulbright Fellowships, sabbaticals, and other creative modalities. This continues to provide Meaningfulworld with a cadre of experienced and available volunteers to serve as disaster team leaders for future catastrophes. It is the hope of establishing and training humanitarian outreach mental health workers that with the combination of research and extensive field experience, future relief will come expeditiously and effectively, even within the limitations of the political climate.

Conclusion

With the increase in globalization, the concern for health and overall well-being of communities around the world continues to grow among social service and health professionals. This is especially true for psychologists who are uniquely trained to acknowledge and respond to the emotional needs of those affected by disasters. In fact, the field of humanitarian psychology is a growing domain that encompasses helping individuals during critical periods after traumatic events, as well as training professionals in their home countries to respond to the chronic effects of trauma. This points to the growing recognition in the field of mental health of the need to treat post-traumatic stress in disaster areas in order to build and support peace in those communities.

Using some traditional models of providing aid to those who have experienced trauma at the individual level, combined with cross-cultural and systemic perspectives that recognize structural challenges, researchers and clinicians are applying their work to global communities where resources for mental health are limited. Meaningfulworld is one such organization that seeks to alleviate human suffering and build peace by offering individuals tangible skills to process emotion, construct meaningful stories, achieve forgiveness, and alleviate the physical effects of traumatic stress. The model of Meaningfulworld's work in humanitarian outreach described in this chapter offers an example of a way in which mental health professionals can provide aid in areas affected by disaster. By sharing our expertise in humanitarian outreach and mental health, we hope to inspire other health professionals to consider why global health matters and to take a global perspective in order to reach the underserved communities and build peace throughout the world.

We give special gratitude to Karolyn Viviana Velaspegui for her assistance with references, to Marian Weisberg, Kathryn Kaze, Karen Gargaryan, Aramazt Kalayjian, and to all the volunteers of Meaningfulworld Humanitarian Outreach teams from 1989-present.

References

American Psychiatric Association. (2013). *Diagnostic and statistical manual of mental disorders (5th ed)*. Washington, DC: Author.

American Psychological Association. (2016). Humanitarian work psychology. *Monitor on Psychology, 47*(4), 61.

Berry, J. W., Worthington, E. L., O'Connor, L. E., Parrott, L., & Wade, N. G. (2005). Forgiveness, vengeful rumination, and affective traits. *Journal of Personality, 73*(1), 183-225.

Carver, C. S. (1999). Resilience and thriving: Issues and models and linkages. *Journal of Social Issues, 54*, 245-266.

Chapman, A. (2007). Truth commissions and intergroup forgiveness: The case of the South African Truth and Reconciliation Commission. *Peace and Conflict: Journal of Peace Psychology, 13*, 51–69.

Cisternas, A., Philip, H., Bousquet, J. C., Cara, M., Deschamps, A., Dorbath, L., Dorbath, C., Haessler, H., Jimenez, E., Nercessian, A., Rivera, L., Romanowicz, B., Gvishiani, A., Shebalin, N. V., Aptekman, I., Arefiev, S., Borisov, B. A., Gorshkov, A., Graizer, V., Lander, A., Pletnev, K., Rogozhin, A. I., & Tatevossian, R. (1989). The Spitak (Armenia) earthquake of 7 December 1988: Field observations, seismology and tectonics. *Nature, 339*, 675–679. doi:10.1038/339675a0

Collie, K., & Long, B. C. (2005). Considering "meaning" in the context of breast cancer. *Journal of Health Psychology, 10*, 843-853.

Deschenie, T. (2006). Historical trauma: Holocaust victims, American Indians recovering from abuses of the past. *Tribal College Journal, 17*, 8 –11.

Dubro, P. P., & Lapierre, D. P. (2002). *Elegant empowerment: Evolution of consciousness*. Boca Raton, FL: Platinum Publishing House.

Fein, E. (1988a, December 9). Toll out in tens of thousands from quake in Soviet Armenia. *The New York Times, 23.*

Fein, E. (1988b, December 10). Soviet aides say deaths in quake may reach 50,000. *The New York Times.*

Figley, C. R. (1985). *Trauma and its wake.* New York: Brunner/Mazel.

Frankl, V. E. (1962). *Man's search for meaning: An introduction to logotherapy*. Boston: Beacon Press (Original work published in 1946).

Frankl's, V. E. (1978). *The unheard cry for meaning.* New York: Simon & Schuster.

Freud, S. (1910). The origin and development of psychoanalysis. *The American Journal of Psychology, 21*(2), 181-218.

Geneva Academy of International Humanitarian Law and Human Rights. (2012). Azerbaijan: The conflict with Armenia. Retrieved from http://www.geneva-academy.ch/RULAC/current_conflict.php?id_state=18

Hong, J., Knapp, M., & McGuire, A. (2013). Income-related inequalities in the prevalence of depression and suicidal behaviour: A 10-year trend following economic crisis. *World Psychiatry, 10*(1), 40-44. doi: 10.1002/j.2051-5545.2011.tb00012.x

Kalayjian, A. (1991a, October). *Genocide, earthquake, and ethnic turmoil: Multiple traumas of a nation.* Paper presented at the 7th Annual Convention of the International Society for Traumatic Stress Studies, Washington, DC.

Kalayjian, A. (1991b, June). *Meaning in trauma: Impact of the earthquake in Soviet Armenia.* Paper presented at the VIII World Congress of Logotherapy, San Jose, CA.

Kalayjian, A. (1994). Mental health outreach program following the earthquake in Armenia: Utilizing the nursing process in developing and managing the post-natural disaster plan. *Issues in Mental Health Nursing, 15*(6), 533-550.

Kalayjian, A. (1995). *Disaster and mass trauma: Global perspectives on post-disaster mental health management.* Long Branch, NJ: Vista Publishers.

Kalayjian, A. (2002). Biopsychosocial and spiritual treatment of trauma. In R. & S Massey (Editors) *Comprehensive handbook of psychotherapy*, Vol. 3, Interpersonal/humanistic/existential. (pp. 615-637). New York, NY: John Wiley & Sons.

Kalayjian, A. (2010). Forgiveness in spite of denial, revisionism, and injustice. In A. Kalayjian & F. R. Paloutzian (Eds.), *Forgiveness and reconciliation: Psychological pathways to conflict transformation and peace building* (pp. 237–250). New York, NY: Springer Media, LLC.

Kalayjian, A. (2015). 7-step integrative healing model: Biopsychosocial and eco-spiritual model for healing, transforming disputes, conflict transformation, peace building, and forgiveness. Retrieved from www.meaningfulword.com

Kalayjian, A., & Eugene, D. (Eds.). (2010a). *Mass trauma and emotional healing around the world: Rituals and practices for resilience and meaning-making* (Vol. 1). Santa Barbara, CA: ABC-CLIO, LLC.

Kalayjian, A., & Eugene, D. (Eds.). (2010b). *Mass trauma and emotional healing around the world: Rituals and practices for resilience and meaning-making* (Vol. 2). Santa Barbara, CA: ABC-CLIO, LLC.

Kalayjian, A., & Paloutzian, R. (2010). *Forgiveness & reconciliation: Psychological pathways to conflict transformation and peace building.* Springer Publishing: New York: NY.

Kalayjian, A., Shigemoto, Y., & Patel, B. (2010). Earthquake in Soviet Armenia: Coping, integration, and meaning-making. In *Mass trauma and emotional healing around the world: Rituals and practices for resilience and meaning-making*, volume 1, 1-21. Santa Barbara: CA: ABC-CLIO, LLC.

Kalayjian, A., & Sofletea, G. (2012). Case study from Sierra Leone. In S. Poyrazli & C. Thompson (Eds.), *International case studies in mental health.* (pp. 33-51). Thousand Oaks, CA: SAGE Publications, Inc.

Kendall-Tackett, K. (2009). Psychological trauma and physical health: A psychoneuroimmunology approach to etiology of negative health effects and possible interventions. *Psychological Trauma: Theory, Research, Practice, and Policy, 1*, 35-48.

Kessler, R. C., Sonnega, A., Bromet, E., & Hughes. M. (1995). Posttraumatic stress disorder in the National Comorbidity Survey. *Archives of General Psychiatry, 52*, 1048–1060.

Kupelian, D., Kalayjian, A. S., & Kassabian, A. (1998). The Turkish genocide of the Armenians. In *International handbook of multigenerational legacies of trauma* (pp. 191-210). Springer US.

Lantz, M. S., & Buchalter, E. N. (2005). Post-Traumatic Stress Disorder: When current events cause relapse. *Clinical Geriatrics, 13*(2), 20-23.

Lee, S., Guo, W., Tsang, A., Mak, A. D. P., Wu, J., Ng, K. L., & Kwok, K. (2010). Evidence for the 2008 economic crisis exacerbating depression in Hong Kong. *Journal of Affective Disorders, 126*(1-2), 125–133. doi:10.1016/j.jad.2010.03.007

Park, C. L., & Ali, A. L. (2006). Meaning making and growth: New directions for research on survivors of trauma. *Journal of Loss and Trauma, 11*, 389–407.

Perry, B. D. (2008). Child maltreatment: A neurodevelopmental perspective on the role of trauma and neglect in psychopathology. In T. P. Beauchaine & S. P. Hinshaw (Eds.), *Child and adolescent psychopathology* (pp. 93–128). Hoboken, NJ: John Wiley & Sons.

Quarantelli, E. L. (1985). An assessment of conflicting views on mental health: The consequences of traumatic events. In C. R. Figley (Ed.), *Trauma and its wake* (pp. 173-215). New York: Bruner-Mazel.

Schaefer, F. C., Blazer, D. G., & Koenig, H. G. (2008). Religious and spiritual factors and the consequences of trauma: A review and model of the interrelationship. *International Journal of Psychiatry in Medicine, 38*, 507–524. doi:10.2190/PM.38.4.i

Skaggs, B. G., & Barron, C. R. (2006). Searching for meaning in negative events: Concept analysis. *Journal of Advanced Nursing, 53*, 559-570.

Staub, E., Pearlman, L. A., Gubin, A., & Hagengimana, A. (2005). Healing, reconciliation, forgiving and the prevention of violence after genocide or mass killing: An intervention and its experimental evaluation in Rwanda. *Journal of Social and Clinical Psychology, 24*, 297–334. doi:10.1521/jscp.24.3.297.65617

Sullivan, H. S. (1953). *The interpersonal theory of psychiatry.* New York: W. W. Norton.

Swart, H., Turner, R., Hewstone, M., & Voci, A. (2011). Achieving forgiveness and trust in postconflict societies: The importance of self-disclosure and empathy. In S. Hermann, R. Turner, M. Hewstone, & A. Voci (Eds.), *In moving beyond prejudice reduction: Pathways to positive intergroup relations* (pp. 181–200). Washington, D. C.: American Psychological Association. doi:10.1037/12319-009

Toussaint, Kalayjian, & Diakonova-Curtis (in press). Forgiveness makes sense: Forgiving others enhances the salutary associations of meaning-making with traumatic stress symptoms. *Peace and Conflict: Journal of Peace Psychology.*

United Nations. (2015). *Transforming our world: The 2030 agenda for sustainable development.* Retrieved from http://www.un.org/ga/search/view_doc.asp?symbol=A/RES/70/1&Lang=E

Van Der Kolk, B. A., & Saporta, L. (1993). Biological response to psychic trauma. In J. P. Wilson & B. Raphael (Eds.), *International handbook of traumatic stress syndromes* (pp. 25-33). New York: Plenum Press.

Ware, R. (1998). Conflict in the Caucasus: An historical context and a prospect for peace. *Central Asian Survey, 17*(2), 337-352.

Wood, P. R., Berrill, J. B., Gillon, N. R., & North, P. J. (1993). Earthquake of 7 December 1988, Spitak, Armenia: Report of the NZNSEE team visit of 1989. *Bulletin of the New Zealand National Society for Earthquake Engineering, 26*(3), 253–283.

World Bank Group. (2014). *Armenia.* Yerevan, Armenia: Author. Retrieved from http://www.worldbank.org/content/dam/Worldbank/document/Armenia-Snapshot.pdf

Worthington, E. L. (2006). *Forgiveness and reconciliation.* New York, NY: Brunner-Routledge.

Wu, N., Schairer, L., Dellor, E., & Grella, C. (2010). Childhood trauma and health outcomes in adults with comorbid substance abuse and mental health disorders. *Addictive Behaviors, 35*, 68-71.

Yehuda, R. (2002). Post-Traumatic stress disorder. *The New England Journal of Medicine, 346*, 108-114.

CHAPTER 10

Community Health Workers as Agents of Change: Case Studies from Haiti, Tanzania, and Burmese Refugees in the United States

Brandon A. Knettel and Shay E. Slifko

The proliferation of community health worker (CHW) programs is one of the greatest trends in public health in the past few decades, and there is mounting evidence to demonstrate the positive potential of CHWs for improving health outcomes in underserved areas. As such, no review of the contemporary footprint of global health efforts would be complete without acknowledging these workers. This chapter will outline CHW programs in three nations: a CHW training program in Haiti, implementation of CHW-led programs in a Burmese refugee community in the United States, and the potential impact of lay workers in a behavioral health program in Tanzania.

CHW programs have become a common approach for improving access to care in Haiti, particularly in rural areas with few trained providers. We will examine a CHW venture by a U.S.-based NGO and the pitfalls and successes of their efforts. Second, the issue of refugee resettlement has taken center stage due to mass migrations stemming from global crises. Meanwhile, past generations of refugees continue to work to make a living and acculturate. We will describe a group of Burmese case aids in Philadelphia tasked with assisting fellow refugees, while at the same time taking their own difficult steps toward independence. Last, in Tanzania, providers in a fledgling mental health system are facing massive demand to address a variety of challenging issues, including substance abuse, sexual violence, and serious mental illness. We will evaluate the potential impact of teachers serving as CHWs to address these concerns by providing basic mental health screening and counseling in Tanzanian schools.

> *"My neighbors were suffering from cholera and I heard about this program. I decided to come here to learn more and be able to help them."*
> *- Haitian Community Health Worker*
> *(personal communication, April 2013)*

Underdeveloped countries with scant health delivery systems frequently face the burden of substantial "treatment gaps," or discrepancies between the medical needs of the population and the availability of providers to treat them (Kale, 2002; WHO, 2016). In response to shortages of trained medical providers, along with common barriers to accessing treatment, community health workers (CHWs) are integrated as an essential link in the chain of access to care in a variety of settings. CHWs are community members who are asked to provide basic health interventions, education, and referral to higher levels of care.

In the greater part of the developing world, and particularly in rural settings, treatments gaps are especially pronounced due to higher burdens of disease and critical shortages of adequately trained health workers. In many of these areas, CHWs are the only health professionals who regularly have contact with large segments of the population. Programs throughout the developing world, including in Haiti, Central America, and sub-Saharan Africa have demonstrated that utilizing CHWs can help improve health outcomes for large populations in underserved regions at reasonable costs (Bhutta, Lassi, Pariyo, & Huicho, 2010). This approach follows a broader trend toward "task sharing" interventions, which involves shifting responsibilities from professional providers to health workers such as nurses, technicians, and CHWs as a means of making more efficient use of limited human resources (Kohrt & Mendenhall, 2015; WHO, 2008).

The proliferation of organized CHW training programs can be traced to the 1978 International Conference on Primary Health Care in Alma-Ata, at which many countries committed to achieving "Health for All" by mobilizing resources to reach the less-developed regions of the world (Perry, Zulliger, Rogers, 2014). This commitment would include the extension of medical services and the promotion of healthy practices and behaviors through education in difficult-to-reach areas. To achieve these lofty goals, conference leaders supported the widespread training and deployment of CHWs, who were introduced as low-cost health workers who could coordinate care, serve as liaisons to formal medical systems, encourage healthy practices, and supplement the deficit of healthcare professionals in areas of need (Perry et al., 2014).

Although the surge in CHW programs can be traced to Alma-Ata, one could argue that the historical background of health workers dates back as far as the medical profession, with lay workers operating alongside and in partnership with the formal medical system. One salient historical example comes from the first half of 20th century in China, where lay health workers known as the Barefoot Doctors assisted the government by recording births and deaths, vaccinating against smallpox, and providing health education (Perry, 2013). This concept continued to grow in the 1960s as more of the world's rapidly expanding population was exposed to the possibility of receiving formal health care, including people living in rural regions of the developing world.

As CHW programs have become more ubiquitous, the titles given to these workers and the ways they have been integrated into communities throughout the world have also expanded. Other names for them include community health aide, health promoter, health care worker, outreach educator, village health worker, community health agent, and health activist (Lehmann & Sanders, 2007). CHWs also vary with regard to their training, available supplies, scope of practice, and oversight, though typical roles include collaboration with the region's existing healthcare system and interaction with other community members in a professional capacity through the use of education, activism, and basic intervention.

Although their titles and roles vary, the definition of these workers, formulated at the 1986 Yaounde Conference (as cited in WHO, 1989), has remained quite consistent. They are "members of the communities where they work, selected by the communities, answerable to the communities for their activities, supported by the health system but not necessarily a part of its organization, and have less training than professional workers" (WHO, 1989, p. 6). They are a diverse workforce of individuals who work outside of formal healthcare facilities, oftentimes within underserved communities, with little formal training in healthcare, a point of debate which we explore in-depth later in this chapter.

There have been remarkable examples of the power CHWs can have when implemented effectively (Perry, 2013). CHW programs have also responded to a call for more definitive and rigorous empirical evidence that they are an effective use of resources. The most ambitious of these efforts was a report prepared for the World Health Organization by Bhutta and colleagues (2010) describing the efficacy of programs in twenty nations, including eight detailed case studies. Among the programs profiled was a large-scale program founded in Pakistan in 1992, which has trained approximately 100,000 women to serve as Lady Health Workers, CHWs who provide support for an estimated 70% of the country's rural residents (Perry, 2013, p. 6). Among the dozens of research studies on this program was a controlled trial by Jhokio, Winter, and Cheng (2005), which explored the Lady Health Workers' impact on maternal and child health. The authors reported a 30% reduction in stillbirths and perinatal mortality, a 39% reduction in hemorrhage-related complications during birth, and a 50% increase in referrals for emergency obstetric care (Jhokio et al., 2005, p. 2095-2098). This is one small example of an impressive body of research that shows positive progress in areas served by CHWs in a majority of the studies currently available (Bhutta et al., 2010).

Despite these examples of the expansion and success of large-scale CHW programs, many initiatives have also met major setbacks or failed entirely due to lack of support (Perry, Zullinger, & Rogers, 2014). CHW programs are typically offered at no charge to the recipients of care and therefore rely entirely on government or charitable support for their operating costs. It is not surprising, then, that the most common challenge for these programs is a lack of sustained funding, which in many cases leads to inconsistent remuneration for CHWs, limited training support, poor oversight of programs, shortages in supplies, and the eventual discontinuation of the program. As past failures have been shared with the international community, a new enclave of smaller-scale programs has arisen with a focus on cost-effectiveness and garnering support within host communities to make them financially sustainable (Bhutta et al., 2010).

Today, there are estimated to be more than five million community health workers functioning in communities worldwide in both developed and developing nations, and the model appears to be here to stay (Perry et al., 2014, p. 400). As a result, there is an ongoing academic and bureaucratic discourse around the role of CHWs in health systems in the coming years (Bhutta et al., 2010). Discussions include advocacy for broadening the roles and reach of CHWs to address a wider variety of health concerns and benefit underserved individuals with limited access to other resources. Although CHWs will certainly play a large role in attempts to address treatment gaps and health disparities, there continue to be unanswered questions surrounding their scope of practice and the level of oversight these programs will require, particularly in areas with dire medical needs.

According to the WHO (2016), CHWs today are better utilized, better trained, and better compensated than they were in the past. As a result, they are more likely to be paid employees who provide treatment, education, counseling, and implementation of preventative measures (Bhutta et al., 2010). National governments and NGOs in Brazil, Pakistan, Ethiopia, India, and Haiti are integrating CHWs to provide a foundation for strengthening health delivery. A key difference between these new national CHW models and the models of the past is that workers are now viewed as a formal part of the health system with established guidelines and standards for effective training, supervision, and feedback (Bhutta et al., 2010; Perry et al., 2014). Ultimately, what sets CHWs apart is their familiarity with the families they serve, which provides an intimate knowledge of the causes of disease and illness. In present-day Haiti, CHWs carry out various tasks including home visits, prenatal and postnatal follow up, education about safe water, and facilitating follow up care for individuals with HIV and other chronic diseases. These community laypersons have become essential links in the chain of access to health care and public health information.

A Training Program in Rural Haiti

'We must have knowledge first. Tools are much more powerful and long lasting if they are paired with strong knowledge."
- Haitian Community Health Worker
(personal communication, April 2013)

Haiti suffers from deficits in both the provision of medical care and the infrastructure needed to access it. This is especially true in the rural areas of the country, where the dire shortage in healthcare resources leaves much of the population without access to adequate facilities, providers, or treatments. The already frail health system has been further debilitated by a series of natural disasters and others challenges, such as the 2010 earthquake, which left 30 hospitals destroyed or damaged, including Haiti's primary teaching hospital and the nation's Ministry of Health (PAHO, 2011, p. 8). Just ten months after the earthquake, Haiti experienced the first cholera outbreak to hit the nation in a century, which was traced to improper sanitation practices by United Nations (U.N.) peacekeepers working in the nation and killed more than 7,000 people in the two years after the disaster (Frerichs, Keim, Barrais, & Piarroux, 2012, p. 158). Most recently, Hurricane Matthew struck the southwestern coast of Haiti in October 2016. The storm destroyed vast numbers of livestock, crops, homes, and medical centers, leaving a significant number of rural residents without basic needs such as food, clean water, shelter, or medical care. The storm has also contributed to a resurgence of the cholera epidemic with more than 1,000 suspected cases in month following the storm (UNICEF, 2016, para. 3).

While affordable health clinics do exist in Haiti, their scarcity means that individuals must make a long and expensive trip to access them, particularly in rural areas of the country. Such a trip may require walking long distances and paying for public transportation, which are not viable options for those with urgent needs such as a serious injury, medical emergency, or labor and delivery. A CHW in rural Haiti shared this example: "In an emergency, we carry people fifty kilometers to the Dominican Republic by stretcher. It takes fifteen people from morning until night" (personal communication, April 2013). The region where this woman received her CHW training was mountainous with no paved roads. The nearest market, where women were spotted daily traversing the steep mountainside loaded with baskets of goods, was a full day's walk from many homes. Thus, imagine the distance, cost, and number of people needed to safely transport a laboring mother to the small clinic in the same village. In this setting, CHWs become a vital resource whose advice may lead to earlier recognition of serious concerns and save lives.

The Training Program

Due to the lack of access to basic resources, proximity to care, and the scarcity of physicians, community-level health interventions have been growing in number in Haiti, particularly those offered by non-governmental organizations (NGOs) (Jerome & Ivers, 2010). As researchers, we (the authors of this chapter) have had the privilege to be granted an inside view into a CHW program in Haiti from its early formation to its recent expansion and the dilemma of seeking ongoing funding to support its operations. What started as a small training program for local, unpaid volunteers has become part of a large, internationally funded network of employed CHWs and supervisors serving over 15,000 vulnerable families in rural Haiti (Pendse & Yu, 2016, p. 12-13). Our role in this program has been to conduct and oversee an objective evaluation of the program to examine its efficacy and to provide recommendations for how it might improve in the future.

The sponsoring NGO for the program originally began working in Haiti in the months following the 2010 earthquake, with the goal of transporting food, water, and medication to those directly impacted by the disaster. However, in response to criticism leveled at many organizations who offered short-term support in the aftermath of the quake and then quickly left, this group resolved to establish a longer-term presence in Haiti with a variety of programs, including the CHW training. In conversations with the Haitian Ministry of Health, the southeast region of the country was identified as an area of high need and thus became the site of the organization's new ventures (Knettel, Slifko, Inman, & Silova, 2017).

In the early years of the CHW program, volunteers and employees from a U.S.-based NGO partnered with a major biomedical technology company to train CHWs in the rural southern region. As researchers, we first conducted an evaluation of this program in 2013, which included 126 Haitian CHW trainees selected from local community federations who took part in one of three identical weeklong training programs. The course instructors were non-Haitian employees of the corporate partner with expertise in medicine and public health. The mean age of the CHW trainees was 37 and the majority were men (64%). Additionally, most had no formal employment; their incomes were based in domestic agriculture such as selling produce or simply growing enough food to support their families (Knettel et al., 2017, p. 5).

The 2013 training covered topics related to prenatal and postnatal health, labor and delivery, managing childhood disease, and family planning. The program's model was to train CHWs to offer health education, monitoring of at-risk families, and referral for higher levels of care when needed. It was hoped that these interventions would replicate the success of other programs in Haiti and elsewhere by reducing the prevalence of morbidity and mortality among pregnant women and children under five in the region. Course content ranged from how to make oral rehydration solution for treating diarrhea to safe birthing methods in the case of a breech delivery. The training program incorporated a training textbook to guide the daily content covering pregnancy, preparation for labor and delivery, care of the newborn in the first 48 hours, sexually transmitted infections, and family planning (Knettel et al., 2017).

Figure 1: A rural, Haitian health clinic

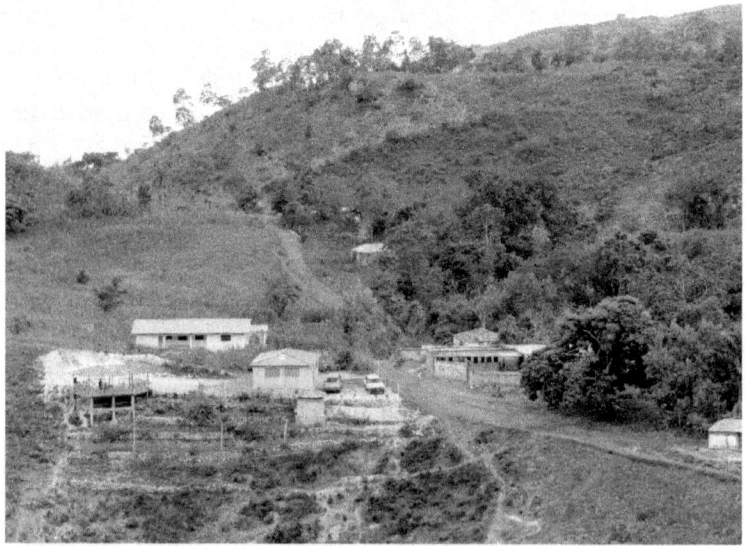

While the evaluation of the 2013 CHW training yielded overwhelmingly positive feedback from the participants on the training content and participants improved significantly on course-related knowledge from pretest to posttest, there were also notable concerns that were both cited by the participants and observed by the evaluators. When participants were asked how the training could be improved, the most common reply was that they desired greater personal support in carrying out their roles. Many noted that being a volunteer CHW came with great personal and economic cost, including lost time and productivity for their other responsibilities, social/emotional stress, and the financial burden of volunteering. These results mirror CHW evaluations conducted in other settings (Kalofonos, 2015; Maes, 2015), which describe the pressure of volunteers to be gracious in their work despite the burdens placed on them.

In our evaluation, female CHWs in particular reported strong cultural norms that they should stay in the home and care for their children, so the prospects of attending a week of training or going out of the home to provide services to families were met with great resistance in their families. Other CHWs requested assistance with transportation to and from the daily training as the average participant travelled 16 kilometers to attend the class, with the majority traveling exclusively on foot (Knettel et al., 2017, p. 5). Finally, CHWs described the burden of missing out on paid work or temporarily overlooking domestic tasks in order to attend the training or dedicate time to their roles as CHWs. This feedback led the program sponsors to provide stipends for participants using the distance they travel as the indicator.

Figure 2: Women walking to the clinic in rural Haiti

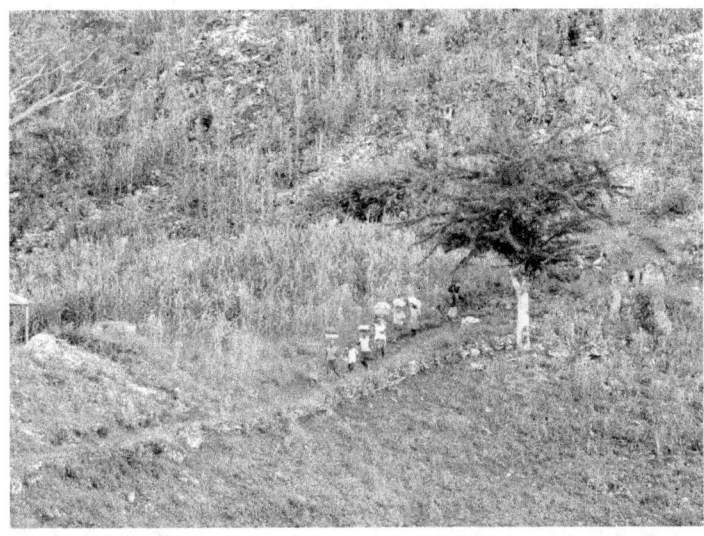

Another primary area of concern identified in the 2013 evaluation was that some CHWs were illegitimately practicing as providers in the community and charging for these services, raising concerns around the level of oversight of the program. For instance, the CHW training program was offered once annually with little supervision of how or whether participants were implementing the training. In light of these findings, we recommended that the sponsoring organizations take a more active role in the supervision of CHWs between training sessions. The evaluation findings also raised questions about whether the CHWs were adequately trained and resourced in a region where there was little to no access to safe and affordable medical care. For example, CHWs were encouraged to recognize signs of emergent medical problems during labor and encourage women in these situations to go to a hospital. However, even if a woman's family could afford to transport her to a hospital in this situation, she would have to survive the long, arduous trip without the support of a medical provider. The unfortunate reality is that the hospital would most likely be ill-equipped to respond to a complicated birth when she arrived.

Finally, given the training organization's stance that health knowledge is the most beneficial tool they can provide for the prevention of health-related concerns, the theme of "tools" was prominent throughout our experience with the CHW training. Trainees frequently voiced their need for tools in order to be of any real help for their community, including medicines and medical equipment. "Knowledge is nothing without the tools to put it to use" (personal communication, April 2013), one CHW shared in a focus group when asked about barriers he faced in meeting his community's needs. Again, in response to this feedback, progress has been made in more recent iterations of the training, as CHWs are now equipped with blood pressure cuffs and stethoscopes. They have also taken steps to overcome their lack of tools and resources through community organization. For example, the CHWs led an "End Open Defecation" program to inspire community members to build their own family latrines. The program, carried out with no external funding or equipment, led to hundreds of additional latrines available to families in the rural southeast of the country.

The example provided here shows that the success of a CHW training program cannot be described only in its effectiveness, but that evaluations should also consider the program's openness to feedback and change. To date, the successes of this program are largely anecdotal as little data exists to identify how effective these workers are in assessing the needs in their region. At the same time, the program has grown immensely since its founding in 2010 and has implemented a variety of changes based on the needs and feedback of its participants. The program leaders understand that everyone stands to gain when CHW programs are effective. Ultimately, with adequate support, CHWs can reach more households to provide essential and sometimes life-saving services.

Implementation and Challenges
in a Burmese Refugee Community in Philadelphia

"The mural shows the whole story of the refugee experience: the country, the mountain, the plane we took to get here. You can see our story from that mural. Have you seen that? It's right there."
— *Karen Youth Program Participant (personal communication, September 2016)*

Like many U.S. cities, Philadelphia has a centuries-long tradition of welcoming immigrants, including refugees, to make a new life and face the many challenges that come with resettlement. As a result, the large refugee community living in Philadelphia today reflects the vibrancy and multiculturalism associated with generational waves of immigrants from every region of the world. In the 2014-2015 fiscal year, resettlement agencies in Pennsylvania served 3,056 newly arrived refugees, with almost 25% of these settling in the Philadelphia area (PRRP, 2016). This is only a small fraction of the 21.3 million refugees worldwide, a number which recently exceeded the years after World War II as the highest in history, largely due to conflicts in Syria, Iraq, the Democratic Republic of Congo, Myanmar, and elsewhere (UNHCR, 2016, p. 6). Despite the residual challenges they face in recovering from traumatic experiences in their home countries, refugees represent a valuable segment of Philadelphia's social fabric. Refugees from Burma (also known as Myanmar) are among the largest groups in the city, with 122 Burmese arrivals in Philadelphia during fiscal year 2014-2015 (PRRP, 2016).

From statistical and epidemiological perspectives, the challenges that face refugees throughout the process of relocation are well-documented. Within each phase of displacement, migration, and resettlement, they experience a unique set of physical, psychological, and social challenges that can have a profound impact on health and well-being (Beiser & Hou, 2016; Summerfield, 1996). Prior to migration, these challenges may include violence or fear of violence, death of loved ones, imprisonment, political instability, poverty, persecution, and disruption of any sense of security or safety. The migratory phase of displacement brings new challenges related to the uncertainty and physical burden of population movement, including the strong potential for further trauma and the lack of basic survival needs such as clean water, food, and shelter, and healthcare (Beiser & Hou, 2016). Finally, in resettlement, refugees face the burden of learning and adapting to a foreign environment, often with few resources and little or no language proficiency (Heptinstall, Sethna, & Taylor, 2004; Rousseau, Drapeau, & Corin, 1997). Together, these many stressors can contribute to the occurrence of "severe and lasting psychological aftereffects" (Porter & Haslam, 2005, p. 602) among refugees in the months and years following their forced relocation, including increased rates of posttraumatic stress symptoms and a variety of other mental health concerns.

Members of Philadelphia's Burmese refugee community have faced several of the aforementioned challenges during all the phases of their relocation. The country of Myanmar struggled through nearly fifty years of brutally oppressive military rule, starting in 1962. This era was marked by civil war and ethnic conflict, leading scholars to describe it as "one of the world's least developed and least free countries" (Barron et al., 2007, p. 1). The Burmese refugee community in Philadelphia has historically been comprised of two minority ethnic groups – the Karen and the Chin. The two groups each traditionally hail from rural, hilly farmlands on opposite ends of Myanmar, and both have been embroiled in decades of conflict with the majority military government. This included the common occurrence of human rights violations including attacks on villages, forced labor, rape, and torture (Barron et al., 2007). Despite the nominal dissolution of the Myanmar's military junta in 2011, steps toward democratization have been slow and challenging, and violent conflict remains widespread in some regions and among some ethnic groups. As a result, refugees continue to leave Myanmar at rates among the highest in the world. The 18,386 Burmese refugees who came to the United States in fiscal year 2015 were more than any other nation (U.S. Department of State, 2015).

The Transition of Refugees to the United States

Historically, most people have agreed that the world's wealthiest nations have a moral imperative to provide asylum and refuge for the worst victims of human rights violations abroad. However, in light of fast-developing political circumstances at the time of this chapter's publication, including efforts by the United States government to temporarily ban refugee resettlement (White House, 2017, sec. 6), it is important acknowledge that the topic of immigration also has had a long and tumultuous history in the U.S. political discourse. Our nation continues to struggle with the issue, sometimes embracing its identity as a "nation of immigrants," or "melting pot," and at other times trending toward xenophobia in efforts to maintain a sense of ethnic, religious, or cultural homogeneity (Murray & Marx, 2013). The tension between these two perspectives has only grown stronger in the recent political climate, including arguments about the implications of high profile terrorist attacks, ongoing conflict in several nations throughout the world, and the refugee crisis resulting from these conflicts (Chebel d'Appollonia, 2012).

To support refugees in their overwhelming transition to a new nation, we rely on governmental agencies, the various subsidiaries of the United Nations, nongovernmental organizations, volunteers, and, most importantly, the efforts of resettlement agencies. Sadly, the international response to human rights violations can be frighteningly slow. The process of a person being exposed to conflict or trauma, fleeing, finding temporary shelter (often in a refugee camp), and attaining permanent residency in another nation may take years or even decades, or may never occur at all. Families are scattered across relocation sites and temporary residences are rife with poverty, disease, crime, and other problems (Agier, 2011). Despite these conditions, the refugees who reside in camps and other relocation sites are filled with hope. In refugee camps, rumors abound that the United States is a place where anyone can receive an education and become successful. For the lucky few who are approved to come to the U.S., the hope they hold is inspiring. They wish for a peaceful life and for their children to have opportunities to learn and grow.

The reality of life in the U.S. for refugees is rarely as bright as the aspirations they hold. Nevertheless, there are systems in place to try to make the transition a success, and refugee resettlement agencies provide the foundation for that transition. These agencies are national non-profit organizations that have historically received modest government funding in exchange for their support in aiding newly arrived refugees. Upon a refugee's arrival in the U.S., resettlement agencies are often the first source of contact in the difficult process of acculturation (Nezer, 2013). These organizations provide links within resettling communities that potentially mitigate the social, psychological, and physical challenges faced by refugees during the post-migration resettlement process (Mott, 2010). According to the U.S. Office of Refugee Resettlement (ORR, 2016, para. 1), there are nine national resettlement agencies currently operating in the United States, with three of these currently offering services in Philadelphia. The largest agency in Philadelphia closed its resettlement program in 2016, citing major shortfalls in funding (Benshoff, 2016).

Resettlement agencies are assigned the immense responsibility of assisting these new residents, many of whom have few possessions and little or no English fluency, in establishing a new life in a new nation. To carry out this incredibly complex task, agencies receive a one-time stipend from the U.S. government of $1800 per refugee arrival (Bruno, 2011, p. 1), which is intended to cover both the basic needs of the person and the operating costs of the agency. Take a moment to consider what this means. Without even considering the burden of traumatic experiences and forced relocation, imagine that all of your possessions are taken from you and you are asked to move with your family to a new country where a new language is spoken. How much would it cost for you to make a reasonable attempt at starting over?

By necessity, resettlement agencies become adept at using multiple resources to assist refugee families in starting their new lives, including the generosity of charitable organizations, volunteers, and government assistance. Nevertheless, a large portion of a refugee's resettlement stipend is typically used for the initial provision of housing, food, clothing, and all other expenses in the first three months after arrival. Refugee families are then expected to be self-sufficient, with little to no additional funds and receiving no special support beyond those offered to the average U.S. citizen. In fact, the cost of the airline tickets to enter the country are offered through interest-free loans from the International Organization for Migration, with repayment starting six months after arrival, so refugees are often already in debt when they arrive in the U.S.

Employment and Access to Government Services

With recent disagreement about the morality of barring refugees from entering the U.S., debates have arisen about nearly every aspect of refugees' lives, including their contributions to U.S. society and the purported burden they place on existing social structures. One of the most common arguments against refugee resettlement is that these individuals struggle to find employment to support their families and therefore place an undue burden on economy and social services offered by the U.S. government. With regard to employment, statistics from the U.S. Office of Refugee Resettlement show that refugees do initially have lower rates (47.4%) when compared to the general population (64.5%) one year after their arrival (ORR, 2017, p. 25). This finding should be unsurprising given the aforementioned challenges of acculturation, language, and skill acquisition in a new nation. Importantly, however, refugee employment quickly and steadily increases over time in the United States and by five years after arrival, the refugee employment rate is equal to that of the general population (ORR, 2017, p. 25).

It is also true that refugees are eligible for many government services, including temporary financial support, medical care, food assistance, case management, and employment programs (ORR, 2017), most of which are facilitated by the resettlement agencies. These services are necessary for temporary support for families with no other resources. Critics of resettlement have expressed concern that refugees' initiation to public services as a means for survival in the weeks and months after their arrival will set the tone for overreliance on government assistance in the years to come. However, similar to employment, the U.S. Bureau of Labor Statistics reports that the overall utilization of government support among refugees is at or below the rates of the general U.S. population (U.S. Department of Labor, 2016), demonstrating that refugees seek alternative means of support as soon as they are able.

In addition to the practical challenges of survival in a new nation, refugees also frequently face various forms of mistreatment upon their arrival in the U.S. These may include exploitation, discrimination, avoidance, or the outright scorn of many U.S. citizens toward those less acculturated. In response to these social stressors, refugee families, especially those without relatives in their new country, tend to rely on an extended social network of fellow immigrants from their home country (many of whom are also poor). They are preyed upon by slumlords, high interest lenders, and exploitative employers who offer low wages or illegal "under the table" payment agreements, no benefits, and poor working conditions, armed with the knowledge that their employees will struggle to find something better.

The Philadelphia Refugee Mental Health Collaborative

Because of their close contact with refugees in the first months after their arrival, resettlement agencies are in a unique position to understand the complexity of the lives of people seeking refuge in a new country. In the best cases, their understanding is transferred to broader programs of care and support beyond simply meeting basic needs. One such example of this type of comprehensive, wellness-based approach is the model adopted by the Philadelphia Refugee Mental Health Collaborative (PRMHC), a program established in 2011 to improve the health care, social support, and acculturation process of refugees during resettlement. The program achieves these aims by linking resettlement agencies with academic and community resources, including health systems, education, NGOs, school systems, arts-based programs, and volunteer networks.

The mutual goal of the PRMHC's diverse partners is to improve the overall health and well-being of refugee families. The program began with a two-part realization. First, social workers and other resettlement agency professionals recognized that they were coming up short in the services offered to refugee families, most often due to financial challenges requiring them to dedicate most of their resources to meeting families' basic needs. Second, as a result of these limitations, they felt incapable of dedicating new resources to support quality of life initiatives in refugee communities. Despite a growing body of evidence showing the value of a comprehensive approach to improving health, well-being, and access to care, as well as increasing interest in these types of support (SAMHSA, 2016), the funds and support to initiate such programs were simply not available. Organizers were fortunate to receive this support from Philadelphia's Department of Behavioral Health and Intellectual Disability Services (DBHIDS), a government organization seeking to establish community collaboratives aimed at tackling the city's most pressing public health issues. With DBHIDS sponsorship, the new refugee health collaborative was funded to operate as a multi-disciplinary coalition of stakeholders interested in refugee mental health with core program partners that included practitioners from medical, resettlement, mental health, and arts organizations.

One of the greatest successes of the PRMHC to date has been the establishment of a community center in the largest Burmese and Bhutanese resettlement neighborhood in Philadelphia. Early iterations of PRMHC programs focused on conventional models of engagement and care through referrals to medical, mental health, government, and other services. However, through a collaborative arts-based research program aimed at using photography to examine and provide support for past trauma (Plumb et al., in press), it became clear that a new approach was needed. The success of that program and its enthusiastic reception in the refugee community, both among participants and the thousands of others who provided support or attended the accompanying gallery events, highlighted the importance of community connection and wellness-based programs in facilitating healing, supporting the process of acculturation, and promoting well-being. To build off this success, the program's organizers created the Southeast by Southeast community center.

Previously a vacant storefront, Southeast by Southeast is now a gathering space and local hub for refugee programs focusing on social connection, cultural preservation programming, community development, and education for both children and adults. Programmatic activities have included workshops on traditional weaving, sewing, dancing, photography, and cooking, as well as daily English as a Second Language (ESL) classes, homework and tutoring support for students, and an elder program focused on mutual social support and education. This vibrant center also serves as an important reminder that providing for basic needs may promote survival, but in order for people to thrive, they must be connected with the things they feel passionate about while surrounded by the people they love most.

Figure 3: A print sale at Southeast by Southeast

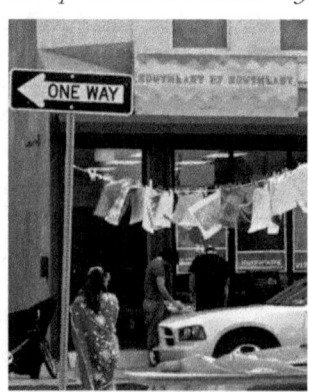

The Refugee Community Case Aides Program

Unfortunately, resettlement agencies are not immune to the plagues of all organizations that rely on private donations and public aid. They are often understaffed, underfunded, and overburdened by the enormous needs of the communities they serve. A single caseworker may carry a caseload of more than 100 refugees representing nations from around the world (M. Fogg, personal communication, September 2016), many of whom speak little English and will initially face multiple challenges to achieving tasks such as attending their appointments or going to the grocery store. The core problems are financial, logistical, social, and cultural. To attend a single meeting with a caseworker, they require the money, support and knowledge to miss work, find childcare, and transport themselves to the appointment. For a family starting with almost nothing, these can be very difficult to accomplish.

Southeast by Southeast is home to a small group of immigrant case aides offering support and education in the local Burmese community. The aides are well-regarded members of the community and were highly trained professionals in their home country, but lack either the English proficiency or the resources to seek similar education and employment in the United States. They have been in U.S. for longer than many of their neighbors, often more than five years, and have obtained many of the skills to thrive in their new home.

The case aides meet all of the criteria to be considered CHWs: they are members of the community; are answerable to the community in their work (in a way that is tightly enforced by the local social structure); are supported by the formal resettlement system but free to represent the community in an independent way; and are previously untrained in the social services, aside from some basic training from the resettlement agencies. The aides were hired in the months following the establishment of Southeast by Southeast to build capacity for the new program. Their roles were to relieve pressure on the overtaxed agency social workers in the neighborhood, to create a new sense of connection and access between the agencies and the community, and to support the process of acculturation for the refugee families. However, the challenges for the aides to implement these goals were immense, as they were now responsible for not only managing the health and well-being of their own families, but also taking on the burdens associated with the struggles of the entire community.

Of course, the case aide model is not without its limitations. As members of the community, aides are frequently unable to hide behind the professional boundaries of the U.S. establishment. Concepts such as a limited scope of practice, setting aside time for administrative responsibilities, or maintaining "normal business hours" are unclear or flatly abandoned. Case aides become true jacks of all trades, managing the distress and confusion of a multitude of families facing a seemingly endless sea of problems. Just as the elders or community leaders in the small communities of their home countries were available during all hours of the day to address difficulties or mediate conflicts, the case aides become the gatekeepers of knowledge and access to a better life. Unfortunately, urban refugee communities in the United States are rarely small and their problems are rarely simple. Case aides may quickly find themselves overburdened by the needs of their neighbors, their own intense longing to be helpful, and their limitations in the skills, knowledge, and resources to cope with the complex issues placed before them.

An Illustration of the Case Aide Approach in Action

The work of a refugee case aide may be best illustrated by describing the roles of two such aides, Moe Yee and Hser Nay (pseudonyms), who are employed part-time by all three resettlement agencies working in a Burmese refugee community in south Philadelphia. Hser Nay is a middle-aged woman who was a nurse in Myanmar and, after many years at a refugee camp in Thailand, worked as a nanny in the U.S. before starting her work as a case aide. She says she enjoys her work, but also faces many challenges and stressors to carry out her roles each day. Moe Yee is younger and feels similarly challenged in her work, particularly because also has a young child who struggles with persistent health concerns.

Hser Nay and Moe Yee are both Karen, an ethnic group from Myanmar that has been entrenched in a half-century of civil war and conflict with the majority ethnic group and the government of the country. They describe their Karen identity as a strength in working with other Karen refugees, but a challenge when they are asked to work with people from other countries or people from other Burmese communities, such as the Chin. Additionally, Moe Yee spent much of her life in a refugee camp, and her inability to speak the Karen language sometimes leaves her feeling disconnected and distrusted by fellow refugees whom she is employed to serve.

In speaking with these remarkable women, seemingly straightforward patterns of need begin to emerge. They often spend 40-50 hours per week on their "part-time" job and feel overwhelmed by the demands of their communities, particularly when they receive phone calls and visits to their homes from early in the morning until late at night, seven days a week. At other times, they accompany a family to a doctor's appointment or government office and act as trip organizer, guide, translator, scribe, and teacher on a trip that could take up most of the day. They assist these families in working with broken government systems and navigating a sea of seemingly arbitrary requirements and paperwork, only to find with disturbing frequency that a key document or piece of information is missing and they will need to return at a later date to start the process all over again.

The case aides also feel overwhelmed in their attempts to complete the documentation and paperwork being asked of them by the agencies; their still-improving English, lack of experience with this kind of protocol, and desire to produce high-quality work frequently prevents them from completing the paperwork in a timely matter. Additionally, working from home leaves them poorly equipped to complete this work, as they lack the computers, software, internet access, printing capacity, and office supplies to complete the administrative tasks being asked of them. They find it hard to justify the time commitment necessary to do such work when the needs of the community are so great, but the agencies persist. It is a frustrating and confusing dance.

A Brief Intervention

Recognizing the immense pressures that the case aides were facing, PRMHC leadership began providing a professional supervision and support group for Hser Nay and Moe Yee in 2013. These sessions were led by a doctoral trainee in psychology and an agency social worker who was also director of the PRMHC. As the group progressed, it became clear that Hser Nay and Moe Yee could benefit from additional resources, both personal and practical, to support their roles. It was also clear that the case aides had become vital receptacles for the vast problems of their community. These women, who, through their intelligence and persistence, had learned to survive and thrive in a new culture, were feeling a constant pull to re-experience the feelings of desperation that embody a new arrival. Moe Yee said it best herself: "We are seeing and feeling the experience of the new refugees every day. We try so hard to help, but sometimes we have our own problems too" (personal communication, May 2013).

From a practical standpoint, the group led to communication about a lack of resources and encouraged the resettlement agency to provide the case aides with access to an office with internet connection and a printer. The supervisors worked with the aides to create and translate a series of electronic and paper forms outlining the steps and requirements involved in key tasks for families in the community, including enrolling child in school, renting an apartment, and applying for a green card. These forms would help the aides to organize their thoughts and place some of the responsibility back on the members of the community to meet various requirements for accomplishing these tasks. The aides also received education and support related to maintaining a good work-life balance and setting professional boundaries. From a more interpersonal standpoint, they were also provided with space to vent their frustrations and discuss the cultural conflicts at play in their professional interactions.

Perhaps the greatest conflicts come from a combination of the urgent cries for help from community members at all hours of the day and night and the case aides' difficulty in asserting their own needs that may inconvenience others. Hser Nay and Moe Yee acutely felt the common internal conflict that arises in public health work – between providing help for the problems in front of you or seeking out those who need help but don't ask. This was only exacerbated by the case aides' collectivistic background and a culturally-informed drive to accept personal inconvenience for the common good.

Overwhelmingly, the aides felt the visible and invisible suffering of their community and they desired to help. As Hser Nay shared, "Our people have no education. They are scared to ask for help but they need it so much" (personal communication, May 2013). Meanwhile, the aides continued to sacrifice their own well-being and the well-being of their families to assist their communities. They seemed impervious to their supervisors' concerns that this way of doing things might not be sustainable. The supervisors continued to push the aides to set professional boundaries by refusing to see families late at night for non-urgent concerns, struggling to understand the message that such rejection would send to a Burmese individual. It was also invalidating to the aids' deep-seated desire to be as helpful as possible. Hser Nay and Moe Yee expressed concern that such steps might be perceived as selfish and uncaring, which might lead to rumors about them in the community and sabotage their relationships with their clients and peers.

Conflicts surrounding assertiveness were also a key topic. One day, for example, Moe Yee shared a story about a woman at a government health care office where many of her clients received their care. This frequently put Moe Yee in contact with an administrative assistant at the office – a woman who often made blatantly racist and disrespectful comments, made mistakes in her work, and lost several important documents belonging to clients. Finally, after a particularly egregious error by the woman, Moe Yee decided to file a formal complaint by calling the woman's supervisor. At a future visit to the office, she found that the woman no longer worked there. Her conviction that she had gotten the woman fired, which might have been perceived as a successful overthrow by many, was deeply disconcerting to Moe Yee: "I think I robbed her of being able to support her family and I am so sorry for that. That was two years ago, but I still think about her and I feel sad" (personal communication, May 2013).

Over time in the group, through compromise, the case aides made small progress. They found the voice to ask for more supplies and practical support, some of which the agency was able to provide and some of which they were not. The aides showed an increased understanding of the difference between urgency and emergency, even asking some of the most frequent offenders to return during normal office hours. Through this sense of empowerment, they also found motivation to share their message with the community in new ways, such as participating in a women's peer mentorship group, starting a social group for community elders, and translating for English language courses. After several months of meeting with the case aides, when asked whether the meetings were helpful for them, Moe Yee replied, "Oh yes. Now we have someone to listen to our hearts, and this is so important for us" (personal communication, May 2013).

Impact of a Behavioral Health Program in Tanzania

"The background of education in Tanzania is very rough. Even the teachers themselves are sometimes very badly educated...They use a lot of corporal punishment - pinching to the point of leaving marks. In many schools they hit them with sticks."
—*Tanzanian School Administrator (personal communication, July 2012)*

"I work to advocate for better treatment. I also coordinate with outside providers and services to meet the needs of the children that we can't provide. This includes many assessments, medical care, medication, imaging tests for the epileptics and the ones with medical problems. We also use art therapy, counseling, play therapy, occupational skills, and health education."
— *Tanzanian School Counseling Trainee and Community Health Worker (personal communication, July 2012)*

Despite vast economic and development challenges placing it among the world's poorest nations, the United Republic of Tanzania has a long history of respect and support for education. As compared to similar nations (both economically and geographically), a large percentage of Tanzanian children attend primary school (Lloyd, Kaufman, & Hewett, 2000), and teachers are often considered respected leaders in Tanzanian communities. The nation's first president, Julius Nyerere, was a former teacher affectionately known as *Mwalimu*, Kiswahili for teacher. The cultural appreciation of education can be (and in some cases already has been) utilized to improve well-being for all students through preventative programming, guidance, and even treatment for mentally-ill youth (Kiweewa, 2015; Mabula & Edna, 2015).

Unfortunately, as the quotations that start this section of the chapter clearly demonstrate, there are contrasting styles at work in the Tanzanian education system. Many educators were brought up in a rigid, lecture-based, and disciplinarian system, that often included the use of corporal punishment, and have continued this tradition in their own classrooms (Feinstein & Mwahombela, 2010). Meanwhile, other educators have come to understand that there are other methods of disciplining children that will

231

allow them to maintain order and promote positive behavior in the classroom without the use of violence. This transition has created space for considering the greater priorities of education overall, including the addition of previously rare supplementary services like guidance counseling, special education, and school psychology (Kiweewa, 2015).

Teachers who take on tasks aimed at supporting children outside of the classroom most certainly fall under the definition of community health workers. They are members of the community, answerable to the community, and while they are not untrained, they are not mental health specialists. By adding these areas of specialization to their skillsets, teachers are capable of creating access to guidance counseling and school psychology, two formal professions with a vast research base of benefit and success in many nations that have simply not been a part of the Tanzanian social fabric to date. The most obvious reason for this absence is financial. In a nation where many families feel fortunate to be able to send their children to primary school, the concept of counseling in school is an unrealistic luxury (Kiweewa, 2015; Mabula & Edna, 2015).

We know from the examples earlier in this chapter that the clinic is absolutely not the only setting for wellness programs and mental health treatment. In fact, in many ways, teachers are particularly well-equipped to provide a variety of services to students, including wellness education, assessment, guidance counseling, and even psychotherapy (Knettel, Rugira, & Tesha, 2016). Teachers typically have a wealth of previous training and experience in childhood development, are immersed in the daily lives of their students, and are thus well-placed to build the trust and rapport that are so commonly predictors of success for positive mental health interventions. Teachers have the capacity and access needed to create a culturally sensitive, non-threatening setting for the assessment and treatment of mental illness from childhood through adolescent and sometimes into early adulthood.

The advancement of mental health capacity among teachers is also an example of wise development. In settings where the creation of new systems and professions is not economically feasible, stakeholders are frequently encouraged to employ task-shifting strategies using existing resources. As previously mentioned, Tanzania has created a powerful and far-reaching network of primary schools across the nation, including rural areas with little access to any other professional services. In areas where even basic medical care is a luxury and which may require hours of travel to access, the prospect of creating a mental health system from the ground up is simply not feasible at this time. However, basic mental health and wellness resources can be incorporated into existing schools at relatively little cost and effort by enhancing the skills of the professionals already working in them.

Figure 4: A Tanzanian primary school

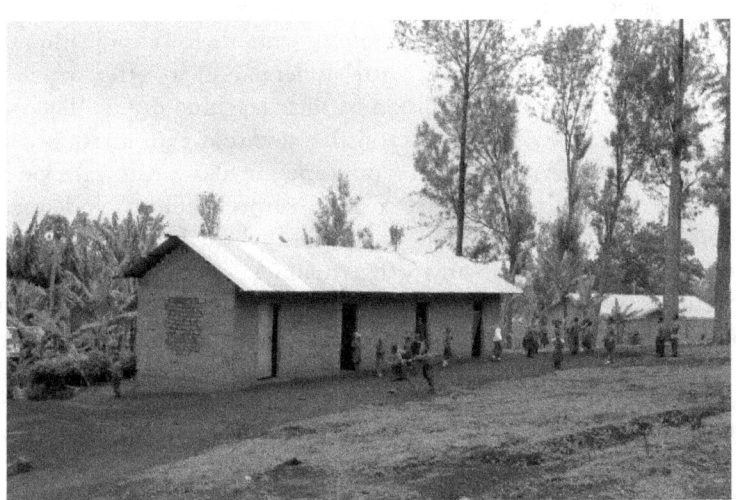

Mount Meru University's Guidance and Counseling Concentration

Some educational programs in Tanzania have already recognized the potential for capacity building via task shifting in school systems. At the university level, some curricula in education now include required courses in special education, guidance counseling, or psychology. This trend can only be viewed as positive – greater education among teachers and administrators can only increase the acceptance of and access to mental health care in Tanzania, including those aimed at serving children with special needs. At least one university has taken this approach a step further, making counseling a formal concentration in one of its degree programs. Mount Meru University (MMU) in Arusha has developed a Guidance and Counseling concentration for students in their Bachelor of Education program, which aims to allow those students to take on the dual role of being an educator and school counselor (MMU, 2016).

Students in the MMU program are most often established teachers who are returning to school to complete their university degrees, as many Tanzanian educators hold only a secondary education. As such, they often have little to no prior knowledge of the field of psychology. After an introductory psychology course, they complete more specialized coursework in the field. This is comprised of twelve courses, which cover topics such as human development, cross cultural psychology, educational psychology, clinical psychology, ethics, and assessment (MMU, 2016). The concentration also includes a capstone research project, although there is no formal practicum component at this time. Despite this limitation, the program provides a strong foundation in the knowledge necessary to provide basic mental health assessment and intervention in a school setting.

Upon selecting the Guidance and Counseling concentration, trainees are encouraged to have a conversation with their school administration about the value of this approach for students and to offer to take on the role of school counselor in addition to their teaching duties. The outcomes for the educators vary: some take on the new role with a reduced teaching load and perhaps even a raise in pay, some are allowed to take on the new role but must maintain their current responsibilities and receive no additional compensation, and some are denied the opportunity to implement their learning in any formal manner.

Students who meet a dead end in their efforts to incorporate their guidance and counseling skills in their current roles as educators typically provide similar explanations for why this is the case: school administration simply did not feel that the benefit of creating a counseling program outweighs the cost of having the teacher take time away from the classroom. Tanzanian schools operate under the pressure of high stakes examinations such as the "Primary School Leaving Exam," which students must pass to advance to secondary education, but which was failed by 49.4% of all examinees in 2013 (Kippenberg, 2014, p. 2). Schools face immense pressure to produce strong results; therefore, a majority of their limited resources are dedicated to preparing students for these exams, often with hour after hour of lectures on common exam content. To date, school leaders rarely make the connection between the well-being of students and their performance on such exams. Consequently, the prospect of a teacher spending several hours per week engaged in promoting student wellness may be viewed as unnecessary or wasteful. Similarly, students with special needs are often viewed as "lost causes" and unlikely to pass the difficult national examinations even with additional support, and thus these students tend to be left unsupported in the education system (Stone-MacDonald & Butera, 2014).

In the face of such strong institutional norms and systemic opposition, it might be understandable for MMU's Guidance and Counseling graduates to simply return to their former roles as teachers. However, this is rarely the case. The trainees continue to advocate for the wellness of students, whether within their institutions or in other roles as community volunteers, local leaders, advocates, educators, or NGO founders. They promote the importance of emotional wellness for young people via research, outreach on social media, and informal conversations with other professionals. In short, their training has unintentionally turned them into a cohort of CHWs, albeit a cohort with no centralized leadership and no formal support. Although no research has been done on the community impact of their work, these educators represent the power of health knowledge in changing community attitudes toward a topic, one small step at a time. They believe that until the educational system is ready to accept them as a valuable resource, they must show their value each day, in any way they can, to help the system change.

Community Health Workers as Agents of Change

It has been reported that the developing world needs 2.4 million additional health workers to fill the current treatment gap and adequately respond to medical needs (WHO, 2008, p.14). Given the geographic realities of the world's poorest nations, with human resource constraints in the area of health care, physicians and other highly skilled health workers are unlikely to fill this gap in the near future. Ultimately, CHWs appear to be a positive response to this need, despite the costs of remuneration, professional development, and other forms of support for these professionals. In multiple settings throughout the world, CHWs engage in task sharing, taking on administrative, social work, and clinical responsibilities typically assigned to specialists.

CHWs relieve burdens that often fall on both members of the general public and the health systems intended to serve them. Individuals who are traditionally disconnected from care by distance, cost, or cultural misunderstanding are able to access advice and referral information from a knowledgeable and familiar face. Medical facilities have the benefits of serving a more well-informed patient population and of more effectively following up with care without dedicating their own precious resources. For these reasons, task sharing via CHW programs is a cost-effective method of scaling up the untapped supply of health workers, relieving the burden on other providers, and bridging the gap between those who do have access to medical care and those who do not.

References

Agier, M. (2011). *Managing the undesirables: Refugee camps and humanitarian government*. Cambridge, UK: Polity.

Barron, S., Okell, J., Yin, S. M., VanBik, K., Swain, A., Larkin, E.,…Ewers, K. (2007). Refugees from Burma: Their backgrounds and refugee experiences. *The Center for Applied Linguistics*. Retrieved from https://cnnc.uncg.edu/wp-content/uploads/2015/06/COR-Burma-Profile.pdf

Beiser, M., & Hou, F. (2016). Mental health effects of premigration trauma and postmigration discrimination on refugee youth in Canada. *The Journal of Nervous and Mental Disease, 204*(6), 464-470. doi: 10.1097/NMD.0000000000000516

Benshoff, L. (2016, April 19). Pennsylvania's largest refugee resettlement agency is shutting down, but pathway to state remains open. *Newsworks*. Retrieved from www.newsworks.org/index.php/local/pa-suburbs/92964-pas-largest-refugee-resettlement-agency-is-shutting-down-but-pathway-to-state-remains-open

Bhutta, Z. A., Lassi, Z. S., Pariyo, G., & Huicho, L. (2010). Global experience of community health workers for delivery of health related Millennium Development Goals. *The World*

Health Organization. Retrieved from
www.who.int/workforcealliance/knowledge/resources/chwreport/en/

Bruno, A. (2011). U.S. refugee resettlement assistance. *Congressional Research Service*. Retrieved from https://fas.org/sgp/crs/row/R41570.pdf

Chebel d'Appollonia, A. (2012). *Frontiers of fear: Immigration and insecurity in the United States and Europe*. Ithaca, NY: Cornell University Press.

Feinstein, S. & Mwahombela, L. (2010). Corporal punishment in Tanzania's schools. *International Review of Education, 56*(4), 399-410. doi: 10.1007/s11159-010-9169-5

Frerichs, R. R., Keim, P. S., Barrais, R., & Piarroux, R. (2012). Nepalese origin of cholera epidemic in Haiti. *Clinical Microbiology and Infection, 18*, 158-163. doi: 10.1111/j.1469-0691.2012.03841.x

Heptinstall, E., Sethna, V., & Taylor, E. (2004). PTSD and depression in refugee children: Associations with pre-migration trauma and post-migration stress. *European Child & Adolescent Psychiatry, 13*(6), 373-380.

Jerome, G., & Ivers, L. C. (2010). Community health workers in health systems strengthening: A qualitative evaluation from rural Haiti. *AIDS, 24*(1), 67-72. doi: 10.1097/01.aids.0000366084.75945.c9.

Jhokio, A. H., Winter, H. R., & Cheng, K. K. (2005). An intervention involving traditional birth attendants and perinatal and maternal mortality in Pakistan. *The New England Journal of Medicine, 352*, 2091- 2099.

Kale, R. (2002). The treatment gap. *Epilepsia, 43*(6), 31-33. doi: 10.1046/j.1528-1157. 43.s.6.13.x

Kalofonos, I. (2015). "We can't find this spirit of help": Mental health, social issues, and community home-based care providers in central Mozambique. In B. A. Kohrt & E. Mendenhall (Eds.). *Global mental health: Anthropological perspectives* (pp. 309-324). Walnut Creek, CA: Left Coast Press.

Kiweewa, J. M. (2015). Integrating guidance and counseling models into teacher training. In A. M. Bwire, M. S. Nyagise, J. O. Masingila, & H. O. Ayot (Eds.), *Proceedings of the 4th International Conference on Education: Building Capacity Through Quality Teacher Education*. Nairobi, Kenya: Kenyatta University.

Kippenberg, J. (2014). Tanzania: Let's tackle the Primary School Leaving Exam. *Human Rights Watch*. Retrieved from www.hrw.org/news/2014/05/13/tanzania-lets- tackle-primary-school-leaving-exam

Knettel, B. A., Rugira, J., & Tesha, F. (2016). *"They Will Start Believing in Counseling": Provider Perceptions of the Presentation and Treatment of Mental Illness in Northern Tanzania*. Unpublished manuscript, Duke Global Health Institute, Durham, NC, U.S.A.

Knettel, B. A., Slifko, S. E., Inman, A. G., & Silova, I. (2017). Training community health workers: An evaluation of effectiveness, sustainable continuity, and cultural humility in an educational program in rural Haiti. *International Journal of Health Promotion and Education*. Advance online publication. doi: 10.1080/14635240.2017.1284014

Kohrt, B. A., & Mendenhall, E. (2015). *Global mental health: Anthropological perspectives*. Walnut Creek, CA: Left Coast Press.

Lehmann, U., & Sanders, D. (2007). Community health workers: What do we know about them? *The World Health Organization*. Retrieved from www.who.int/hrh/documents/community_health_workers.pdf

Lloyd, C., Kaufman, C., & Hewett, P. (2000). The spread of primary schooling in sub-Saharan Africa: Implications for fertility Change. *Population and Development Review, 26*(3), 483-515.

Mabula, N., & Edna, K. (2015). Is it not now? School counselors' training in Tanzanian secondary schools. *Journal of Education and Practice, 6*(19), 160-169.

Maes, K. (2015). Task-shifting in global health: Mental health implications for community health workers and volunteers. In B. A. Kohrt & E. Mendenhall (Eds.). *Global mental health: Anthropological perspectives* (pp. 291-307). Walnut Creek, CA: Left Coast Press.

Mott, T. E. (2010). African refugee resettlement in the U.S.: The role and significance of voluntary agencies. *Journal of Cultural Geography, 27*(1), 1-31. doi: 10.1080/08873631003593190

Mount Meru University (MMU). (2016). *The prospectus, 2014-2017*. Retrieved from www.mmu.ac.tz/uploads/prospectus.pdf

Murray, K. E., & Marx, D. M. (2013). Attitudes toward unauthorized immigrants, authorized immigrants, and refugees. *Cultural Diversity and Ethnic Minority Psychology, 19*(3), 332-341. doi: 10.1037/a0030812

Nezer, M. (2013). *Resettlement at risk: Meeting emerging challenges to refugee resettlement in local communities*. Hebrew Immigrant Aid Society (HIAS). Retrieved from www.hias.org/uploaded/file/Resettlement_at_Risk.pdf.

Office of Refugee Resettlement (ORR). (2016). *Voluntary agencies*. Retrieved from www.acf.hhs.gov/orr/resource/voluntary-agencies

Office of Refugee Resettlement (ORR). (2017). *Annual report to congress: Fiscal year 2015*. Retrieved from www.acf.hhs.gov/sites/default/files/orr/arc_15_final_508.pdf

Pan American Health Organization (PAHO). (2011). *Earthquake in Haiti – One year later: PAHO/WHO report on the health situation*. Retrieved from www.paho.org/disasters/index.php?option=com_content&view=article&id=1088

Pendse, A., & Yu, X. (2016). *Healthy people, healthy community: Evaluation of a train-the-trainer program on water, sanitation, and hygiene in southeast Haiti*. Unpublished manuscript, College of Education, Lehigh University, Bethlehem, U.S.A.

Pennsylvania Refugee Resettlement Program (PRRP). (2014). *Demographics and arrival statistics*. Retrieved from www.refugeesinpa.org/aboutus/demoandarrivalstats/ index.htm

Perry, H. (2013). A brief history of community health worker programs. *USAID Maternal and Child Health Integrated Program*. Retrieved from www.mchip.net/sites/ default/files/mchipfiles/02_CHW_History.pdf

Perry, H. B., Zullinger, R., & Rogers, M. M. (2014). Community health workers in low-, middle-, and high-income countries: An overview of their history, recent evolution, and current effectiveness. *Annual Review of Public Health, 35*, 399-421. doi: 10.1146/annurev-publhealth-032013-182354

Plumb, E. J., Knettel, B. A., Fogg, M., Owens, E. M., Walinsky, S., Brawer, R., & Plumb, J. (in press). Envisioning home: The Philadelphia Refugee Mental Health Photovoice Project as a story of effective relationship building. In M. Capous-Desyllas & K. Morgaine (Eds.). *Creating social change through creativity: Anti-oppressive arts-based research methodologies*. London: Palgrave Macmillan.

Porter, M., & Haslam, N. (2005). Predisplacement and postdisplacement factors associated with mental health of refugees and internally displaced persons. *The Journal of the American Medical Association, 294*(5), 602-612. doi: 10.1001/jama.294.5.602

Rousseau, C., Drapeau, A., & Corin, E. (1997). The influence of culture and context on the pre- and post-migration experience of school-aged refugees from Central America and Southeast Asia in Canada. *Social Science & Medicine, 44*(8), 1115-1127.

Stone-MacDonald, A., & Butera, G. (2014). Cultural beliefs and attitudes about disability in East Africa. *Review of Disability Studies, 8*(1), 62-77.

Substance Abuse and Mental Health Services Administration (SAMHSA). (2016). *SAMHSA's wellness initiative: Connecting all aspects of behavioral health*. Retrieved from www.samhsa.gov/wellness-initiative

Summerfield. D. (1996). The psychological legacy of war and atrocity: The question of long-term and transgenerational effects and the need for a broad view. *The Journal of Nervous and Mental Disease, 184*, 375-377.

United Nations High Commissioner for Refugees (UNHCR). (2016). *Global trends 2015: Forced displacement hits a record high*. Retrieved from www.unhcr.org/en-us/ global-trends-2015.html

United Nations International Children's Emergency Fund (UNICEF). (2016). *Hurricane Matthew one month on: More than 600,000 children still in need of aid.* Retrieved from www.unicef.org/media/media_93040.html

U.S. Department of Labor (2016). Labor force characteristics of foreign-born workers summary. *Bureau of Labor Statistics.* Retrieved from www.bls.gov/news.release/forbrn.nr0.htm

U.S. Department of State. (2015). Fiscal year 2015 refugee admission statistics. *Bureau of Population, Refugees, and Migration.* Retrieved from https://2009-2017.state.gov/j/prm/releases/statistics/251285.htm

White House Office of the Press Secretary (2017). *Executive order protecting the nation from foreign terrorist entry into the United States.* Retrieved from www.whitehouse.gov/briefing-room/presidential-actions/executive-orders

World Health Organization (WHO). (1989). *Strengthening the performance of community health workers in primary health care.* Retrieved from http://apps.who.int/iris/handle/10665/39568

World Health Organization (WHO). (2008). *Task shifting: Global recommendations and guidelines.* Retrieved from www.who.int/workforcealliance/knowledge/resources/taskshifting_guidelines/en/

World Health Organization (WHO). (2016). *MHGAP intervention guide: For mental, neurological, and substance use disorders in non-specialized health settings.* Retrieved from www.who.int/mental_health/mhgap/mhGAP_intervention_guide_02/en/

CHAPTER 11

The Utilization of the Biopsychosocial Model for Disease Prevention and Global Health Promotion

Samara Lipsky and Marissa Vishnu Mack

Smoking is the number one preventable cause of death globally and is estimated to cause six million deaths a year (CDC, 2015a, para. 6). Smoking contributes to the following non-communicable diseases: cancer, heart disease, stroke, lung diseases, and diabetes (CDC, 2015). According to the World Health Organization's (WHO) World Health Report (2002), an individual can reduce his/her risk factors by eliminating tobacco use, limiting alcoholic beverage consumption, eating healthily, engaging in physical activity, and adhering to medication. A combination of biological (genetic, gender, stress reactivity), psychological (personality, behavior, emotions, coping skills, trauma) and social (culture, family circumstances, relationships) factors contribute to an individual's health and well-being. This chapter will discuss a global treatment program that will utilize the biopsychosocial model to assist in the prevention of chronic diseases while promoting global health.

Across the globe, there are challenges to an individual's mental, physical, and emotional health. According to the WHO (1978), the definition of health includes "state of complete physical, mental, and social well-being and not just the absence of infirmary" (p. 1) Health is no longer understood by using a unidimensional model, but instead by utilizing a multidimensional model that encompasses different factors of health. Beaglehole and Bonita (2010) discuss global health as being a collaborative, trans-national research and action for promoting health for all. When illnesses are combined, they account for 15% of the total global burden of disease (Patel, 2012, 1:23). The four main types of non-communicable diseases (cancer, diabetes, cardiovascular disease, and chronic lung disease) account for over 30 million (Kim & Oh, 2013, p. 165) deaths a year and are the leading causes of death in most low- and middle-income countries (Kim & Oh, 2013). This chapter will discuss interventions and programs based on the biopsychosocial model that are aimed at preventing non-communicable diseases and helping to promote global health.

Treating an individual includes addressing a combination of biological, psychological, and social components. Biological factors that contribute to disease include genetics, gender, and stress reactivity. There are many psychological contributors to health and disease as well, such as behavior, emotions, coping skills, and personality. These behavioral factors contribute to diseases such as heart disease, diabetes, and cancer. Social factors, such as family and friends, relationships, and culture, also impact an individual's health. When exploring health on a global scale, it is important to have cultural awareness and sensitivity regarding Western and non-Western beliefs, attitudes, and values, all of which impact an individual's decision-making. Recognizing the importance of using a multidimensional model, such as the biopsychosocial model, to assist in global health prevention and promotion will be the main theme throughout this chapter.

The WHO defines health as a multidimensional concept that contains three sets of domains to describe health: (1) core domains of health that are the direct measures of health (e.g. affect, pain, cognition, and mobility), (2) additional domains of health that are the direct measures of health (e.g. vision, hearing, sleep, and energy), and (3) indirect measures of health (e.g. self care, and daily activities) (Chatterji, Ustun, Sadana, Salomon, Mathers, & Murray, 2002).

Being such a complex term, it is imperative to have a clear definition of the word "health." The WHO (1948) defines health as "a state of complete physical, mental, and social well-being and not merely the absence of disease or infirmity" (para.1). To expand on this definition, health is defined as the absence of (1) objective signs that the body is not functioning properly, and (2) subjective symptoms of disease or injury (Lu, 2002). The focus of health, based upon this definition, is on an individual's physical symptoms. There are other definitions that encompass different areas of health.

The psychological concept of health encompasses life stresses, mental illnesses, affect, and life satisfaction (Lu, 2002). According to the WHO (2016) mental illness is characterized by "a combination of abnormal thoughts, perceptions, emotions, behavior, and relationships with others" (Key facts, para. 1). Research findings have shown that there are approximately 450 million people across the globe affected by mental illnesses (Patel, 2012,1:27) which are amongst the leading causes of disabilities.

The socio-cultural concept of health proposes that disease is a disturbance of an individual's ability to perform tasks. Health is socially defined as an individual's well-being that is separate from physical and mental health. According to Lu (2002) as cited by Wright (1990), an individual's perception of health is defined as, "health as being, health as doing, and health as having" (Lu, 2002, p. 2). According to Myers and colleagues (2000), wellness is defined as being "a way of life oriented toward optimal health and well-being in which body, mind, and spirit are integrated by the individual to live more fully within the human and natural community" (Myers, Sweeney, & Witmer, 2000, p. 252). According to this definition, changes in one area of wellness can impact other areas of life in both positive and negative ways.

There have been numerous research studies exploring the methods in which different cultures view health. For example, a qualitative study conducted in Taiwan that consisted of 201 undergraduate students (ages19-25 years-old) and 45 community female adults, found that health was viewed as the absence of physical, mental, and behavioral deviations (Lu, 2002). The three components to functioning were found to be: (1) normal physical functioning (absence of physical disease or symptoms), (2) normal mental functioning (absence of mental illness or symptoms), and (3) normal behavioral functioning (absence of bad habits). Health was viewed as being more than freedom from disease. Instead, it encompassed many hierarchical components: (1) clinical components (overall health and personal happiness), (2) role components (social functioning in society and relationships), (3) adaptive components (personal equilibrium in a stressful situation), and (4) well-being components (content and having positive beliefs and values and pursuing goals) (Lu, 2002).

The way in which individuals subjectively define their health depends on their culture and sociodemographic variables (Lu, 2002). This includes gender and cultural differences in areas of wellness (Myers et al., 2000). Diverse cultural groups have different belief systems, including the way in which they view heath and disease. For example, non-Western cultures that believe in using non-Western healing art focus on psychosomatic harmony and utilize a holistic understanding of health. The Yin-Yang theory proposes that health is a state of physical and spiritual harmony. This theory transforms into an individual's beliefs, traditions, and attitudes in Chinese culture (Lu, 2002).

Belief systems vary between different cultures. There are four types of belief systems regarding attribution of disease: (1) factors within the individuals themselves, (2) factors within the natural environment, (3) factors associated with others, and (4) supernatural factors. Individuals in

Western countries are more likely to attribute a disease to individuals themselves or to the natural environment, whereas non-Westerns are more likely to attribute disease to social or supernatural circumstances (Vaughn, 2010).

One popular belief is the connection between mind and body, otherwise known as monism vs. dualism (separation of the mind and body). According to Resnick (1997) there is an increasingly strong connection between mind and body. For example, integrated care practices that include psychological services can be successful in improving an individual's mental and behavioral health (Dale & Lee, 2016). There are multiple necessary steps to increase the diversity in developing group practices of psychologists. The first step is to establish strong links with health care providers, which will lead to the next step, developing and creating multidisciplinary group practices. The final step is to create and implement an integrated health care delivery systems (Vaughn, 2010).

Locus of Control

Global health beliefs are also characterized by an individual's internal vs. external locus of control. One has an external locus of control if one perceives a reward to be based on luck, chance, fate, or based on other powers. In other words, an individual with external locus of control believes the event happens by a means outside of his/her control. On the other hand, one has an internal locus of control if one believes that an event happens due to his/her own behaviors. In this situation, the individual believes that it was his/her actions that caused the event to happen. When comparing interval vs. external locus of control, there is a difference in an individual's behavior in a situation that is chance-determined, as opposed to skill-determined, respectively. Since an individual's health belief can lead to individual differences within a situation, behavioral outcomes can lead to different behavior choices (Rotter, 1960).

Models of Health

There are many diverse models of health that consider different cultural factors. Vaughn (2010) discusses two important models of health and factors that impact an individual's health. The first model is The Mandala of Health Model (Hancock & Perkins, 1985) which contains four factors that influence an individual's health: (1) human biology, (2) personal behavior,(3) psychosocial environment, and (4) physical environment. In addition, family, lifestyle, the medical care system, community, biosphere, and culture impact an individual's health. Another multidimensional model by Geiger and Davidhizar (1985) discusses six cultural variables that are used to view healthcare and disease prevention: (1) environmental control,

(2) biological variables, (3) social organization, (4) communication, (5) space, and (6) time orientation.

The model is like Western models, depicting a multidimensional model with four aspects of health, but differs culturally in the importance of social roles, such as interpersonal relationships and maintaining a harmonious social network. The focus is on an interdependent society that emphasizes the collective society over the individual society. There is the desire to achieve homeostasis between Yin and Yang. Furthermore, illnesses and wellness are not separate but overlap as is the case in the biopsychosocial model (Lu, 2002).

Another multidimensional model of health is The Hispanic Health Protection Model (HHPM), which includes cognitive, psychological, and physiological factors. This model can be used with non-communicable diseases, such as diabetes. The cognitive component of HHPM is the way in which the individual understands diabetes, the psychological component explores the individual's quality of life (QOL) with diabetes, and physiological component is focused on reducing an individual's hemoglobin A1c (Latham & Calvillo, 2009).

Biomedical Model

The biomedical model, as known as the "disease" model, revolves around the physical state of an individual's body in health and illness (Lu, 2002) and is the main model used in Western medicine (Engel, 1980). According to Engel (1977), as cited by Lu (2002), the model proposes that all diseases and physical disorders can be explained by disturbances in physiological processes, which in turn lead to injuries, imbalances, and infections.

Engel (1979) proposes that Western medicine is based on dualism (separation from mind and body) and reductionism (life and biological phenomena, behavior, and mental processes, as studied and explained by chemistry and physics). Reductionism is a linear, cause-and-effect relationship that regards disease as discrete entities that can be eliminated by discovering the cause of the disease. The biomedical model is disease-oriented and not patient-centered. For the model to become patient-centered, it would need to encompass a psychosocial component. The biomedical model has been helpful in the development of antibiotics, has assisted with a decline in infectious diseases, increasing life expectancy. It is through the biomedical model that many infectious diseases are no longer the primacy causes of death in developed countries (Johnson, 2013).

Although the biomedical model has helped with physical diseases, the model lacks in its ability to address mental health problems, as it is only concerned with a biological approach to healthcare. Its effort is exclusively on disease. This model defines disease as a biologic defect (Johnson, 2013).

The model is focused on biological factors and not on psychological, social, or environmental factors. The model utilizes mind-body dualism (Johnson, 2013) and considers disease to be separate from the psychological and social processes (Lu, 2002). Research on the biomedical model shows that it is less successful in treating chronic diseases. This has led to a shift from the biomedical to the biopsychosocial model of health and disease (Johnson, 2013).

Biopsychosocial Model

Pilgrim (2015) discusses the strong legitimacy of utilizing the biopsychosocial model in researching health and illness. The biopsychosocial model consists of genetic, environmental, and social factors. In the biopsychosocial model, health, function, and well-being are the outcomes, in addition to disease. The premise of the biopsychosocial model is that physical health and well-being are shaped by the interactions between biological, psychological, and social factors. The model utilizes intra- and inter systemic harmony (Engel, 1979) and rejects the separation of mind and body, as it is focused on the theory of holism. Treatments can be behavioral, biologic, or environmental (Johnson, 2013).

The biopsychosocial model is a scientific model that takes into consideration what the biomedical model is missing (Engel, 1980). The model focuses on patient-centered integrated care in which the patient is viewed as a whole person. According to the biopsychosocial model, this viewpoint will lead to better quality of care, access to care, reduced stigma, lower costs, and better patient satisfaction (Johnson, 2013). In addition, the model emphasizes the importance of collaboration with health professionals from different disciplines who are competent in diverse areas of healthcare (Engel, 1979). Schwartz (1982) discusses that improved diagnosis and better predictions about treatment should occur as a medical diagnosis in conjunction with the biopsychosocial model, which considers the importance biological, psychological, and social factors.

There is a global need to utilize the biopsychosocial model in both Western and non-Western countries. The integrated care mode in the United Kingdom (U.K.) includes developing psychological and behavioral roles within primary care. This includes creating a primary care team of both medical and non-medical members to work together to treat medical, social, and psychological/behavioral issues. Creating a multidisciplinary team would lead to better prevention, intervention, and decreased hospital visits (Dale & Lee, 2016).

In addition to the U.K., there have been other countries throughout the world that have utilized a multidisciplinary team for health and well-being. For example, countries with higher economies, such as Germany, Australia, and Singapore, have utilized integrated care teams that include a behavioral component and collaboration among different health professionals. The United States (U.S.) has utilized a multi-disciplinary team in the Veterans Health Administration that has incorporated telemedicine among other treatments (Dale & Lee, 2016). The success of implementing a multidisciplinary team has been confirmed by research studies that have used a combination of healing methods. For example, Vaughn (2010) cites a research study by Willems and St. Pierre-Hansen (2008) that found that integrative medicine utilizes the body's own natural healing ability to incorporate beliefs, attitudes, and culture into treatment decisions that include complementary and alternative medicines.

The impact of an individual's culture and belief system varies. The ethno-biopsychosocial model acknowledges the part that indigenous culture plays in human rights. It recognizes the role that spirituality plays in a holistic approach. The model is based on human rights and psycho-spiritual perspectives. There are nine dimensions in the model: (1) sickness conception, (2) body function beliefs, (3) well-being criteria, (4) causal/healing beliefs, (5) health practice efficacy beliefs, (6) recognition of health need, (7) reliance on self-treatment, (8) acceptance of suggestion for health care, and (9) cooperation with health advice (Alladin, 2009). These components are important to take into consideration when working with individuals who believe that spirituality is an important factor for health.

Other important contributing factors for health are biological factors and social factors such as family circumstances and relationships. When exploring the biological contributions to disease, the following lifestyle and psychological factors should be included: (1) diet and nutrition, (2) obesity, (3) alcoholic intake, (4) psychosocial stress, (5) occupational and environmental exposures, and (6) other diseases. The impact that these factors have on the relationship between observed tobacco exposure and health-related tobacco outcomes among racially classified social groups was explored (RCSCG) (Fernander, Shavers, & Hammons, 2007).

Triggers

Diet and Nutrition

Diet and nutrition are important elements of human health throughout the world. Tilman and Clark (2014) discuss that many of the world's most impoverished individuals have diets that are inadequate. If their diets were inclusive of essential fatty acids, minerals, vitamins, and other nutritionally appropriate sources, they would have much improved health. Diet also varies by gender and culture. For example, a survey conducted by Wardle and colleagues (2004) in 23 countries, consisting of 20,000 university students, found that women engaged in healthier eating habits (p. 109).

They ate fewer fats, and consumed more fruit and fiber in comparison to men (Wardle, Haase, Steptoe, Nillapun, Jonwuites & Bellisle, 2004).

Tillman and Clark (2014) posit that countries such as China, India, Mexico, Nigeria, and Tunisia are in the midst of "increasing disease incidence" (Tillman & Clark, 2014, p. 521). Unless changes in nutrition practices occur, individuals in these countries will be prone to chronic diet related non-communicable diseases, such as diabetes and chronic heart disease. Due to this dominant burden in terms of global disease, "poorer members of poorer nations will be affected, whereby healthcare is unavailable" (Tillman & Clark, 2014, p. 521).

When utilizing the biopsychosocial model to encompass diet and nutrition, these risk factors that contribute to non-communicable disease consist of a biological, and specifically, a genetic component. According to Morrison (2008), obesity appears to be a product of genetic vulnerability as well as a combination of maladaptive and environmental factors. However, due to the exorbitant increases in obesity rates, genes cannot be the sole explanation. If a person engages in physical activity with the incorporation of a healthy diet, genetic tendencies can be limited. Obesity is also linked to connections among friends. Christakis and Fowler (2007) conducted a study over the span of 32 years, which showed that if an individual had an obese friend, that individual would be more likely to be obese. If the friend is a close friend, the odds are then tripled.

Fruits and vegetables help protect against many cancers, while, red meat has been found to be a predictor of cancer. Dietary factors may modulate DNA methylation in the following four ways: (1) they may influence the supply of methyl groups, (2) they modify the use of methyl groups for process, (3) they influence DNA demethylation, and (4) they may impact response of bioactive food component. Nutrition is also part of the social factor of the biopsychosocial model, specifically the environment that a child is raised in, as it has been found that early life nutrition has a big impact on diseases in the future (Fernander, Shavers, & Hammons, 2007).

Obesity

When discussing obesity, it is important to note that cultures view obesity differently. Although some countries look fondly on obesity, it is a risk factor for disease (Fernander, Shavers, & Hammons, 2007). According to Jansen (1983) (as cited by Vaughn [2010]), obesity is viewed as a health problem in the West, but in African cultures, it is a sign of wealth and prestige. Excessive obesity was at one time considered a problem in the U.S. and other high-income countries of the Western world, but it has now become a major contributor to the global burden of disease (Malik, Walter, Willett & Hu, 2013). For example, Calle and colleagues (2003) (as cited by Fernader and colleagues [2007]) argue that U.S. obesity accounts for 14% of cancer deaths in males and 20% of cancer deaths in females (Fernander et al., 2007, p. 48).

Obesity is not just a problem in the U.S., but is a global health epidemic. According to the WHO (2016d), there are 1.9 billion adults who are overweight (BMI >= 25) and 600 million adults are obese (BMI >=30) (Facts about overweight and obesity, para. 1); 11% of men and 15% of women are obese (Facts about overweight and obesity, para. 2), and 38% of men and 40% of women are overweight (Facts about overweight and obesity, para. 3). Obesity not only negatively affects adults – children are not immune from gaining an unhealthy amount of weight. Globally, there are 41 million children under five years old who are overweight or obese (Key facts, para 5).

When examining the causes of obesity, it is important to consider the biopsychosocial model. Obesity is caused by a change in diet and exercise, such as eating high fat foods and decreasing physical activity. There are many ways to prevent obesity (WHO, 2016d). Research has found that the prevention of obesity needs to occur in infancy. Infant obesity and unusually fast weight increases are related to obesity in later childhood. An obese child is more likely to become an obese adult (Sarafino & Smith, 2014). This leads to the belief that the social component of the biopsychosocial model that is a contributor to obesity is the environment in which the child is raised. A study conducted by Cartwright and colleagues (2003) sampled 4,320 schoolchildren who completed questions based on stress and eating habits. The children who reported the highest levels of stress were less likely to engage in healthy eating behaviors. This study shows that unhealthy eating behaviors are triggered by stress.

Even if an individual is obese or overweight, there are many behavioral changes that he/she can make to lose weight and lead a healthier lifestyle. According to The Center for Disease Control and Prevention (CDC, 2015c), maintaining a healthy weight is a lifestyle change that consists of healthy eating and physical activity. The first step is to use screening tools to assess an individual's weight. This is typically done by calculating the Body Mass Index (BMI) and waist circumference. An individual's BMI should ideally be 18.5-24.9. Individuals who are overweight have a BMI of 25.0-29.9. A BMI higher than 30 is considered obese (CDC, n.d.a, Adult body mass index or BMI, para. 1). In addition, if the waist circumference is greater than 40 inches for a male and 35 inches for a female, it can put the individual at a greater risk for high blood pressure, Type 2 Diabetes, and coronary artery disease (CDC, n.d.a, Waist circumference, para. 2). Making these behavioral changes utilizes the psychological component of the model.

Obesity is a risk factor for health. Obesity can lead to non-communicable diseases such as cardiovascular disease (CVD) (heart disease, and stroke), diabetes, musculoskeletal disorders, and some cancers (colon, prostate, gallbladder, and liver). Children in low- and middle-income countries are more susceptible to obesity, since nutrition intake is worse. Foods in their geographic area may cost less, but also have less nutritional value (high sugar and sodium content) (WHO, 2016d). Obesity is best prevented in children by implementing behavioral changes such as healthy eating and an increase in physical activity, which can lead to weight loss and a healthier lifestyle.

Alcoholic Intake

According to the WHO (2015a), alcohol is related to 3.3 million deaths a year and is a causal factor for over 200 diseases and injuries (Key facts, para. 1). For individuals aged 20-39, alcohol is the cause of 25% of deaths (Key facts, para. 4). There is a causal relationship between alcohol use and a range of mental and behavioral illnesses. In addition, harmful use of alcohol can also impact an individual socially and economically. The context in which the individual is drinking can have an impact on this. There are also differences in alcohol consumption by gender. Alcohol is related to 7.6% of male deaths and 4% of female deaths (WHO, 2015a, Factors affecting alcohol consumption and alcohol related harm, para. 6). Alcohol consumption is two-dimensional: (1) total volume of alcohol that the individual consumes and (2) the individual's drinking pattern.

There are many negative impacts to health and well-being that drinking an excessive amount of alcohol can cause. For example, high levels of alcohol consumption has been found to be related to CVD. In addition, heavy drinkers are more likely to smoke cigarettes, which can lead to a range of other non-communicable diseases. Chronic alcohol consumption is a risk factor for cancer in the larynx, throat, and liver (Fernander, Shavers, & Hammons, 2007).

Alcoholism not only has underlying psychosocial and sociocultural factors, but a biological one as well. According to Wallace (1990), alcoholism is a biopsychosocial disease that encompasses the mind, body, and society, and must be viewed as a human problem. Wallace (1990) summarizes research on genetics and alcoholism and found that environment also plays a role in causation because not all individuals who abuse alcohol have a family history of alcohol abuse. Culture and society also influence drinking habits. There are genetic predispositions, risk factors, and vulnerabilities that impact alcohol use. Individuals with a specific gene pattern tend to experience stronger cravings for alcohol after one drink compared to individuals who do not have this gene pattern. The role of stress in consuming alcohol is also strong for people with gene patterns that promote heavy drinking (Hutchinson, McGeary, Smolen, Bryan, & Swift, 2002).

Psychosocial Stress

There are many psychosocial stresses that can lead to negative health and disease. For example, immigrants have psychosocial factors that may impose stressors in children, including mental health issues due to relocation, adaptation issues, and a lack of strong support networks from their country of origin. One factor that impacts the health of immigrants that migrate to the U.S. is poverty. This often manifests itself in substandard housing, which can lead to stress and illness. It is important to reduce the risk factors that can lead to a non-communicable disease. For example, an unhealthy diet can lead to obesity, diabetes, and cancer (Li & Pawlish, 1998). Tobacco, alcohol, and drugs can also lead to health problems (Vaughn, 2010).

Mental health disorders are triggered by stress, genetics, nutrition, perinatal infections, and exposure to environmental toxins (WHO, 2016c). In low- and middle-income countries, 76-85% of individuals with mental illnesses are not receiving treatments. In high-income countries, around 35-50% of individuals with mental illnesses are not receiving treatments (WHO, 2016c, Health and support, para. 1). Furthermore, those who do receive treatment are not always receiving the best quality of care (WHO, 2016c).

Psychosocial stress might influence disease and onset, such as in cardiac health. Studies have shown that men and women who experience chronic high levels of anger, depression, or anxiety are more prone to suffer from heart disease. Additionally, individuals who receive high levels of emotional support are less likely to suffer from coronary disease (Sarafino & Smith, 2014). Stress does not only have psychological and social components, but there is a biological component as well. Being prone to stress earlier in life can influence the formation of the hippocampus and hypothalamic-pituitary-adrenal cortical axis, which can damage cardiovascular health (Fernander, Shavers, & Hammons, 2007).

Occupational and Environmental Exposure to Tobacco

Tobacco is the "biggest cause of non-communicable disease" and is responsible for more deaths than obesity both in high-income countries (such as the U.S.) and globally (Jha, Phil, & Peto, 2014, p. 61). Fernander and colleagues (2007) define tobacco use as being characterized by rates of smoking and cigarette consumption patterns. However, there are challenges with using this definition – for example, on average, African American's smoke fewer cigarettes, yet have more diseases that are tobacco-related. Smoking topography is defined as an individual's puffing and inhalation during smoking; it measures their exposure to smoke ingredients. This includes the frequency, duration, and volume. Tobacco has over 4000 chemicals, of which 250 are harmful and 50 have been found to cause cancer (WHO, 2016e, Second-hand smoke kills, para. 1).

According to the WHO (2016e), each year, tobacco kills around six million people worldwide (Key facts, para. 2). Of those deaths, 600,000 people died due to second-hand smoke (Key facts, para. 2). Second-hand smoke causes cardiovascular and respiratory diseases (CHD and lung cancer) in adults and sudden death syndrome in infants. In 2004, children were the victims in 28% of second-hand smoke-related deaths (Second-hand smoke kills, para 2). The CDC (2015b) states that smoking causes about 90% of lung cancer deaths in the U.S. (para. 4) and about 80% of deaths due to chronic obstructive pulmonary disease (COPD) (para. 5). Tobacco is responsible for approximately 20% of cancer deaths (WHO, 2015b, Key Facts, para. 6). If smoking was eliminated, then one out of every three cancer deaths in the U.S. would not happen (CDC, 2015b, Smoking and cancer, para. 3). Smoking is also a cause for Type 2 Diabetes and rheumatoid arthritis. It can increase an individual's risk of cataracts, bone health, oral health, and can cause inflammation (CDC, 2015b, Modifying and avoiding risk factors, para. 2).

There are one billion smokers worldwide, and approximately 80% of those smokers reside in low- and middle-income countries (WHO, 2016e, para. 2). There were 5.8 trillion cigarettes smoked in 2014 (The Tobacco Atlas, 2015, para. 1). While there was a significant decrease in smoking in the U.K., Russia, Brazil, and Australia, there was an increase in tobacco use in China. Two of the countries with the highest rates of tobacco use are Russia and the U.S. Other countries, such as Africa, lack cigarette smoking policies and preventions and are in danger of losing more people to the negative effects of tobacco use (The Tobacco Atlas, 2015). In addition to the social and cultural components mentioned, there are behavioral and biological components to tobacco use – smoking behavior and nicotine dependence are influenced by genetics (Fernander, Shavers, & Hammons, 2007).

The World Health Assembly in 2013 sought assistance from governments to reduce the prevalence of smoking by about a third by 2025 (Jha et al., 2014). It has been found that smoking cigarettes is associated with lower socioeconomic status (The Tobacco Atlas, 2015). Jha and colleagues (2014) discussed that smoking accounts for 12-25% of deaths among males in countries such as China, India, Bangladesh, and South Africa. In most countries around the world, smoking by young adults shortens their lifespans by a decade (Jha et al., 2014, p. 64).

Other Diseases

Diabetes is a public health concern globally, as the number of people affected by diabetes has risen from 180 million in 1980, to 422 million in

2014 (WHO, 2016b, Key facts, para. 1). In the U.S., 29.1 million adults (9.3% of the population) have diabetes (CDC, 2014, para. 1). Most individuals (90%) with diabetes have Type 2 Diabetes (Rock, 20003, p. 137)), which is characterized by obesity, insulin resistance, or deficiency. Being diagnosed at a younger age can lead to more complications and an earlier death (Rock, 2003).

There are also genetic factors that predispose some individuals to be diagnosed with Type 2 Diabetes. Diabetes affects Hispanics at double the rate as compared to other ethnicities. Mexican Americans in the U.S. have the highest rate of diagnosis at approximately 24% (Clark, Vincent, Zimmer, & Sanchez, 2009, p. 382) and the highest rate of complications due to their diagnosis (Clark, Vincent, Zimmer, & Sanchez, 2009).

Risk factors for diabetes are composed of biological, psychological, and social components. Factors related to diabetes are genetics, obesity, proteinuria, glucose intolerance, lack of physical activity, and social factors such as acculturation, income, support, and education (Latham & Calvillo, 2009). Diabetes is also associated with complications such as cardiovascular disease, kidney disease, neuropathy, sexual dysfunction (Segal, Leach, May, & Turnbull, 2013), blindness limb amputations, and organ transplants (Rock, 2003). Effective diabetes care is influenced by "health literacy, physical limitations, mental well-being and nonnative language proficiency" (Segal, Leach, May & Turnbull, 2013, p. 1898).

Another non-communicable disease is CVD which encompasses CHD (myocardial infarction and angina pectoris), high blood pressure, cardiac arrest, and ischemic heart disease. CVD is the number one cause of death globally (WHO, 2016a, key facts, para. 1), and according to Lloyd-Jones and colleagues (2009), as cited by Shields and colleagues (2012), it is responsible for one out of every 2.9 deaths in the U.S. It affects African American males the most, then Caucasian males, African American females, and Caucasian females (Shields, Finley, Chawla, & Meadors, 2012, p. 268). Over 75% of CVD deaths occur in low- and middle-income countries (WHO, 2016a, Key facts, para. 3), which is due to the lack of integrated primary health care programs and services. Individuals living in poverty suffer the most (WHO, 2016a). Risk factors for CHD include smoking, hypercholesterolemia, and hypertension. Additional risk factors are obesity, a lack of physical activity, and psychosocial factors (Karner et al., 2005).

Another type of non-communicable disease is chronic lung disease, which includes chronic obstructive pulmonary disease (COPD), asthma, lung diseases, respiratory allergies, and pulmonary hypertension (WHO, n.d.b). Over 60 million individuals have COPD (WHO, n.d.b, main facts, para. 1). It is expected to be the third leading cause of death by 2030 (WHO, n.d.a, Facts, para. 1). Risk factors are tobacco, pollution, chemicals, and childhood respiratory infections (WHO, n.d.a). There are over three million deaths a year due to COPD (WHO, n.d.a, Facts, para.1) 90% of which are from low- and middle-income countries (WHO, 2015c, Key facts, para. 3). Although these diseases are not curable, there are treatments that can help to control symptoms and improve QOL (WHO, n.d.c).

According to the WHO (2015b), there are 8.2 million people who die each year from cancer, over 14 million cases (Key facts, para. 1), and over 100 types of cancers (para. 1). Around 70% of cancer deaths occur in low- and middle-income countries and over 60% of new cases are from Asia, Africa, and Central and South America (WHO, 2015b, Key facts, para. 8). The five most common types of cancer that men die from are lung, stomach, liver, colorectal, and esophagus (WHO, 2015b, Key facts, para. 3). For women, the most common are breast, lung, stomach, colorectal, and cervical cancer (WHO, 2015b, Key facts, para. 4). Cervical cancer is the most common cancer in many developing countries, and up to 20% of these deaths are due to HBV/HPV infections, which can be prevented by immunizations (WHO, 2015b, Modifying and avoiding risk factors, para. 2). Twenty percent of all cancers are caused by a chronic infection (WHO, 2015b, Modifying and avoiding risk factors, para. 2). Breast, cervical, and colorectal cancer can be cured if detected early and treated.

The Role of Behavior and Risk Factors in Disease Prevention

A global health intervention using the biopsychosocial model can be utilized to help reduce the risk factors associated with non-communicable diseases. This can be accomplished by modifying behavior. Most U.S. Americans die from a chronic disease (7 out of 10 deaths) (CDC, n.d.b, para. 2), and almost 50% of adults have at least one chronic disease (CDC, n.d.b, para. 1). The WHO's World Health Report (2002) stated the following as risk factors for non-communicable diseases: (1) tobacco use, (2) alcohol consumption, (3) being overweight, (4) physical inactivity, (5) high blood pressure, and (6) high cholesterol. For example, tobacco use has been the greatest contributor to non-communicable diseases in Korea (Kim & Oh, 2013). Most CVD can be prevented by smoking cessation, physical activity, curbing alcohol use, healthy eating (reducing sodium intake and eating fruits and vegetables), and controlling body weight (WHO, 2016).

McGinnis and Foege (1993) propose that certain behaviors lead to non-communicable diseases, such as smoking, nutrition, lack of physical activity, and substance abuse. For example, smoking was linked to many diseases and was the cause of many deaths (Johnson, 2013). The types of lifestyle and behavior changes for non-communicable diseases overlap. The role of behavior in disease management for diabetes includes medication adherence, diet and exercise, and physiological assessments (taking blood sugar) (Johnson, 2013). Behavioral changes for CVD include physical activity, medications, and dietary modifications (Shields, Finley, Chawla, &

Meadors, 2012). Behavioral changes for diabetes self-management include eating healthily, engaging in physical activity, adhering to medication, and monitoring blood sugar levels (Clark et al., 2009). There is a similar lifestyle change that can be implemented to reduce risk for certain cancers – over 30% of cancers (WHO, 2015b, Modifying and avoiding risk factors, para. 1) can be prevented by making the following lifestyle changes: (1) not smoking tobacco, (2) eating healthily, (3) engaging in physical activity, and (4) limiting the use of alcohol. On the other hand, smoking, drinking alcohol, and having high body mass index, a lack of physical activity, and a diet that is low in fruits and vegetables increases one's risk of being diagnosed with cancer. Strategies to prevent cancer include vaccinations, controlling occupational hazards, and reducing exposure to ultraviolet radiation (UVR) and radiation. In addition to being a preventative measure, screening for certain cancers is crucial for early diagnosis (WHO, 2015b).

The Importance of Education

It is imperative that a greater emphasis be put on disease prevention and health promotion. In particular, there is a need to educate individuals in both Western and non-western countries about the dangers of tobacco use and excessive drinking and the benefits of healthy eating and engaging in physical activity. According to Vaughn (2010), there are cultural differences regarding health beliefs and practices.

A study conducted in China in 2009 found that 38% of smokers were knowledgeable that smoking causes CHD, and 27% knew that it causes stroke (WHO, 2016e, Tobacco users need help to quit, para. 1). Furthermore, while most smokers who are aware of the dangers of smoking want to quit, many do not have the means to quit. In 25% of low-income countries, there is no assistance for those who desire to quit smoking (WHO, 2016e, Tobacco users need help to quit, para. 4).

The sooner these behavioral changes are made, the sooner they can positively impact health. For example, quitting smoking reduces an individual's risk of a heart attack significantly after one year, his/her risk of cancers of the mouth, throat, esophagus, and bladder by 50% within five years, and his/her risk of developing lung cancer by 50% within 10 years. Furthermore, the individual's risk of having a stroke decreases to that of a nonsmoker 2-5 years after quitting smoking (CDC, 2015, Quitting and reduced risks, paras. 1, 3, & 4).

According to Fernander and colleagues (2007), there is evidence that suggests that tobacco-related deaths are not distributed equally. CVD due to tobacco use is more prevalent among African Americans and Latinos. Tobacco-related cancers such are colon/rectal cancer are higher among both male and female African Americans.

In addition to making behavioral changes with regard to tobacco use, it is important to reduce other risk factors, such as obesity. Malik and colleagues (2013) discuss the need for an increase in global awareness to combat high rates of obesity and, more specifically, the need for high-level policy changes from the international community to help governments create guidelines and health outcome surveillance systems. Due to high rates of obesity, it is imperative for low- and middle-income countries to create health systems to deal with chronic diseases. Caregivers should model health-promoting behaviors to assist youth in adopting healthier nutritional choices. The U.S., Canada, and Brazil have adopted nutritional and agricultural policies to prevent obesity. For example, they require nutritional labels to list trans fat amounts (Malik, Willett, & Hu, 2013). Countries such as Brazil, Argentina, Chile, and South Africa have made great strides in eliminating trans fat from food. These behavioral changes can reduce non-communicable diseases and save lives.

Lifestyle Changes

For the changes to have a long-term effect, they must coincide with one's culture and beliefs. A study conducted by Karner and colleagues (2005) consisted of interviewing 113 participants who had a cardiac event and found that there are four main qualitative categories for facilitating lifestyle changes: somatic incentives, social/practical incentives, cognitive incentives, and affective incentives. In addition, individuals made lifestyle changes by increasing their physical activity, eating more healthily, seeking treatment for drug use, and decreasing stress levels and cigarette smoking.

The first category is somatic incentives, which consists of different types of physical symptoms of an illness. This includes direct signals, which increase the individual's awareness of the biological state of his/her body, and indirect signals, which include test results indicating health difficulties. The direct signals can be negative (e.g. reducing pain) and positive signals that increase an individual's well-being (e.g. lifestyle changes). These negative and positive signs can lead to health promoting behavior (Karner, Tingstrom, Abrandt-Dahlgren, & Bergdahl, 2005).

Social/practical incentives are environmental in nature and are comprised of three subcategories: (1) shared concerns (a social network of family and friends that provides support), (2) changed conditions (behavioral change), and (3) external environmental factors (safe and easy access to services). It is more likely that one will change one's behavior if one has positive social support. Safe neighborhoods and access to places where individuals can engage in physical activity also positively influence behavior change. Social/practical incentives mostly affect behavior changes like smoking cessation and increasing physical activity. (Karner, Tingstrom, Abrandt-Dahlgren, & Bergdahl, 2005).

Cognitive incentives are thoughts and beliefs about making lifestyle changes. They include decision making, reflecting, and insights. Active decision-making is when an individual uses his/her insight to make decisions about lifestyle changes. It was found that individuals who made an active decision (as opposed to a passive one) and appropriated the knowledge into their lifestyle were more likely to engage in the behavior change. For example, individuals who were knowledgeable about the positive impact that smoking cessation has on their health were more likely to make behavior changes (Karner, Tingstrom, Abrandt-Dahlgren, & Bergdahl, 2005).

Emotions also play a role in lifestyle changes, and these are called affective incentives. There are three subcategories of affective incentives: (1) fear/reluctance (if needs and safety are not met), (2) self-esteem and limitations, and (3) immediate satisfaction of needs (inability to resist needs and break lifestyle patterns). Of all the three subcategories, fear motivates individuals the most to engage in smoking cessation and physical activity (Karner, Tingstrom, Abrandt-Dahlgren, & Bergdahl, 2005).

Diverse Global Treatment Programs

When creating a health promotion and intervention program it is important to be culturally aware and sensitive to the various methods used to treat psychological illnesses. Hales (1996), who studied beliefs in West Africa regarding mental illness, found that treatment for mental illnesses consisted of (1) confession of what they did to "deserve" the mental illness, (2) removing the spirit, and (3) prevention of an inherited illness (Vaughn, 2010).

Interventions in Western countries would involve a Behavioral Health Consultant (BHC) who assists with communication, particularly motivational interviewing and decision-making. Utilizing BHCs increases patient accessibility and treatment expedience. In addition, this method helps to reduce stigma, which leads to greater patient trust (Dale & Lee, 2016). Although this is primarily a Western method, BHCs that have cultural awareness and sensitivity can be implemented globally.

Training in cultural competency models that address attitudes, knowledge, and skills can be used globally. The first method, an attitudinal approach, respects cultural differences, appreciates diversity, and includes individual self-reflection (regarding biases, thinking, culture, etc.). The next method, a knowledge approach, emphasizes multicultural differences, and each group is examined with respect to its attitudes, values, beliefs, and behaviors. The last method is the skills-based behavioral approach, which emphasizes communication skills and ways to interview that can be generalized across different cultural groups. This approach focuses on beliefs about healing, decision-making, and family dynamics (Betancourt,

2003). These multicultural approaches can be implemented in global health promotion programs and interventions for non-communicable diseases.

Understanding different cultures is important when working with adults with Type 2 Diabetes. For example, in Mexican American culture, concepts play a role in self-management beliefs, and behaviors. These factors include family support (familismo), stress, and smooth social relationships (personalsimo). Self-management needs to focus on stress, depression, and fatigue. Recommendations from the study are to manage emotions and stress (Clark et al., 2009). Psychologist Kelly McGonigal discusses a study that was conducted at Harvard University in which participants were exposed to a social stress test, but were taught to rethink their stress response as being helpful. Participants who viewed their stress as helpful found their blood vessels were more relaxed, and their heart had a much healthier cardiovascular profile (McGonigal, 2013).

Another stress reduction approach that is appropriate in diverse cultures is mindfulness. According to Chelsea and Malinowski (2011), the use of mindfulness is a powerful stress reduction tool. Studies have shown that individuals who embed the use of mindfulness have displayed lowered cortisol responses and lower levels of negative emotion to a laboratory task. Other benefits that were found from meditating are lowered blood pressure and lowered anxiety levels. Mindfulness-based stress cognitive therapy (MBCT), which uses neuroimaging, increases activity in the frontal cortex, which leads to emotional regulation in the amygdala. This type of therapy exhibited an increase in tissue density in the hippocampus and other structural changes (Hozel et al., 2011). The structural changes in the hippocampus due to MBCT possibly reflect improvements in emotional regulation.

Stress reduction techniques have been used on participants with non-communicable diseases. For example, a study on 240 participants of Mexican or North Central American descent with Type 2 Diabetes found that lifestyles, health beliefs, and acculturation impacted perceptions of self-efficacy. For example, social support impacted satisfaction with self. Participants in the study believed they were in control of their own health and utilized Western medicine (Latham & Calvillo, 2009).

These studies portray the importance of cultural sensitivity and the utilization of cross-cultural communication when treating individuals with different backgrounds. Clinicians should focus on interventions that enable individuals to focus on their health and wellness. Furthermore, cross-culturally relevant health measures need to be developed (Lu, 2002).

Smoking Cessation

It is important to tailor interventions to an individual's specific risk factors for non-communicable disease and to reference studies that have used smoking prevention strategies. For example, Patkar and colleagues (2003) cite the U.S. Public Health Program smoking interventions, which include the five R's: (1) relevance (why quitting smoking is important), (2) risk (harmful effects of smoking), (3) rewards (from quitting smoking), (4) roadblocks (barriers to quitting), and (5) repetition (why not try again).

Addressing Obesity

Lifestyle interventions that combine physical activity, a healthy diet, behavioral interventions, and caregivers can reduce obesity levels (Straub, 2014). To prevent obesity, individuals need to engage in healthy eating and physical activity. Past interventions have focused on changing an individual's behavior and not on environmental factors (Kumanyika, Jeffery, Morabia, Ritenbaugh, & Antipatis, 2002).

A study conducted by Gittelsohn and colleagues (2006) used environmental factors to develop a food-store-based intervention in the Marshall Islands. Although this is a developing country, it has become more westernized. The goal of this intervention was to improve diet and decrease obesity. The program emphasized label reading, which was taught by handing out information, by having the interventionists explain it, and via comic strips in the newspapers. The program also emphasized diabetes prevention.

There were five in-store components to the intervention: (1) cooking demonstrations and taste tests, (2) recipe cards, (3) stocking of key foods, (4) shelf labels for promotional foods, and (5) posters reiterating key messages. The intervention contained three mass-media components: (1) newspaper ads containing cooking demonstrations and taste tests, (2) radio announcements discussing the importance of eating healthily, and (3) videos of cooking demonstrations (Gittelsohn, Dyckman, Tan, Boggs, Frick, Alfred, et al., 2006).

There are five major areas of wellness that should be included in interventions. The first is spirituality, which is a force that gives a sense of wholeness and represents an individual's beliefs and values. Lightly (1966) (as cited by Myers and colleagues [2000]) proposes that well-being and resistance to stress incorporates positive thoughts, hardiness, generalized self-efficacy, and optimism. Positive thoughts and optimism are components of spirituality.

The second is self-direction, which is the way an individual carries out obligations and pursues goals. Self-esteem is a stronger predictor of satisfaction in individualistic cultures, as opposed to collectivistic societies, where relationship harmony is more important. Higher levels of perceived self-control predict healthier behaviors. Having realistic beliefs, perceiving things accurately, and having positive emotional awareness, strong coping skills, and a sense of humor are all important components to an individual's well-being. Other areas in which an individual can carry out his/her goals to improve his/her health include: (1) nutrition, (2) physical activity, (3) self-care (e.g. safety habits, checkups, and avoiding harmful substances), and (4) stress management (e.g. biofeedback, relaxation techniques, social support, and behavioral/environmental efforts). Cultural identity is important in goal-setting, since the concept of health varies across cultures. In Western cultures, happiness is correlated with having an internal locus of control and being independent, but in non-Western societies it is correlated with relationship harmony and interpersonal commitments (Myers et al., 2000).

The third component is work and leisure. Work satisfaction and competence is a predictor for longevity and QOL. Leisure, such as physical, social, and volunteer activities, has a positive impact on self-esteem. Leisure activities like exercise reduce stress.

The fourth component is friendship. Individuals with strong social relationships are more likely to avoid damaging behaviors. Friendship is correlated with physical and mental health and helps with stress (Myers et al., 2000)

The final component is love, which consists of intimacy, trust, affection, care, stability, and physical intimacy. Mortality rates are higher for single and divorced individuals. Individuals who are in an unhappy marriage are less healthy than those who are not attached. Divorced individuals have higher rates of non-communicable diseases and poorer immune systems. This is regardless of gender or culture (Myers et al., 2000).

This study found that exposure to the intervention was related to an increased knowledge in diabetes and label-reading. The intervention was associated with an increased purchase of some nutritional foods (e.g. oatmeal, fish, and vegetables) and with an increase in adoption of healthier food preparation techniques (Gittelsohn, Dyckman, Tan, Boggs, Frick, Alfred, J., et al., 2006). Furthermore, Willoughby and colleagues (2000) based their study on previous research that found that psychosocial factors (such as problem-focused/cognitive coping strategies and greater social support) had a positive adjustment for women with diabetes.

Individuals at risk for Type 2 Diabetes can help prevent the disease by losing weight and increasing their physical activity (Rock, 2003). Rock (2003) cites McKinlay and Marceau (2000), who posit that social structure (e.g. age, gender, race/ethnicity, and socioeconomic class), environmental influences (e.g. geographic, occupation, housing, and access to services), lifestyle influences (e.g. smoking, nutrition, physical activity, and psychosocial factors), and physiological influences (e.g. blood pressure, cholesterol, and obesity) have different levels of causation and need different interventions.

Another trigger for non-communicable diseases is alcohol abuse, which can be modified with lifestyles changes. When designing a program to help women with alcoholism, it is important to be sensitive to racial, ethnic, and cultural factors (Wardle, Haase, Steptoe, Nillapun, Jonwutiwes, & Belliisle, 2004). It is imperative to raise awareness to public health problems caused by alcohol use. For individuals with alcohol-related problems, treatment programs must be accessible and affordable. Health services should include procedures that screen for alcohol problems and provide brief interventions (WHO, 2015a).

The World Health Assembly (2010) created a global strategy to reduce the use of alcohol that consisted of the following 10 recommended target areas: (1) leadership, awareness, and commitment, (2) health services response, (3) community action, (4) drink-driving policies, (5) availability, (6) marketing, (7) pricing, (8) reducing negative consequences, (9) reducing public health impact, and (10) monitoring and surveillance (WHO, 2015).

Global Health Intervention

The intervention for global health primarily consists of providing patient-centered care and integrating a holistic approach. Johnson (2013) discussed the importance of comprehending the culture of the population being attended, as well as integrating both a mental health and health care team in a "non-stigmatizing environment" (Johnson, 2013, p. 316). The biopsychosocial model certainly encourages the use of an interdisciplinary team to share diverse areas of expertise and to strategize health promotion, disease treatment, and prevention. It is imperative to conduct behavioral screenings and provide counseling recommendations (this has been supported though scientific evidence).

Vaughn (2010) posits the importance of culturally competent communication and how this can be impacted in terms of patient culture and beliefs. Banerjee (2015) discusses that health, illness, and healthcare are interconnected as meanings are embedded in that particular cultural context. Culture plays a vital role in the comprehension of health-related concepts such as management of illness and the promotion of health-related beliefs and behavior. In a global health intervention, it is imperative to be cognizant of provider bias and beliefs.

Frankel and Quill (2005) discuss the importance of patient-centered care to address psychosocial and biological aspects of patient concerns. Utilizing such an approach will improve the initiation of treatment for psychosocial problems and enhanced screening. To deliver best-care practice for diabetes care, the intervention must include delivering advanced education to persons of all ages and learning abilities diagnosed with diabetes and must use appropriate learning techniques. The care team should discuss diabetic complications, blood glucose monitoring, and germane self-care practices such as exercise. Segal and colleagues (2013) again stress the importance of a multidisciplinary team inclusive of nursing, optometry, mental health, pharmacy, and indigenous or ethnic-specific health workers, depending on the population. Public perceptions in terms of belief of health interventions, etiology, and prognosis influence health-seeking behaviors. A household survey conducted in Kenya discussed the importance of aligning health interventions/promotions with the public's concept of mental illness (Muga & Jenkins, 2008). A global intervention plan would need to consider the fact that many individuals rely on traditional and religious healers.

Malik and colleagues (2013) discuss the positive effects of lifestyle counseling to promote motivational behavioral change. A project in Finland, the North Karelia project, exhibited community-based interventions to reduce cardiovascular disease. The project consisted of community education and raising awareness of CVD by including community leaders, schools, health services, non-governmental organizations (NGOs), the local media, and supermarkets. Malik and colleagues also discuss a program in France, parts of Europe, and South Australia called EPODE, which seeks to fight obesity in children. This program was executed on a community level and consisted of actions such as removing vending machines from schools, promoting physical activity in schools and families, education campaigns, and limiting the consumption of beverages and unhealthy foods. The towns that have adopted EPODE have seen significant reductions in childhood obesity.

Conclusions and Future Recommendations

This chapter discusses a global treatment and health prevention program that utilizes the biopsychosocial model to assist in reducing risk factors associated with non-communicable diseases. An individual can decrease his/her risk factors of developing cancer, Type 2 Diabetes, CVD, or lung diseases by eliminating tobacco use, limiting alcoholic beverages, eating healthy foods, and increasing physical activity. Furthermore, individuals need to be educated on the dangers of their behavior (including the risks posed by tobacco use), and a global health intervention program using the biopsychosocial model needs to be created.

For any health-based program to be successful, it must be a community-based intervention, and culture must be considered. Tilman and Clark (2014) hold that dietary choices are influenced by culture. However, due to rapid globalization, obesity has increased across the globe, in part because populations have access to low-cost foods that have minimal nutritional value. Sarafino and Smith (2014) explain that eating patterns are hard to change due to an inability to control one's "antecedents and consequences in their environment" (Sarafino & Smith, 2014, p. 214). They reference a pioneering study conducted by Richard Stuart, which involved lifestyle interventions through the incorporation of behavioral methods.

The lifestyle intervention projects have been shown to reduce body weight by 7-10% in the first four months (p. 214).

Straub (2014) says that individuals who displayed "hardiness" were more apt to living healthier lives. These individuals approached life with enthusiasm, were committed to their families, and had a sense of control over their lives. Hardy individuals were less likely to be upset during a stressful situation. Segerstrom (2006) also found that individuals who display a more optimistic lifestyle lead longer, healthier lives. Studies have also shown that individuals who exhibit feelings of helplessness tend to engage in self-defeating behaviors that can be life-threatening. Williams (2003) says that in Westernized cultures, men tend to be socialized to achieve and to be competent in all aspects. When this does not occur (due to discrimination as or economic marginalization), their self-efficacy can be impacted. Social support plays a significant role in combatting stress and depression, and those with it are as less likely to suffer from heart attacks (Straub, 2014).

The application of cognitive behavioral therapy (CBT) can assist in changing an individual's mindset, which in turn can assist in the reduction of environmental stressors. MBCT can help people with high levels of stress by providing preventative coping strategies. Community-wide health interventions are crucial on a global level in order to promote healthy behaviors. Multifaceted, community approaches that occur through schools, governmental agencies, and non-governmental agencies allow for higher levels of success in terms of adopting healthier lifestyles.

In any culture, it is imperative to gain a comprehensive understanding of what the targeted health problems are and to create a health education program that is centered on these issues. The North Karelin Project, adopted in Finland, would be a great success story of a community-wide international intervention that significantly lowered rates of CHD despite previously having the highest rates in the world. According to Sarafino and Smith (2014), deaths from heart disease in Finland decreased by 85% (p. 368). Straub (2014) stresses the importance of community-based health interventions that motivate individuals to change unhealthy behaviors, as trying to change alone can be daunting.

Future recommendations include community engagement in discussions with governments, ensuring QOL promotion, addressing disparities in health equity, and creating physical and social environments that promote healthy living. The studies cited in this chapter demonstrate the need to utilize a multidimensional model of health that encompasses biological, psychological, and social/cultural factors to implement lifestyle changes and to improve health, well-being, and overall QOL.

References

Alladin, W. (January 01, 2009). An ethno biopsychosocial human rights model for educating community counselors globally. *Counseling Psychology Quarterly, 22*(1), 17-24.

Banerjee, B. (2015). Impact of culture in caregiving experiences in the context of mental illness: A brief review. *Journal of the Indian Academy of Applies Psychology, 41*(2), 272-281

Beaglehole, R., & Bonita, R. (2010). What is global health? *Global Health Action. 3*, 5142. DOI: 10.3402/gha.v3i0.5142

Betancourt, J.R. (2003). Cross-cultural medical education: conceptual approaches and frameworks for evaluation. *Academy Medicine, 78*(6), 560-69.

Cartwright, M., Wardle, J., Steggles, N., Simon, A., Croker, H, Jarvis, M.J. (2003). Stress and dietary practices in adolescents. *Health Psychology, 22*(4), 362-369

CDC. (n.d.a) Assessing your weight. Retrieved from http://www.cdc.gov/healthyweight/assessing/index.html

CDC. (n.d.b). Chronic disease overview. Retrieved from http://www.cdc.gov/chronicdisease/overview/

CDC. (2014). 2014 National diabetes statistics report. Retrieved from http://www.cdc.gov/diabetes/data/statistics/2014statisticsreport.html

CDC. (2015a). Health effects of cigarette smoking. Retrieved from https://www.cdc.gov/tobacco/data_statistics/fact_sheets/health_effects/effects_cig_smoking/

CDC. (2015b). Smoking and tobacco use. Retrieved from http://www.cdc.gov/tobacco/data_statistics/fact_sheets/fast_facts/

CDC. (2015c) Strategies to prevent obesity. Retrieved from http://www.cdc.gov/obesity/strategies/

Chatterji, S., Ustun, B.L., Sadana, R., Salomon, J.A., Mathers, C.D., & Murray, C. (2002). The conceptual basis for measuring and reporting on health. In *Global Programme on Evidence for Health* Policy *Discussion Paper No. 45*. World Health Organization, Geneva.

Chelsea, A., Malinowski, P. (2011). Mindfulness-based approaches: Are they all the same? *Journal of Clinical Psychology, 67*, 404-424.

Christakis, N.A., Fowler, J.H. (2007). The spread of obesity in a large social network over 32 years. *New England Journal of Medicine, 357*, 370-379.

Clark, L., Vincent, D., Zimmer, L. & Sanchez, J. (2009). Cultural values and political economic contexts of diabetes among low-income Mexican Americans. *Journal of Transcultural Nursing, 20, 4*, 382-394.

Dale, H., & Lee, A. (January 01, 2016). Behavioural health consultants in integrated primary care teams: a model for future care. *Bmc Family Practice, 17*.

Engel, G.L. (1980). The clinical application of the biopsychosocial model. *The American Journal of Psychiatry, 137*(5), 535-544.

Engel, G.L. (1979). The biopsychosocial model and the education of health professionals. *General Hospital Psychiatry, 1*(2), 156-165.

Fernander, A. F., Shavers, V. L., & Hammons, G. J. (January 01, 2007). A biopsychosocial approach to examining tobacco-related health disparities among racially classified social groups. *Addiction (abingdon, England), 102*, 43-57.

Gittelsohn, J., Dyckman, W., Tan, M. L., Boggs, M. K., Frick, K. D., Alfred, J., Winch, P. J., ... Palafox, N. A. (2006). Development and implementation of a food store-based intervention to improve diet in the Republic of the Marshall Islands. *Health Promotion Practice, 7*(4), 396-405.

Hozel, K., Carmody, J., Vangel, M., Congleton, C., Yerramsetti, G., Lazer, W. (2011). Mindfulness practice leads to increases in brain grey matter density. *Psychiatry Research: Neuroimaging, 91*(1), 36-43.

Hutchinson, K., McGeary, J., Smolen, A., Bryan, A., Swift. R. (2002). The DRD4 VNTR polymorphism moderates craving after alcohol consumption. *Health Psychology, 21,* 139-146.

Johnson, S. B. (January 01, 2013). Increasing psychology's role in health research and health care. *The American Psychologist, 68*(5).

Kärner, A., Tingström, P., Abrandt-Dahlgren, M., & Bergdahl, B. (2005). Incentives for lifestyle changes in patients with coronary heart disease. *Journal of Advanced Nursing, 51*(3), 261-275.

Kim, H. C., & Oh, S. M. (2013). Non-communicable diseases: current status of major modifiable risk factors in Korea. *Journal of Preventive Medicine and Public Health = Yebang Uihakhoe Chi, 46*(4), 165-72.

Kumanyika, Jeffery, Morabia, Ritenbaugh, Antipatis, & Correspondence. (March 01, 2002). Obesity prevention: the case for action. *International Journal of Obesity, 26*(3), 425-436.

Latham, C.L., & Calvillo, E. (2009). Predictors of successful diabetes management in low-income Hispanic people. *Western Journal of Nursing Research, 31*(3), 364-388.

Lu, L. (June 01, 2002). A preliminary study on the concept of health among the Chinese. *Counseling Psychology Quarterly, 15*(2), 179-189.

Malik, V., Willett, W., Hu, F. (2013). Global obesity: trends, risk factors and policy implications. *Endocrinology, 9,* 13-27.

McGonigal, K. (2013). How to make stress your friend. Ted. Retrieved from: https://www.ted.com/talks/kelly_mcgonigal_how_to_make_stress_your_friend

Morrison, C.D. (2008). Leptin resistance and the response to positive energy balance. *Physiology and Behavior, 94,* 660-663.

Muga, F., Jenkins, R. (2008). Public perceptions and explanatory models and service utlisation regarding mental illness and mental health care in Kenya. *Social Psychiatry Epidemiology, 43,* 469-476.

Myers, J.E., Sweeney, T.J., & Witmer, J.M. (2000). The wheel of wellness counseling for wellness: A holistic model for treatment planning. *Journal of Counseling & Development, 78*(3), 251-266.

Patel, V. (Vikram Patel) (2012, June). Mental health for all by involving all. Retrieved from: https://www.ted.com/talks/vikram_patel_mental_health_for_all_by_involving_all

Patkar, A. A., Vergare, M. J., Batra, V., Weinstein, S. P., & Leone, F. T. (January 01, 2003). Tobacco smoking: current concepts in etiology and treatment. *Psychiatry, 66*(3), 183-99.

Resnick, R. J. (January 01, 1997). A brief history of practice— expanded. *American Psychologist, 52,* 4, 463-468.

Rock, M. (2003). Sweet blood and social suffering: Rethinking cause-effect relationships in diabetes, distress, and duress. *Medical Anthropology, 22*(2), 131-174.

Rotter, J. B. (1966). *Generalized expectancies for internal versus external control of reinforcement.* Washington: American Psychological Association.

Sarafino, E., & Smith, T. (2014). *Health Psychology. Biopsychosocial interactions.* 8th Ed. New Jersey: Wiley Press.

Schwartz, G. (1982). Testing the biopsychosocial model: The ultimate challenge facing behavioral medicine? *Journal of Consulting and Clinical Psychology, 50,* 1040-1053.

Segerstrom, S.C. (2007). Stress, energy and immunity: An ecological view. *Current Directions in Psychological Science, 16,* 326-330.

Segal, L., Leach, M., May, E., Turnbull, C. (2013). Regional primary care team to deliver best-practice diabetes care. *Diabetes Care, 36*(7), 1898-1907.

Shields, C. G., Finley, M. A., Chawla, N., & Meadors, W. P. (2012). Couple and family interventions in health problems. *Journal of Marital and Family Therapy, 38*(1) 265-80.

Straub, R. (2014). *Health Psychology: A biopsychosocial approach.* 4th Ed. New York: NY. Worth Publishers.

The Tobacco Atlas. (2015). Cigarette use globally. Retrieved from http://www.tobaccoatlas.org/topic/cigarette-use-globally/

Tilman, D., & Clark, M. (2014). Global diets link environmental sustainability and human health. *Nature. 515*, 518– 522.

Vaughn, L. (2010). *Psychology and culture: Thinking, feeling, and behaving in global contexts.* England: Psychology Press.

Wallace, J. (1990). The new disease model of alcoholism. *The Western Journal of Medicine, 152*(5), 502-505.

Wardle, J., Haase, A.M., Steptoe, A., Nillapun, M., Jonwutiwes, K., & Belliisle, F. (2004). Gender differences in food choice. The contribution of health beliefs and dieting. *Annals of Behavioral Medicine, 27*, 107-116.

Williams, D. (2003). The health of men: Structured inequalities and opportunities. *American Journal of Public Health, 93*(5), 724- 731.

Willoughby, D. F., Kee, C., & Demi, A. (2000). Women's psychosocial adjustment to diabetes. *Journal of Advanced Nursing, 32*(6), 1422-1430.

World Health Organization (n.d.a). Chronic obstructive pulmonary disease. Retrievedfrom http://www.who.int/respiratory/copd/en/

World Health Organization. (n.d.b). Chronic respiratory diseases. Retrieved from http://www.who.int/respiratory/about_topic/en/

World Health Organization. (n.d.c.). Chronic respiratory diseases. Retrieved from http://www.who.int/respiratory/en/

World Health Organization. (1948). WHO definition of health. Retrieved from http://www.who.int/about/definition/en/print.html

World Health Organization. (2002). World Health Report 2002: Reducing Risks, Promoting Healthy Life. Retrieved from http://www.who.int/whr/2002/en/whr02_en.pdf?ua=1

World Health Organization, (2015a). Alcohol. Retrieved from http://www.who.int/mediacentre/factsheets/fs349/en/

World Health Organization. (2015b). Cancer. Retrieved from http://www.who.int/mediacentre/factsheets/fs297/en/

World Health Organization. (2015c). Chronic obstructive pulmonary disease (COPD). Retrieved from http://www.who.int/mediacentre/factsheets/fs315/en/

World Health Organization. (2016a). Cardiovascular disease. Retrieved from http://www.who.int/mediacentre/factsheets/fs317/en/

Word Health Organization (2016b). Diabetes. Retrieved from: http://www.who.int/mediacentre/factsheets/fs312/en/

World Health Organization. (2016c). Mental disorders. Retrieved from http://www.who.int/mediacentre/factsheets/fs396/en/

World Health Organization. (2016d). Obesity and overweight. Retrieved from http://www.who.int/mediacentre/factsheets/fs311/en/

World Health Organization. (2016e) Tobacco. Retrieved from http://www.who.int/mediacentre/factsheets/fs339/en/

CHAPTER 12

Promoting Global Mental Health through Counselor Education

Amy Nitza, Kerrie Fineran, and Lidija Hurni

One glance at any national or international news outlet reveals the striking need for interventions to relieve the physical and emotional suffering of many people around the world. As with many issues of global disparity, individuals in low-resource settings bear a disproportionate burden of this suffering. The same disparities often prevent these individuals from receiving the support services that they need. The availability and quality of mental health services in particular is an area of inequality on a global scale.

Global mental health prioritizes improving health and achieving equity in health for all people around the world (Koplan et al., 2009). As delineated by Patel (2014), global health is in part defined by its emphases on equity, justice, and fairness in the distribution of health, and on "what all countries can learn from each other and do together to address the health of all the peoples who must share our planet," (p. 778) rather than what can be taken from the "developed" world and applied in the "developing world."

Fortunately, global mental health is increasingly recognized as an important target for global development efforts. The United Nations Millennium Development Goals (MDGs), which guided global development policy from 2000 to 2015, placed little direct emphasis on mental health. Correspondingly, improvements in mental health did not keep pace with other improvements in global health during the tenure of the MDGs (McGovern, 2014). However, the post-2015 development agenda reflects a heightened awareness that global health and economic development goals will only be achieved if mental health goals, particularly for vulnerable populations, are included as a core component of the agenda (McGovern, 2014).

In advancing mental health within the global development agenda, one important step forward must be a consideration of how best to train the next generation of mental health practitioners to think about their profession and their work in a global context. Global mental health is a multidisciplinary approach that includes diverse mental health professions in collaboration with community-based organizations and prioritizes social justice (Patel, 2014). As such, professional counseling is one discipline that fits well within the field of global mental health. This chapter will consider how counselor education can best prepare professional counselors to promote global mental health, reduce disparities, and improve the lives of individuals around the world.

Professional Counseling

In the United States, counseling is a field of study that encompasses a broad range of specialties, typically involves advanced training and the procurement of a master's degree, is represented by various professional organizations, is governed by both state law and codes of ethics outlined by professional organizations, and is subject to various national and state requirements for accreditation, licensure, and certification.

According to the American Counseling Association (ACA), counseling is a process that incorporates mental health, psychological, and human development principles (Remley & Herlihy, 2010). The field of professional counseling is often one that struggles to accurately define itself in light of the varied specialties, unique work environments, and competing related fields; therefore, strengthening professional identity has been a goal of the ACA in recent years. In partnership with the American Association of State Licensing Boards (AASCB), the ACA engaged in creating a strategic plan focused on promoting the growth and sustainability of the counseling profession, entitled "20/20 Vision for the Future of Counseling." This multi-year program strives to create picture of the future of counseling that involves a unified identity for the counseling profession, specifically including a consensus on the definition of counseling, clarification of the roles of professional counselors, plans for strengthening the profession, and specific plans for how to move the field forward by the year 2020. Through this process, the ACA and its associates defined counseling as "a professional relationship that empowers diverse individuals, families, and groups to accomplish mental health, wellness, education, and career goals" (American Counseling Association as cited in Kaplan, 2014, p. 1). Creating this definition was not meant to supersede all other definitions, but rather to be a building block upon which specialty fields within the counseling field could define themselves. It also serves as a concise description of the profession that is easily communicated to those who may be unfamiliar with the field.

History of Professional Counseling in the United States

The roots of professional counseling can be tied to social work, psychology, assessment, humanism, medicine, and multiculturalism (Pope, 2004a). The counseling profession in the United States developed primarily due to the demands of urbanization and industrialization on the population (Glosoff and Schwarz-Whittaker, 2013). In the late 19th century, school curriculums changed, and there were more career options available to students. This, in turn, necessitated assistance in navigating the new career landscape, a need which led to the development of counseling and guidance programs in schools. The new science of psychology began in Europe, and this studying of individual psyches led to an increased interest in using strategies to assist people with psychological problems. When counseling psychology developed as a specialty within the psychology profession, the counseling profession began to emerge as a unique alternative (Goodyear, 2000). Counseling psychology was quite different in that it focused on developmental stages and career concerns rather than on pathology, which was typically the emphasis in the psychology field. This switch from stressing pathology to working within a normal, developmental framework changed the scope of practice for counseling psychologists and, in combination with the growth of school counseling and federal funding for vocational guidance services, provided the impetus for an entirely new field (Remley & Herlihy, 2010).

The historical foundations of the modern counseling profession expanded in the 1950s in response to a need for a larger and more diverse population of counseling professionals (Pope, 2004b). Throughout the second half of the 20th century, various legislative actions helped to support the development of the counseling field in the United States (see Glosoff and Schwarz –Wittaker, 2013). As the field grew, so did associated organizations related to professional development, licensing, and accreditation.

The largest professional organization of counselors is known today as the American Counseling Association (ACA), although at its inception in 1952, it was known as the American Personnel and Guidance Association (APGA) (Glosoff and Schwarz-Wittaker, 2013). The ACA is made up of a general membership of professional counselors and counseling students and also serves as the umbrella organization for a variety of more specialized divisions (e.g. Association for Specialists in Group Work, Association for Counselor Education and Supervision, Counselors for

Social Justice, International Association of Addictions and Offenders Counselors, etc.). The association provides a Code of Ethics, annual conferences, legislative advocacy for the field, and professional development opportunities and trainings and promotes the practice of counseling.

In the United States, counselor licensure is a credential that is granted by governments of each individual state. Licensure is designed to provide quality assurance for clients and helps to regulate the practice within established frameworks. Certification is carefully delineated from licensure and is typically granted to individuals from various professional bodies. The National Board of Certified Counselors (NBCC) is the body in the United States that offers national certification to counselors (allowing them to be identified as Nationally Certified Counselors, or NCCs). In order to be nationally certified, counselors must hold a master's degree or higher with significant study of counseling that includes at least forty-eight credit hours, demonstrate that they took coursework in various identified areas, have completed a supervised field experience, provide at least two professional endorsements, and pass a national examination.

Because licensure and certification in the United States requires a master's degree, counselor education programs are designed to help students develop knowledge and skills related to the practice of professional counseling. Some amount of consistency in training is desirable to contribute to professional identity and establish basic educational requirements for all counselors-in-training. To this end, the Council for Accreditation of Counseling and Related Educational Programs (CACREP) was developed to provide accreditation of counselor education programs. CACREP (2015) accredits doctoral programs in counselor education and master's programs with specialties in School Counseling, Clinical Mental Health Counseling, Addiction Counseling, Career Counseling, Clinical Rehabilitation Counseling, College Counseling and Student Affairs, and Marriage, Couple, and Family Counseling. The mission of CACREP is to develop competent professional counselors by providing a set of preparation standards that counselor preparation programs can utilize which are comprised of expected common curricular experiences and professional practice guidelines.

Development of Professional Counseling Internationally

Although counseling clearly developed within a Western context, much progress is being made, and counseling practice is developing rapidly in many areas of the world. For many countries, the proliferation of the counseling field begins with the establishment of counseling in schools and the development of a school guidance curriculum. Therefore, the schools serve as the main base for providing many mental health and social needs services to both students and communities at large. From there, school counselors are able to advocate for the expansion of additional resources outside the school setting can provide more specialized mental health services.

The development of counseling as a professional field internationally has many challenges. First, education and training are significant barriers in many countries. In many locales, the need for professionals who are able to provide mental health services far outpaces the ability to train providers; many countries do not have the resources available to establish counseling training programs. Relatedly, many countries do not have governmental recognition or regulation of the counseling field, as this is not widely practiced outside the United States. This is a barrier, according to Gazzola and Smith (2007), who have noted that recognition and regulation by governmental bodies may play a part in the accessibility of services through specific definition of the field and regulation of training and services. For those countries that do adopt practices common in the United States, some translation of these activities must occur so that they fit governmental structures and diverse cultural traditions.

The Current Role of Counselors in Global Mental Health

One organization specifically related to the counseling field and global mental health is a division of the National Board for Certified Counselors (NBCC), the NBCC International (NBCC-I). It was established in 2003 with the goal of advocating for and collaborating on the worldwide development of counseling as a profession as well as increasing the availability of counseling services to underserved areas of the globe. Specifically, NBCC-I promotes the following: a) quality assurance in counseling practice, b) the value of culturally sensitive counseling, c) public awareness of counseling quality, d) professionalism in counseling,and e) leadership in credentialing (NBCC-I, 2016).

NBCC-I has strong partnerships with both the World Health Organization (WHO) and the United Nations Educational, Scientific, and Cultural Organization (UNESCO), which has designated NBCC-I as a partnering nongovernmental organization (NGO). These relationships allow them to both access and develop relationships with new and existing regional and national counseling organizations around the world. One aspect of cultural competence that is specifically present in their mission is the demonstration of respect for the lived realities (social, cultural, political, and economic) of the areas they visit and serve by taking a collaborative, partnering view rather than one of consultation.

NBCC-I is a significant source of support for professional counselors who are interested in getting involved with the promotion of the profession internationally and for areas of the world that desire to develop more and varied mental health services. NBCC-I offers training institutes and conferences for professional counselors in various areas of the world, including Rwanda, Italy, France, Malawi, and Uganda. NBCC-I also providse Mental Health Facilitator (MHF) training, which is customizable to the needs and cultural values of the communities that request it. This training is designed to increase and improve access to mental health treatment in a community by educating individuals from various backgrounds to recognize mental health needs, offer support, work with existing health resources, and make referrals to higher levels of care as necessary. NBCC-I also strives to provide support and training to potential leaders in the counseling field from non-U.S. counseling organizations or universities through an appointment with NBCC-I as a Counselor-in-Residence (CIR). This person works with the members of the organization to share information about counseling practice, the status of the counseling field, and opportunities for the expansion of counseling and credentialing in his or her nation and region. Similarly, the NBCC International Fellows program sponsors the professional development of counselors who may assume leadership positions in a growing international counseling profession. One of the goals of this program is to provide a platform for developing international relationships between counseling professionals, which can lead to enhanced counseling knowledge that can be brought into the fellows' home communities and may promote engagement in cross-national counseling research.

Another counseling organization with an international mission is the International Association for Counselling (IAC). It is an NGO with international association status headquartered in Belgium. The goal of the organization is to serve the counseling field by "advancing culturally relevant counselling practice, research and policy to promote well-being, respect, social justice, and peace worldwide" (IAC, 2016, paragraph 2). Since the inception of the IAC in 1966, the organization has arranged for over thirty international counseling conferences which have taken place in over twenty countries. These conferences typically involve an international research seminar, presentations by representatives from the host country and other international NGOs, and educational sessions and discussions which take place in smaller working groups. Additionally, the organization has founded the *International Journal for the Advancement of Counselling* which publishes original articles and research papers related to international counseling topics.

Global Mental Health Training in Counselor Education

With increased recognition of the need for mental health services within the global development agenda, an established professional identity, and related organizations that have begun the work of global collaboration, it is imperative that counselor education promote the development of a global perspective in its training of new professionals. Yet to date, no broadly accepted curriculum for global mental health training for counselors exists. In this section, we highlight major concepts that can comprise a global mental health training agenda within existing counselor education programs.

Culture

Training in the role culture plays within mental health must be the cornerstone of global mental health education for professional counselors. As described by Kirmayer and Swartz (2014), culture impacts all aspects of mental health, including:

- Learning skills of active listening so family and friends can vent their feelings as well as being able to express one's own needs
- Learning stress management skills and cognitive behavioral strategies for addressing helplessness and negative thinking.
- Offering support services where on the grassroots level, refugees can restore self and the community through being able to be of help to others
- Perception and experience of symptoms, suffering, and well-being
- Modes of expression of distress
- Explanations, interpretations, or causal attributions of symptoms and illness
- Patterns of coping and help-seeking
- Strategies for healing and treatment intervention
- Expectations of illness course and outcome
- The social consequences of symptoms, functional impairment, and diagnostic labels

Counselors must thus be able to identify how to work appropriately with the cultural frameworks that are intertwined with the mental health of individuals and communities. Counselors must thus be able to identify, consider, and where appropriate work from within the cultural frameworks that are intertwined with the mental health of individuals and communities.

The initial (and arguably most important) component involves counselors developing an awareness of the ways in which their own culture(s) impact their views, assumptions, and understanding of the world generally and mental health specifically. Awareness is also essential because it is not possible for students to learn the nuances of every culture they might encounter; rather, students must be able to approach any cultural setting with an understanding of their own cultural assumptions and a mindset of curiosity about the culture with which they are engaging in order to understand it on its own terms.

In addition to cultural self-awareness, in order to work effectively in a global context, counselors must have knowledge of, and able to work effectively with, a wide range of cultural differences. While not an exhaustive list, counselors should have knowledge of differences between individual and collective worldviews and the crucial role of interdependence in collective societies, different family structures and hierarchies, tribal loyalties and identities, differences in communication patterns (such as high-and low-context communication styles), spiritual beliefs (including the crucial role of ancestors in many belief systems), and traditional helping practices. To intervene effectively, counselors must recognize the culture-bound nature of many Western theories and techniques and be able to adapt to the needs of different populations. They must also be able to incorporate aspects of traditional healing practices and/or collaborate with traditional healers when appropriate. Finally, the ability to work appropriately with interpreters is essential in many settings.

Cultural competence is necessary but not sufficient for counselors working in global mental health. Also essential is the promotion of cultural safety, or "the need to address the legacy of colonialism and ongoing issues of power and discrimination that make clinical settings unsafe" (Kirmayer & Swartz, 2014, p. 50). There is danger associated with counselors working in post-colonial countries; without a thorough understanding of the history and modern day consequences of colonialism in such settings, counselors can perpetuate social injustices through maintaining the status quo. At an individual level this may occur through power dynamics in relationships between Western counselors and their international clients or colleagues. This may also occur on a larger scale through the promotion of Western ideas and interventions through what Bemak and Chung (2015) have termed "mental health colonialism and imperialism" (p. 11). To avoid such dangers and promote cultural safety, careful attention to social justice and issues of power and oppression as applied to the long history of colonialism throughout the world must be included alongside other issues of culture.

Global Mental Health Systems

A second major construct in training professional counselors is helping them to situate their own work in the context of global mental health systems and to understand the ways in which these systems are shaped by forces like historical background, political and economic context, and the dynamics of power and oppression. In many settings, there may be no existing mental health system or infrastructure in place, and learning to operate effectively within such settings is of key importance.

Some models for conceptualizing mental health services within a global context have emerged; such models can serve as useful frameworks for training students to contextualize their work as embedded in larger systems.

One such model is the Global Mental Health Action Plan, developed by the Harvard Program in Refugee Trauma (HPRT; Mollica, 2011). This framework includes eight dimensions linked to mental health and trauma recovery, including mental health policy and legislation, financing, science-based mental health services, building an ongoing program of mental health education, coordination of mental health activities among local and international agencies, linkage of mental health to economic development, linkage of mental health to human rights, and research, evaluation, and ethics. The HPRT uses this eight-dimensional framework in its work with Ministries of Health around the world to assist them in improving their mental health policies and response planning, as well as to train practitioners in working effectively in a global context. The eight dimensions are used as a framework for case studies of both broad policy questions and clinical cases. As such, it serves as a useful model for considering how best to assist counselors in developing a global perspective for their work.

Evidence-Based Practices

Counselors must be able to use the best available evidence to guide their decisions about which interventions to use in any given situation; however, at present, there is an insufficient body of research evidence to support the implementation of mental health and social support activities in many non-Western settings. In such settings, counselors must draw upon other resources to guide their work, including the most current global guidelines. These include the World Health Organization's Mental Health Gap Action Program guidelines and evidence resource center (WHO, 2010) and the Interagency Standing Committee Guidelines on Mental health and Psychosocial Support in Emergency Settings (IASC, 2007). In referring to such documents, counselors can ensure that their work is consistent with identified global standards drawn from the best available scientific evidence.

At the same time, counselors also need to consider alternative forms of evidence that may be more appropriate and/or practical in non-Western settings in which the scientific paradigm used by Western researchers is not consistent with the worldview of the people. As asserted by Chilisa (2012):

> ...current academic research traditions are founded on the culture, history, and philosophies of Euro-Western thought and are therefore indigenous to the Western academy and its institutions. These methodologies exclude from knowledge production the knowledge systems of formerly colonized, historically marginalized, and oppressed groups, which today are most often represented as Other. (p. 1)

Chilisa's assertion is an important caution to professional counselors – indeed, to anyone working in global mental health – to maintain an awareness not only of whether there is evidence to support a given intervention, but also of what sources of evidence are appropriate for the cultural context in which it is being applied.

Hanlon, Fekadu and Patel (2014) suggested one set of factors to be considered when applying Western interventions in non-Western settings. These included feasibility, equity, sociocultural acceptability, contextually acceptable outcomes, and affordability. Feasibility involves ensuring that the intervention can be implemented and sustained appropriately with the existing mental health resources available in a given location. Equity refers to the importance of making services available to vulnerable and disadvantaged groups so as not to reinforce the inequalities that exist between and within communities. This may necessitate moving beyond what is convenient in order to overcome barriers to services for these groups.

Sociocultural acceptability involves considering how the intervention fits, or does not fit, with the worldview of the people involved, including their conceptualization of the causes of disorders, patterns of help-seeking, and modes of intervention and healing. Relatedly, contextually acceptable outcomes refers to targeting the interventions toward outcomes that are meaningful and important to the people being helped; that is, while symptom reduction is often the focus of Western-designed interventions, this may be less important to the people receiving the intervention than other potential outcomes such as improved social relationships, poverty reduction, etc. Finally, affordability in terms of both direct and indirect costs to individuals, caregivers, and health systems should be considered.

Adaptations in Service Provision

Counselors trained in global mental health must be able not only to conceptualize their work in different ways, but to be flexible enough to alter the actual practice of their work according to the demands of the context. In many settings, particularly in those without an existing mental health infrastructure, the most useful and practical role for mental health counselors may not be that of direct service providers. Rather, a number of other roles may be more appropriate.

Task Shifting

In many low-resource settings with a shortage or absence of mental health professionals, task shifting, or training lay and community health workers to provide specific, first-line, psychological interventions, is a necessity if services are to be made available to all those who need them. Increasingly, task shifting is being used to deliver interventions for a range of problems, including providing psychoeducational programs for caregivers of the mentally ill and survivors of disasters and providing specific manualized interventions such as group interpersonal therapy and cognitive behavioral therapy (Kakuma, Minas, & Dal Poz, 2014). Evaluations of these interventions generally support their effectiveness, and best practices in implementing task shifting programs are beginning to emerge (Patel, 2012). Roles for professional counselors may include providing clinical care to more severe cases that are referred by lay health workers and providing these workers with training, supervision, and support for self-care.

Disaster Mental Health and Humanitarian Response

The first practical introduction of many Western counselors to mental health services in non-Western countries may come in a post-disaster (or other humanitarian response) situation. At the same time, these situations may be the first exposure of those in non-Western settings to Western mental health services. The importance of specific training for humanitarian response is highlighted by Mollica (2011) who described the current situation in many disaster settings:

> It is common now for hordes of humanitarian aid workers mostly from Western countries outside of the devastated country to flood in during the emergency phase of a disaster/conflict… But unfortunately, these life-saving attempts to relieve the physical and emotional suffering of traumatized persons have also become linked to intrusive practices that invade the privacy and undermine the dignity of survivors. Western aid workers can unintentionally break cultural taboos as they aggressively "pry" into the lives of survivors in order to help relieve their suffering. And survivors because of their vulnerability often cannot resist this type of assistance. (p. 17)

Fortunately, many of the mistakes and pitfalls associated with untrained individuals moving into the field of humanitarian response can be avoided with proper training. In addition to the issues of culture described above, Halpern and Tramontin (2007) identified several training considerations for counselors in adapting their work to disaster response settings; these adaptations may apply in any settings in which there is not an established mental health infrastructure or a norm of using professionals for mental health services.

Nontraditional Service Settings and Arrangements

Counselors must be able to work beyond their traditional office settings and be ready to provide services in whatever space is available. This might include churches, schools, or other community settings; it might also include outdoor spaces that lack both comfort and privacy. Particularly in times of disaster, services are likely to be needed in settings that are chaotic, noisy, and otherwise not conducive to services being provided. Using maximum flexibility along with good judgment to adapt and improvise as situations change is essential.

One-Shot Interventions

For a number of reasons, counselors working in many global mental health settings may only have the opportunity to see clients once and need to be able to adapt their work accordingly. For example, individuals in some cultures may value and be seeking practical solutions and advice and might expect a counselor to be able to provide these things in a single session. They may see little purpose in the kind of rapport-building and "intake assessment" activities that make up the initial stage of many Western counseling models. Clients may also have traveled a long distance to seek professional help and may not have the time or resources to engage in a series of sessions or interventions over time. In disaster situations, one-shot interventions with clients who may be experiencing extreme distress are often necessary and require "instant rapport" and rapid assessments in order to proceed effectively (Halpern & Tramontin, 2007).

Clients not Actively Seeking Therapy

In some situations, counselors may be in the position of making services available to individuals, groups, or communities who are not actively seeking mental health interventions or support. This may be the case for many reasons. There may be cultural norms against seeking professional help or disclosing emotional distress with strangers. Mental health may not be a priority when individuals are struggling with basic needs and practical concerns. Clients may not be aware that such services exist or are available. In humanitarian or disaster work, clients may be overwhelmed with intense emotions and/or frenzied activity, but not necessarily aware of their emotional state or their need for support.

Ethics

Ethics links all of these concepts in global mental health. Counselor education for global mental health must be able to train counselors in the ethical standards of their own profession while simultaneously encouraging them to consider the cultural limitations of these standards and helping them develop the decision-making processes necessary to work ethically in any setting.

The ACA Code of Ethics (ACA, 2005), while providing clear expectations and decision-making processes for professional counselors and giving attention to issues of culture, is nonetheless rooted in a Western worldview in which individualism and autonomy are prioritized. As such, there are important additional ethical considerations for counselors working in more collectivist cultural contexts. For example, as described by Kirmayer and Swartz (2014):

> Imposition of individualistic norms of practice on societies that embrace collectivist values may constitute an inappropriate form of cultural imperialism. People may seek help and healing as groups rather than as individuals, and decisions about consent and autonomy may be negotiated within a group context. (p. 51)

Similarly, ethical guidelines regarding the termination of the counseling process and dual relationships do not fit neatly with the collectivist belief that once developed, relationships never end (Nitza, Chilisa, & Makwinja-Morara, 2010). Thus, as with other aspects of culture, counselors must develop an awareness of their own ethical "worldview" and the limitations therein and be able to respond and adapt appropriately to avoid situations of mental health colonialism and imperialism (Bemak & Chung, 2015).

The core principles of the Interagency Standing Committee (2007) offer a starting point for considering the ethics of practicing in a global context. These principles include promoting human rights and equity, providing for full participation of local populations in planning and implementation efforts, doing no harm, building on available resources and capacities, integrating support systems, and offering multilayered supports. Miller (2012) has proposed two additions to these principles, which include stressing cultural responsiveness and maintaining organizational responsiveness.

Best Practices for Incorporating a Global Mental Health Perspective in Counselor Education

We would like to propose a few best practices related to promoting global mental health for counselors and counselor educators. First, dedicating oneself to further education about the topic of global mental health may be warranted as well as adopting those perspectives and lifestyles which actively demonstrate a commitment to social justice, diversity, equality, and equal access to mental health care for all people (O'Donnell, 2012). As a starting point, it may be helpful to identify sources for ongoing updates about global mental health; this may involve joining professional organizations that are either international by design or promote global perspectives. Additionally, incorporating global mental health topics and international viewpoints in the counselor education curriculum is vital to raising awareness about the importance of global mental health for counselors-in-training. Given the many requirements for credit hours, training standards, and clinical practice for accredited counselor education programs, incorporating additional global mental health training into existing programs will require commitment and intentionality on the part of counselor educators. Nevertheless, such training is essential for individual counselors and vital for the profession as a whole.

Incorporating Global Mental Health Perspectives into Theoretical Training

Many post-modern counseling theories have a focus on equity, diversity, and social justice. Counselor educators who teach theory may consider adopting a social justice pedagogy (Adams, Bell, & Griffen, 2007) in which students are encouraged to develop a sense of shared responsibility for advocating for the equitable sharing of resources and opportunity. When considering various theories, it could be powerful to have students analyze them according to principles of social justice, reflect on the application of the theory with diverse populations, and investigate ways in which the theoretical lens may propagate equality or oppression. Additionally, educators may investigate ways to include teaching lesser known theories which embody significant global, multicultural, and social justice perspectives into their curriculum.

One theory that may be lesser-known in counselor education is that of Liberation Psychology, which was first articulated by Martín-Baró (1994). In developing this theory, he posited that in order for psychological treatment to be relevant to all mental health needs, it must be focused on the lived experience of those who live in the most extreme conditions (Tate, Torres Rivera, Brown, & Skaistis, 2013). A very rough outline of this treatment philosophy includes the idea of recovering historical memory for oppressed populations, challenging the realities of history established by dominant forces of government and media that are both intentionally and unintentionally oppressive, and focusing on the strengths of the oppressed population.

When clients and practitioners are able to view problems in this light rather than through the dominant narrative, they are able to develop a new understanding of their problems and plight, which can and should lead to personal and social action. Counselors who practice from this theoretical base must also be agents of change and advocate for these steps with and for their clients. The foundational perspective of Liberation Psychology blurs the lines between counseling and social action and provides what is often a very new perspective for counselors-in-training that can lead to a revolution in treatment and the counseling field. Such new perspectives may be particularly applicable to the development of a global perspective.

Incorporating Global Mental Health into the Curriculum

In addition to the need for students to develop a global lens through which to consider theory, global mental health concepts are relevant to and can be infused into all aspects of a counselor education curriculum. In its current accreditation standards, CACREP (2016) includes eight common core areas they define as the foundational knowledge required of all entry-level counselors, regardless of specialty. These core areas include Professional Counseling Orientation and Ethical Practice, Social and Cultural Diversity, Human Growth and Development, Career Development, Counseling and Helping Relationships, Group Counseling and Group Work, Assessment and Testing, and Research and Program Evaluation. Each core area in turn includes eight to fourteen standards, all of which must be specifically addressed within the curriculum of accredited programs. These core areas and standards can be used as a guide to organize the incorporation of global mental health content into a program's curricular map.

There are multiple ways to conceptualize the mapping of global mental health concepts onto CACREP standards. Table 1 (see Appendix A*) provides one example. As is clear from this table, some of the concepts are more closely linked to current standards than others. CACREP multicultural and diversity standards are closely linked to global mental health, and many global mental health concepts can be covered through the careful selection of readings, films, examples, case studies, and role play scenarios into a multicultural counseling course. Global mental health systems, while not directly addressed in the standards, could be taught as an extension of the standards related to the roles and responsibilities of counselors in working within larger systems and in interdisciplinary capacities. Doing so would likely necessitate the inclusion of additional readings and assignments beyond what is typically covered in these standards. Additional global mental health systems content can be linked to standards related to identifying the systemic and contextual influences on individuals and communities and those related to social justice and advocacy.

Evidence-based practices for global mental health can be considered in any course in which the evidence base for counseling interventions is covered, including theories courses, multicultural courses, and research courses. Students can be required to incorporate empirical articles from other countries into any assignment, conduct literature reviews of the outcome research related to specific countries or cultures, or critique the applicability of Western-based empirical articles to other contexts. Issues of culturally appropriate research methodologies and the sociocultural acceptability of outcomes and evidence from different worldviews are addressed in depth in the book *Indigenous Research Methodologies* (Chilisa, 2012).

---

*Appendices for this chapter can be found at: http://tinyurl.com/wghm-attachments

Adaptations in service provision are unevenly addressed in CACREP's core areas.

Task shifting is not covered directly and would require specific inclusion, perhaps in combination with coverage of global mental health systems, in coverage of standards related to the roles and responsibilities of counselors working within larger systems and in interdisciplinary capacities. The supervision standard refers to the role of supervision in counseling, but students do not typically receiving training in conducting supervision themselves; this is an area that would require the inclusion of additional content and learning experiences. The standard related to consultation offers an opportunity to consider task shifting through that lens. Disaster mental health and humanitarian response are directly targeted in the standards and can include a global emphasis through intentional selection of readings, examples, and case studies. Adaptations in service settings and arrangements do not appear to fit directly within CACREP's core area standards and might be better addressed in clinical training.

Training in ethics is a clearly articulated standard, but this standard refers to training students to apply existing ethical codes and does not specify the need for counselors to be able to critique the cultural relevance of these codes to the global environment. This is an area in need of further attention within the counseling profession as a whole.

Stand-alone courses may be the best option for some global mental health content such as global ethics. Stand-alone courses also allow students to synthesize their learning in other courses or can serve as an introduction to the topic onto which other content can be built. Courses in global mental health and/or disaster mental health (which often serves as an introduction to global mental health) are currently offered in a few counselor education programs in the United States. The Psychology Department at SUNY New Paltz, in collaboration with the Institute for Disaster Mental Health there, offers an elective course in disaster mental health that also serves as an introductory course for their Advanced Certificate Program in Trauma and Disaster Mental Health. Students enrolled in this course explore the impact of disasters on individuals and communities globally as well as options for providing acute, intermediate, and long-term interventions. The final project in the course involves an analysis of a disaster situation and the development of a mental health response plan within the cultural context of the disaster.

Similarly, the Disaster Mental Health Institute at the University of South Dakota offers a disaster mental health course that is both a supplemental for counseling students and a required course for their Disaster Mental Health Graduate Certificate. The master's program in International Disaster Psychology at the University of Denver, which leads to license eligibility as a professional counselor in Colorado, includes required courses in both global mental health systems and disaster mental health, among other courses with global content infused.

Incorporating Global Mental Health into Clinical Training

While clinical training is the foundation of counselor education, it can be challenging to provide students with clinical experiences in global mental health. Creating opportunities for students to gain experience in adapting service provision to meet situational demands is a particular challenge. A commitment to incorporating a global mental health perspective must be weaved into accreditation standards for clinical training as well as state licensing standards and must also be shaped in such a way as to meet the developmental needs of counselors-in-training.

The Counselor Education program at Indiana University-Purdue University Fort Wayne (IPFW) has worked to provide global mental health training to its students and address real needs in the community by partnering with a local not-for-profit agency to provide no-cost, student-led counseling services to immigrant and refugee families. The challenges faced by the IPFW program in this endeavor are informative.

As described above, providing culturally and logistically appropriate services requires a great deal of flexibility and the ability to adapt quickly to the needs of particular clients. At the same time, accreditation and licensing standards are highly prescriptive regarding clinical training and leave little room for flexibility. For example, clinical training sites must be open to the recording of sessions and/or live observation by supervisors. While this is challenging for many sites, it creates a particular barrier in attempting to provide services to clients native to cultures for which there is a heavy stigma around mental illness and that do not regularly use professional mental health services. Individuals who are undocumented or who have fled regimes/settings in which authorities cannot be trusted are necessarily and understandably very cautious. The requirement of being recorded or observed may keep them from receiving the help they need and also inhibit students from gaining direct experience with this population.

A related limitation is that engaging successfully with hesitant clients takes time. Cultural sensitivity has necessitated outreach and rapport-building with cultural groups, such as the Burmese and several Arabic-speaking groups in the Fort Wayne community, in order to establish ongoing relationships and be viewed by individuals (especially the leaders within those groups) as trustworthy. This process, although imperative, can be time-consuming and cumbersome. State licensure standards are typically very strict in terms of what types of services or time spent with clients are eligible for approval. Students faced with pressures to meet licensure requirements, even when they have a particular interest in work with immigrant and refugee populations, have been reluctant to engage in the time-consuming process of rapport-building necessary to build up a client load because the time spent in that process does not count toward licensure.

Finally, among the additional skills needed to do clinical work in global mental health is the ability work effectively with interpreters in a mental health care setting. Learning the complexities of language interpretation among and within cultures is necessary in a profession that so reliant on dialogues as a means of processing and healing invisible wounds. Incorporating this training into an already jam-packed curriculum is a notable challenge and one with which the IPFW program faculty continues to wrestle.

Another set of challenges faced by the IPFW Counselor Education program in its attempts to integrate global mental health practices into its training has been the tension between the developmental needs of counseling students and the needs of clients from non-Western settings. In the early stages of their development, students typically require a greater level of structure and predictability as they learn the processes of conceptualization and intervention. At the same time, conceptualizing and intervening with clients from non-Western settings often requires a high level of cognitive flexibility and tolerance of ambiguity. A developmental approach to counselor training suggests that the early stages of development are characterized by high anxiety and a need for structure and vigilance for doing the "right" thing (which makes creativity and adaptability difficult at this stage). Thus, the program's faculty supervisors are constantly reviewing and considering the best placement of global mental health into clinical experiences and how to balance students' developmental needs with the more practical concerns of providing these experiences.

Promoting Global Mental Health through Cultural Immersion

An additional option for providing students with both content knowledge and clinical skills in global mental health is cultural immersion. By studying multicultural content while being immersed in an unfamiliar culture, students have the opportunity to gain a deeper understanding of how culture mediates relationships, attitudes, values, and behaviors. Such immersion experiences also provide a learning context for students to become more critically conscious of global and societal dynamics of power and privilege. International immersion offers a different method of achieving the desired outcomes outside the traditional class structure. The "dissonance" involved in a cultural immersion experience promotes a heightened opportunity for experiential learning to occur.

Important aspects of student learning that can be more readily provided through international immersion include: the affective experiences that come with being immersed in an unfamiliar culture, making sense of and accommodating cultural differences, the opportunity to compare and contrast their home and host cultures, societal structures, and relative privilege and oppression, and the experience of being seen and treated as "other." By processing these experiences, students will be prompted to examine how their own culturally-imbedded perspectives lead to the construction of what is understood as general knowledge (Banks & Banks, 2004). The cognitive shifts that occur through these learning experiences have been repeatedly linked to multicultural sensitivity and cultural competence in counselor training (Garcia, Kosutic, McDowell, & Anderson, 2009; McDowell, Storm, & York, 2007).

The efficacy of this type of learning experience is supported by a recent study of multicultural counseling competencies in international immersion courses (McDowell et al., 2012). Student learning outcomes in this study included changes in important aspects of personal transformation (awareness), social awareness and knowledge, and professional development (skills), including an enhanced ability to think contextually and systemically and to work cross-culturally.

Conclusion

Looking forward, issues of forced migration, refugees and internally displaced persons, chronic political conflict, and climate change are among the growing threats to mental health on a global scale (Halpern & Vermeulen, 2017). The expansion of global mental health training in counselor education is one way to address these coming threats and support the overall global mental health agenda of ensuring that all people have access to effective and equitable mental health care. Global mental health training is not currently a standard part of most counselor preparation programs, but there are several options for incorporating such training in counselor education theory, curriculum, and clinical experiences. The addition of stand-alone courses and cultural immersion experiences are other options that have been used successfully. It is our hope that the ideas proposed in this chapter will spark further conversation, innovation, and action to promote global mental health through counselor education.

References

Adams, M., .Bell, L. A., &.Griffin, P. (2007). *Teaching for diversity and social justice* (2nd ed.). New York. NY: Routledge

American Counseling Association (2005). ACA code of ethics. Alexandra, VA: Author.

Banks, J. A. & Banks, C. A. M. (Eds.). (2004). *The handbook of research on multicultural education* (2nd ed.). San Francisco: Jossey-Bass.

Bemak, F. & Chung, R. C-Y. (2015). Critical issues in international group counseling. *The Journal for Specialists in Group Work, 40*(1), 6-21. doi: 10.1080/01933922.2014.992507

Chilisa, B. (2012). *Indigenous research methodologies.* Thousand Oaks, CA: Sage.

Council for Accreditation of Counseling and Related Educational Programs (CACREP). (2016). 2016 CACREP Standards. Retrieved from: http://www.cacrep.org/for-programs/2016-cacrep-standards/

Council for Accreditation of Counseling and Related Educational Programs (CACREP). (2015). Areas/Specializations. Retrieved from: http://www.cacrep.org/glossary/specialty-areasspecialization/

Garcia, M., Kosutic, I., MdDowell, T., & Anderson, S. (2009). Raising critical consciousness in family therapy supervision. *Journal of Feminist Family Therapy, 21*(1), 18-38.

Gazzola, N., & Smith, J. D. (2007). Who do we think we are? A survey of counsellors in Canada. *International Journal for the Advancement of Counselling*, 29(2), 97-110. doi:10.1007/s10447-007-9032-y

Glosoff, H. L., & Schwarz-Wittaker, J. E. (2013). The counseling profession: Historical perspectives and current issues and trends. In D. Capuzzi and D. R. Gross (Eds.). *Introduction to the Counseling Profession* (6th ed.) (pp. 30-76). New York: Routledge.

Goodyear, R. K. (2000). An unwarranted escalation of counselor-counseling psychologist professional conflict: Comments on Weinrach, Lustig, Chan, and Thomas (1998). *Journal of Counseling and Development, 78*, 103-106. doi: 10.1002/j.1556-6676.2000.tb02566.x

Halpern, J. & Tramontin, M. (2007). *Disaster mental health: Theory and practice.* Belmont, CA: Thomson Brooks/Cole.

Halpern, J. & Vermeulen, K. (2017). *Disaster mental health interventions: Core principles and practices.* New York, NY: Routledge.

Hanlon, C., Fekadu, A., & Patel, V. (2014). Interventions for mental disorders. In V. Patel, H. Minas, A. Cohen, & M. Prince (Eds.), *Global mental health: Principles and practice* (p 252-276). New York, NY: Oxford University Press

Interagency Standing Committee (IASC). (2007). *IASC Guidelines on Mental Health and Psychosocial Support in Emergency Settings.* Geneva, Switzerland: IASC International Association for Counselling. (2016). IAC Mission and Vision. Retrieved from: http://iac-irtac.org/?q=node/36.

Kakuma, R. Minas, H., & Dal Poz, M R. (2014). Strategies for strengthening human resources for mental health. In V. Patel, H. Minas, A. Cohen, & M. Prince (Eds.), *Global mental health: Principles and practice* (p 193-223). New York, NY: Oxford University Press

Kaplan, D. (2014). 20/20: A vision for the future of counseling: The new consensus definition of counseling. *Journal of Counseling and Development, 32*, 366-372. doi: 10.1002/j.1556-6676.2014.00164.x

Kirmayer, L. J., & Swartz, L. (2014). Culture and global mental health. In V. Patel, H. Minas, A. Cohen, & M. Prince (Eds.), *Global mental health: Principles and practice* (p 41-62). New York, NY: Oxford University Press

Koplan, J. P., Bond, T. C., Merson, M. H., Reddy, K. S., Rodrigues, M. H., Sewankambo, N. K., et al. (2009). Towards a common definition of global health. *Lancet, 373*(9679), 1993-1995. doi: 10.1016/S01406736(09)60332-9

Martín-Baró, I. (1994). *Writings for a liberation psychology.* A. Aron & S. Corne (Eds.). Cambridge, MA: Harvard University Press.

McDowell, T., Goessling, K., & Melendez, T. (2012). Transformative learning through international immersion: Building multicultural competence in family therapy and counseling. *Journal of Marital and Family Therapy, 38*, 365-379. doi: 10.1111/j.1752-0606.2010.00209.x

McDowell, T., Storm, C., & York, C. (2007). Multiculturalism in couple and family therapy education: Revisiting familiar struggles and facing new complexities. *Journal of Systemic Therapies, 26*, 75-94.

McGovern, P. (2014). Why should mental health have a place in the post-2015 global health agenda? *International Journal of Mental Health Systems, 8* (38), 1-4. doi: 10.1186/1752-4458-8-38

Miller, J. L. (2012). *Psychosocial capacity building in response to disasters.* New York, NY: Columbia University Press.

Mollica, R. (2011). Introduction. In R. Mollica (Ed.), *Global mental health: Trauma and recovery* (p. 13-44). Cambridge, MA: Author.

National Board for Certified Counselors International. (2016). Mission Statement. Retrieved from http://www.nbccinternational.org/Who_we_are/Mission_Statement

Nitza, A., Chilisa, B., & Makwinja-Morara, V. (2010). *Mbizi:* Empowerment and HIV/AIDS prevention for adolescent girls in Botswana. *The Journal for Specialists in Group Work, 35*(2), 105-114. doi:10.1080/01933921003705990

O'Donnell, K. S. (2012). Global mental health: A resource primer for exploring the domain. *International Perspectives in Psychology: Research, Practice, Consultation, 1*, 191-205. doi: 10.1037/a0029290

Patel, V. (2014). Why mental health matters to global health. *Transcultural Psychiatry, 51*(6), 777-789. doi: 10.1177/1363461514524473

Patel, V. (2012). Global mental health: From science to action. *Harvard Review of Psychiatry, 20*(1), 6-12. doi: 10.3109/10673229.2012.649108

Pope, M. (2004a). Counseling psychology and professional school counseling: Barriers to a true collaboration. *The Counseling Psychologist, 32*, 253-262. doi: 10.1177/0011000003261370

Pope, M. (2004b). Professional counseling and Dr. Glasser: A relationship based on reality and choice. *The Family Journal, 12*(4), 345-349. doi: 1177/1066480704268422.

Pressly, P. K., Parker, W. M., & Jennie, J. (2001). Actualizing multicultural counseling competencies: A multifaceted course approach. *International Journal for the Advancement of Counselling, 23*, 223-234.

Remley, T. P., & Herlihy, B. (2010). *Ethical, legal, and professional issues in counseling* (3rd ed.). Upper Saddle River, NJ: Pearson Education, Inc.

Tate, K., Torres Rivera, E., Brown, E, & Skaistis, L. (2013). Foundations for liberation: Social justice and Liberation Psychology. *Interamerican Journal of Psychology, 47*, 373-382.

World Health Organization. (2010). *mhGAP intervention guide for mental, neurological and substance use disorders in non-specialized health settings: Mental health Gap Action Programme (mhGAP).* Geneva, Switzerland: Author.

CHAPTER 13

PTSD in Ugandan Refugees: Establishing a Peer-Counseling Program with a Global Health Partner

Kenneth H. Kessler

Rosalind Franklin University of Medicine and Science (RFUMS) is a health sciences university. We train students at the graduate level for various careers in health care including medicine, psychology, physical therapy, and pharmacy. Because of its commitment to service learning, the university administration established an Office of Global Health. Through the Office of Global Health, students from a variety of disciplines can complete service learning rotations in places outside the United States. By doing so, students not only help those in need, but also learn about themselves, health care delivery outside the United States, and the challenges faced by people from other cultures and financial backgrounds. Students completing global health rotations may do so at partner organizations where there is an established relationship, curriculum, and protocol, or, with the appropriate approvals and after the establishment of educational goals, they can complete their rotation at a non-partner site. This chapter will focus on the establishment of a university relationship with a regular partner agency in a third-world county, and how student and faculty volunteers from a health sciences university can provide needed (and requested) services to a partner agency in a way that minimizes disruption to the agency's day-to-day activities and can also take away important lessons that will advance themselves as individuals and as health care providers.

It all began one day ever so innocently. We were nearing graduation time, and the faculty and students of the university had assembled for the annual awards ceremony that occurs the day before graduation. Shortly before, the Director of the Global Health Office, Inis Bardella, had approached another member of the faculty, who was doing some global health work in Mexico, about the possibility of completing some additional work in Uganda, Africa. It turns out that Bolingo Ntahira, the executive director of our partner agency in Uganda, Hope of Children and Women Victims of Violence (HOCW, HOCWUG.NET), had asked Dr. Bardella about the possibility of RFUMS creating a program for the treatment of Post-Traumatic Stress Disorder (PTSD) 'in its refugee clients. That particular faculty member was not interested in doing so, but introduced Dr. Bardella to me (the author of this chapter) at that awards ceremony. The introduction went something like this, "Dr. Bardella, meet Dr. Kessler. He likes places where you can't drink the water, where there is no electricity, and where there are many mosquitoes. I think he is a natural for Africa." He was referring to my love of the woods of northern Minnesota and my annual treks with my family to the Boundary Waters Canoe Area Wilderness. The introductions were made, and thus the love affair with global health and the people of Uganda began.

Dr. Bardella explained the nature of the problem. Our global health partner in Uganda was in need of additional services. Students had been going to HOCW for the past few years and were teaching health and wellness classes, organizing HIV screening clinics, and volunteering at Zanta clinic (the local level IV governmental health care clinic in the village of Ndejje, which is near Kampala). Yet there was an unmet need. Refugee clients of HOCW were often limited in making progress in their training at HOCW because of rampant symptoms of PTSD. Some clients of the organization were essentially unable to leave their homes due to symptoms that included panic, anxiety, and flashbacks. Others had sporadic attendance, and many had poor attention and concentration due to internal distractions resulting from severe symptoms of PTSD. Could a sustainable program be created to serve this dire need in the face of few to no mental health services in a country where even basic health care provisions are quite scarce?

The challenge had been set: Create an effective PTSD treatment program that could sustain itself in a third-world environment with scarce resources and few (if any) trained mental health professionals. I confided to my colleague that all I knew about Uganda was that it is in Africa and that I had no idea how to proceed with developing such a program – but I committed to looking into what could be done.

The main issue was that unlike providing educational programming, vaccine clinics, or surgery clinics, the intervention would need to occur over a significant period of time – about four to six months from beginning to end of treatment. Not only was it impossible for any of us to stay that long, but even if we could, that type of program was not sustainable. The minute we left Uganda, the program would cease. Furthermore, the patients we treated would be left without a provider with whom they could follow up. So, that issue became our first challenge to solve. Could a program be developed that would outlast our stay in Uganda?

I was assigned a team of four fourth-year medical students and one second-year clinical psychology student. The six of us were to work together to determine if such a program could be created and, if so, to do what was needed to implement the program in the one month we would collectively spend in Uganda at the HOCW program. We began by going to the literature. Much to our surprise, we learned that a treatment program, known as Narrative Exposure Therapy (NET) (developed by Shauer, Neuner, & Elbert), had been used in northern Uganda. Furthermore, it was meant to be taught to and implemented by lay counselors. So there was hope!

Our team began to meet regularly to learn about the NET treatment program and to determine how we would best teach it to the trainees in Uganda in order to implement it. We had about six months to prepare ourselves for this task. One of our biggest challenges was that we did not know what level of training the counselors would already have. We also had no way of knowing the various social and cultural considerations that would be at play during the training or that would affect the response of the clients whom the counselors would ultimately serve. However, two of the medical students had been to HOCW as first-year students, so we were not completely blind to all of the challenges we would be facing. We planned as best we could and prepared ourselves for the likelihood that we would have to adjust our plans as we went along. In addition to preparing a variety of presentations, we purchased NET manuals for ourselves as well as for each of the counselors we were to train.

Upon arriving at HOCW, we met with the executive director to review our planned program and seek his input. We were very concerned about the fact that we were from a completely different country and culture and were cognizant of the fact that we might inadvertently violate a multitude of cultural norms and customs. We also discussed with him the fact that, for the most part, we were unaware of what resources were available locally. After we made some revisions based on his feedback, he approved our general training program and we embarked on daily meetings with the volunteers who were to become counselors.

We began by making an assessment of what the trainees knew about mental health, the functioning of the brain, confidentiality, mental status, etc. What we found was a willing, caring, bright, and highly-motivated group who had little information on which to build. We needed to start at the beginning! Some counselors had university training and others had, for one reason or another (usually financial hardship or civil unrest), not completed high school. Our idea of handing out the NET manuals to everyone and asking them to read a chapter and come back to discuss it in daily sessions was not going to work. Our training team met that first evening and we discarded a good amount of what we had originally planned. We stayed up late and came up with a "Plan B" that would meet our trainees where they were – at the beginning, in a culturally and educationally relevant manner.

We continually had to spend a good deal of time and effort encouraging the trainees to talk and share their thoughts on various matters relevant to the training at hand. One of the hurdles we had to overcome was empowering the trainees to share their opinions and, most importantly, to tell us when something was not making sense or when something was unlikely to work with people from their culture. There was a strong cultural propensity for the training recipients to listen and nod politely, even when they didn't understand or agree with the lesson. They were afraid to share negative information with us for fear that it would show lack of respect and/or that we would give up on the program and withdraw our resources. Time and again, we had to reinforce that we could not properly train them or evaluate the program overall if we did not have honest feedback from them. We repeatedly instilled in them that honest feedback was the foundation upon which we would build. We positively reinforced the trainees for bringing up the smallest concern. We feel that eventually we succeeded, for the most part.

We also were keenly aware of the cultural differences between Uganda and the U.S. A Ugandan counselor or refugee client might see something completely differently than we would as U.S. American volunteers. We continually sought feedback from the trainees in this regard. We often found ourselves saying, "This is how we would do it in the U.S. What would work here?" By asking that and other open-ended questions, we avoided yes-or-no answers and opened the opportunity for dialogue. With time, the trainees felt more and more comfortable sharing their thoughts and opinions with us. We then could modify the program and procedures accordingly – in ways that were consistent with the empirically-based methodology that was informing our program, but also in ways that were culturally and socially meaningful.

We covered the basics of the etiology and symptoms of PTSD, how to determine who met diagnostic criteria, how to use NET to treat PTSD, and also broader topics, such as active listening, the importance of confidentiality, how to build rapport, what to do with clients who might become suicidal, how to keep clients engaged, and what to do when they weren't. As our training progressed, the counselor trainees asked more and more questions. Some of the questions were on topics that we judged as possibly controversial (e.g., those involving family values and sexuality). We determined that answers to those questions would be deferred until the next day. Those became "Bolingo questions." Each evening at dinner, we would speak with Bolingo, the Executive Director, about the questions that we were not sure how to answer. We would explain how we thought we should answer and what the facts were to support our answer. After some thought he would either say, "It's okay," or would help us formulate an answer that was factual and also culturally informed.

Knowing we only had a month total, we had the trainees start seeing clients under our supervision at the beginning of the third week. We provided more feedback and engaged in more problem solving. After the first week of supervised sessions, we had a feeling that time was short but that we were close to having our team of trainees being minimally competent. We made plans for ongoing consultation and supervision via email and recurring Skype sessions. We concluded the week with a graduation ceremony for the newly trained counselors. The entire refugee-client community was invited to the celebration. This was important for two reasons: the counselors could feel proud and accomplished and the community could recognize the counselors as leaders and helpers. We were quite surprised and encouraged when some of the most private and severely-traumatized refugees, who were now clients, showed up at the ceremony. The ceremony had begun the process of destigmatizing psychological difficulties in the HOCW refugee community.

Challenges We Faced and What We Learned

As outsiders, we see a need and we want to help. One of the problems with outside help is that it must be sustainable. Most of the needs in third-world countries are large and ongoing, and few needs can be addressed in a one-shot manner. The counseling program, as designed, seemed to be self-sustaining. We would train the counselors, and, with their new training, they would remain on-site while we went back to our homes and lives. There were several problems we did not consider. First, the counselors were voluntary participants in the training. They were selected by HOCW as individuals who had characteristics that would make them good counselors: bright, caring, patient, etc. They came from varied backgrounds and spoke various languages, and some were even former refugees themselves. However, the volunteer counselors needed to make ends meet. They had families to feed and expenses of their own so it was not sustainable for them to remain as volunteers forever. A funding source would need to be found in order to retain the newly-minted counselors, otherwise they would move on when an opportunity arose for them to take work that would enhance their financial well-being. (N.B.: In the end, the administration of RFUMS elected to provide an annual grant to fund the counselors' salaries. This grant continues to-date in spite of some changes in administration, including the appointments of a new global health director, Catherine "Cat" Myser, Ph.D.)

Ongoing consultation was also an issue of sustainability. From previous reports, things had improved with regard to internet communication at the facility. Furthermore, nearly everyone in Uganda has a cell phone, and most have some type of smart phone that allows for use of various apps such as Facebook, Skype, and Whatsapp in addition to email. Counselors could email or message us questions after we left for very little cost. We set up monthly video-conference consultation and supervision sessions in order for counselors to have a forum to continue to develop their skills. At times, even with the improved internet functionality, the video conference (and even an audio-only conference) had to be foregone. Quality, high-speed internet capabilities exist, but it is yet another issue of funding. A high-speed, unlimited bandwidth connection could cost $200-300 U.S. dollars per month. That's expensive even by U.S. standards, but equivalent to the monthly salary of at least one full-time employee in Uganda. When money is short, another employee or two is more important than continual high-speed internet connectivity.

Different cultural standards in health care policies were quite striking. For example, in the U.S., provider-patient confidentiality is a cornerstone of care which helps patients feel safe and comfortable. However, it is often non-existent in third-world countries. We witnessed medical visits at the local clinics occurring with several other patients in the room as they inched their way through the line, into the examination room, and up to the providers' desk. The providers spoke in a hushed voice in some attempt to shield the private conversation from others, but to little avail. Considering the close proximity of people in third-world countries combined with open-air offices, there is little in the way of routine confidentiality. We had to spend a great deal of time talking about the importance of confidentiality, particularly when dealing with mental health issues and issues of a traumatic nature. We, along with the counselor trainees, structured many policies and procedures that were designed to enhance confidentiality. We had to structure a counseling office in such a way that confidentiality could be reasonably assured (e.g., making sure counseling occurred at a time when no classes were going on right outside the room, making sure no one was sitting on the door step outside, waiting for an appointment or for another class to begin, etc.). We also learned that there was no secure place to store patient records, so we arranged to purchase a file cabinet – which was delivered via motorcycle taxi, of course.

Although the stigma of mental health issues still exists to some degree in the U.S., we have made great strides in making mental health less of a taboo subject with the American public. This is still not the case with Ugandans and most people from third-world countries. Mental illness and mental health problems are to be kept private and are certainly not to be freely discussed with others. Having a behavioral health problem is seen as a weakness or sometimes even as some type of spirit-based phenomenon. Problems are typically not discussed because knowledge of their existence can be used against the individual. We had to work with the trainees to ensure the establishment of policies and procedures that would establish a safe, confidential environment in which the clients could seek care. Together with the counselors, we also had to undertake a bit of a public relations campaign in the client-community in order to explain what we were doing and how the program worked.

One of the issues our team had to contend with was that for all intents and purposes, there was no higher level of care for patients who really required 24-hour care or who became suicidal during treatment. Our team quickly discovered that there were no resources like ambulances or inpatient psychiatric facilities. The local people told us that the one inpatient psychiatric facility that existed was more dangerous than the prison. Nevertheless, the fact remained that we needed some kind of plan for patients who were not safe alone. Together with Director Bolingo and the local counselors, we devised a protocol for suicidal patients that included the community and members of the patient's family (if there were any locally – often our patients were the sole survivors of their family unit) coming together to care for the individual 24 hours a day until the individual had stabilized. By western cultural standards, such a care plan was fraught with liability and concerns; however, by local customs and resources, this was the best plan that could be implemented. Fortunately, to date, we have only had to enact the protocol once and it worked well.

Clients of the treatment program are often limited in time and money. Even though the program is free, money is still a limiting factor. Many clients are trying to work a job, often for very little pay, in order to survive in their new country. Money is more than tight. It is often non-existent. Consequently, a client's work takes precedence over attending counseling appointments. Similarly, money for transportation is an issue. Even though it might only cost one U.S. dollar to go to and from the appointment by taxi bus, those funds could mean the difference between eating that day or not. So, when push comes to shove, clients often cancel appointments or simply fail to show up due to work or issues related to transportation funds.

Since we trained lay counselors to administer this program, we had to make sure to have a plan in place for on-going supervision and skill development. Although the counselors could communicate with us using the internet (when it is working adequately) or via a text message app, we determined that more was necessary. Therefore, at least one of us visits annually to provide on-going training, case management, and in-person supervision of cases. This is an important commitment of time and resources in order to ensure the program progresses and maintains its fidelity to empirically-supported methodologies. Ongoing support is necessary for the program's success. Arguably, without ongoing support and training, the program could even become harmful. Without continuous oversight, even the most well-intentioned trainees could easily drift away from their training. We see this in all settings, but in particular, in those in which trainees are isolated from professional development resources and opportunities.

In spite of many challenges, I believe our multispecialty-team succeeded in its mission. We have been collecting outcome data for the past two-and-a-half years of the program, and our preliminary analysis suggests that clients are improving. Approximately forty individuals have completed the program in its entirety, and all have shown a significant reduction in symptoms. All but two are reporting PTSD symptoms that are below the threshold for diagnosis on our PTSD screening assessment instrument. Some challenges remain to be solved (the internet connectivity issue and continued funding of the counselor salaries), but these seem relatively easy to solve in comparison to the establishment of the entire program. Another sustainability problem that we discussed is how to plan for attrition of the counselors. Inevitably, some will move on. We have lost two of the original group already, but as luck would have it, a colleague from the U.K., Ellen Watkins, Ph.D., volunteered at HOCW for several months the year after our program was established. She is not only a psychologist, but was already trained in NET. She provided an invaluable amount of training to all the counselors during that summer, but also trained two new replacement counselors during her stay. We realize opportunities like that do not come along very often; thus, we have begun talking about having trainee-counselors being involved with our current program so they can learn from those who have become experts. Since the counselors have only been trained to treat PTSD in adults, we have also begun discussing the possibility of expanding services – either to other diagnoses, like depression or anxiety disorders, or to other age groups, such as treating PTSD in adolescents or children. As we solve some of the connectivity and funding challenges HOCW faces, we feel confident that we can eventually expand the training of the HOCW counselor group.

CHAPTER 14

PTSD Unites the World:
Prevention, Intervention, and Training
with the Therapeutic Spiral Model

Kate Hudgins

Trauma is a normal occurrence for many, and as Post-Traumatic Stress Disorder (PTSD) burgeons globally, mental health providers have long sought a system of training, education, and research. While initiatives in global health exist from micro-to macro-interventions, this chapter describes one small, private organization, Therapeutic Spiral International (TSI) from the United States, and its impact on trauma work at therapeutic and structural levels of change. Over twenty-five years, TSI has partnered with individuals, groups, organizations, NGOs, universities, and businesses to promote international training of trauma workers across cultures and languages. I (the author of this chapter) present the therapeutic spiral model (TSM) as a research-supported system of experiential change that is rooted in the theories of interpersonal neurobiology and experiential therapy (Hudgins and Toscani, 2013). TSM derives from classical psychodrama and modifies its concepts and techniques for clinical safety and effectiveness for use with traumatized persons. It is the first-ever clinical map for trauma treatment translated into simple role theory terms, providing an easy-to-use guide for all experiential methods of change with trauma (Hudgins, 2015, 2007b, 2002). Included here are examples of TSI's global health initiatives showing its applicability from the individual to the collective. Stories range from the beginning of TSM in 1992, with small, clinical groups of sexual abuse survivors, to its current global expansion in therapeutic and structural intervention and training. Additionally, I present TSI's international certification program for healthcare training, affording a path for sustainability across generations of TSM practitioners, as well as continued expansion into new areas of trauma repair.

Introduction

Post-traumatic Stress Disorder (PTSD) (APA, 2013) is rampant in today's world of global terrorism, health crises, ethnic wars, family disruption, and other multi-causal effects of both violence and witnessing violence on others (Atwoli, Stein, Karestan, & McLaughlin, 2015). The previously mentioned study by Atwoli et al. (2015) also holds that there are long-term individual and family health consequences from trauma on physical and mental health, resulting in decreases in morbidity and increases in substance use disorders. Although its symptoms had long been known by other names (such as soldier's heart and battle fatigue) (Tick, 2011), PTSD was added as a psychiatric disorder to the DSM-III (APA, 1980) following the Vietnam War. Friedman (2015) presents a historical, epidemiological, and cross-cultural description of the development of PTSD as a diagnosis of a psychological problem in Western medicine.

Interestingly, Shallcross (2012) and White, et al. (2014) show that in many developing countries, PTSD is still considered a foreign diagnosis, as it is in China where I have worked for 15 years. Recently, in an online course in China, students and I discussed the reasons for this viewpoint. The focus of a traumatic impact on the individual is not consistent with their view of community culture, nor is the idea that parental behavior can negatively impact a child. Another possible reason for many global mental health providers' hesitancy to use a PTSD diagnosis is the traditional parent-child relationship, which requires filial loyalty and submission of individual wants for communal values. This is also true in Egypt where Ben Rivers (personal communication, August 2013) has developed a diploma program in the therapeutic spiral model (TSM), thereby leaving the bio-medical model behind to concentrate on social and political determinants that hold the deepest wounds of trauma. Yet, when the actual symptoms of PTSD from the DSM-5 (APA, 2013) are described, many people recognize themselves, their families, and their societies in how they live their day to day lives.

From my experience in 30 countries, I suggest that a diagnosis of PTSD is one that carries across cultures and languages when behaviors are described rather than labels applied. What makes a diagnosis of PTSD user-friendly is that its main criterion is that something bad has happened to a person and not that they were born mentally ill. This allows them to see the possibility of change. Thus, it follows that if something bad changed the patient's personality, health, and life, then something good can do the same. Therefore, viewing many global problems using the lens of PTSD provides a worldview that unites people across cultures.

In this chapter, TSM is anchored into current research on interpersonal affective neurobiology, showing that the impact of trauma shapes not only a person's social and cultural world, but his/her actual brain development and neuroplasticity as well (Cozolino, 2014). TSM is also firmly seated in the decades-long psychological process research on experiential psychology as a method of therapeutic change (Klein, Kiesler, & Coughlin, 1961; Hudgins and Kiesler, 1987). Specific studies to post-traumatic stress, anxiety, and depression helped further refine TSM as a solid psychological theory and method of treatment (Elliott, Watson, Greenberg, Timulak, & Friere, 2013). Classical psychodrama (Moreno & Moreno, 1969) is the cradle that supports the generation of spontaneity and creativity to build new productive roles following the experience of trauma and violence, helping people to find quicker and more effective post-trauma responses.

TSM is a system of clinically modified psychodrama for people who have suffered from traumatic stress and/or violence in their lives (Hudgins, 1998, 2002, 2000). TSM uses Terr's (1991) definition of trauma as "an external blow or series of blows rendering the person temporarily helpless and breaking past ordinary coping and defensive operations" (p. 12). This inclusive definition is based on how a person actually experiences a traumatic event, not on what caused the stress or what diagnostic label they have. Thus TSM bridges the gap between the Western world of PTSD diagnoses (which is considered individualistic) and offers many ways to see the effects of trauma that relate to a more communal and even global frame of mind. Case examples in this chapter show adaptations of TSM to culturally specific examples.

Across both therapeutic and structural interventions, TSM's unique contribution is its all-important clinical map to guide experiential trauma work in the global arena, including theoretical orientations, principles of change, and its operationalized clinical action intervention modules. Case examples show just how far one small organization with dedicated professionals and volunteers can bring therapeutic and structural support well beyond its own borders.

Interpersonal Neurobiology

When TSM was initially developed from clinical practice in psychodrama, sociometry, and group psychotherapy from 1992 to1995, little was conclusively known about the neurobiology of trauma. In 1996, the first MRI of a traumatized brain (Rausch et al.) demonstrated what TSM had developed clinically: more containment of affect was needed for trauma repair. By 1995, Toscani and Hudgins had developed the trauma survivor's intrapsychic role atom (TSIRA), which is described in this chapter as showing both a clinical map and experiential interventions. Now, neurobiology and role theory come together in the TSIRA to support self-soothing, self-regulation, safe expression of affect, and integration of left and right brain modes of functioning for new meaning-making to guide the future. Keltner and Edman (2015) point out that research on neurobiology has even made it into popular culture with the movie *Inside Out*.

In this brief overview to the neurobiology of trauma and repair, I present the structural view of the brain and its evolution to what is now called the "social brain" (Cozolino, 2014, 2016), which is inextricably linked to interpersonal emotional experiences.

Structural View of the Brain

In 1996, Rausch et al. published a radical study using MRIs to show a map of three consistent and profound structural brain changes in people recalling or re-experiencing traumatic events that they had written down. The amygdala, visual cortex, and emotional centers of the brain were lit up on the MRI, while the hippocampus and Broca's speech center in the left brain were almost totally dark. In basic terms, these early brain scans proved that when a person recalls or re-experiences a traumatic event, their brain is dominated by right brain structures related to sensations, images, feelings, and survival responses, while left brain structures are relatively immobile. This scientific proof of the effect of trauma on the brain has profoundly affected the way in which professionals view persons with PTSD or other trauma-induced conditions.

Since these early MRIs, knowledge of the brain has expanded exponentially and has revealed the complexity of its neurobiology and its connection to all body-based systems and social relationships. The brain itself can no longer be reduced to anatomical structures that show cause and effect. Many brain structures, such as the amygdala, actually are connected to the right and left brain functions. Far from being static, they are in a state of ever changing flux and learning through experience (Cozolino, 2014; van der Kolk, 2014).

Poly-Vagal Theory and the Importance of Attachment

Poly-vagal theory (Porges, 2011) provides a foundation to conceptualize three phylogenic systems within the brain: the dorsal vagal complex, the sympathetic nervous system, and the ventral vagal system, which is also known as "the smart vagus." The first to develop evolutionarily was the dorsal vagal system, which facilitates our immobilization or "freeze" responses to danger. Later, the sympathetic system emerged to provide an option for mobilization of a fight or flight response. Most recently, the smart vagus has been shown to self-regulate, using social engagement before reverting to more primitive responses. The smart vagus is essential in our development of social connection, as it is sensitive to nonverbal and paralanguage cues, such as facial expressions, voice tone, and other interactive behaviors related to self-organization and attachment. The functions of the smart vagus and its capacity for self-regulation are at the core of psychotherapy findings that the therapeutic relationship is a most important factor for change (Cozolino, 2016; van der Kolk, 2006).

Interpersonal and Affective View of the Brain

Concurrent with the first MRI studies, Siegel (1999, 2007) and Shore (1994) examined the development and neurobiology of attachment. Today, these two strands of exploration intertwine to create the newer field of interpersonal neurobiology, sometimes called affective neurobiology (Panksepp, 1998). Regardless of the term, current research emphasizes the constant interaction of interpersonal experience at the intersection of biological and social factors (Cozolino, 2002, 2014; Siegel, 2010, 2012). Two findings are particularly important to this chapter. First, interpersonal neuroscience demonstrates the significance of new experience to change the impact of trauma, promoting rapid and effective brain plasticity. Second, the fact that human brains interact with each other demonstrates that interpersonal interactions have an impact on their neurobiology. It is at this nexus that experiential methods of change (TSM in particular) meet the call for rigorous systems that can be replicated for sustainability in trauma work in clinical and structural settings.

Neuroplasticity of the Brain

As shown in numerous MRI studies over the past two decades of research, the brain has billions of neurons and trillions of connections among different structures, and it functions through synaptic connections, chemical signals, blood flow, and other autonomic nervous system functions (Cozolino, 2014). Cozolino (2014) showed clearly that each experience, whether it is an old, repeated behavior or a new, creative action, is directly correlated with the firings of neurons in patterns in the brain. More interesting and relevant to this chapter is the fact that the social brain is in constant interaction with other brains, influencing and changing or reinforcing current states of brain development.

The brain, therefore, has the ability to change throughout life through new social interactions that help provide regulation, containment, nurturance, and further growth. Neuroplasticity of the brain allows it to learn and grow through direct experience, bringing hope for change in interpersonal relationships for individuals, families, groups, societies, and cultures following trauma. A direct quote from Cozolino (2016) states:

The social synapse is the space between us— a space filled with seen and unseen messages and the medium through which we are combined into larger organisms such as families, tribes, societies, and the human species as a whole. Because our experience as individual selves is lived at the border of this synapse, and because so much communication occurs below conscious awareness, this linkage is mostly invisible to us. (p. 3)

It is here, at the social brain, that the bio-medical model of treating PTSD as an individual problem can be expanded to include social relationships as part of healing, even when the trauma is from social, political, racial, or other structural violence, as shown in the examples below.

In 1999, David Read Johnson, a drama therapist, called for a structured model of experiential therapy to treat PTSD, as clinical examples showed its effectiveness using action techniques and expressive arts therapy methods. TSM is such a system of experiential change with limited but definite research to support its efficacy and sustainability (Hudgins, Culbertson, & Hug, 2009; Hudgins & Drucker, 1998; Hudgins, Drucker, & Metcalf, 2000; McVea & Gow, 2006; McVea, Gow, & Lowe, 2011; Perry, Saby, Wenos, Hudgins, & Baller, 2016). As a clinical system of experiential psychotherapy integrating psychodrama, Gestalt therapy (Perls, Hefferline, & Goodman, 1951), and Gendlin's (1996) Focusing, TSM has been operationalized, researched, and used multi-culturally (Hudgins, Cho, Lai, & Ou, 2005; Hudgins, 2007a; Lai, 2013), in therapy offices (Chimera, 2013; Cox, 2013; Drucker, 2013; McVea, 2013), community applications (Salole, Forst, & Goodwin, 2013), and with structural changes (Baim, 2013; Carnabucci and Fullin, 2013; Rivers, 2015).

Experiential Psychotherapy

While research and written literature on TSM has mainly been within the fields of psychodrama, drama therapy, and expressive arts therapy, TSM has always been rooted in the psychological and clinical research on experiential change (Hudgins, 2007a). Experiential therapy was first included in *The Handbook of Psychotherapy and Behavior Change* in 1998 (Greenberg, Watson, & Lietaer), clearly showing several decades ago that experiential psychotherapy is equal to and at times superior to psychodynamic and cognitive behavioral treatments in the areas of depression, anxiety, and trauma (Elliott, Davis, & Slatick, 1998; Elliott, Greenberg, & Lietaer, 2005). In 2013, Greenberg summarized the research on experiential therapies, including psychodrama and TSM, within the broader psychological literature, concluding that there is great promise in TSM's effectiveness. He also suggested that more research is needed, particularly controlled comparison studies, which are now being conducted (Perry, Saby, Wenos, Hudgins, & Baller, 2016).

TSM has always been grounded in three concepts that define experiential therapies in the psychological literature: 1) self-organization, 2) active experiencing of the felt sense, and 3) active therapist interventions (Hudgins, 2007b). Using these parameters, TSM adds a clinical map to guide the safe use of all experiential methods when working with trauma at any level of change.

Self-Organization

Affective neurobiology now describes emotional regulation as a here-and-now interplay among various brain structures and functions, creating a neural net that becomes embedded over time through interpersonal interactions (Badenoch, 2008; Cozolino, 2014). Experiential psychotherapy has long-described the same behaviors clinically and in much the same way. The concept of the self in experiential methods of change is as an ever-changing, fluid, here-and-now flow of awareness among thoughts, feelings, defenses, and behaviors as people interact with others and their environment (Elliott, Watson, Greenberg, Timulak & Freire, 2013). This increased knowledge in the neuroplasticity of the brain corresponds to the clinical picture experiential therapists have always had of their patients' self-organization and ability to change. What Toscani and Hudgins wrote about the clinical map of a trauma survivor's intrapsychic role atom (TSIRA) in 1995 is now supported by two decades of research on the neurobiology of the brain (Dayton, 2016; Hug, 2013).

Active-Experiencing of the Felt Moment

Rogers' (1951) triad of therapy conditions of empathy, unconditional positive regard, and congruence has long been accepted as necessary for any therapeutic or structural change to occur. However, the early experiential therapists added a description of what is needed from the person who wants to change: an active experiencing of their own self-organization and their interaction with the world (Klein, Kiesler, & Coughlin, 1961). Interestingly, this early definition relied heavily on nonverbal awareness and cues that can now be explained by the neural changes in the brain during human interactions (Eckman & Friesen, 1978).

Gendlin (1957) was the first to name the "felt experience" of this internal active experiencing of self and the environment. He described an early view of an experiential sense of self as a process of directed attention, trust in the natural healing capacity of humans, and a system of nonverbal, affective awareness of self-organization and new cognitive meanings in a system he calls "Focusing," which is still taught around the world (Gendlin, 1996). Affective neurobiology now challenges people to become aware of unconscious, autonomic brain functions, such as breathing and nonverbal behaviors, facial recognition, paralanguage, and other interactive aspects of interpersonal relationships related to emotional experiencing and attachment (Siegel, 2012).

TSM's entire clinical map is designed to help increase active experiencing inside the window of tolerance (Siegel, 1999) so that traumatized persons and groups can become more empowered in making psychologically healthy decisions for new and creative responses to trauma.

Active Therapist Interventions

A final element of the psychological definition of any experiential method of change is that it includes active therapist interventions. Therapist- or trauma-worker-initiated interventions target individual and communal experiences through increased awareness of active experiencing. These include directed attention, sensory and somatic awareness, imagination, enactment, and the expressive arts, along with the newer individualized trauma therapies in the West, like EMDR (Shapiro, 2012) and Somatic Re-experiencing (Levine and Frederick, 1997). Both of the latter experiential methods rely heavily on technique-driven interventions for quick and efficient changes in self-regulation, resource building, and conscious re-experiencing, but have not yet been translated into use outside of individual therapy settings. Research support for mindfulness-based practices show how powerful a simple act of spending 10 minutes a day in a meditative state can be (Siegel, 2007, 2010) and begin bridging Eastern and Western methods of active experiential interventions.

In the case of TSM, the TSIRA operationalizes clinical action intervention modules for use as a protocol for prevention, intervention, education, research, and training in trauma work (Hudgins, 2002; Hudgins & Toscani, 2013). This means that TSM has active therapist interventions that are divided into various steps guided by the clinical map, making each an intervention module directly targeted at a specific psychological function. TSM provides the base map of therapeutic and structural change and of experiential change modules that are operationalized for sustainable training and research in global health.

Classical Psychodrama

I want to personally thank Zerka T. Moreno (1969), my mentor, friend, and psychodrama teacher for her support of TSM as I learned the concepts and methods of classical psychodrama, the seminal method of action change developed by J.L. Moreno. I also want to thank Dale Richard Buchanan, Ph.D., TEP who directed the National Institute for Mental Health (NIMH) internship program at St. Elizabeth's Hospital on psychodrama, sociometry, and group psychotherapy during my year-long internship there (Buchanan, In Press). Three concepts integrated into the theoretical orientations of TSM are: 1) spontaneity and creativity, 2) role theory, and 3) surplus reality.

In his 1953 work, *Who Shall Survive?*, Moreno was prescient, predicting that only the spontaneous will survive. After his death, Zerka Moreno (2012) continued to develop and spread psychodrama worldwide, bringing together many cultures under the banner of spontaneity and creativity as curative for today's ills. As psychodrama continued to expand, she taught the concept of surplus reality, awakening interest in internal self-organization, and the interactive roles of self (Moreno, Blomkvist, and Rützel, 2000). The compilation of decades of her research is shared in a book by Moreno, Horvatin, and Shreiber (2006), showing the Morenos' early dedication to research to prove that the changes they saw in people, as they developed psychodrama, were true and replicable.

Wieser (2002, 2011) presents an ever-increasing body of research on the use and effectiveness of psychodrama across many settings – from education to therapy and from small groups to large, cultural issues. Stadler, Wieser, & Kirk (2016) demonstrate psychodrama's effectiveness across settings, populations, languages, and cultures. While some studies show the specific effects of psychodrama with different populations, there is research on trauma related improvement in mental health, such as addictions (Cox, 2013), Dissociative Identity Disorder (Altman, 2000; Leutz, 2000), and sexual offenders (Baim, 2013). Rezacian, Mazumdar, & Sen (1997) did a comparison study on depression and found that psychodrama was more effective than a standard talk therapy psychiatric group. On the other hand, Ragsdale, Cox, Finn, & Eisler (1996) found mixed results when studying a group of inpatients in a psychodrama-based program. As noted above, research studies on TSM specifically show effectiveness in both individual and group therapy, clinical treatment, and psycho-educational programs; results of additional research on structural interventions currently in place in China and Egypt will be available soon.

Spontaneity and Creativity Theory

Spontaneity and creativity theory is the life-blood of TSM. It is what truly embodies the model, drawing on the spirit of trauma healing across all cultural applications (Hudgins, 2015; 2013a). Corey (2013) states that classical psychodrama is unique in its goal of experiential change to increase spontaneity and creativity in order to develop new roles in the present moment. Spontaneity itself is defined as an adequate response to a new situation or a novel response to an old behavior, making it an ideal match to what is needed to counter traumatic experiences with new healing interpersonal experiences.

When trauma happens, survival modes of coping (such as fight, flight, or freeze) lock into both neurobiology and social roles, thus inhibiting the development of new, more spontaneous and creative actions in the present. Old behavior patterns, or "old neural firings," were not able to keep a catastrophe from happening. Therefore, the goal of classical psychodrama and TSM is to regain a sense of personal vitality and connection to others, called spontaneity and creativity, in order to make new narratives for the future. TSM takes this goal of achieving a state of psychological health and defines it further in terms of role theory, presenting the prescriptive roles of the TSIRA as the operationalized definition of spontaneity in action.

Role Theory

Blatner (2000, 2013b) describes the importance of role theory to the psychodramatic concept of healthy self-organization and reiterates Moreno's (1953) teachings that the self develops from and through the roles we enact. Simple role terms such as mother, father, aunt, uncle, teacher, doctor, cab driver, farmer, daughter, or son are easily understood to people who are not psychologically sophisticated. They are also easily understood across cultures and languages, though how these roles are defined in healthy functioning certainly varies by culture (Hudgins, 2015). However, using role theory helps people easily understand the impact of trauma at all levels of health care, from survival needs to post-trauma recovery and sustainability.

In TSM, role theory further delineates and, in fact, operationalizes the roles needed for healthy psychological functioning, the roles that are internalized from trauma, and the new and creative transformative roles that emerge from trauma repair. The TSIRA takes the more complex view of an experiential sense of self and simplifies it according to psychological functions through the three categories of the prescriptive, trauma-based, and transformative roles (Hudgins and Toscani, 2013; Toscani and Hudgins, 1995). This role definition of the self has made TSM highly applicable to trauma work around the globe, including natural disasters, family violence, torture, and trauma from war and resettlement, as well as for education, conflict resolution, and peace-building.

Surplus Reality

The third contribution of classical psychodrama that informs TSM is the concept of surplus reality. Moreno, Blomkvist, & Rützel (2000) describe surplus reality as the internal experience that goes on continuously in every person's body, mind, heart, and spirit. In psychodrama, this is expressed externally by concretizing the internal experience through roles, dialogues, dramas, and techniques of psychodrama. Making these experiences tangible is particularly useful for trauma survivors who often try to hide their internal chaos by externalizing their thoughts, feelings, defenses, and behaviors, so that they can view them from a place of observation and begin to make changes.

In TSM, it is the surplus reality of the actual brain processes that are concretized in clinical and therapeutic interventions. The TSM leader prepares the trauma survivor to go more deeply into the internal chaos of the past or present by building up the prescriptive roles that define spontaneity, as defined above. This then allows them to re-experience, safely and consciously, the memories, flashbacks, body memories, and intense emotions of PTSD in order to transform the old survival powers into new, healthy patterns of living.

The Therapeutic Spiral Model to Treat PTSD

TSM is now presented in its fullness as a clinical system of experiential change through the description of the TSIRA, which guides all interventions with trauma, whether therapeutic or communal. TSM began in 1992 as a model of clinically-modified psychodrama that focused specifically on small groups of trauma survivors diagnosed with complex PTSD, Dissociative Identity Disorder, and Borderline Personality Disorder. However, the TSI global initiatives described below also show how well this clinical map can guide change in education, social, and even political arenas, broadening its application to meet the new findings in neurobiology that show there is a social brain.

The TSIRA: The clinical map of experiential change

TSM's clinical map, the TSIRA, was conceived and defined as a guide for experiential interventions and garnered from years of work with people experiencing the symptoms and effects of PTSD (Toscani and Hudgins, 1995). Through observation of therapeutic changes, this role atom was envisaged as an intrapsychic role diagram of a trauma survivor's self-organization. The roles that presented were in continual interaction, flux, ascendancy, and descendancy, much like what is now known about interactive neuronal firings during interpersonal interaction. As the years and the work progressed, the TSIRA became a comprehensive working system that is inclusive and multi-dimensional. Because of its essential flexibility, it is a clinical map that is broad but specific enough to accept overlays and techniques from other psychological and therapeutic modalities. Its use has been expanded to become a template for multi-cultural work with traumatized individuals, groups, and cultures.

In the previous literature on TSM, the main focus has been on the specific roles and action interventions that make up the TSIRA for use in psychodrama, drama therapy, and other expressive arts therapies (Hudgins and Toscani, 2013). In order to explain its roots in psychological methodology, it is important to focus on the psychological function of each of the role categories that define the TSIRA through the use of clinical and structural global initiative examples.

Prescriptive Roles of TSM: A State of Spontaneous Learning

Hermann (1992) first detailed therapy models for trauma, showing they all have stages of self-regulation and strength building, trauma work and repair, and integration and meaning-making. The TSIRA starts out with prescriptive roles, roles that a psychologist or trauma worker deems necessary for self-regulation and resource installation, just as a physician prescribes medicines that are needed to restore physical balance (Blatner, 2013a). A TSM leader then guides the protagonist, client, or group to use these prescriptive roles to increase observation, resilience, and safety, thus establishing a state of spontaneous learning.

Observation: The Observing Ego Role

The first psychological function that the TSIRA focuses on is increasing conscious awareness of what is actually being experienced in the moment so that trauma responses can be seen and hopefully changed. Therefore, the very first role that is enacted in any setting using the TSIRA is that of the internal observing ego (OE), a necessary developmental role for psychological awareness and active experiencing in all situations. In TSM terms, the OE role holds the psychological function of accurately and neutrally seeing and labeling behavior in the here-and-now to increase conscious awareness.

This might appear to be a simple function, but a trauma survivor's internal structures are filled with negative messages, horrific images, unmanaged affect, and chaotic or non-existent relationships. Therefore, most traumatized persons and groups of any size actually find it difficult to maintain an accurate, non-judgmental, and neutral record of what is happening at a behavioral and interpersonal level. As this role develops internally, the client or group is then able to sustain an emotional distance and neutrality (not dissociation) that is necessary before any real change can take effect.

In the beginning of TSM in the U.S., in individual and small group therapy, the role of the Observing Ego was developed through the simple use of inspirational cards that people pick that have words or pictures on them to help provide the strength to see themselves in a neutral way. In later experiences, I found that this role can also be held by an external documentarian on a large project, essentially an OE of the group. This evaluator helps clients, students, or community workers to internalize the role through interpersonal interaction (Hudgins, Culbertson, & Hug, 2009). Additionally, the OE can play a role in a theater performance or other communal activity dedicated to trauma repair (Rivers, 2015)

In 2002, TSI worked extensively in Ivory Park, South Africa with a non-profit organization (NGO) called "ACTING THRU UKUBUYISELWA." *Ukubuyiselwa* is a Zulu word that means to gain back your dignity. The importance of the OE role, this time to a culture, became immediately obvious in this racially mixed group of African tribal leaders, immigrant social workers, and Western TSI team members. The TSI trainer chose not to use American inspirational cards, which group members could not afford to purchase or have reproduced by local funding. Instead, participants drew their own OE roles in the dirt with sticks outside the venue. After drawing their images, a tribal leader spontaneously jumped onto a bench, saying that she was the village's scout. The group could see that she was looking out over the Savannah watching for danger, thereby making herself the OE for her community. She called out information, in her own tribal language, about what she saw. When it became obvious, nonverbally, that she was saying it was safe, the TSI trainer asked her to translate the last words, which were: "It is safe. The animals are quiet. Everyone can go to sleep". The group responded with cheers and others began to enact their images as well, demonstrating a wealth of creative resources many Westerners might have thought impossible under such conditions of poverty and lack of health care.

Restoration: Strength Roles

The next psychological function of the prescriptive, clinical roles of the TSIRA is to install and instill roles of internal, interpersonal, and transpersonal strengths. Since by nature, trauma, overwhelms a person's coping ability, trauma survivors are in desperate need of having their internal strengths rebuilt as soon as possible. Thus, the TSIRA places an immediate emphasis on calling up courage, determination, resilience, and other internal strengths by creating experiences in which people can reclaim their dignity and compassion through clinically modified psychodramatic methods of change.

In addition to personal strengths, interpersonal supports must be established for trauma survivors to feel positive connections to others, to organizations, and to governments that support their healthy psychological functioning. Important, new experiences that encourage brain plasticity can only be accomplished when supportive roles are present to do so. The restorative roles of the TSIRA reinforce positive attachments and help prevent an ever-widening epidemic of global PTSD by changing interpersonal interactions.

In Taiwan, the first Asian culture in which TSM was taught and practiced, I had an on-going discussion with a local psychologist about how to internalize personal and interpersonal strengths. This conversation was, in short, an East-West dialogue of cultural applicability. The Circle of

Strengths, a clinical safety action structure (Cox, 2001) which often begins a TSM workshop with colored scarves representing personal strengths, was challenged as being too individually centered. Instead, Lai Nien-hwa, Ph.D, TEP suggested a more culturally sensitive method in which people pick up scarves to represent another person's strength and to mirror the strengths back to them, thereby creating an interpersonal connection. TSM's emphasis of internalizing cultural/communal support follows the recommendation of affective neuroscience, showing that new experiences reinforce the restorative roles through positive interpersonal interactions.

For many people and societies, a transpersonal strength is either the first or the last one they call on during times of crisis, chaos, and the stress that creates PTSD. Since PTSD is defined as something that overwhelms the coping strategies of humans, TSM maintains that there is a need for resourcing through spiritual aspects of life. The TSIRA includes a transpersonal strength that can include all religions, but can also be described simply as something beyond one human being or group, such as a nature or art. It can also be culturally specific where people share stories of what brings them strength as a family, a group, a country, or a culture.

A poignant example happened in 1996 while training refugee counselors at the New South Wales Service for the Treatment and Rehabilitation of Torture and Trauma Survivors (STARTTS) in Sydney, Australia. The embodiment of the role of Allah as a transpersonal support for a Muslim Bosnian woman became a teaching and learning moment for this multi-cultural training group. As she could barely say the name of her God, much less pick someone to enact Allah in a group, the TSI trainer asked her what qualities her God brought to help her through dark times. By removing the focus from Allah per se, she was able to experience an overall felt sense of calm knowing that the new focus relieved anxiety and gave her strength. When asked to choose someone in the group who could represent that quality, she chose a man from Cambodia who, interestingly, was a Buddhist. Throughout the telling and enactment of a traumatic, brutal scene of ethnic genocide, her transpersonal strength sat quietly and radiated a knowing love to which she looked, and from which she took strength. This role superseded all religious, cultural, familial, and personal boundaries and limitations, and thus became a touchstone for everyone throughout the training from 1996-2000.

Containment: Body Double, Containing double, and Manager of Defenses Roles

The third psychological function of the prescriptive roles focuses on providing self-regulation and containment of dissociation, emotional volatility, and the rigid defenses that always follow trauma. The TSIRA describes three roles that are clinical action intervention modules of containment: the body double (BD) (Hudgins and Ciotola, 2003), the containing double (CD) (Toscani and Hudgins, 1993), and the manager of defenses (MD) (Toscani and Hudgins, 1995). Together these three roles help create a bridge from the immobility of destructive behaviors that are often a response to trauma to the spontaneity and creativity that is the goal of all TSM intervention modules.

The BD was first developed when working in homogeneous clinical groups of Western women who had been sexually abused and who were suffering with long-term eating disorders. The BD was created by Burden and Ciotola (2002) to become an inner voice that is dedicated to self-soothing, self-regulation, and here-and-now awareness of bodily cues and nonverbal behaviors. The BD picks up on autonomic experiences such as facial expressions, breathing, and proprioception to help people with a traumatized brain begin to self-modulate their unconscious responses to trauma. The BD has become a mainstay to prevent dissociation, to stabilize, and to help form a spontaneous and creative self-organization, even under the most acute or chronic states of PTSD. It has been clinically hypothesized as bringing the amygdala online so that it can learn from positive experiences and repair the smart vagus (Carnabucci and Ciotola, 2013; Hudgins, 2008).

Another variation of the psychodramatic double, the CD (Toscani and Hudgins, 1993), developed as the second prescriptive role after the OE for the purpose of providing safety for those who are caught in the throes of PTSD. It has become the foundation of all adaptations and expansions of TSM over the 25 years of its development from a model of therapy to a system of structural change around the world (Hudgins and Toscani, 2013). The CD has been compared to the corpus callosum, which connects the right and left hemispheres of the brain, because its clinical goal is to balance thinking and feeling, which are generally left and right brain functions. To do this, the CD has a three-part structure: to establish safety by containing affect (hold and steady), to verbalize the present confusion and gain some awareness (anchor or ground), and to connect with the broader, interpersonal world and promote safe and rational action (lead forward).

To honor the original participants, I give the following example from 1992 in which the CD first developed clinically in a client group at the Psychodrama Theatre of Protection in Black Earth, Wisconsin. In a TSM drama, while the protagonist was telling her story of childhood abuse, a TSI team member saw that another group member was beginning to dissociate and regress. This group member had been triggered into her own childhood trauma of being locked in a refrigerator. The terror was palpable and the team member stayed with her using "I" statements to increase her cognitive functions, since she was in a feeling regression: "I am scared and I can still breathe. I can breathe and calm myself. I can lift my eyes slowly and see that I'm not alone; I'm not in the refrigerator but in a drama with so-and-so. I can breathe and witness her work." Eventually, the panicked breathing and terror subsided and the team member helped lead this client back to the drama that was unfolding, still using "I" statements. The director seamlessly wove the two dramas together, giving the group member who had been "in the refrigerator" a supportive companion role with the original protagonist. In processing the drama afterwards, the TSI team knew that a new kind of double had emerged, one which was necessary for containment, safety, and small forward action, affirming that change can happen. This role was called the containing double and henceforth was prescribed for every drama that would include trauma.

Additionally, the CD has been a major crossover experiential intervention in settings other than therapy groups. The motto of a TSI collaboration with the University of Virginia's Foundation for the Humanities was, "Out of the therapy office and into the streets." Here, the CD was used in combination with literature, poetry, and public speaking as a bridge to the community to support first responders to the U.S. Pentagon crash in 2001 (Hudgins, Culbertson, & Hug, 2009). Rivers (2015) even uses the CD as part of theatre performances in Egypt that directly target the social and political traumas that are both historical and current in the Middle East.

The final clinical intervention module of the TSIRA that fulfills the psychological function of containment is the MD. The defenses of fight, flight, or freeze are neurobiologically programmed to operate in the face of trauma, and these responses then become internalized into rigid defense structures and trauma-based roles. Thus, before the trauma worker can move to address the strong defenses that surround trauma in any situation, the role of a manager must be established.

A group of Protestants and Catholics in Derry, Northern Ireland had come together in 2006 for a TSM residential training on conflict resolution with the non-profit organization from Belfast, Breaking the Silence. As soon as some of the Catholics walked into the church that was the venue for the workshop, several people immediately experienced PTSD body memories and flashbacks from having been there when the church was bombed by Protestants a few years before. Putting in CDs for individuals still left many reeling from the bombardment of past experience, while interpersonal suspicion, projections, and avoidance began to swirl around the room. It became clear the MD was needed.

The concretization of an MD role was necessary to hold the triggers that were going off among members of this committed but fragile group of collaborators from different sides of the Troubles. Many of the normal roles that people create in TSM dramas to manage defenses (e.g., solders, police, organized authority) were immediately discarded because they were contaminated by group members' real experiences of corruption, betrayal, and violence. So the TSM leader asked the group, "If we can't meet safely in this room, where can we meet? In TSM psychodrama we can set the scene anywhere we need it to be." Helping people warm up to their spontaneity through the surplus reality of imagination led the group to the enactment of a neighborhood pub where people could have a pint, watch sports, and chat in a friendly environment. Here in the less-charged atmosphere of a metaphorical space, the director also established a special containment circle that was designated as the MD, into which people could name and place a scarf to label their triggered defenses. Thus, their survival skills would still be available if needed, but they could come into this "Peace Building Pub" with more trust and hope in the moment.

Defenses: Survival, Control, and Compensation

The TSIRA clearly names the defenses that arise at the time of trauma and thereafter. Survival states are experienced and then repeated so they become rigid, engrained roles in the self-organization of a trauma survivor and in the neurobiology of their brain. This chapter briefly examines the three psychological functions of various defenses that surround trauma within a taxonomy that was derived from decades of clinical experience worldwide.

Survival

While the brain seems to have three main survival strategies of fight, flight, or freeze at the time of trauma, the psychological defenses that are used can be further delineated. However, if the person cannot fight overwhelming odds during a traumatic experience (e.g., natural disaster, entrenched oppression), the survivor will naturally use regression, splitting, and even multiple states of consciousness to flee the trauma internally and interpersonally. If even those defenses are not enough, the survivor will rely on denial and dissociation as a freeze response. While the brain and the mind are quite adaptive to using these survival defenses at the actual time of trauma and during acute post-trauma response, they can become embedded in the self-organization and then appear automatically long after they are no longer needed. In the case of structural violence and oppression, these defenses may simply become a way of life in order to survive.

Control

This second psychological function of defenses comes into play when the survival defenses are no longer working, so the trauma survivor needs to turn to a more complex set of behaviors to hold back the frightening PTSD symptoms of body memories, sensory flashbacks, intense feelings, and images of the past. In this case, trauma survivors use obsessions, compulsions, addictions, and eating disorders to attempt to control these lingering impacts of trauma, further complicating the picture of repair in the present.

Compensation/Coping

The final psychological function of the TSIRA's categorization of defenses is named compensation and coping because these roles generally reflect a higher order of functioning (although they are still dysfunctional at times). Some roles that help people cope with trauma are those of people-pleasing, a need for extreme control, or a necessary submission to oppressive authority, often reflecting cultural norms and nuances.

Trauma-Based Roles: Internalization of Experience

The second category of roles in the TSIRA is trauma-based roles, and they represent the internalization of victim, perpetrator, and abandoning authority arising from any traumatic experience, whether individual or societal. The TSIRA's addition of the abandoning authority role to the picture of a trauma survivor's psychological functioning is a unique contribution to the understanding of trauma responses. Most systems of trauma look at the internalization of the victim and perpetrator experiences, but do not pay attention to the fact that trauma can only happen when an authority abandons their role to stop abuse, neglect, or oppression. While this is first an interpersonal role that was originally absent, the abandonment becomes internalized through destructive behaviors or through failing to acknowledge on-going traumatic situations or their aftermath. This also happens when a group collectively denies or disregards the reality of organized and oppressive violence (e.g., during ethnic cleansing and refugee displacement).

Communication of Trauma: The Victim Role

In the TSIRA, the main psychological function of the victim role is to hold and communicate the experience of what actually happened during trauma. Right brain functions communicate fragmented body memories and flashbacks that hold important information about both context and details of actual neglect, abuse, or violence. The limbic system expresses the unprocessed, often intense and dissociated feelings of horror, terror, rage, grief, and despair that could not be experienced at the time of trauma. The clinical goal of conscious re-experiencing of the victim role is to move it from a static state of self-organization to the role of the wounded child who can now create a narrative of what happened.

TSM has the power to bring together human rights, racial equality, and the healing of victimization. During a TSM drama enacted on the last day of training at the previously-mentioned global initiative in South Africa, two women, one an African tribal leader and one a Caucasian Australian immigrant, joined together to heal the wounds of being sexually abused at eight years old. For the first time in this mixed race group, tribal leaders, social workers, and TSI team members saw the two protagonists pick people for the roles of restoration across races. Banding together as women whose human rights had been violated, they jointly decided to bring their perpetrators to justice by concretizing a tribunal similar to Mandela's Truth and Reconciliation Commission (1996). Playing the role of judge, each protagonist expressed her own sentencing to right the wrongs done by their individual perpetrators and by society. It was interesting to note that neither of these women took the role of perpetrator in response, but instead demonstrated the role of an appropriate authority, reflecting the cultural changes that Nelson Mandela had brought to South Africa.

Keeping Trauma Unconscious: The Perpetrator Role

The psychological function of keeping the trauma unconscious and at bay is at the core of the persistence of the perpetrator role. As many of the survival defenses demonstrate, identifying with the role of perpetrator can feel powerful and life-saving following trauma. In fact, individuals, groups, societies, and even cultures can live in a chronic state of perpetration, disguising their own feelings of victimization and fear. Learning to accept this role as part of self-organization or a cultural norm is often difficult but necessary in order to fully understand the impact of traumatic situations around the world.

An interesting use of the perpetrator role emerged during the TSI global initiative to provide resources to the 3rd Military Division of the Chinese Army in Chengdu, China following the 2008 earthquake. Twelve Chinese psychologists trained in TSM and I formed a TSI team and donated six weeks of our time to prevent secondary PTSD in the first responders, including Army officers, physicians, psychologists, social workers, educators, and volunteers. In the case of such a natural disaster, the perpetrator becomes Nature or Mother Earth, which is totally out of control and creates apparent meaningless violence.

Identification of Lack of Safety: Abandoning Authority

The psychological function of the abandoning authority role in the TSIRA is to provide trauma survivors with information about the original disruption in attachment and the fact that, in their past experiences, they were fully abandoned to neglect or violence. In other cases, abandonment and the lack of help for even basic necessities continue to play out in current lives, particularly for those ravaged by war or turned away from safe harbors. This missing role was identified early in the development of the TSIRA when the original TSI training group noticed that many clients could not mobilize new and creative responses, even when resourced by the prescriptive roles. During small, residential workshops, clients' recounted stories of sexual abuse, and the TSI leaders repeatedly saw the absence of any external authority to stop the abuse. This led to a clinical emphasis on developing the function of the appropriate authority (which is distinct from a single strength as it is a role cluster of many positive roles, as seen below in the transformative roles).

The TSM Trauma Triangle

The TSM trauma triangle deserves attention because it is a clinical action structure that weaves together the trauma-based roles and represents a closed circuit of energy embedded in the self-organization and neurobiology of those who have survived cruelty or trauma. The three trauma-based roles—victim, perpetrator, and abandoning authority—while discreet in their meanings and psychological functions, are collaborative in trapping a trauma survivor into a destructive cycle of repetition at all levels of society and culture. Together these interactions create an often subtle web that can be hard to identify and pinpoint because these roles are fluid and changeable. The TSM trauma triangle is used as a clinical action intervention module to identify old patterns of behaviors while providing role development for new, spontaneous, and creative actions of personal and group authority.

In 2008, we presented this concept to the student advisors at Hua Qiao University in Quangzhou, China, where I have been helping to build their first mental health center from 2004 to the present. The TSI team created a triangle made of scarves on the floor in a large auditorium space; each corner of the triangle was designated as one trauma-based role and was held by a team member. The victim role position was styled as fearful and sad, a place of immobilization; the perpetrator was violent and angry with triggered, unmoderated mobilization; the abandoning authority was the "not there" spot – dreaming, blissed out, blind, and deaf, relying on survival defenses.

Undergraduate students were then directed to choose the role they most identify with when they find themselves in a difficult situation doing peer counseling at their university. As each participant went to the place of the marked role, they were directed to stay in that role and give voice to it by calling out, "I feel like a failure. I hate myself! I hate that teacher. He doesn't like me. No one cares. I might as well give up." Spontaneously, for most participants, after a few moments, the roles shifted, and they identified the next step of their trauma pattern (e.g., going from perpetrator position to abandoning authority). As director of this 250-person student training, I asked people to move about and find their own insight and feelings, which they then shared with another person.

This action example has been replicated in many settings and has yielded much insight and useful information for trauma workers by showing clearly that, while the roles themselves are rigid, the triangle energy is not static. This awareness allows for the eventual movement out of this closed circuit of energy, with a follow-up exercise directing participants to use one or more of the prescriptive roles to help break into the destructive pattern. The role that often emerges to rescue or break the pattern is the appropriate authority that holds the clarity (observation), strength, and support (containment) of the prescriptive roles.

Transformative Roles

As a result of the interaction of the prescriptive and the trauma-based roles, the transformative roles of the TSIRA naturally develop. From early clinical experiences with PTSD, the transformative roles emerged to implement the psychological functions of autonomy, connection, and integration for developmental trauma repair. These roles represent the third stage of all good trauma work in which the emphasis is on stable self-organization, healthy attachments, and new narrative labels to guide future spontaneous and creative actions.

Autonomy: The Sleeping-Awakening Child

The first psychological function of the transformative roles is to build autonomy to foster a stable self-organization and the ability to make integrated decisions in the here-and-now. While there are generic roles of the manager of healthy functioning and the change agent, a unique role called the sleeping-awakening child emerged spontaneously in a drama, which initiated TSM's early development (Hudgins and Kiesler, 1987). This role is said to hold intact a person's innate potential, creativity, and gifts at the time of birth, which stay protected without dissociation and other necessary defenses until they can be reclaimed once safety is established.

Connection: The Good-Enough Roles

When trauma happens, it always causes disruptions in attachment to others, both personally and collectively. For full symptom repair of PTSD, interpersonal roles of safety, nurturing, and boundary setting must become internalized as well as externalized. In a therapeutic drama, clients easily see the need for a good-enough parent who can listen, support, contain, and guide self-organization in an uncertain world. At the cultural level, one often seeks a good-enough government to support post-trauma repair in the form of both humanitarian aid and changes in policy.

As noted, since 2008, I have been training the first generation of Chinese psychologists at Hua Qiao University in Quangzhou, China. Here, university counselors learn how to provide the reparative good-enough mother and father roles to students who are often far from home and in a new environment. In many cases, receiving this role gives students their first experience of an authority figure who is not demanding perfection, nor physically abusive, nor attempting to motivate them through fear. It is clear that this good-enough connection to a safe attachment figure allows students to settle into university life and connect with others more easily.

Integration: Appropriate and Ultimate Authority Roles

The final psychological function of the transformative roles is to integrate all that has come before in TSM initiatives in prevention, intervention, and training. As neurobiological research shows, it is only when the unprocessed trauma is consciously experienced and expressed that the neural firings associated with the trauma can be integrated into a new narrative. There are two roles that developed in this area: the appropriate and ultimate authority roles.

The Appropriate Authority Role

The appropriate authority role has been mentioned above in contradistinction to the abandoning authority (the role that was absent when trauma happened). Its psychological function is to stand up to a traumatic situation and stop the neglect or abuse, whether on behalf of an individual or a culture. When the appropriate authority appears, it helps to transform worthlessness into self-worth with the subsequent changes in self-sabotaging behavior at all levels. In clinical cases, the appropriate authority can appear as an interpersonal or internal rescuer, can have a profound and lasting effect on the self-organization of the protagonist to correct the trauma picture, and can transform the chaos into a cohesive story. In other initiatives, the appropriate authority comes from an external situation, in which a structural intervention stops oppression at social, political, and cultural levels.

For example, in a particular TSM drama with trauma survivors in Australia, the stage was filled with roles that were fighting, rescuing, and arguing, and the protagonist was in a child role being nurtured and protected in the arms of her good-enough mother. After making a safe space for the wounded child role, the person playing the role of the mother suddenly stood up and declared that she had seen enough; she would correct what she should have done years previously. She took charge and, in righteous rage, called a halt to the abuse. She then addressed her child, apologizing for what she wasn't able to do 20 years earlier. At that moment, the protagonist stood up, clasped the hand of this appropriate authority, and faced her abusers herself. With her transformed mother beside her, she spoke with self-confidence and righteous anger, her internal psychological structure having changed from a victim mentality to one of her own personal authority.

As noted here and in the example from South Africa, the appropriate authority does not seek vengeance, but justice, not punishment, but balance. As people, groups, societies, and cultures gain a corrected experience of an appropriate authority, they can become authors of their own script, not dependent on previous fears nor submerged in self-sabotaging behaviors.

The Ultimate Authority Role

With the appropriate authority integrated, there is just one more small, yet profound step to the final transformative role – the ultimate authority. In this role, individuals, families, groups, and cultures rise from their own dysfunction and operate from more than their personal power – they operate from a transformative role that connects directly to a transpersonal strength or belief. The ultimate authority is driven from a teleological perspective. It is not propelled from personal initiative alone, but operates from a collective purpose and is dedicated to a comprehensive plan. When this role is internalized into self-organization or into an organized system, all feel less anxiety regarding their objectives and more centered in their actions. Identity and self-worth are no longer tied to personal or societal accomplishment, but are subsumed into an overarching principle. Integrating this role is ideal for therapists, health care workers, educators, community workers, and others whose work outcomes depend on factors beyond their control. Through this role, persons and governments assume responsibility for themselves, for others, and even for the condition of the world while maintaining a sense of balance and equanimity.

In New Zealand, a TSI leader worked with a group of therapists and community workers whose clients had experienced terrible sexual abuse, including cult and international pedophile ring-related abuse. Most of the therapists were themselves sexual abuse survivors and were highly committed to making a difference. The protagonist for a drama, which was about the global nature of the abuse, explained that she had always felt isolated and alone in her work. Her identity was tied closely to a martyr complex, and she was angry, even enraged, at the apparent lack of commitment, as she saw it, from other trauma workers, thus creating a palpable divide in the group.

During a TSM drama, she asked which group members would be committed to the overwhelming task of confronting the global rings of abuse. This was acknowledged as a very profound and powerful question, requiring a thoughtful, sincere, and balanced answer from each participant. After hearing their responses, she calmly declared that if anyone wanted to join her, she would welcome them. She also stated plainly that she no longer had any rancor toward those who did not want to do this dangerous work. She understood that for her to commit to a global mission was her choice, it was not foisted upon her to take up by herself. Her psychological structure had been transformed from an angry isolate identifying with the victim to an active advocate and aide. Follow-up reports found her committed to her work with a peace she had not experienced before – a straightforward example of taking on the mantle of the ultimate authority.

A cultural example of the ultimate authority comes from the TSI initiative in Chengdu, China following the earthquake of 2008. While working with the army of first responders, the TSI trainer and Chinese psychologists saw in action how the Communist government of China became an ultimate authority by bringing in all resources to provide immediate assistance to persons displaced by the earthquake. While this might appear to be the appropriate authority role, it took on an ultimate authority quality. The first responders, as well as the government itself, were able to transcend cultural and ideological differences in the perception of PTSD as an individual diagnosis. Instead, they saw its cause as a natural disaster and responded with food, water, shelter, and humanitarian aid. They also tended to the psychological state of the first responders. Without obstruction, they addressed the on-going demand for integrating orphans and other displaced family members into new schools and homes.

Conclusion

Examples throughout this chapter show that Therapeutic Spiral International (TSI) is a small organization that has had larger-in-results leverage. In 1992, the Therapeutic Spiral Model (TSM) was first developed as a system of experiential psychotherapy, using clinically modified psychodrama to treat sexual abuse survivors, who in many cases were diagnosed with complex PTSD, Borderline Personality Disorder, or Dissociative Identity Disorder. Group therapy vignettes demonstrate the power of TSM as it evolved in the Western world based on clinical wisdom a few years before the Rausch et al. (1996) study showed the impact of trauma on the neurobiology of the brain. Many of the prescriptive roles of the TSIRA and active intervention modules emerged directly from observing sexual abuse survivors' needs for self-soothing, contained expression of intense dissociated affect, and increased meaning making. Later, the abandoning authority was added as a unique contribution to trauma work in the global community. Finally, the transformative roles were created as TSI leaders helped clients move from surviving trauma to thriving in their lives.

As advances in neurobiology point to the existence of the neuroplastic social brain that can change through positive interpersonal experiences, TSM becomes even more relevant to all areas of trauma work and global health. Being an experiential method of change, TSM is embedded in actively experiencing the internalization of new interpersonal roles that provide for refinement of self-organization following trauma, and also reaches into structural interventions in prevention, education, conflict resolution, and peace-building. Prevention of PTSD is shown in the collaborative project with the University of Virginia using TSM and the humanities following 9/11. Creative ways to reach conflict resolution are seen in Derry, Ireland where TSM united persons from both sides of the Troubles through the use of metaphors and active experiencing of alternative realities. The project to prevent PTSD in first responders following the Chengdu earthquake details how TSM has expanded into global initiatives from a model of experiential psychotherapy.

TSI has trained mental health professionals in 30 countries over the past 25 years through the International Certification Training Program in Trauma Therapy, which includes theory, practice in a setting of your choice, and supervision to apply the TSIRA and to use the active therapist interventions for both therapeutic and structural interventions. Certification requires four levels of competency: 1) Trained auxiliary ego, 2) Assistant leader, 3) Team leader, and 4) TSI trainer (Hudgins, 2013b). There are currently over 1000 people trained in at least one of these levels – there are TSI Trainers in Australia, Bali, Canada, China, Egypt, England, Germany, South Africa, Taiwan, and the U.S.

TSM trained professionals, including myself, have produced a large body of published works which support sustainability through the written word. In addition to writings noted throughout, Alers (2008, 2013, 2014) writes about the use of TSM with underserved populations in South Africa. She also developed a course at the University of the Witwatersrand, Johannesburg, following several TSM workshops in Ivory Park. Cossa (personal communication. March, 2016) describes a program for youth in Bali that integrates TSM with classical psychodrama and drama therapy.

Currently, sustainability in China is being directly addressed by professors and scholars at Hua Qiao University in Quanzhou, China, who submitted a proposal for approval of the TSI International Certification Program to the government's Psychodrama Association in Fujian Province. With this approval, they will use their TSM training to meet some of the requirements of this governmental, nation-wide regulating body, and hope to increase the number of indigenously trained TSI trainers and team leaders every year.

TSI's efforts in China speak most effectively to the power of TSM to bridge the gap between Eastern and Western ways of thinking while presenting post-traumatic stress as more than an individual diagnosis. Using TSM to educate student advisors and psychologists at Hua Qiao University in Quanzhou, I found that individuals, families, and the culture itself is still impacted by the effects of the Cultural Revolution. Symptoms of PTSD are rampant, but are often identified as depression and lack of motivation.

The most profound TSM program of sustainability to date was created by Ben Rivers, a Registered Drama Therapist and graduate of the TSI International Certification in Trauma Therapy. Rivers not only utilizes TSM in therapeutic settings, but also reports on its use as a structural intervention in a TSI Diploma Program in TSM in Cairo, Egypt. Since 2012, Rivers has worked extensively in Egypt, forming partnerships between TSI and a number of local institutes, organizations, and associations (e.g., the Studio Emad Eddin Foundation, Orient Productions, and the Egyptian Association for Group Therapies & Processes). The program, now in its final year, offers training in TSM, psychodramatic group work, and somatic approaches to trauma healing and psychotherapy. Fourteen Egyptian and Lebanese practitioners from the fields of psychiatry, psychotherapy, education, and community work, apply TSM in a range of settings including hospitals, community centers, psychiatric clinics, and private practice. Under Rivers' direction, trainees also participate in TSM teams to work with communities impacted by state violence and forced displacement, including Syrian refugees and other groups.

Previous to his work in Egypt, Rivers worked in the West Bank as an applied theatre practitioner with The Freedom Theatre, a Palestinian cultural organization based in the Jenin Refugee Camp. Collective trauma in Palestine occurs within the context of Israel's ongoing military occupation, settler colonialism, and apartheid policies (Veronese, Fiore, Castiglioni, Kawaja, and Said, 2013; White et al., 2014). Therefore, a biomedical approach to trauma, with its de-politicized emphasis on individual pathology, was deemed an inappropriate paradigm for TSI programs. Instead, Rivers' curricula take into account the social and political determinants that underpin collectively held experiences of hardship, oppression, and adversity. Throughout these programs, prescriptive roles emerged that pay tribute to the importance of familial bonds, social networks, and the greater struggle for a sustainable peace grounded in principles of freedom, justice, and equality. Social relations and coherent meaning systems, recognized as protective factors against the development of trauma (Veronese, et al., 2013), are clearly apparent and then elaborated as personal, interpersonal, and transpersonal strengths. For a full description of the depth and breadth of Rivers' ongoing work, readers may visit the Facebook page of Dawar for Arts and Development: www.facebook.com/DawarEgypt.

Finally, I want to thank the many people who have donated their time to the early efforts of TSM as a clinical method of experiential psychotherapy, as well as to the structural interventions mentioned above. First and foremost is Francesca Toscani, M.Ed., TEP, who is both the original co-developer of TSM and an editor for this chapter. She is joined by Mimi Cox, LSCW, TEP and Cathy Wilson, RN, MSN, CP, as the first TSI team to take TSM globally and expand its application beyond sexual abuse. Additionally, Vivyan Alers in South Africa, Professor Zhao Bingjie at Hua Qiao University, and Professor Zhao Shulan in Chongqing are recognized for their work in developing countries. Most recently, Scott Giacomucci, LSW, CTTS, CET II has joined the team, bringing his knowledge of brain neurobiology and trauma to the mix. Most of all, I thank the many people touched by TSM's experiential healing for sharing their stories.

References

Alers V.M. (2008). Proposing the social atom of occupational therapy: Dealing with trauma as part of an integrated inclusive intervention. *South African Journal of Occupational Therapy, 38*(3), 3 – 10.

Alers, V.M. (2013). The therapeutic spiral model perspective from South Africa—The rainbow nation. In K. Hudgins & F. Toscani (Eds.), *Healing world trauma with the therapeutic spiral model* (pp. 285-300). London: Jessica Kingsley Publishers.

Alers, V.M. & Crouch, R. (2014). Trauma and its effects on children, adolescents and adults. *Occupational Therapy in Psychiatry and Mental Health,* 337-355. doi:10.1002/9781118913536.ch2.

American Board of Examiners in Psychodrama, Sociometry, and Group Psychotherapy approved training programs: Training program resource. Retrieved from. https://www.uclartsandhealing.net/view_trainingprogram.aspx?rid=15.

American Psychiatric Association (1980). *Diagnostic and statistical manual of mental disorders,* (3rd ed.). Washington, DC: Author.

American Psychiatric Association (2013). *Diagnostic and statistical manual of mental disorders,* (5th ed.). Washington, DC: Author.

Altman, K. P. (2000). Psychodramatic treatment of dissociative identity disorder. In P. F. Kellerman & M. K. Hudgins (Eds.), *Psychodrama with trauma survivors: Acting out your pain* (pp. 176-186). Philadelphia: Jessica Kingsley Publishers.

Atwoli, L., Stein, D. J., Koenen, K. C., & McLaughlin, K. A. (2015). Epidemiology of posttraumatic stress disorder. *Current Opinion in Psychiatry, 28*(4), 307-311. doi:10.1097/yco.0000000000000167.

Badenoch, B. (2008). *Being a brain-wise therapist: A practical guide to interpersonal neurobiology.* New York: W.W. Norton and Company.

Baim, C. (2013). Footsteps on the moon: Using therapeutic spiral model concepts with offenders who have unresolved trauma. In K. Hudgins & F. (Ed.), *Healing world trauma with the therapeutic spiral model* (pp.317-332). London: Jessica Kingsley Publishers.

Blatner, A. (2000). *Foundations of psychodrama: History, theory, and practice.* New York: Springer Publishing Company.

Blatner, A. (2013a). Forward: Therapeutic spiral model as a type of psychotherapeutic "heart surgery". In K. Hudgins & F. Toscani (Eds.), *Healing world trauma with the therapeutic spiral model* (pp.9-14). London: Jessica Kingsley Publishers.

Blatner, A. (2013b). Psychodrama: Beyond psychotherapy (Psikodrama: Psikoterapinin Otesi) *International Group Psychotherapies and Psychodrama E-Journal, 1*(1), 8-10. http://www.istpsikodrama.com.tr/mainpage/.

Buchanan, D.R. (In Press). Forty years of psychodrama training at St. Elizabeths Hospital. In *Journal of Psychodrama, Sociometry and Group Psychotherapy.*

Burden, K. & Ciotola, L. (2002). The body double: An advanced clinical action intervention module in the therapeutic spiral model to treat trauma. Retrieved from www.vsjournals.de/pdf/body-offener-beitrag-032007.pdf Accessed on September, 2016.

Carnabucci, K. & Fullin, K. (2013). Two programs: The therapeutic spiral model in domestic violence work with perpetrators and survivors. In K. Hudgins & F. Toscani (Eds.), *Healing world trauma with the therapeutic spiral model* (pp. 317-332). London: Jessica Kingsley Publishers.

Carnabucci, K., & Ciotola, L. (2013). *Healing eating disorders with psychodrama and other action methods: Beyond the silence and the fury.* London: Jessica Kingsley Publishers.

Chimera, C. (2002). The yellow brick road. In A. Bannister & A. Huntington (Eds.), *Communicating with children and adolescents: Action for change* (pp. 175-190). London: Jessica Kingsley Publishers.

Chimera, C., (2013). Seeing the wizard: The therapeutic spiral model to work with traumatised families. In K. Hudgins & F. Toscani (Eds.), *Healing world trauma with the therapeutic spiral model* (pp. 317-332). London: Jessica Kingsley Publishers.

Corey, G. (2012). *Theory & practice of group counseling.* Belmont, CA: Brooks/Cole, Cengage Learning.

Cozolino, L. J. (2002). *The neuroscience of psychotherapy: Building and rebuilding the human brain.* New York: W.W. Norton & Company.

Cozolino, L. J. (2014). *The neuroscience of human relationships,* (2nd Ed). New York: W.W. Norton & Company.

Cozolino, L. J. (2016). *Why therapy works: Using our minds to change our brains.* New York: W.W. Norton & Company.

Cox, M. (2013). Learning to remember: Applications of the therapeutic spiral model with addictions. In K. Hudgins & F. Toscani, (Eds.). *Healing world trauma with the therapeutic spiral model* (pp. 225-237). London: Jessica Kingsley Publishers.

Cox, M. (2001). Therapeutic spiral international - The six safety structures. Retrieved from http://www.drkatehudgins.com. Accessed September, 2016.

Dayton, T. (2016). Neuropsychodrama in the treatment of relational trauma: Relational trauma repair—An experiential model for treating posttraumatic stress disorder. *The Journal of Psychodrama, Sociometry, and Group Psychotherapy, 64*(1), 41-50. doi:10.12926/0731-1273-64.1.41.

Drucker, K. (2013). Psychodrama and the therapeutic spiral model in individual therapy. In K. Hudgins & F. Toscani, (Eds.). *Healing world trauma with the therapeutic spiral model* (pp. 225-237). London: Jessica Kingsley Publishers.

Ekman, P. & Frisen, W.V. (1978). *Facial action coding system.* (2nd ed.). Salt Lake City, UT: Research Nexus E-book.

EMDR International Association. (2016). What is EMDR therapy? Retrieved from http://www.emdria.org/?page=2. Accessed September 2016.

Elliott, R., Davis K.L. & Slatick, E. (1998). Process-experiential therapy for posttraumatic stress difficulties. In L.S. Greenberg, J.C. Watson & G. Lietaer (Eds). *Handbook of psychotherapy and behavior change* (4th Ed) (pp. 239- 271). New York: Guilford Press.

Elliott, R., Greenberg, L.S., & Lietaer, G. (2005). Research on experiential psychotherapy. In M. Lambert, A. Bergin & S. Garfield (Eds.), *Handbook of psychotherapy and behavior change* (5th Ed) (pp. 493-540). New York: Wiley & Company.

Elliott, R., Watson, J., Greenberg, L.S., Timulak, L., & Freire, E. (2013). Research on humanistic-experiential psychotherapies. In M. Lambert, A. Bergin, & S. Garfield (Eds.), *Handbook of psychotherapy and behavior Change.* (6th Ed) (pp. 495-538). New York: Wiley & Company.

Friedman, M. J. (2015). Overview of posttraumatic stress disorder (PTSD). *Posttraumatic and Acute Stress Disorders* (6th Ed), 1-8. doi: 10.1007/978-3-319-15066-6_1

Gendlin, G.T. (1996). *Focusing-oriented psychotherapy: A manual of the experiential method.* New York: Guilford Press.

Gendlin, E.T. (1957). A descriptive introduction to experiencing. *Counseling Center Discussion Papers, 3* (25). Chicago: The University of Chicago.
http://www.focusing.org/gendlin/gol_primary_bibliography.htm -. Accessed September 2016.

Greenberg, L.S. (2013). Anchoring the therapeutic spiral model into research on experiential psychotherapies. In K. Hudgins, & F. Toscani (Eds.), *Healing world trauma with the therapeutic spiral model: Stories from the front-lines* (pp. 132-148). London: Jessica Kingsley Publishers.

Greenberg, L. S., Watson, J. C., & Lietaer, G. (1998). *Handbook of experiential psychotherapy.* New York: Guilford Press.

Hudgins, M.K. (1998). Experiential pyschodrama with sexual trauma. In L.S. Greenberg, J.C. Watson, & G. Lietaer (Eds.), *Handbook of Experiential psychotherapy* (pp. 328-348). New York: Guildford Press.

Hudgins, M.K. (2000). *The therapeutic spiral model to treat PTSD in action.* In P.F. Kellermann, & M.K. Hudgins (Eds.). *Psychodrama with trauma survivors: Acting out your pain* (pp. 229-254). London: Jessica Kingsley Publishers.

Hudgins, M.K. (2002). *Experiential treatment of PTSD: The therapeutic spiral model.* New York: Springer Publishing Company.

Hudgins, M.K. (2007a). Building a container with the creative arts: the therapeutic spiral model to heal post-traumatic stress in the global community. In S. Brooke (Ed). *The use of creative therapies with sexual abuse* (pp. 280-300). Springfield, IL: Charles C. Thomas Publishers.

Hudgins, M.K. (2007b). Clinical foundations of the therapeutic spiral mode: Theoretical orientations and principles of change. In C. Baim, J. Burmeister, & M. Maciel (Eds.) *Psychodrama: Advances in theory and practice* (pp. 175-188). London: Routledge Press.

Hudgins, M.K. (2008). Nourishing the young therapist: Action supervision with eating disordered clients using the therapeutic spiral model. In S.L. Brooke, (Ed.). *The creative therapies with eating disorders* (pp 254-262). Springfield, IL: Charles C. Thomas Publishers.

Hudgins, K. (2013a). The spirit of healing trauma: The Therapeutic Spiral Model. In S.B. Linden (Ed). *The heart and soul of psychotherapy: A transpersonal approach through theater arts.* (pp. 361-370). North America: Trafford Publishing.

Hudgins, K. (2013b). Therapeutic spiral international: International certification training standards. Retrieved from http://www.drkatehudgins.com.

Hudgins, K. (2015). Spiral healing: A thread of energy and connection across cultures. In S.L. Brooke & C.E. Myers (Eds). *Therapists creating a cultural tapestry: Using the creative therapies across cultures* (pp. 260-281). Springfield, IL: Charles C. Thomas Publishers.

Hudgins, M.K. & Ciotola, L. (2003). The body double: An experiential intervention for eating disorders. *IADEP Connections Newsletter.* August, 2003.

Hudgins, M.K. & Drucker, K. (1998). The containing double as part of the therapeutic spiral model for treating trauma survivors. *The International Journal of Action Methods, 51*(2), 63-74.

Hudgins, M.K., & Kiesler, D.J. (1987). Individual experiential psychotherapy: An initial validation study of the intervention module of psychodramatic doubling. *Psychotherapy, 24*, 245-255.

Hudgins, K. & Toscani, F. (2014). Containment = Safety with action methods. *The Journal of Psychodrama, Sociometry and Group Psychotherapy, 62*(1), 105-110.

Hudgins, K. & Toscani, F. (Eds.) (2013). *Healing world trauma with the therapeutic spiral model: Stories from the front-lines.* London: Jessica Kingsley Publishers.

Hudgins, M.K., Culbertson, R., & Hug, E. (2009). Action against trauma: A trainer's manual for community leaders following traumatic stress. Charlottesville, VA: University of

Virginia, Foundation for the Humanities, Institute on Violence and Culture. Retrieved from www.lulu.com/action-against-trauma-a-trainers-manual/6009176.

Hudgins, M.K., Drucker, K., & Metcalf, K. (2000). The containing double: A clinically effective psychodrama intervention for PTSD. *The British Journal of Psychodrama and Sociodrama, 15*(1), 58-77.

Hudgins, M. K., Cho, W. C., Lai, N. W., & Ou, G. T. (2005) *The therapeutic spiral in Taiwan 2000-2005.* Paper presented at the Pacific Rim Conference for the International Association of Group Psychotherapy, Taipei, Taiwan, June 2005.

Hug, E. (2013). A Neuroscience perspective on trauma and action methods. In K. Hudgins, & F. Toscani (Eds.), *Healing world trauma with the therapeutic spiral model* (pp. 111-131). London: Jessica Kingsley Publishers.

Johnson, D.R. (1999). *Essays on the creative arts therapies: Imaging the birth of a profession.* Springfield, IL: Charles C. Thomas Publishers.

Keltner, D., & Ekman, P. (2015). The science of 'Inside Out'. Retrieved from http://www.nytimes.com/2015/07/05/opinion/sunday/the-science-of-inside-out.html.

Klein, M. H., Kiesler, D. J., & Coughlan, P. M. (1961). *The experiencing scale.* Madison, WI: Madison Psychiatric Institute.

Lai, N.W. (2013). A workshop using the therapeutic spiral model and art therapy with mothers and children affected by domestic abuse in Taiwan. In K. Hudgins & F. Toscani (Eds.), *Healing world trauma with the therapeutic spiral* (241-265). London: Jessica Kingsley Publishers.

Lewis, P., & Johnson, D. R. (2000). *Current approaches in drama therapy.* Springfield, IL: Charles C. Thomas Publishers.

Leutz, G. A. (2000). Appearance and treatment of dissociative states of consciousness in psychodrama. In P. F. Kellerman, & M. K. Hudgins (Eds). *Psychodrama with trauma survivors: Acting out your pain.* (pp. 187-197). Philadelphia: Jessica Kingsley Publishers.

Levine, P. A., & Frederick, A. (1997). *Waking the tiger: Healing trauma: The innate capacity to transform overwhelming experiences.* Berkeley, CA: North Atlantic Books.

McVea, C. (2013). The therapeutic alliance between protagonist and auxiliary. In K. Hudgins & F. Toscani (Eds.), *Healing world trauma with the therapeutic spiral model* (pp. 168-182). London: Jessica Kingsley Publishers.

McVea, C. & Gow, K. (2006). Healing a mother's emotional pain: Recall of a therapeutic spiral model session. *Journal of Psychodrama, Group Psychotherapy and Sociometry, 59*(1), 3-2.

McVea, C., Gow, K., & Lowe, R. (2011). Corrective interpersonal experience in psychodrama group psychotherapy: A comprehensive process analysis of significant therapeutic events. *Psychotherapy Research, 21*(4), 416-429.

Moreno, J. L. (1953). *Who shall survive? Foundations of sociometry, group psychotherapy and sociodrama.* Beacon, NY: Beacon House.

Moreno, Z. T. (2013). A life in psychodrama. In K. Hudgins, & F. Toscani (Eds.), *Healing world trauma with the therapeutic spiral* (pp.33-48). London: Jessica Kingsley Publishers.

Moreno, Z.T. (2012). *To dream again: A memoir.* Catskill, NY: Mental Health Resources.

Moreno, J.L. and Moreno, Z.T. (1969). *Foundations of psychodrama.* (Volume 1I). Beacon, NY: Beacon House Press.

Moreno, Z. T., Horvatin, T., & Schreiber, E. (2006). *The quintessential Zerka: Writings by Zerka Toeman Moreno on psychodrama, sociometry and group psychotherapy.* London: Routledge Press.

Moreno, Z. T, Blomkvist, L.D., & Rützel, E. (2000). *Psychodrama, surplus reality and the art of healing.* London: Routledge Press.

Panksepp, J. (1998). *Affective neuroscience: The foundations of human and animal emotions.* New York: Oxford University Publishing.

Perls, F.S., Hefferline, R.F., & Goodman, P. (1951). *Gestalt therapy.* New York: Julian Press.

Perry, R., Saby, K., Wenos, R., Hudgins, K., & Baller, M. *(2016)*. Psychodrama intervention for female service members using the therapeutic spiral model. *The Journal of Psychodrama, Sociometry, and Group Psychotherapy, 64*(1), 11-23.

Porges, S. W. (2011). *The polyvagal theory: Neurophysiological foundations of emotions, attachment, communication, and self-regulation.* New York: W.W. Norton & Company.

Ragsdale, K.G., Cox, R.D., Finn, P., & Eisler, R.M. (1996). Effectiveness of short-term specialized inpatient treatment for war related posttraumatic stress disorder: A role for adventure-based counseling and psychodrama. *Journal of Traumatic Stress, 9*, 269-283.

Rausch, S.L., van der Kolk, B., Fishler, R.E., & Alpert, N.M. (1996). A symptom provocation study of post-traumatic stress disorder using positron emission tomography and script- driven imagery. *Archives of General Psychiatry, 53*(5), 380-387.

Rezacian, M.P., Mazumdar, D.P.S., & Sen, A.K. (1997). The effectiveness of psychodrama in changing the attitudes among depressed patients. *Journal of Personality and Clinical Studies, 13,* 19-23.

Rivers, B. (2015). Mobilizing aesthetics in psychodramatic group work. *Drama Therapy Review, 1*(2), (161–171).

Rogers, C. R. (1951). *Client-centered therapy: Its current practice, implications, and theory.* Boston: Houghton Mifflin.

Salole, R., Forst, M., Goodwin, R., (2013). The application of the therapeutic spiral model in the Men and Healing Programs, In K. Hudgins & F. Toscani, (Eds.)., *Healing world trauma with the therapeutic spiral model* (pp.303-316). London: Jessica Kingsley Publishers.

Schore, A.N. (1994). *Affect regulation and the origins of the self: The neurobiology of emotional development.* Hillsdale, N.J.: Erbium Press.

Shallcross, L. (2012). Where east meets west. *Counseling Today.* Retrieved from http://ct.counseling.org/2012/10/where-east-meets-west/_15.

Shapiro, F. (2012). *Getting past your past: Take control of your life with self-help techniques from EMDR therapy.* Emmaus, PA: Rodale Books.

Siegel, D. (1999). *The developing mind: Toward a neurobiology of interpersonal experience.* New York: Guilford Press.

Siegel, D. (2007). *The mindful brain: Reflection and attunement in the cultivation of well-being.* New York: W.W. Norton & Company.

Siegel, D. (2010). *The mindful therapist: A clinician's guide to midnight and neural integration.* New York: W.W. Norton & Company.

Siegel, D. (2012). *Developing mind: How relationships and the brain interact to shape who we are.* New York: Guilford Press.

Stadler, C., Wieser, M., & Kirk, K. (Eds.). (2016). Psychodrama: Empirical research and science 2. Psychodrama. Empirische Forschung und Wissenschaft 2 (Zeitschrift fuer Psychodrama und Soziometrie ed. Vol. 15, 1 supplement). Wiesbaden: Springer VS. http://link.springer.com/journal/11620/15/1/suppl/page/1

Terr, L. (1991). Childhood traumas: An outline and overview. *American Journal of Psychiatry, 148*(1), 10-20. doi:10.1176/ajp.148.1.10.

Tick, E. (2005). *War and the soul: Healing our nation's veterans from post-traumatic stress disorder.* Wheaton, IL: Quest Books.

Toscani, M.F. & Hudgins, M.K. (1993). *The containing double.* Workshop Handout. Madison, WI: The Center for Experiential Learning.

Toscani, M. F., & Hudgins, M.K. (1995). *The trauma survivor's intrapsychic role atom.* Workshop Handout. Madison, WI: The Center for Experiential Learning.

van der Kolk, B. A. (2006). Clinical implications of neuroscience in PTSD. *Annals of the New York Academy of Sciences, 1071*(1), 277-293.

van der Kolk, B. A. (2014). *The body keeps the score: Brain, mind, and body in the healing of trauma.* New York: Viking Press.

Veronese, G., Fiore, F., Castiglioni, M., el Kawaja, H., & Said, M. (2013). Can sense of coherence moderate traumatic reactions? A cross-sectional study of Palestinian helpers operating in war contexts. *British Journal of Social Work*, *43*, 651–666.

Volkas, A. (2003). Armand Volkas keynote address. *Dramascope: The Newsletter of the National Association for Drama Therapy, 23*(1), 6-9.

Volkas, A. (2009). Healing the wounds of history: Drama therapy: Collective trauma and intercultural conflict resolution. In D. Johnson & R. Emunah (Eds.), *Current approaches in drama therapy* (pp. 145-171). Springfield, IL: Charles C. Thomas Publishers.

Wieser, M. (2007). Studies on treatment effects of psychodrama psychotherapy. In C. Baim, Clark, J. Burmeister, & M. Maciel, Manuela (Eds.) *Psychodrama: Advances in theory and practice* (pp. 271-292). New York: Routledge/Taylor & Francis Group.

Wieser, M. (2011). Studies on treatment effects of psychodrama psychotherapy. In C. M. D. Sales, G. Moita, & J. Frommer (Eds.), *Methodological diversity in psychotherapy and counselling research: Qualitative-quantitative approach.* (pp. 37-40, 111-124). Lisbon: Universidade Autónoma de Lisboa.

White, J. L., Fodor, K. E., Unterhitzenberger, J., Chou, C., Kartal, D., Leistner, S., & Alisic, E. (2014). *Is traumatic stress research global? A bibliometric analysis.* https://www.ncbi.nlm.nih.gov/pubmed/24563730. Accessed August, 2016.

CHAPTER 15

Amaudo Itumbauzo – Settlement of Peace: A Collaborative Approach to Community-Based Psychosocial Service Provision in Sub-Saharan Africa

Adeyinka M. Akinsulure-Smith, Enyi Anosike, and Kenneth Nwaubani

Introduction

As the global burden of disease attributed to neuropsychiatric disorders has continued to rise, mental health has become a critical international health concern (Prince et al., 2007). Despite efforts in the global health field to develop efficacious pharmacological and psychosocial mental health interventions in low- and middle-income countries (LMIC), these findings are often not readily translated into clinical practice (Madon, Hofman, Kupfer, & Glass, 2007; Sussman, Valente, Rohrbach, Skara, & Pentz, 2006; Tansella & Thornicroft, 2009).

Studies indicate that mental health problems are salient in Sub-Saharan Africa, where the need for services is great (Fournier, 2011; Ehiemua, 2014; Okasha, 2002) yet overlooked, and mental illness is undertreated. To date, there is limited data about effective psychosocial services developed and delivered in Sub-Saharan African settings (Cohen, 2001; Jenkins et al., 2010; Patel et al., 2007). Within the Sub-Saharan African context, efforts to increase and improve the availability of mental health services remain severely hampered by a range of difficulties, including the prevalence of conditions due to conflict (Okasha, 2002), the lack of physical and mental health infrastructure (Jenkins et al., 2010), cultural beliefs about mental illness, and, within the majority of subcultures, the severe stigmatization of the mentally ill and of mental health services (Gureje & Alem, 2000; Hugo,

Boshoff, Traut, Zungy-Dirwayi, & Stein, 2003; Kabir, Iliyasu, Abubakar, & Aliyu, 2004). Information is essential not only for understanding mental health needs, but also for developing and monitoring culturally-informed, cost-effective interventions (Cohen et al., 2012; Jenkins et al., 2010).

The extent of this problem has been highlighted by Lora et al. (2012) in a study exploring mental health service accessibility, treatment gaps, and service utilisation of individuals with schizophrenia in 50 low- and medium-income countries. Among other findings, this study revealed that 35% of those needing treatment for schizophrenia in Nigeria do not receive any (Lora, et al. 2012, p. 54B). Scholars have expressed concern about the situation in West Africa and frequently argue that there is a mental health crisis, specifically regarding a lack of services, that needs to be addressed (Carey, 2015, Eaton, Des Roches, Nwaubani & Winters, 2015).

Nigeria: An Overview

As is typical of countries in Sub-Saharan Africa, Nigeria struggles to provide effective and population-centered mental health services. Located in West Africa, Nigeria has a surface area of 923,768 sq km, a population of 177.2 million, and a gender ratio of 1.04 males/female (Central Intelligence Agency [CIA], 2016, Geography section, subsection Area). Nigeria is Africa's most populated country and home to 250 ethnic groups. The most populous of its ethnic groups are the Hausa and the Fulani (29%), Yoruba (21%), Igbo (18%), Ijaw (10%), Kanuri (4%), Ibibio (3.8%) and Tiv (2.5%) (CIA, 2016, People and Society section, subsection Ethnic groups). While Nigeria's official language is English, Hausa, Yoruba, Igbo, and over 500 other indigenous languages are also spoken. (CIA, 2016, Population section, subsection Languages). With a life expectancy of 52 years, Nigeria hosts a youthful population – 62% are below the age of 25, and only 3% are over 65 years (CIA, 2016, Population section, subsection Age structure). According to data from 2008-2012, its total adult literacy rate is 51.1% (UNICEF, 2012, Basic Indicators section). The total expenditure on health as a percentage of Gross Domestic Product by the Nigerian Government in 2014 was 3.7% (CIA, 2016, People and Society section, subsection Health expenditure).

Mental Health Services

Nigeria's healthcare system has been plagued by a multitude of difficulties, particularly inadequate service provision and inefficient management systems. While some hospitals in Nigeria provide psychiatric services, eight regional psychiatric hospitals and the departments of psychiatry in twelve medical schools (Ayonrinde, Gureje, & Lawal, 2004) provide most of the mental health services. Despite the clear need to address mental health, there are limited options for care.

Many of these services are in urban centers in the southern region of the country. Such locations restrict accessibility to mental health services for individuals in other regions or rural areas. A 2006 report by the World Health Organization (WHO) assessing the mental health system in Nigeria revealed that the ratio of mental health professionals (specifically psychologists) with at least one year of training in mental health care was estimated at 0.02 to 100,000 persons throughout the country (WHO-AIMS Report, 2006, p. 28).

As is the case throughout Sub-Saharan Africa, Nigeria's limited mental health care provision is further compromised by stigma and negative attitudes and beliefs regarding mental illness within the larger Nigerian society (Adewuya & Makanjuola, 2008; Gureje, Lasebikan, Ephraim-Oluwauga, Olley, and Kola, 2005). This is further aggravated by media stereotypes regarding mental illness and treatment options (Aina, 2004). Attempts at managing mental disorders have led to shackling, beating, and confinement of individuals with mental illness (Carey, 2015, Eaton et al., 2015). Given the limited mental health treatment options in Nigeria (as in the rest of Sub-Saharan Africa), there is need for alternate treatment interventions and settings to provide desperately needed services.

This chapter introduces and describes the development of and services provided by Amaudo Itumbuazo (AI), a community-based, psychosocial service located in a rural setting in Southeastern Nigeria. In a country with very limited mental health resources, AI stands out in the Nigerian mental health care system because of its community-based approach to service provision for the mentally-ill homeless and because of the nature of the relationships AI has developed both within its community and among governmental and non-governmental agencies in the larger society. This presentation of AI highlights ways in which key collaborative partnerships can support and sustain mental health service provision, thereby offering directions for future mental health intervention and services in LMICs.

Sources of Information

With the approval of the Board of Directors of the Methodist Church Nigeria (MCN), which oversees AI, and in partnership with the director of AI (the third author, Reverend. Nwaubani), information for this chapter was gathered in a pre-evaluation visit to AI during which the site was reviewed, processes were observed, and semi-structured individual and group interviews were conducted with program administrators, staff (past and current), and residents (past and current). The first and second authors reviewed and collected as many available documents about AI as possible to serve as additional sources of information, including a publication (Onyekwere, 2000), independent evaluations and reports (CBM [formally Christian Blind Mission], 2013a; CBM, 2013b; CBM, 2011), chart notes, AI admission and discharge records, and documentaries (Methodist Church Nigeria Amaudo Itaumbauzo Centre, 2011; Methodist Church Nigeria Amaudo Itaumbauzo Centre, 20113). Table 1 (Appendix A*) provides an at-a-glance view of AI and what it does.

Amaudo Itumbauzo: History, Mission, and Evolution

"We made it an open [emphasis added] community, without any fences around it…we don't need to lock these people up in locked wards - in psychiatric hospitals. We can actually live with them in a place without [emphasis added] walls and locks and gates around us, and maybe they won't run away, maybe they can stay and root themselves somewhere, and of course, it happened."
— R. Colwill, AI founder (personal communication, April 26, 2014)

Established in 1989, the Amaudo Itumbauzo Center for Mentally-Ill Destitutes is located in a rural setting in Abia State, Nigeria. The center was founded by social worker Rosalyn Colwill with the support of the MCN in response to the increasing number of mentally-ill, homeless people found in the streets of urban towns in Southeast Nigeria. With no mental health services and limited support from their families and communities, these individuals had become increasingly isolated and were living on the edge of society (R. Colwill, personal interview, April 26, 2014; Onyekwere, 2000).

Armed with the knowledge that service provision for the mentally ill in Nigeria occurred in asylum-like psychiatric hospitals in which treatment often consisted of physical and social restriction and minimal stimulation (Ayorinde et al; 2004; Onyekwere, 2000), Colwill sought to develop and implement an alternative approach to mental health service provision, one that would take into account both the lack of information about mental illness within Nigerian communities and the associated stigma that resulted in mentally-ill individuals experiencing a profound loss of a sense of self and identity – a loss that only worsened with their increased isolation, diminishing their overall prognosis (R. Colwill, personal interview, April 26, 2014; Onyekwere, 2000). Colwill conceptualized a psychosocial intervention that would draw on the African concept of community to promote healing. In essence, AI would support emotional wellness through the re-establishment of community ties while providing services and living in a strong, vibrant, and caring community.

---

*Appendices for this chapter can be found at: http://tinyurl.com/wghm-attachments

The Residents of Amaudo Itumbauzo

Admission to AI

In keeping with AI's mission to care for the destitute mentally ill, AI staff routinely admits between 8-13 mentally-ill individuals (depending on the number of beds available), who are drawn from the streets of urban towns in Abia, Anambra, Ebonyi, and Imo states (Onyekwere, 2000) twice a year. These individuals are removed from the chaos and overstimulation of living on the streets in urban towns and are provided with the tranquil, rural community of AI.

> *"I was taken to several hospitals...They said I had depression, they just gave me drugs...Finally, I was taken to Amaudo."*
> — *AB, Former AI resident (personal communication, December 6, 2014)*

Resident Demographics

Amaudo Itumbauzo started in 1989 with the admission of two residents and has since hosted over 833 homeless individuals from Abia, Anambra, Ebonyi, and Imo States and beyond. Today AI can house up to 65 residents at any given time. While AI is located in the southeast Nigeria and the majority of the residents are Ibo and Christian, some of Nigeria's other ethnic groups (e.g., Yoruba, Hausa, Efik, and Igala) have been represented among the residents, along with a Ghanaian and a Cameroonian (Onyekwere, 2000). Residents range in age from their early 20s to mid-60s, and the average age is 30. Over the years, the male residents have slightly outnumbered the female residents. Incoming residents typically present with a range of chronic, pervasive mental illnesses, including schizophrenia, affective disorders (bipolar and clinical depression), and substance abuse. The length of stay for a typical resident at AI can range from six months to two years.

The Amaudo Itumbauzo Approach to Community-Based Psychosocial Services

> *"I ended up on the streets of Lagos, I lost my senses, I was what people termed as a 'mad man.'"*
> — *BF, Former AI resident*
> *(personal communication, December 6, 2014)*

Amaudo Itumbauso's approach to mental health care draws primarily on the recognition of the critical roles that community and community life play in facilitating physical, emotional, and spiritual well-being within Sub-

Saharan African cultures. Thus, a vital part of the healing process draws on social and collateral ties that are critical to the African traditions of hospitality and community (R. Colwill, personal communication, April 26, 2014; Makgoba, 1997).

Life for residents at AI is comprised of a structured daily program (Table 2 in Appendix B) which is infused with community life and communal activities aimed at providing residents with a renewed sense of belonging and community. This happens through integration of therapeutic services (e.g., spiritual, individual, and group counseling), vocational/skills training (e.g., hair braiding/barbering, sewing/tailoring, jewellery making), and recreation (e.g., music, indoor and outdoor games, gardening) to facilitate healing within a nurturing, rural community setting. Staff and residents live, eat, work, and learn together. This provides residents with a network of positive relationships within the immediate community.

When a resident is admitted to AI, the treatment process occurs in sequenced phases, including cleansing, stabilization and observation, treatment, and eventual discharge of the individuals to their families and communities. Progress through each phase and the length of stay varies.

During their first few hours at AI, new residents are observed as they are groomed (hair and nails cut), bathed, given clean clothing, and fed. They adjust to their new surroundings, and the initial phase is complete when the newly admitted residents are placed in gender-specific dormitories, under the care of trained house parents. AI has seven houses and seven house parents who take care of eight clients per house. While some residents present with challenging behaviors at the time of admission, AI does not use chains or locks to restrain residents (unlike other facilities). There are no fences or walls around AI's compound. While some residents have expressed suicidal or homicidal ideation at some point in their treatment, there have been no suicide or homicide attempts to date.

During the second phase, the observation and assessment of the new residents continues with a more formal evaluation, including a review of the individual's current mental state and as much history and information as the individual is willing to disclose or can provide. A psychiatric nurse, with observations from the assigned house parent, conducts the evaluation. This initial assessment allows the treatment team (comprised of nurses, house parents, and counselors), to develop a working diagnosis, an initial treatment plan, and decisions regarding psychotropic medication.

In addition, the process of "home tracing" (the search for the resident's family in order to gain a more detailed history and background information and to initiate family and community reconnections) begins. Once the family is located, they become part of the treatment. The resident's family receives psychoeducation regarding mental illness and care, and thereby become an integral part of the resident's support community. Over the next few days, an individualized treatment plan is put in place, which integrates therapeutic (spiritual counselling, both individual and group), vocational (e.g., hair braiding, sewing, carpentry), and recreational elements (e.g., soccer, gardening). Multidisciplinary resident reviews, during which treatment plans are reviewed, occur once a week at AI. Each resident case is presented to the treatment team once a month. This individual review encompasses every aspect of the resident's life, including psychopharmacology, counseling, occupational skills, spiritual care, and nutritional needs. Every staff member involved in the resident's care takes part in the review, thereby allowing for robust information sharing and informed decision making.

Once the treatment team has determined that the new resident has been stabilized, the process of therapeutic treatment begins fully. AI's holistic approach to care includes a gradual reintroduction into community life with the aid of psychopharmacology, counseling, spiritual activities, vocational skills training (e.g., farming, carpentry, tailoring, jewellery making, and hair dressing/barbering), recreational activities, and visits to their families and communities of origin for increasing periods of time.

Over time, residents begin to demonstrate increasing levels of self-awareness and community awareness and improved psychosocial functioning and interpersonal relationships. When the time is right, AI's treatment team gradually prepares both the residents and their families for the residents' integration into family and larger community life.

With input from the treatment team (e.g., nurses, house parents, counselors) and community members (noted interactions with peers, observations by other staff) regarding the resident's emotional stability, interpersonal interactions, and overall cognitive and emotional functioning, trial home visits begin. At first, these only last a few hours, but the duration is gradually increased to overnight visits and then to a few days. Residents and their families begin to prepare for discharge and the residents' eventual re-entry into their former home and community life. The vocational skills learned at AI provide the residents with a means of sustainable livelihood, so they can become financially independent. AI hosts a special "Discharge Ceremony" for residents which typically occurs in December. During the ceremony, family and members of the community are invited to attend and celebrate the individual's recovery and return to community life. Prior to discharge, AI works extensively with the families through multiple home visits and workshops to prepare them for family reunification. Once the residents have been discharged from AI's grounds, they are referred to one of the 73 satellite community clinics established by AI. This allows them to receive follow-up care, thereby preventing relapse.

Program Administration

AI has an organizational structure that provides for oversight and creates opportunities to evaluate its processes. The MCN takes ownership of AI and through their appointed Board of Trustees, makes final decisions regarding AI's overall strategic direction, and hires the project director. AI's project director reports directly to MCN's Board of Trustees, and as such, he or she is responsible for the day-to-day running of the AI. Within the AI chain of command, all staff report to the project director. For example, house parents are answerable to supervisors, who then provide feedback to the project coordinators, who in turn share information with the project director during weekly meetings. The clinical staff (i.e., the mental health nurses, volunteer psychiatrist, and outreach workers) also have weekly rounds with the project director present.

The Evolution of AI

In the course of establishing the project, it was noted that there was a group of mentally-ill persons who were unresponsive to treatment. The chronicity of their illness and the attendant disability they suffered alerted AI to the necessity of a long stay unit, Amaudo Ntalakwu, to accommodate them and to provide treatment and rehabilitation more suited to their needs. In addition, Project Comfort was established to enable persons with learning disabilities to acquire skills to best manage their disabilities to allow for functioning in the wider community.

Unsurprisingly, a subsequent assessment of community mental health care uncovered a significant need for a service that catered to individuals that were still under the care of their families, but had nowhere to go for much-needed mental health care. AI therefore expanded its services to include the Community Psychiatric Programme (CPP), which was set up in partnership with regional state governments to take services to people where they reside at an affordable cost (CBM 2013a; Onyekwere, 2000). This involved setting up satellite outpatient clinics (currently 73 in number) which can be accessed by the patients and their families. The 1991 enactment by the federal government of Nigeria of the National Mental Health Policy, which saw the inclusion of mental health care as part of primary health care, served as added justification for the creation of CPP (Gureje, Kola, & Fadahunsi, 2006). The availability of a large pool of trained psychiatric nurses made it operationally possible to establish CPP. In effect, the state governments employ the nurses and send them on secondment to work at these clinics, and AI provides their transportation.

In 2007, AI collaborated with CBM, an international development organization catering to persons with disabilities, to establish the Community Mental Health Programme (CMHP), which is essentially a consolidation of the structure and functions of CPP. Next, the Mental

Health Awareness Programme (MHAP) was created with the support of CBM and with funding from the Australia Agency for International Development (AusAID). MHAP has invested in educating communities about mental health by improving knowledge, changing attitudes, and reducing discrimination against persons with mental illnesses. MHAP has also worked to increase the number of persons with mental illness diagnoses who access their local primary care clinics and has improved its overall management through the establishment of self-help groups.

AI is currently proposing a comprehensive community mental health program which would enable AI to strengthen its advocacy arm while addressing issues like youth and gender as they pertain to mental health.

Collaborative Partnerships: Practicalities and Implications

Although AI initially began as a psychosocial service for 65 residents, the organization has strived to be innovative and has been successful in this regard, both in in terms of the services it provides and in terms of the partnerships it has built over the years. These innovations have proved to be important as AI works to extend mental health care beyond the Itumbauzo community to additional communities in four Nigerian states. AI's longevity and commitment have given it the opportunity to build meaningful working relationships with other stakeholders. The challenge, however, lies in the quality, extent, and sustainability of these collaborations.

Partnership with the Local Community

The Itumbauzo community of Southeastern Nigeria, which provided the land on which AI is built, continues to be involved in the delivery of AI's objectives in ways that are mutually beneficial for AI and the community. AI consistently engages the community in mental health awareness education and employs the services of local contractors from the community to work within the project. AI relies on the community to alert it when its mentally-ill patients have strayed into the wider community.

Another demonstration of AI's investment in the community is a "helping hands" school which educates children from the greater community. This nursery through elementary school was started by AI in 1996 with the support of local and international volunteers. The growth and development of this school has been facilitated in collaboration with the Eze, or chief, of the village and local community leaders. It has served to foster community ownership and maintain a good relationship between AI and the community over the years. Teachers are sourced from the local community and the school serves as the mainstay institution of learning for the children of the local community.

Partnership with State and Local Governments

AI's partnership with the state and local governments that represent the population AI serves is also quite robust. The government of Abia State, where AI is based, gives AI a monthly subvention to help support the project's work. This subvention is a recurrent budgetary allocation that automatically leaves the coffers of the government at a set date every month. This money constitutes about half of AI's monthly budget and is usually enough to pay staff salaries. In addition, the state Ministry of Women's Affairs supports AI with gifts of money and foodstuffs, as does Abia State Ministry of Health.

AI's CMHP engages the four states and their local governments in a partnership that has made it possible to set up 73 satellite clinics in the local communities. The local governments provide office space and furniture, and the state governments send nurses, employed and paid by them, to staff these clinics. Through other partnerships detailed later, AI is able to provide required medications and motorbikes on which the nurses travel to clinics and to patients in their communities. AI also provides supervisors to the states who capture the number and nature of referrals, monitor patient attendance at clinics, and monitor nurse attendance. From an oversight standpoint, the nurses report to the supervisors, who in turn report to an overall coordinator appointed by AI. The coordinator reports to the AI project director bi-weekly (and informally as needed).

Information from structured interviews and review of AI documents reveals that the challenges AI encounters while partnering with local governments to provide follow-up care in rural communities include:

- Inability to guarantee adequate number of nursing staff in rural community clinics
- Shortage of supervisors in the states where the clinics are situated
- Shifting local government priorities which impact availability of services
- Inadequate resources to maintain motorbikes, which quickly deteriorate because of bad roads

Some clinics are better staffed than others. This discrepancy results in varying quality of care and varying quality of attendance data collated from these clinics. As noted by the acting national coordinator for CMHP, "Nurses are sometimes requested by their direct employers to attend meetings. When they do, they can't be accessed and statistics are not collected" (personal communication, December 1, 2014). The same individual said, "I work with nurses. Apart from when doctors did attend the AI clinic from the neuro-psychiatric hospital, they have not come for a long time," (personal communication, December 1, 2014).

Community clinics are nurse-led and have very little input from trained psychiatrists (aside from volunteers, who are few and far between).

Interviews with nurses and the AI director revealed that a volunteer psychiatrist supports AI in the community clinics once every 3-6 months on average. This has implications for the quality control of service provision in these clinics.

Due to a socio-political landscape that is sometimes unstable, AI has taken precautions to work with state security services to guarantee the safety of its staff and collaborators. There have been no incidents that have put AI staff or collaborators in harm's way.

Community Volunteers

AI successfully harnesses the commitment of volunteers as it seeks to expand the work of Project Comfort to rural communities. This is done with the support of community leaders. These volunteers are native to their communities, live within them, and "speak the language" of the community (i.e., they have a comprehensive understanding of societal norms and practices). AI provides these volunteers with basic training in sign language, physiotherapy, and the use of disability aids (e.g., canes for the blind). They know the villages and can penetrate where others cannot, and thereby promote follow-up and reduce noncompliance. Twice a week, they go house-to-house, visiting clients who suffer from physical and learning disabilities. Additionally, some volunteers donate items to these clients from their own limited resources. Once a month, they report to a supervisor who reviews their cases and assesses their service delivery needs. The challenges they encounter include working with children with multiple disabilities and a frequent rate of transportation problems.

Volunteer recruitment can be difficult because they are asked to provide totally voluntary services and time. However, as stated by one volunteer, the motivation for doing the work is that it is in keeping with Christian principles. "My motivation for doing this is that it is God's work" (Project Comfort volunteer, personal communication, December 3, 2014). For Project Comfort and MHAP volunteers, conducting their duties takes away from providing for themselves and their families. This sacrifice has implications for the sustainability of their volunteer roles in their communities (CBM, 2013b).

Relationship with Local Pharmaceutical Companies

AI makes medication available to the clinics through its revolving drug fund. Via this mechanism, medication is sold at cost to mentally-ill members of local communities. The money generated from the sale of medication at cost is used by AI to procure more medication. Medication is procured from locally based pharmaceutical companies that guarantee quality and prompt delivery. The success of this system stems from the fact that the fund is protected and not accessed for any other purpose. AI provides medication to poor patients who otherwise cannot afford the medication at all. There is, however, no clearly articulated strategy that underpins free medication provision, including how it is funded or for how long.

Collaborations with Faith-Based Entities

Apart from the MCN, which takes ownership of the project and oversees it, occasional support also comes from other faith-based organizations such as the Catholic Church, the Presbyterian Church, Winners' Chapel (a prominent Pentecostal church), and women's groups. Individuals also periodically donate money to support AI's services.

Media and Communications

Despite a lack of a clearly defined media strategy, AI enjoys a good relationship with local media organizations. This relationship started at the inception of AI, when Colwill employed the support of local media organizations to lobby the state government to garner more financial support for the work (R. Colwill, personal communication, April 26, 2014). The Broadcasting Corporation of Abia State regularly airs phone-in programs anchored by the AI director. Through the use of a question-and-answer format, the programming educates the public about AI's work. Additionaly, AI can put out press releases about its activities free of charge. Other media organizations that have aired programs educating the public about the project's work include Pacesetter FM, Vision Africa FM, and Radio Nigeria.

Partnerships with International Organizations

Over the course of its existence, AI has developed strong working relationships with several overseas organizations, including Amaudo UK, CBM, AusAID, Transpetrol Switzerland, the Vitol Foundation, and The Akabusi Charitable Trust (TACT). Collaborating with these organizations at critical phases in its development has enabled AI to improve its model of community mental health care and create room for new ideas.

Amaudo UK is a United Kingdom-based charity that was founded in 2003 by former AI volunteers. For more than 10 years, it has supported AI by raising funds from individuals and donor organizations, including the British Lottery Fund. It has also actively supported the project by organizing volunteers to support specific AI projects and transfer much needed skills to AI staff. Amaudo UK trustees and staff make planned visits to AI every year to provide training for its health workers and administration staff, provide mentoring, and advocate. We noted however, that training is ad hoc at times and is not always guided by a training needs assessment. Furthermore, training is not always evaluated in terms of its impact on the quality of service provision.

The working relationship between CBM and AI started in 2007 when CBM provided support to strengthen AI's CMHP. Between 2009 and 2013, CBM supported AI's efforts to set up the MHAP with funding sourced from AusAID, the Australian Government agency that has responsibility for managing Australia's overseas aid program. To guarantee quality program delivery, CBM also worked closely with Amaudo UK to improve the skills of AI staff, especially in report writing, and to provide a mid-term evaluation of the program. An end-of-program evaluation of MHAP revealed that in terms of training trainers and village health workers in mental health awareness, MHAP largely met its objectives and, in some cases, moderately surpassed expectations (CBM, 2013b). MHAP also achieved its goals related to its support work for CMHP. AI came up short, however, in its role as champion of MHAP, in the areas of documentation of work and prompt sharing of information with key stakeholders (CBM, 2013b; CBM, 2013c). A mid-term evaluation of MHAP revealed that, in accommodating the needs of MHAP, the resources of AI's CMHP were sometimes stretched too thin – community-based nurses were required to facilitate training in mental health awareness in addition to being involved in monitoring and evaluating MHAP (CBM, 2011).

CBM has also actively supported AI's efforts to improve staff knowledge. In 2015, CBM partially funded the project director's enrollment in a postgraduate diploma course in mental health and human rights (remaining funding was provided by Amaudo UK). We (the authors) expect that the knowledge acquired from attending the course will be harnessed to further expand AI's services, especially in mental health advocacy and mental health and human rights.

The Akabusi Charitable Trust (TACT) has worked closely with Amaudo UK to support AI's efforts to train mental health workers in Imo State and has provided funds over a two-year period. TACT was founded by Kriss Akabusi, a former British track and field athlete of Nigerian descent. One of its main objectives is to support individuals and groups with mental health problems. Providing funds for training in just one state, however, has negative implications for quality, balanced, and sustainable training being cascaded to all of AI's operations. "Training was done for Imo State because Kriss Akabusi hails from Imo state. Imo State was therefore a little bit ahead of every other state, and they were more exposed to current trends" (Acting national coordinator for CMHP, personal communication, December 2, 2014).

The Vitol and Transpetrol Foundations have provided funding for AI to acquire vehicles, including motorbikes, to enable effective delivery of its CMHP. The Vitol Foundation, which was established in 1986, provides grants to projects which support children living in deprivation. The Transpetrol Foundation supports social welfare projects that aim to improve the lives of deprived and disadvantaged persons around the world. The support both foundations provide to AI is on-going.

Table 3 (Appendix C) is a chart detailing a Strengths, Weaknesses, Opportunities and Threats (SWOT) analysis carried out by the authors of this chapter. It identifies the key internal and external factors at play as AI attempts to harness resources, support, and collaborative partnerships in order to achieve its objective of providing affordable and population-centered mental health care in an environment replete with challenges as well as opportunities. Interviews with key stakeholders and examination of policy and process documents have informed this SWOT analysis.

Recommendations

AI can demonstrate its success in several ways: 1) the number of individuals who continue to receive services from AI, 2) the number of programs that have evolved because of AI's work, and 3) AI's extensive local, national, and international collaborations. In addition, the fact that several schools of nursing in Southeast and Southern Nigeria (e.g., School of Psychiatry and Mental Health Nursing Calabar; Cross River State, School of Nursing Federal Medical Center Umuahia, Abia State; School of Nursing Amigbo, Imo State; and School of Nursing Abia State University Uturu, Abia State) have chosen AI as the site for their nursing students' community mental health experience speaks to AI's reputation, ability, and potential to provide practical, competent, hands-on training to the next generation of psychiatric nurses.

From our preliminary observations, however, including information gleaned from interviews and records, for AI to continue to provide a full range of psychosocial, community-based care to this underserved and overlooked population, there are four areas that need ongoing attention/strengthening: 1) Residents' Care/Service Provision, 2) Staff Support, 3) Documentation, and 4) Resources/Infrastructure.

Resident's Care/Service Provision

While AI continues to provide services and works to increase the number of mentally ill served, there are areas that could use further improvement in order to enhance resident psychosocial health. Interviewed house parents reported that as residents' mental health improved, they increasingly challenged AI's somewhat rigidly-structured treatment system. This suggests that AI should consider incorporating a more flexible regimen, thereby supporting the drive for independence that comes with improved emotional and psychological functioning. Similar considerations should ideally be put in place for resident discharge decisions. Currently residents are discharged once a year, during the December Discharge Ceremony. If residents have shown all signs of being fully stabilized months prior to the ceremony, it may well not be to their advantage to remain at AI until December, although they can still return for the celebration.

Finally, while AI attends well to many aspects of residents' lives, one area that warrants more attention is resident nutrition. AI's grounds can perhaps be enhanced to better serve as an abundant natural resource to improve nutrition for residents. It would be beneficial to AI's holistic model to include a nutritionist on the treatment team to ensure that residents' diets are more varied and nutritious than the standard gari and sauce or beans that are typically offered.

Staff Support

While the AI staff – past and present – have spoken proudly of deep professional satisfaction derived from seeing residents stabilized and reintegrated into their families and communities, these staff repeatedly commented on the fact that they are severely underpaid. AI staff have long days, are on-call around the clock (even on weekends), and for many, their lives are tied to AI's expectations of dedication. Furthermore, they all described working with a challenging population and living in a limited social environment. AI staff reported that, on average, their remuneration packages were significantly lower than other professionals working in government establishments. "Salary is so poor, can't sustain a family…Salary is so meagre…before the end of the month will run out, you will see people borrowing money" (AI Staff member of 14 years, personal communication, April 24, 2014).

It must be noted, however, that due to inflationary pressures inherent in Nigeria's economy, AI's best efforts at subsidizing staff salaries through the provision of free amenities and food while they work do not go far enough to bridge the relative poverty gap experienced by AI staff. A low staff turnover was reported. The reasons staff stay despite low wages ranged from "the community living" to "It is the work of the Lord." Across the spectrum of AI jobs, those interviewed expressed a strong sense of job satisfaction. Former staff who were interviewed also spoke very positively of their time at AI.

Given the extensive demands on staff, it is important to find ways to increase staff remuneration and improve working conditions. While in the past AI has offered staff periodic specialized skills training (e.g., computer skills, drug management, communication skills, motivation skills), additional relevant, culturally informed clinical trainings could serve as further incentives to boost staff skills and morale. Furthermore, additional training in clinical and administrative roles would allow AI staff to take on more leadership positions and strengthen service provision.

There are certain key staff roles that could be adjusted to improve services at AI. For example, AI's project director has many roles and duties (including the supervision of trainees, administrative duties, grant writing, reporting, and recruitment, hiring, and management of all staff) that take away from his time, which might be better used elsewhere. With staff trained to function more independently, the project director could use his time more strategically to meet the administrative and development needs of the project. Currently, there is only one volunteer psychiatrist who visits AI once a month. For a program like AI, in which psychiatric services play a key role in achieving wellness, a more permanent clinical supervisory presence is needed.

Although none of the staff interviewed mentioned burnout or compassion fatigue, and while there is a low turnover rate at AI, it is important for AI to address such areas so that neither the well-being of the staff nor the care of the residents is compromised. Despite these challenges, there is a sense among residents that the staff at AI "have a passion for what they are doing...they care" (BF, Former AI resident, personal communication, December 6, 2014).

Documentation

As part of the pre-evaluation visits undertaken by the first and second authors, AI's information system and client records were reviewed. While we could examine some statistics on the sociodemographic and clinical characteristics of clients, there were striking gaps regarding interventions and how often clients accessed services and treatments. Our overall sense was that AI significantly underreported the services provided and the number of recipients of those services. We noted that this "data failure" was largely due to inefficiency, poor record keeping, lack of physical space, outdated computers and software programs, viruses damaging data, and limited internet access. Modern computers/software and staff trained in documentation and good recordkeeping are necessary.

Limited Resources/Infrastructure

As stated earlier, there are many advantages to AI's rural location; however, the bad condition of the roads that lead to AI is a major disadvantage. AI staff repeatedly ranked the poor roads among their top stressors. To access AI's services, one must drive on terrible roads that worsen during the rainy season. The roads cause significant wear and tear on the few available vehicles. While repairing the roads to AI is outside of the project's capacity, these roads significantly affect the project's functioning by restricting staff movement and hindering fieldwork and provision of critical services to residents. AI also struggles with inconsistent electricity provision and aging buildings that need significant repair.

Reflections and Implications for the Future

While this chapter presents a description of AI and discusses the significance of key collaborative partnerships critical to sustaining and enhancing AI's psychosocial services, we recognize the need for a comprehensive evaluation of AI's clinical care and service delivery and are in the process of conducting such an evaluation.

In the meantime, AI's commitment to sustainable rural community mental health care provision appears to have enabled AI to acquire useful experiences. These experiences, along with program process improvements, could make AI's model an invaluable contributor, not just to community mental health care, but also to community care in general, as it affects other healthcare disciplines in LMICs.

Mental health care provision is very low priority on the list of public health priorities in LMICs, and this has negative consequences on investments and funding in this field (Saraceno et al., 2007). Despite this challenge, AI has increased community engagement and has leveraged partnerships at local, national, and international levels.

AI's psychosocial, community-centered approach, its focus on human rights, and its efforts to achieve the restoration of patient productivity with the support of patients' families and communities, make the project a potentially useful contributor to the conversation surrounding the Comprehensive Mental Health Action Plan 2013- 2020 (WHO, 2013). However, this would require better and more sustainable collaborative working with partners, especially governments. A more-integrated and better-funded Nigerian health care system that invests strategically in primary health care should certainly create an opportunity to harness AI's community care experience. This would strengthen primary health worker knowledge, attitudes, and practice in the mental health field.

AI would need investments in staff training and a robust system of data collection and utilization to improve its processes. We expect that achieving this on a sustainable basis would promote an even better understanding of mental health and disability, especially as it affects individuals in LMICs.

"Amaudo allowed me to recover the dream I had before the break...most mental patients don't get that back."
- BF, Former AI resident (personal communication, December 6, 2014)

References

Adebowale, T.O., & Ogunlesi, A.O. (1999). Beliefs and knowledge about aetiology of mental illness among Nigerian psychiatric patients and their relatives. *African Journal of Medicine and Medical Sciences, 28*(1-2), 35-41.

Adewuya, A. O., & Makanjuola, R. O. (2008). Lay beliefs regarding causes of mental illness in Nigeria: pattern and correlates. *Social Psychiatry and Psychiatric Epidemiology, 43*(4), 336-341.

Aina, O. F. (2004). Mental illness and cultural issues in West African films: implications for orthodox psychiatric practice. *Medical Humanities, 30*(1), 23-26.

Ayonrinde, O., Gureje, O., & Lawal, R. (2004). Psychiatric research in Nigeria: Bridging tradition and modernization. *British Journal of Psychiatry, 184*, 536-538.

Carey, B. (2015, October 11). The chains of mental illness in West Africa. *The New York Times.* Retrieved from http://www.nytimes.com/2015/10/12/health/the-chains-of-mental-illness-in-west-africa.html.

Central Intelligence Agency. (2016). The world factbook. Retrieved from https://www.cia.gov/library/publications/the-world-factbook/geos/ni.html

CBM (2011). *Amaudo Mental Health Awareness Programme: Mid-term evaluation.* Umuahia, Abia State, Nigeria: Christian Blind Mission Country Office

CBM (2013a). *Mental health awareness programme: End of programme evaluation.* Umuahia, Abia State, Nigeria: Christian Blind Mission Country Office

CBM (2013b). *Report of Partner Assessment of Amaudo Itumbauzo.* Umuahia, Abia State, Nigeria: Christian Blind Mission Country Office

Cohen, A. (2001). *The effectiveness of mental health services in primary care: The view from the developing world.* Geneva, Switzerland: World Health Organization.

Cohen, A., Eaton, J., Radtke, B., De Menil, V., Chatterjee, S., De Silva, M., & Patel, V. (2012). Case study methodology to monitor & evaluate community mental health programs in low-income countries. Retrieved from http://www.cbm.org/article/downloads/54741/Case_Study_Methodology_to_Monitor___Evaluate_Community_Mental_Health_Programs_in_Low-Income_Countries__CBM-LSHTM_.pdf

Dovi, M. (2013). The silent crisis: Mental health in Africa. Retrieved from http://www.consultancyafrica.com/index.php?option=com_content&view=article&id=1213:the-silent-crisis-mental-health-in-africa&catid=61:hiv-aids-discussion-papers&Itemid=268

Eaton, J., Des Roches, B., Nwaubani, K., & Winters, L. (2015). Mental health care for vulnerable people with complex needs in low-income countries: Two services in West Africa. *Psychiatric Services, 66*(10), 1015-1017

Ehiemua, S. (2014). Mental disorder: Mental health remains an invisible problem in Africa. *European Journal of Research and Reflection in Educational Sciences Vol, 2*(4), 11-16.

Fournier, O. (2011). The status of mental health care in Ghana, West Africa and signs of progress in the Greater Accra Region. *Berkeley Undergraduate Journal, 24*(3), 8-34.

Gureje, O., Kola, L., & Fadahunsi W. (2006). *WHO-AIMS report on mental health system in Nigeria.* Retrieved from http://www.who.int/mental_health/evidence/nigeria_who_aims_report.pdf

Gureje, O., Lasebikan, V.O., Ephraim-Oluwanuga, O., Olley, B.O., & Kola, L. (2005). Community study of knowledge of and attitude to mental illness in Nigeria. *British Journal of Psychiatry, 186*, 436-441.

Hugo, C.J., Boshoff, D.E., Zungu-Dirwayi, N., & Stein, D.J. (2003). Community attitudes toward and knowledge of mental illness in South Africa. *Social Psychiatry and Psychiatric Epidemiology, 38*(12), 715-719.

Jenkins, R., Baingana, F., Belkin, G., Borowitz, M., Daly, A., Francis, P., … Sadiq, S. (2010). Mental health and the development agenda in sub-Saharan Africa. *Psychiatric Services, 61*(3), 229-234.

Kabir, M., Iliyasu, Z., Abubakar, I.S., & Aliyu, M.H. (2004). Perceptions and beliefs about mental illness among adults in Karfi village, northern Nigeria. *BioMed Central International Health and Human Rights, 4*, 3.

Lora, A., Kohn, R., Levav, I., McBain, R., Morris, J., & Saxena, S. (2012). Service availability and utilization and treatment gap for schizophrenic disorders: a survey in 50 low-and middle-income countries. *Bulletin of the World Health Organization, 90*(1), 47-54B.

Madon, T., Hofman, K.J., Kupfer, L., & Glass, R.I. (2007). Public health: Implementation science. *Science, 318*, 1728-1729.

Makgoba, M.W. (1997). *MOKOKO, the makgoba affair: A reflection on transformation.* Florida Hills, RSA: Vivlia Publishers and Booksellers.

Mbatia, J., & Jenkins, R. (2010). Development of a mental health policy and system in Tanzania: An integrated approach to achieve equity. *Psychiatric Services, 61*(10), 1028-1031.

Methodist Church Nigeria Amaudo Itumbauzo Centre (2011). *Basic skills in management and support for people with mental health problems in community.* Nigeria: Ntaco Creation Digital Video.

Methodist Church Nigeria Amaudo Itumbauzo Centre (2013). *Picking exercise of 13 mentally ill destitutes.* Nigeria: Ezechukwu Adimoha, Broad casting Corporation of Abia State.

Okasha, A. (2002). Mental health in Africa: The role of the WPA. *World Psychiatry, 1*, 32-35.

Onyekwere, R. (2000). *Heads, hearts, and humans, the Amaudo model; A holistic approach to mental health management.* Nigeria: Precision Press.

Oyefeso, A.O. (1994). Attitudes towards the work behavior of ex-mental patients in Nigeria. *The International Journal of Social Psychiatry, 40*, 27-34.

Patel, V., Araya, R., Chatterjee, S., Chisholm, D., Cohen, A., De Silva, M., … van Ommeren, N. (2007). Treatment and prevention of mental disorders in low-income and middle-income countries. *Lancet, 370*, 991-1005.

Prince, M., Patel, V., Saxena, S., Maj, M., Masekdo, J., Philips, M.R., & Rahman, A. (2007). No health without mental health. *Lancet, 370*, 859-876.

Rudolf, J. (2013, November 1). Where mental asylums live on. *The New York Times.* Retrieved from http://www.nytimes.com/2013/11/03/opinion/sunday/where-mental-asylums-live-on.html?_r=0

Saraceno, B., van Omerren, M., Batniji, R., Cohen, A., Gureje, O., Mahoney J., Underhill, C. (2007). Barriers to improvement of mental health services in low-income and middle-income countries. *The Lancet, 370*(9593), 1164-1174.

Sussman, S., Valente, T.W., Rohrbach, L.A., Skara, S., & Pentz, M.A. (2006). Translation in the health professions: Converting science into action. *Evaluation & the Health Professions, 29*, 7-32.

Tansella, M., & Thornicroft, G. (2009). Implementation science: Understanding the translation of evidence into practice. *British Journal of Psychiatry, 195*, 283-285.

UNICEF data (2012). At a glance: Nigeria. Retrieved from http://www.unicef.org/infobycountry/nigeria_statistics.html

World Health Organizatin (2006). WHO-AIMS Report on Mental Health System in Nigeria. Retrieved from http://www.who.int/mental_health/evidence/nigeria_who_aims_report.pdf.

World Health Organization (2013). Mental health action plan 2013-2020. Retrieved from http://apps.who.int/iris/bitstream/10665/89966/1/9789241506021_eng.pdf

PART 3

APPROACHES AND STRUCTURAL SOLUTIONS

CHAPTER 16

International Disaster Preparedness and Response

Stephanie Benjamin

Introduction

Disasters appear to be occurring with increasing frequency around the world. At best, they are isolated incidents that fade away over time and are given little attention and concern. At worst, a select few will snowball into catastrophic disasters – incidents such as the Haiti Earthquake in 2010, the Syrian Refugee Crisis, and the Ebola Virus Disease outbreak. These events leave an indelible imprint on the countries in which they occur and require extraordinary time and effort to recover. Large-scale disasters often necessitate coordinated responses from providers around the world. The increasing frequency of terrorist attacks, pandemics, and natural disasters require well-laid plans and rapid mobilization of responders. However, coordinating individuals and teams in a safe and efficient manner that is respectful of the country in which the disaster is occurring is an intricate process rife with complicated practical and ethical issues.

This chapter will provide an overview of the issues relevant to the United States' role in international disaster preparedness and response. Topics to be covered include disaster preparedness, mobilization of people and resources, ethical issues involved in disaster response, and the potential long-term impact on the mental health of responders. The end of the chapter will provide ways in which lay people and healthcare providers can get more involved. Each topic presented has many additional components and nuances that out of necessity have been culled to only the pertinent points. The goal of this chapter is to lay a foundation of knowledge that will entice readers to become more involved on a personal level with international disaster preparedness and response in the future.

Disaster Preparedness

A disaster is any unanticipated event that causes destruction, which results in the local infrastructure and healthcare resources of a system to be overwhelmed. An international disaster is an event in which the resources of an entire country are overwhelmed and international aid is required in order to recover (Koenig and Schultz, 2016). Preparing for a disaster is essentially trying to make an educated guess about the future by considering all the ways that it could possibly go wrong. Predictions are based on prior events but must also consider a wide variety of scenarios that may never happen. Some threats can be anticipated more easily than others; for instance, yearly weather patterns cycle through different countries in predictable ways, but terrorist attacks occur sporadically throughout the world. In the past few decades, there has been increasing interest in studying patterns of disasters and responses to them in order to improve preparedness and mitigate the consequences of such events (Haddow, Bullock & Coppola, 2014).

There are different types of disasters that can be categorized in various ways such as whether the incident is an isolated or an ongoing disaster. These events are often broadly defined as being terrorist attacks, pandemic outbreaks, technological disasters, or natural disasters. In each of these events, there is typically a sudden and unexpected inciting incident that disrupts and overwhelms a region. After the initial event is over, the country enters a post-impact phase of recovery. The rebuilding may take years, but the disaster itself is a contained event with a definite start and end time.

Unfortunately disasters that stem from a single incident often parlay into multiple subsequent disasters. One example of this is the Haiti Earthquake in 2010 that devastated the area around the capital city of Port-au-Prince and affected millions of people (Millar, 2010, para. 8). During the aftermath, while citizens were cramped in tent cities and subject to poor sanitary conditions, a cholera epidemic broke out, which resulted in many additional casualties (Al Jazeera, 2010). Another example is the Japan Earthquake and Tsunami that occurred in 2011. Those two events resulted in a radiation leak caused by a nuclear reactor breech, essentially creating three different disasters that occurred all at once (Koenig and Schultz, 2016).

Another type of disaster is referred to as a Complex Humanitarian Emergency (CHE). A CHE is an ongoing disaster that develops slowly over time, is often generated and propagated by human behavior and actions, and has many components and overlapping issues (Haddow et al., 2014;

Koenig and Schultz, 2016). The origin of a CHE involves a combination of deterioration of government authority, a deeply rooted and often violent civil conflict, massive dislocation of a population, devaluation of the economy (often resulting in market collapse), and an overall decline in food security with associated malnutrition and starvation (Koenig and Schultz, 2016). CHEs are fundamentally different than isolated events because they stem from a multitude of compounding issues; they often involve chronic political instability and government oppression, and there is rarely a defined starting point or endpoint to the disaster.

While preparedness for such horrific and damaging events would ostensibly seem like an area of great concern, to many nations, it is often necessarily overlooked in favor of more active issues such as healthcare, education, and defense. Disasters are relatively rare events that are hard to predict, and setting aside funding for a "what if" event can be especially challenging (Haddow et al., 2014; Koenig and Schultz, 2015). As reported in Haddow et al. (2014), developing nations with per capita income levels below $760 per year are subject to 90 percent of disaster-related morbidity and mortality (p. 263). Developing countries have less available funds to allocate towards preparedness and are also more likely to have suboptimal infrastructure that cannot withstand the impact of a disaster. Since they have fewer economic resources, there is a huge economic burden created during the recovery phase (Kreps et al., 2006).

Due to the variety of catastrophic events that can occur, the approach to disaster preparedness involves incorporating different resources such as infrastructure, national security, and education. Instead of putting disasters in categories such as natural disasters or pandemics, there is now a trend towards creating unified disasters plans. This "all-hazards" approach works from the same central protocol regardless of the type of incident (The United Nations, n.d.; Koenig and Schultz, 2016). The benefit is that instead of trying to imagine every possible emergency and associated response, one creates a comprehensive system that is adaptable to a variety of needs. An example of this in the United States is the new "Emergency Preparedness Requirements for Medicare and Medicaid Participating Providers and Suppliers." These new guidelines aim to ensure continuity of patient care at both inpatient and outpatient facilities in the face of any type of domestic disaster (Centers for Medicare and Medicaid, 2016). Even though this would seem to be a logical and beneficial advancement in disaster preparedness, there was still a lot of pushback. According to a New York Times article by Dr. Fink, some saw the new regulations as too costly, while others simply thought the new disaster preparedness standards to be unnecessary (September 9, 2016a). Since disaster preparedness involves planning for events that will likely never occur, it can be very difficult to get people from different fields to agree on how limited resources should be allocated.

Interdisciplinary cooperation is key to disaster preparedness, and "mitigation" is a new buzzword within the field that aims to bring together different viewpoints. The concept of mitigation focuses on risk reduction and decreasing vulnerability to disasters by implementing sustainable technology and infrastructure. Mitigation involves surveyors, engineers, disaster preparedness experts, and other people and groups involved in city planning. The overall goal is to decrease the impact a disaster has on the infrastructure and healthcare of a society (Koenig and Schultz, 2015). An example of risk reduction is retrofitting a building to meet new earthquake codes or moving back-up generators from the ground floor to a higher floor to decrease risk of damage by flooding. In the United States, interventions are often guided with the help of a tool called the Federal Emergency Management Association (FEMA) Risk Mapping, Assessment and Planning (FEMA, 2016). Mitigation specialists help to create sustainable and economically secure communities. Another way to decrease the negative impact of a disaster is to encourage healthcare providers to participate in disaster drills and exercises. There are different types of drills ranging from tabletop scenarios to immersive mass casualty incident scenarios complete with moulaged actors. While beneficial to participate in, they can be expensive and difficult to coordinate. The geographic and linguistic barriers as well as other practical obstacles can prevent an international training drill from being feasible. Drills need to be generic enough that they can be applied to a variety of different situations. Countries may not agree on what type of disaster they should focus on or they may not agree how the response should be implemented.

On September 7th and September 8th, 2016 the Indian Ocean Wave Tsunami Exercise took place. It was dubbed IOWave2016 and is possibly the largest disaster drill ever undertaken (Indian Ocean Wave Tsunami Exercise (IOWAVE), 2016; Baker, 2016). For this drill, an estimated three thousand volunteers executed the two-day event, which tested tsunami warning systems and included evacuations of entire villages (IOWave, 2016). Overall, this exercise involved approximately 50,000 people from 24 countries along coastal regions of the Indian Ocean (Baker, 2016, para. 5; IOWave, 2016, p. 1). The extraordinary coordination and cooperation required for this drill was in response to the devastation caused by the 2004 earthquake centered near Sumatra, Indonesia. That 9.2 earthquake triggered multiple tsunamis, resulting in the deaths of 230,000 people and causing catastrophic devastation to regions throughout 14 countries (Baker, 2016, para. 14). Back in 2004, there were no coordinated warning systems in place to respond to a tsunami threat. As mentioned earlier, it can be difficulty to allocate money and resources towards a hypothetical future event. In this case, the lack of preparedness contributed to massive casualties. Since that disaster in 2004, the Intergovemental Oceanographic Commission (IOC) began holding tsunami drills and they have grown exponentially in scale. The 2016 drill was considered a qualified success and helped the participating countries better evaluate their earthquake and tsunami plans.

One alternative to live drills is to use technology to run simulated drills in which individuals can participate remotely from all over the globe. One company that is dedicated to developing such computer simulation exercises is iNovaria, which originated in Italy (iNovaria, 2013). They currently have three computer programs available for international disaster training drills: the Inter-active Simulation Exercise for Emergencies (ISEE), the Disaster Simulation Suite (DSS), and a 3D virtual reality simulator called XVR (iNovaria, 2013). Each is an interactive software program in which participants are in charge of a mock disaster response. The simulator allows players to have control over resources and virtual response personnel. Success is determined by how well the gamers contain the incidence and treat the victims. There are a variety of scalable catastrophic situations, so responders can practice disaster management in a variety of events (iNovaria, 2013). Perhaps in the future there will be additional technological developments using multiplayer platform gaming to provide individuals around the world the chance to practice working together in real time on mock disaster drills. However, even with the best laid plans and in depth drills, disasters will still strike.

Disaster Has Struck! ... Now What?

In the wake of a disaster, a neighboring country or agency cannot barge in and demand to provide assistance. The ruling government where the disaster occurred must first agree to accept any offered aid, and they can create boundaries that all relief groups must respect. This concept is referred to as sovereignty of state, and it prevents foreign countries from making decisions in a country that may not be welcomed or warranted (Haddow et al., 2014). Specifically, this means that international aid groups cannot interfere with domestic issues unless the local government has given them explicit permission to do so. However it can be difficult for a developing country that is relying on external assistance to maintain its authority over the wealthier countries that are providing such aid. Contrasting views between countries on how aid should be distributed can lead to a subpar disaster response. Ideally, before a disaster response is launched, the needs of the country are fully assessed and the aid is provided in coordination with their stated needs (Koenig and Schultz, 2015). Aside from sovereignty of state, there are also issues around respecting customs of different countries. Responders who have never been to a particular region may benefit from cultural tutoring prior to deployment in order to avoid accidentally insulting or aggravating locals who are already under a tremendous amount of stress.

Once a foreign nation has declared a disaster and they have formally requested aid, the United States must agree whether or not aid will be provided. If yes, then the United States mobilizes assistance through the Office of the U.S. Foreign Disaster Assistance (OFDA) by working directly with the U.S. Embassy and the ambassador of the impacted country (Haddow et al., 2014; The Office of U.S. Foreign Disaster Assistance (OFDA), 2016). The OFDA is a branch of the United States Agency for International Development (USAID), which oversees international disaster response (USAID, 2016). One of the first tasks USAID/OFDA will undertake is assembling a Disaster Assistance Response Team (DART) to deploy to the country in need, assess the damage, and coordinate the initial disaster response plans. These specialized DARTs are composed of crisis response experts, humanitarian specialists, healthcare providers, hydro-meteorological advisors and logisticians, as well as other specialists that may be beneficial to helping the particular country in need (OFDA, 2016). This multifaceted approach allows DARTs to be rapidly deployed to a variety of disasters. USAID/OFDA works with other international agencies as well to provide a comprehensive approach to the disaster. In addition to medical needs, a country will also need financial support, various engineers, access to clean water, nutrition, temporary housing, and sanitation.

One of the key organizations during an international disaster is the United Nations (U.N.), which has several branches that help coordinate distribution of resources. The central hub that oversees all U.N. and non-U.N. agencies is the Inter-Agency Standing Committee (IASC) (Koenig and Schultz, 2015; Haddow et al., 2014). The IASC provides a framework and objectives that other organizations can reference when developing their own disaster response (Haddow et al., 2014). The IASC works with other international relief agencies to streamline the disaster response and rapidly distribute needed aid. The U.N. Emergency Relief Coordinator oversees IASC and all disaster-relief efforts. The U.N. refers to this coordinated response as a "cluster approach to humanitarian assistance" (Humanitarian and Disaster Relief Assistance, n.d.) The joint goal of the U.N. and IASC is to create a dynamic web that has a high level of communication between multiple different agencies.

For those who have been displaced from their homes, the Office of the U.N. High Commissioner for Refugees (UNHCR) and the International Organization for Migration (IOM) help to set up refugee camps and shelters. Nutritional support is provided by The World Food Programme (WFP) and the Food and Agriculture Organization of the U.N. (FAO). For issues that directly impact children, there are the specialized organizations such as the United Nations Children's Fund (UNICEF) and Save the

Children (Humanitarian and Disaster Relief Assistance, n.d.). Some of the non-U.N. organizations that frequently work with IASC include the International Committee of the Red Cross (ICRC) and the International Save the Children Alliance (Kreps et al., 2006).

The branch of the U.N. that is dedicated to healthcare is the World Health Organization (WHO), which has offices in over 150 countries (The World Health Organization, 2016, para. 1). Within the WHO, there is a branch specifically devoted to preparedness, surveillance, and response. Some of their specific tasks include risk assessment, monitoring health situations, and delegating supplies and other resources to countries during emergencies. In the aftermath of a disaster, they help to monitor unsanitary conditions and any subsequent disease outbreaks (The World Health Organization, 2016; Haddow et al., 2014).

There are numerous medical and humanitarian societies providing care in limited-resource areas. Some well-known organizations include Amnesty International and Doctors Without Borders (Kreps et al., 2006). For a veritable who's who of newer organizations, one can reference The New Humanitarians, a three-volume compendium highlighting aid work that is taking place all over the world (Stout, 2009). The volumes contain information profiling about three dozen unique organizations around the world, ranging from Flying Doctors of America, which carries out medical missions in remote regions of the world, to Endeavor, which helps small businesses within disaster areas transition from recovery to rebuilding after a catastrophe, to the Marjorive Kovler center in Chicago, which provides mental health aid and resources to refugees who are survivors of torture.

The International Federation of Red Cross and Red Crescent societies (IFRC) is the largest humanitarian relief organization in the world (IFRC, 2016b). The IFRC, which provides medical relief to victims of violence and disasters, is an active proponent of international humanitarian law. They have established offices throughout the world, which allows for rapid activation and deployment of personnel and relief supplies when the need arises. According to their mission statement, their goal is to focus on four core areas of relief: promotion of humanitarian values, disaster response, disaster preparedness, and health and community care (IFRC, 2016b). The IFRC contributes to disaster response by assembling and disseminating Emergency Response Units (ERUs), which are specialized teams that are always on call and ready to respond to disasters. Each ERU is a comprehensive entity comprised of people with extensive specialized disaster training, as well as readily available equipment and relief supplies to keep the unit self-sustainable and functional for one to four months (IFRC, 2016a). The ERUs come in different varieties depending on the requested resources (e.g., a water and sanitation ERU, a logistics ERU, or a hospital

ERU). Since they are prepackaged and ready for action, an ERU can be deployed to an affected area rapidly (IFRC, 2016a).

Financial aid during and after a disaster plays an integral role in international disaster response. The World Bank, established in Europe after World War II, exists to help countries recover financially after a disaster (World Bank, 2016). Since poorer countries are disproportionately affected by disasters and have fewer available funds for relief efforts, these countries tend to suffer greater financial hardship after a disaster has occurred (Haddow et al., 2014). Approved loans of various types are implemented under the guidance of the World Bank financial planners. Each loan must meet certain criteria in order to be awarded. Prospective loans must outline how the funds will be used to mitigate future disaster risk and to increase productivity of the nation. Additionally, they offer risk assessment analysis to help determine a country's level of preparedness for subsequent disasters (Koenig and Schultz, 2015).

The International Monetary Fund (IMF) is another organization that provides financial assistance to help reestablish economic stability throughout the recovery period. As with the World Bank, the IMF requires that countries requesting aid comply with certain parameters regarding the ways in which the money must be used. In addition to loans, the IMF also provides macroeconomic guidance to help a country regain control over its finances post-disaster (Kreps et al., 2006; Koenig and Schultz, 2015).

Ethics

In theory, the mix of organizations mentioned above (as well as a multitude of others that were not mentioned) all work together in harmony and without any conflict. In reality, even during the most well-intentioned and well-coordinated responses, disasters are rife with practical and ethical issues. The topic of medical ethics during and after a disaster response is a complicated subject that can be debated and discussed for hours on end. Provided here are just a few examples of the many pertinent issues one can expect to arise in the aftermath of a typical disaster.

One of the first issues to address is distribution of medical care in the immediate aftermath of a disaster. In terms of those affected by an incident, a "patient" is someone who is injured and requires medical care, and a "victim" is someone who experienced the disaster but does not require any acute medical interventions (Benjamin, 2016). Ideally, physicians act in the best interest of their patients, with the ethos of "do no harm." Disasters and mass casualty incidents do not change this, but instead of focusing on the individual, a health care worker often must focus on doing the most good for the greatest number of people. In the immediate aftermath of a disaster, a triage system is employed whereby patients can be rapidly assessed. Typically, this system involves labeling patients by severity of injury. One example of a triage method is the Simple Triage and Rapid Treatment (START) system that is utilized by many Emergency Medical Services in the U.S. during mass casualty incidents. Adult patients are each given a triage tag and assigned to a severity group (Minor/Green, Delayed/Yellow, Immediate/Red or Expectant/Morgue) representing acuity of injury. Categories are assigned on the basis of a 30 second or less assessment of airway, respiratory rate, capillary refill/radial pulse and mental status only (Benjamin, 2016). After all the patients have been triaged they are then treated according to severity group, starting with the "Immediate" group, then the "Delayed" group, then the "Minor" group. Patients in the "Expectant" group are left where they are until such as a time when the morgue or burial personnel can collect them.

The "Expectant" patients are those with injuries that are not compatible with life given the available medical supplies and personnel. Patients with injuries that require extensive care and continuous attention (such as someone requiring chest compressions or rescue breathing) will often be overlooked in favor of patients with less severe injuries. The reasoning behind this is that one single patient consuming a lot of attention and resources could distract responders from dispersing medical treatment among the larger group and potentially saving multiple lives. If that particular patient were injured under other circumstances and he were the only patient around, then he might have survived his injuries. However, under mass casualty triage protocol, he would necessarily be left alone or only provided palliative care measures such as pain control. Medical personnel may understand the concept of "saving the most lives" intellectually but still face incredible difficulty when they approach a living person whose medical needs outweigh the medical availability, and the patient must be left behind to die. The lasting impact of having to make such difficult decisions will be discussed later in the chapter.

It is possible that a provider may feel the need to perform duties outside of their educational level in order to help a patient. For example, a medical student who is volunteering abroad during a crisis may find herself with a lot less supervision than usual. As Dr. Gawande elegantly discusses in his book, *Complications* (2002), medical students and residents travel a long road to attain the status of attending physician, and there are a lot of mistakes along the way. Is it ethical for a student to attempt to provide care that is above their level of training when the alternative may be no care at all for a particular patient? Is sub-par care better than no care? People may argue either way. Additionally, should an unsupervised medical student acting in the best interest of the patient be held responsible for any negative outcomes? An alternative scenario to consider would be an experienced physician or surgeon who provides care without the sterilization techniques, medications, and equipment that is available when practicing at home. Can the physician then be blamed for any subsequent infections? Who determines what risk is acceptable, and who accepts the blame for the negative consequences? Negative outcomes may be likely to occur in either scenario.

Another issue that is germane to international disaster medicine is determining who gets care and in what order. As an Emergency Medicine Physician in the U.S., there is rarely a need to ration the everyday care of my patients. All those who enter the hospital at which I work will be treated and cared for regardless of their socioeconomic status, gender, age, criminal background, or any other defining characteristic. On the contrary, equitable division of relief assets can be very difficult to implement when in a disaster zone (Koenig and Schultz, 2015). In regions where certain populations are marginalized, particular groups may face difficulty in accessing needed relief provisions. Societal barriers such as gender, religion, or class inequality create vulnerable groups among women, those at extremes of age, and those of low socioeconomic status (Koenig and Schultz, 2016; Kreps et al., 2006). Children are more vulnerable to diseases, malnutrition, and environmental exposure, leading to increased rates of injury, illness, and death. Societal barriers can make it especially hard for women, children, and the elderly to seek aid (Haddow et al., 2014; Koenig and Schultz, 2015). Women may especially have more difficulty accessing aid if they live in a gender-biased society. The increasing hardships during a disaster can result in women turning to desperate measures in order to provide for themselves and their families. If a woman is desperate enough for essentials such as food, water, or medical care, she may turn to prostitution in exchange for those items, thus putting her at increased risk for sexual violence and sexually transmitted infections (Herman, 1997; Koenig and Schultz, 2016).

Another issue related to distribution of care is discrimination stemming from sharply divided societal groups. According to a 2001 Human Rights Watch report, after India was struck by a devastating earthquake in 2001, there was uneven distribution of resources because of the caste system. Although the government reportedly distributed aid and relief money equally, upon investigation, it was found that the higher castes were living in nicer camps with access to clean water and electricity, while the lower castes received almost no supplies from the government and were living in squalor. As an outsider, it can be difficult to understand these deeply engrained beliefs about social hierarchies.

When humanitarian workers are deployed to a disaster site, the goal is to provide relief to all those affected by the incident. However, it is important to keep in mind that not all individuals will want the help provided by outside nations. Some may not trust foreigners either from fear, misinformation, or prior negative experiences with people from outside their neighborhood or society. In Haiti, during the cholera outbreak that occurred after the 2010 earthquake, some believed that relief workers intentionally brought cholera into the country. This resulted in anti-U.N. riots and the murder of 45 individuals who were accused of using "black magic" to spread the disease (Al Jazeera, 2010, para. 1).

It is imperative to keeping responders safe during incidents such as the one in Haiti. Based on provisions originating at the Geneva Convention of 1949 and then developed by the ICRC, medical personnel are supposed to be protected in areas of war and conflict (Koenig and Schultz, 2014). Specific clauses note that medical personnel should never be targeted or punished for provided medical care, hospitals and civilians shall not be directly targeted, and non-medical humanitarian workers must be protected as well. Intentionally violating these clauses violates international law (Koenig and Schultz, 2014). However, in the past two years alone, there have been approximately 1,000 individuals that have been killed at healthcare facilities around the world, while another 1,500 have been injured (Danilova & Keaton, 2016, para. 2). According to a quote in the WHO's "Reports on Attacks on Health Care in Emergencies," "patients are shot in their hospital beds, medical personnel are threatened, intimidated or attacked, hospitals are bombed" (2016, p. 4). Preliminary data notes that about half of the attacks targeted hospitals or other healthcare facilities, while another quarter of the attacks specifically targeted healthcare providers (Danilova & Keaton, 2016, para. 3). These incidents are more than ethical violations – they are war crimes. Unfortunately, they appear to be increasing in frequency, and their long-term effects have yet to be realized (The World Health Organization, 2015). The only recommendation made to humanitarian aid workers so far is to keep recording and reporting these attacks, as there is no solution to this dilemma at the moment (The World Health Organization, 2015).

As a disaster progresses, resources dwindle, medications run out, equipment fails, and sometimes even basic necessities like gloves and running water disappear. When this occurs, difficult decisions must be made about resource allocation. An article on this topic by Dr. Sheri Fink was recently published in The New York Times (2016b). Her article discusses not only the issues that exist regarding the rationing of care and resources, but also the American public's thoughts on resource allocation. The state of Maryland is currently holding open forums for the public to come together and debate such issues. The goal is for lay people to provide input regarding guidelines that physicians would then be able to reference in the event of a limited resource disaster. A multitude of differing viewpoints have been debated during these meetings. Some of the participants felt that medical care should be first-come, first-serve while others suggested having a lottery for resources. Still others believe that medical care should be allocated towards those most likely to survive the event, and others thought that resources should be directed towards children first (Fink, 2016b). Although no one enjoys thinking about these types of disastrous events, the guidelines may help unburden physicians from having to make life-or-death choices without any input on the matter. These guidelines would not mandate what physicians and other healthcare providers would have to do in these types of events. Rather, it would provide healthcare workers with collected information about how the community feels about resource allocation.

The Aftermath

In the aftermath of a disaster, a country will enter the reconstruction phase. The goal of reconstruction is to have the country once again function independently. The country or region receiving help needs to be left with a plan for how to continue their recovery efforts once the international aid has stopped. Temporarily providing support and then suddenly leaving would not help the country in the long run. As mentioned earlier, there are ongoing issues that both individuals and the local government will be facing, including financial strain, infrastructure issues, and housing concerns.

In the aftermath of a disaster, it can be difficult to determine whether or not a disaster response was actually effective. Historically, disaster responses were not subject to a "good" versus "bad" analysis because all help was deemed humanitarian and thus should not be criticized. The Humanitarian Practice Network, however, lays out three reasons why a disaster response should be evaluated (1995). Their first point explains that given the life or death situations that disasters create, a systematic review of the effectiveness should be implemented. If a particular method of response is not working well, it may need to be altered in order to decrease overall morbidity and mortality. Since the annual financial investment in disaster medicine and response can run in the hundreds of millions of dollars, a country providing resources should be privy to results of their investment. Their last point posits that evaluating a disaster response can help to ensure accountability to the population that is being helped (Humanitarian Practice Network, 1995).

Even with the best intentions of evaluating a disaster, there are many roadblocks. Individuals and families can be hard to track over time due to evacuations and multiple subsequent relocations (Koenig and Schultz, 2015). Population fluidity makes it difficult to track medical care and ongoing rehabilitation needs. Communication is often limited, which decreases responder's ability to share real-time information regarding the effectiveness of certain interventions. Keeping current records of relief provided can quickly fall by the wayside if a responder is overwhelmed by their duties. Also, different relief organizations may care about different metrics. A housing organization may concern themselves with the cost and amount of materials used, while a medical relief group may worry about overall infection rates and post-disaster disease outbreaks. Retrospective evaluation of a disaster can be helpful, but as in all scientific inquiries, prospective analysis would likely provide better data.

Another issue regarding evaluating relief success is that although the disastrous event may be over, some of the victims may have ongoing medical needs. Patients who have lost a limb, burn victims, or someone who sustained a traumatic brain injury may require months of rehabilitation and intensive medical care and monitoring (Koenig and Schultz, 2015). The growing field of Disaster Rehabilitation, a subspecialty within Physical Medicine & Rehabilitation, is dedicated specifically to this issue. Disaster Rehabilitation focuses solely on helping individuals with traumatic injuries sustained during disasters regain functionality and independence (Koenig and Schultz, 2015). This growing field will hopefully provide additional insights into the ongoing medical needs of disaster survivors.

The U.N. Development Program (UNDP) helps transition countries into the recovery and rebuilding phase. Some of the UNDP activities include performing post-disaster needs assessments (PNDAs), helping to return displaced persons, supporting economic recovery, and focusing on infrastructure issues. PDNAs assess the damage caused by a disaster, provide a comprehensive overview of a disaster response, and allow countries invested in the recovery effort to follow progress that is being made (UNDP, 2015). Ideally, PDNAs involve the collected effort of the U.N., various governmental associations, and disaster response specialists. Special training is offered which certifies individuals as disaster response experts. However, the PDNA guidelines are also available online for free, so any individual evaluating a recovery effort can utilize them. If all PDNAs are amassed and the results shared, then a meta-analysis of the collected data could potentially provide valuable insights into the process of disaster recovery.

Disaster medicine is a relatively new field and the majority of information amassed thus far is a compilation of personal experiences and field notes, rather than information gathered from scientific research studies (Koenig and Schultz, 2015). Fortunately, this is starting to change. The WHO and the Belgium Government created the Emergency Events Database (EM-DAT) to monitor disasters around the world (EM-DAT, 2016). EM-DAT studies the epidemiology of disasters with the goal of mitigating the impact on affected populations. When a disaster occurs, EM-DAT tracks the number of individuals affected by the disaster and estimates the relief cost. Currently, they have collected data on over 22,000 mass disasters that have occurred around the world since 1900 (EM-DAT, 2016, p. 3). By analyzing data from prior incidents, they are able to provide countries and regions with specific information regarding likely disasters and thus influence disaster preparedness for that particular region.

Another active organization that is amassing and disseminating information about worldwide disaster risks and their aftermath is the Regional Disaster Information Center (CRID). They have collected over 12,000 articles, interviews, and records relevant to disaster preparedness and response on their website (CRID, 1999, p. 3). Topics range from tsunami and earthquake preparedness to epidemiology of recent disasters and from risk management to articles and information about global warming and rising sea levels. Their focus is mainly on Latin America and the Caribbean though the depth and breadth of information available on their website is an invaluable resource to any individual involved in disaster response and disaster epidemiology (CRID, 1999). The articles are free of charge, the only caveat being that they are not necessarily peer-reviewed. The website also contains links to related agencies such as the United Nations Office for Disaster Risk Reduction, which issues warnings about current disaster activity, links to disaster preparedness courses and events being held around the world, as well as ways to get involved with disaster response and humanitarian aid work (CRID, 1999).

The Knowledge Center on Public Health and Disasters is another comprehensive website that collects and disseminates information on disasters (The Knowledge Center, 2016). One of the ways they are expanding is by sharing links to disaster sites that are recommended by individuals that visit their website. Additionally, readers can sign up for their biannual newsletter to receive up-to-date information about topics trending in international disaster preparedness and response (The Knowledge Center, 2016).

While the victims of the disaster undoubtedly had their lives changed, it is important to note that humanitarian aid workers are bearing witness to a tremendous amount of trauma and suffering. A humanitarian aid worker may respond to only one disaster, but within that crisis, he or she witnesses the pain and trauma of many individuals. Often aid workers go on different missions, the cumulative effect of which puts them at higher risk for mental health issues (Antares Foundation, 2012; Erich 2014). According to an article by McFarlane (2010), "Combat and emergency service work involves repeated activations of the fear and stress systems that are then prone to present as future dysregulation over time" (Triggering and Sensitization section, p. 3). Upon returning from deployment, some of them may face ongoing mental health issues.

After a traumatic event, during which there was the actual or perceived risk of harm to oneself or to others, a person is at risk for posttraumatic stress disorder (PTSD) (Sadock & Sadock, 2007). This is true of responders who have secondary trauma by bearing witness to the disaster and those directly affected by it. According to the Antares Foundation (2012), approximately 30% of international aid workers suffer from significant PTSD (Humanitarian aid and development workers section, p.1). Posttraumatic stress disorder results in a variety of psychological and physical symptoms. Mental health issues include persistently re-experiencing the event via intrusive thoughts and memories, and there are often nightmares and other sleep disturbances involved such as insomnia. Biologically, dysregulation of the hypothalamic-pituitary-adrenal (HPA) axis and the autonomic nervous system results in a variety of physiological symptoms (McFarlene, 2010; Sadock & Sadock, 2007). Patients may exhibit persistent hyper arousal, elevated heart rates, elevated blood pressure, palpitations, flushing, and sweating. In the short term, the combination of mental and physical issues results in poor sleep architecture, an elevated fear response, agitation, difficulty concentrating, and poor memory. Correlations have also been made between PTSD and long-term health issues. People with PTSD may be at increased risks for medical issues such as obesity, hypertension, metabolic syndrome, hyperlipidemia, cardiovascular disease, and coronary artery disease (McFarlane, 2010). Other psychosomatic symptoms such as abdominal pain or headaches that do not have an apparent underlying cause may manifest themselves in both the short and long term (McFarlane, 2010).

People with PTSD are more prone to developing comorbid psychiatric conditions such as depression, panic disorder, generalized anxiety disorder, and/or substance abuse disorders. The most devastating outcome is when a responder suffers so severely that he or she commits suicide (Erich, 2014). Humanitarian workers may feel that since they are helping with the relief effort, they themselves should not then need help. Wanting to appear strong and not ask for help while repeatedly being exposed to trauma on subsequent missions can compound a person's emotional suffering (Erich, 2014). If responders are unfamiliar with mental health and the warning signs of PTSD, they may not understand why their job has become more difficult, or why they are feeling more moody or emotional than usual (Antares Foundation, 2012).

One resource for healthcare workers is the First Responder Support Network, a website developed and run by and for first responders. They offer mental health support groups and a 24-hour crisis hotline, and they coordinate wellness retreats for healthcare workers (First Responder Support Network, 2015). Another foundation that is actively working to decrease the mental health impact on humanitarian workers is the Antares Foundation. Their goal appears to be to caring for the caregivers, and they provide a multitude of resources on their website. According to the guidelines Antares Foundation published in 2012 regarding the care for humanitarian aid workers, an important first step is to destigmatize the need for mental health care. Early and targeted interventions to debrief and support returning aid workers should be a requisite part of all international missions. Responders should be provided with mental health resources and should be informed that PTSD and other mental health issues may arise upon their return. International aid workers and those who organize missions may want to familiarize themselves with these guidelines for managing stress. Proper debriefing after spending time in a disaster zone is recommended to help ensure proper reintegration to life at home. Responders may be helped by psychotherapy, joining a support group, participating in art therapy, or starting medication if necessary. Other interventions specific to PTSD such as eye movement desensitization and reprocessing (EMDR) and neurofeedback have also shown promising results (Sadock and Sadock, 2007; MacFarlane, 2010).

Get More Involved

The ongoing devastation from a disaster is far-reaching. At the national and regional level, there will be a long-lasting economic impact commensurate to the magnitude of the disaster. According to the United Nations Food and Agriculture Organization (FAO), natural disasters alone caused over $1.5 trillion in damage between the years 2003 and 2013 (FAO, 2015, para. 2). The devastation of a disaster can seem overwhelming, and it can be difficult to know where to start when it comes to helping out. Outlined below are some initial steps to take. This is not meant to be a comprehensive to-do list; rather, it is meant to be a starting point for those interested in becoming more involved with disaster preparedness and in volunteering with relief groups abroad.

At the most fundamental level, disaster preparedness starts at home. Learn which types of disasters are most prevalent in your area by checking out local neighborhood and city websites. Next, consider transportation, as being able to safely travel to and from work during a disaster is essential. Map out several routes to all local hospitals in case you become ill or injured during a disaster and the major roads are blocked from hazards such as rubble or fallen electrical lines. Have another method of transportation available, such as a bike, in case your vehicle is damaged. Additional information about basic disaster preparedness can be found at the website for the Department of Homeland Security and the Red Cross.

While people may get excited to help out and want to immediately hop a plane or bus over to a disaster site, this is not recommended. One should never arrive at a disaster site without being accepted by a volunteer organization or before going through proper training. Keep in mind that every volunteer who arrives at a disaster site is another body that will need food, water, security, and a sanitary living space. A well-meaning person who is not prepared for a particular situation may end up being a victim him/herself and merely add to the disaster burden. Additionally, an unprepared person, no matter how well-intentioned, may be at increased risk for mental health issues if they are not properly prepared to enter a disaster zone.

There are different types of organizations with which one can volunteer. Some volunteer programs are based in the United States while others are stationed abroad. Groups that are designated as non-governmental organizations (NGOs) are not affiliated with any particular country or government. Others may have religious affiliations or focus their work in a particular region of the world.

If you are looking to get involved right away, consider registering with local and national volunteer disaster relief registries. The USAID Center for International Disaster Information is a U.S. database that provides information about prospective volunteers to various international relief agencies. By registering with them, various disaster organizations around the world will have access to your profile and a list of your qualifications. While it may not guarantee deployment to a particular site, you may increase your chances of being contacted when a relief organization is looking for help.

For humanitarian workers in the field, there are a few general tips to keep in mind. Since your goal is to provide care, minimizing temperature exposure, hunger, and fatigue will help you stay on task. Having extra layers of clothing and a headlamp can be invaluable if you find yourself working in a makeshift area that is not climate controlled or well-lit. If possible, having your own cache of food and water will minimize your reliance on relief provisions. There are many additional items recommended by countless disaster preparedness website and books, but these are some basics.

Joining an international relief group right away may be too big of a commitment for people first learning about humanitarian aid work. Consider expanding your practical skills or broadening your knowledge base first. To start getting your feet wet, consider joining a local relief effort. Research your regional volunteer groups such as the Red Cross or United Way. Spending a day volunteering helps the community and also helps determine in which area of volunteer or aid work you prefer to participate. There are numerous opportunities regardless of whether your area of expertise is medicine, construction, education, or any other field. For those less physically-able, there are options to help out behind the scenes by participating in fundraisers or event planning.

Participating in a local mass casualty incident (MCI) disaster training drill combines volunteering one's time with gaining practical disaster response experience. Learning the MCI managing process is useful knowledge to have if you plan on volunteering abroad one day. Disaster drills are typically only one day but involve a combination of different community and government agencies. Paramedics, park medics, police, fire crews, and other healthcare providers are often needed. There are different roles assigned to responders during MCI drills, including the Incident Commander (IC), who is in charge, and assisting roles such as Triage and Extrications Leaders (Benjamin, 2016; United States Department of Labor, n.d.). During the drill the IC and supporting Leaders are generally assigned to experienced first responders. New participants may be assigned to shadow different roles. For individuals not in medicine, there are plenty of other disaster drill roles. Consider being a patient or victim during the drill and observe how the day is run. If you are an artist, consider volunteering to provide moulage for the fake victims to enhance the visual reality of the day. A photographer may be welcomed to document the day and provide images to the media to help spread awareness about disaster preparedness. These drills can be scaled from small, five-person MCIs to large incidents involving thousands of people (Benjamin, 2016).

To broaden your medical knowledge base, there are a multitude of courses available. Some courses are online, and some are classroom-based; different courses are available to meet any individual's level of training. The most basic medical courses are First Aid and CPR/AED (cardiopulmonary resuscitation/automatic external defibrillation) courses. Having a basic grasp on wound care and learning what to do when someone has a cardiac arrest are life-saving skills (American Red Cross, 2016). For additional training, one could take a two-week course and become an Emergency Medical Responder (EMR). For outdoorsy people, another option would be to take the ten-day Wilderness First Responder (WFR) course, offered through organizations such as the National Outdoor Leadership School (National Outdoor Leadership School, 2016).

For those who are already in medicine, public health, or hospital administration, consider getting additional training specifically in disaster medicine, mass casualty training, or disaster preparedness. Koenig and Schultz (2015) suggest learning about pre-hospital emergency plans, how a disaster impacts public health, nutrition, and food supply, mass casualty management, and management of donations. The Federal Emergency Management Institute (FEMA) offers over 200 free classes online for qualified providers and public health officials as part of their Independent Study Program. Once a student registers with FEMA, they are given a Student Identification Number and can access and keep track of all of their courses. Categories within their online curriculum include: Mitigation, Preparedness and Technology, Professional Development, Disaster Operations and Recovery, and Integrated Emergency Management. Within those categories, course topics include managing disasters as an Incident Commander, handling specific incidents (e.g. earthquakes, tsunamis, biohazards, terrorist attacks), protecting small businesses and places of worship, and keeping animals safe during disasters. College students may even be able to earn credit for completing these courses. While deployed, it is essential to know how to use your available medical equipment in multiple ways. Training in limited resource medicine or wilderness medicine enables people to improvise and alter available equipment for a needed purpose, not necessarily its intended purpose. There are a multitude of wilderness medicine courses and conferences offered around the world throughout the year.

The American College of Surgeons offers a Disaster Management and Emergency Preparedness (DMEP) course. The day-long course starts with the epidemiology and history of disasters and goes through post-disaster assessment and recovery. The course has been taught in six countries and is designed to be applicable to any type of disaster, whether local or international (American College of Surgeons, 2016). Lastly, fellowship training is available for board-certified Emergency Medicine Physicians in areas such as Emergency Medical Services, Disaster Preparedness, and Disaster Response.

Summary

This chapter provides a foundation for understanding some of the complex issues germane to international disaster response. One of the underlying themes is that greater disaster preparedness will lead to improved disaster response. Mitigation is a key topic and a rapidly growing specialty within the field of disaster preparedness. Increased planning that is done beforehand results in improved response times and decreased morbidity and mortality when disasters strike.

Having an appreciation of the ethical conundrums surrounding international disaster response is key. While humanitarian aid work is often well-intentioned, it is not always welcomed. Being sensitive to a country's unique culture and respecting their sovereignty of state can help mitigate stressful ethical issues that are prone to arise.

In the aftermath of a disaster, humanitarian aid workers can develop PTSD, compassion fatigue, burnout, and other mental health issues. Proper training beforehand and debriefing afterwards can be protective against some of these mental health issues. Disaster relief workers should be made aware of these issues and given access to mental health resources upon their return home.

One way to start getting involved with international disaster response is to expand one's skills and knowledge base at home by participating in drills, volunteering locally, and taking classes relevant to disaster management. Remember to register with a relief group – do not show up at a disaster site without proper training.

As discussed, there are multiple benefits to quantifying the success of a disaster response. Hopefully, there will continue to be systematic reviews of disaster management that will improve efficiency and effectiveness in the future. Demonstrating a decrease in projected lives lost and a decreased in negative financial impact could encourage countries to invest more in disaster preparedness and disaster drills. Ideally, a greater understanding of the issues discussed in this chapter will improve response times, minimize waste of resources, and enhance global healthcare outcomes for all victims and humanitarian aid workers involved in future disasters.

References

Al Jazeera. (2010, December 31). Haiti's cholera deaths increase. Retrieved from http://www.aljazeera.com/news/americas/2010/12/201012314485023394.html

American College of Surgeons. (2016). Disaster management and emergency preparedness course. Retrieved from https://www.facs.org/quality%20programs/trauma/education/dmep

American Red Cross. (2016). Red Cross training- Get trained and certified. Retrieved from http://www.redcross.org/ux/take-a-class

Antares Foundation. (2012, March). Managing stress in humanitarian workers- Guidelines for good practice (3rd ed). Retrieved from https://www.antaresfoundation.org/guidelines#.WA0YYNxW04o

Baker, N. (2016, September 8). Tsunami drill tests real-time preparedness. *The World Health Organization*. Retrieved from http://www.mmtimes.com/index.php/national-news/22374-tsunami-drill-tests-real-time-preparedness.html

Benjamin, S. (2016). National park service multi-casualty incident drill manual. Retrieved from http://www.fresno.ucsf.edu/em/parkmedic/downloads/NPS%20MCI%20Drill%20Manual.pdf

Centers for Medicare and Medicaid. (2016, September 8). CMS finalizes rule to bolster emergency preparedness of certain facilities participating in Medicare and Medicaid. Services. Retrieved from https://www.cms.gov/newsroom/mediareleasedatabase/press-releases/2016-press-releases-items/2016-09-08.html

Danilova, M. & Keaton, J. (2016, May 26). WHO: Nearly 960 killed in attacks on hospitals in 2 years. *The Washington Times*. Retrieved from http://m.washingtontimes.com/news/2016/may/26/who-some-1000-killed-in-attacks-on-hospitals-in-2-/

Department of Homeland Security. (n.d.). Make a plan. Retrieved from https://www.ready.gov/

EM-DAT: The OFDA/CRED International Disaster Database. (2009). *Welcome to the EM-DAT website. Université Catholique de Louvain, Brussels, Belgium.* Retrieved from www.emdat.be

Erich, J. (2014, November 1). Earlier than too late: Stopping stress and suicide among emergency personnel. Retrieved from http://www.emsworld.com/article/12009260/suicide-stress-and-ptsd-among-emergencypersonnel

Federal Emergency Management Association (FEMA). (2016, May 2). Federal risk mapping, assessment and planning (Risk MAP). Retrieved from https://www.fema.gov/risk-mapping-assessment-and-planning-risk-map

Food and Agriculture Organization of the United Nations. (2015, November 26). Surge in climate change-related disasters poses growing threat to food security. Retrieved from: http://www.fao.org/news/story/en/item/345727/icode/

Fink, S. (2016a, September 9). Health care providers scramble to meet new disaster readiness rule. *The New York Times*. Retrieved from http://www.nytimes.com/2016/09/10/us/medicare-requirements-disaster-readiness.html?_r=0

Fink, S. (2016b, August 21). Whose lives should be saved? Researchers ask the public. *The New York Times*. Retrieved from http://www.nytimes.com/2016/08/22/us/whose-lives-should-be-saved-to-help-shape-policy-researchers-in-maryland-ask-the-public.html?_r=0

First Responder Support Network. (2015). Frequently asked questions. Retrieved from http://www.frsn.org/about/faq

Gawande, A. (2002). *Complications: A Surgeon's Notes on an Imperfect Science*. New York, NY: Picador.

Haddow, W., Bullock, J., & Coppola, D. (2014). *Introduction to Emergency Management* (5th ed). Oxford: Elsevier.

Human Rights Watch. (2001, September). Caste discrimination: A global concern. Retrieved from https://www.hrw.org/reports/2001/globalcaste/caste0801-03.htm#P133_16342

Humanitarian Practice Network. (1995). Accountability in disaster response: Assessing the impact and effectiveness of relief assistance. Retrieved from http://odihpn.org/magazine/accountability-in-disaster-response-assessing-the-impact-and-effectiveness-of-relief-assistance/

Indian Ocean Wave Tsunami Exercise 2016 (IOWave2016). (2016). Twenty-four Indian Ocean countries participated in IOWave16 tsunami exercise. Retrieved from http://iowave16.org/press-media/24-indian-ocean-countries-participated-iowave16-tsunami-exercise/

iNovaria. (2013, August 28). Our products. Retrieved from https://www.inovaria.com/inovaria/?lang=en

International Committee of the Red Cross. (2010, October 29). Mandate and mission. Retrieved from https://www.icrc.org/eng/who-we-are/mandate/overview-icrc-mandate-mission.htm

International Federation of Red Cross and Red Crescent Societies (IFRC). (2016a). Emergency response units. Retrieved from http://www.ifrc.org/eru

International Federation of Red Cross and Red Crescent Societies (IFRC). (2016b). Our vision and mission. Retrieved from http://www.ifrc.org/en/who-we-are/vision-and-mission/

The Knowledge Center on Public Health and Disasters. (2016). Publications and resources. Retrieved from http://www.saludydesastres.info/index.php?option=com_recursos&view=&Itemid=479&lang=en

Koenig, K.L. & Schultz, C.H. (Eds.). (2016). *Disaster medicine: Comprehensive principles and practice* (2nd ed). New York, NY: Cambridge University Press.

Kreps, G.A., Berke, P.R., Birkland, T.A., Chang, S.E., Cutter, S.L., Lindell, M.K., Olson, R.A., Ortiz, J.M., Shoaf, K.I., Sorensen, J.H., Tierney, K.J., Wallace, W.A., and Yezer, A.M. (2006) *Facing hazards and disasters: Understanding human dimensions*. Washington, D.C.: The National Academies Press.

McFarlane, A. C. (2010, January 28). The long-term costs of traumatic stress: intertwined physical and psychological consequences. *World Psychiatry, 9*(1), 3–10.

Millar, L. (2010, January 17). Tens of thousands isolated at quake epicenter. Retrieved from http://www.abc.net.au/news/2010-01-17/tens-of-thousands-isolated-at-quake-epicentre/1211748

National Outdoor Leadership School. (2016). About us. Retrieved from
  http://www.nols.edu/about/

Office of U.S. Foreign Disaster Assistance (OFDA). (2016, March 14). Who we are.
  Retrieved from https://www.usaid.gov/who-we-are/organization/bureaus/bureau-
  democracy-conflict-and-humanitarian-assistance/office-us

Regional Disaster Information Center (CRID). (1999). International strategy for disaster
  reduction: Latin America and the Caribbean. Retrieved from
  http://www.eird.org/eng/revista/No15_99/pagina25.htm

Sadock, B.J., & Sadock, V.A. (2007). *Synopsis of psychiatry* (10th Ed.). Philadelphia, PA:
  Lippincott, Williams & Wilkins.

Stout, C.E. (Ed.). (2009). *The new humanitarians: Inspirations, innovations, and blueprints for
  visionaries.* [Three volumes]. Westport, CT: Praeger Publishers.

The United Nations. (n.d.). Humanitarian and disaster relief assistance. Retrieved from
  http://www.un.org/en/globalissues/humanitarian/

The United Nations Development Program (UNDP). (2015). UNDP and EU partnership
  for resilient recovery. Retrieved from
  http://www.undp.org/content/brussels/en/home/partnerships_initiatives/results/E
  U-UNDP-PDNA.html

United States Department of Labor. (n.d.). What is an incident command system. Retrieved
  from https://www.osha.gov/SLTC/etools/ics/what_is_ics.html

The World Bank. (2016). About the World Bank. Retrieved from
  http://www.worldbank.org/en/about

The World Health Organization. (2016). About the World Health Organization: What we
  do. Retrieved from http://www.who.int/about/what-we-do/en/

The World Health Organization. (2015). Reports on Attacks on Health Care in Emergencies.
  Retrieved from http://who.int/hac/techguidance/attacksreport.pdf?ua=1

CHAPTER 17

A Curriculum for Increased Psychological Well-being Worldwide

Barbara Lutz and Nausheen Pasha-Zaidi

In September 2015, mental health and substance abuse were included in the Sustainable Development Agenda adopted at the United Nations General Assembly. Thus, psychological concerns will likely become part of international development plans and the focus of development assistance. To improve mental health services for global populations, we must consider the history of colonialism and the limitations of a Western ethnocentric approach. Mental health planners and practitioners must be provided with training opportunities to acclimate themselves to a collaborative, community-oriented approach, rather than the dominant expert ideology. Methodologies and ethics based on the International Bill of Human Rights can begin to balance individual rights, community responsibility, and government interests. A rights-based approach creates a humanistic force to counter the predominantly economic definition of globalization. However, the conceptual tools, training, research, and interventions in the field of mental health still lack the community orientation that is needed to collaborate effectively in addressing global concerns. This chapter draws from the traditions of international psychology, community psychology, and the human rights movement to highlight the possibilities of a rights-based curriculum for global mental health.

Introduction

The importance of introducing a human rights-based curriculum for psychological well-being goes hand in hand with the inclusion of mental health in the United Nation's Sustainable Development Goals for 2030. The third goal, "good health and well-being," includes the following subsection (3.4): "by 2030, reduce by one third premature mortality from non-communicable diseases through prevention and treatment, and promote mental health and well-being" (United Nations Department of Economic & Social Affairs, 2015, "Rubric: Targets and Indicators," 3.4). While this short phrase seems not to do justice to the wide range of mental health issues (Carriere, personal communication, August 27, 2016), the first step toward an increased focus on psychological well-being worldwide has been taken. The mission statement of the Division for Sustainable Development indicates the wide-ranging implications of this:

> The work of the Division translates into six core functions: (1) support to UN intergovernmental processes on sustainable development; (2) analysis and policy development; (3) capacity development at the request of Member States; (4) inter-agency coordination; (5) stakeholder engagement, partnerships, communication and outreach; and (6) knowledge management. (United Nations Department of Economic & Social Affairs, 2015, "Rubric: About," para. 2)

Each of these functions provides options for addressing psychological well-being based on the 2013 Mental Health Action Plan of the World Health Organization (WHO). The four main objectives of the action plan are to:

> (1) strengthen effective leadership and governance for mental health; (2) provide comprehensive, integrated and responsive mental health and social care services in community-based settings; (3) implement strategies for promotion and prevention in mental health, and (4) strengthen information systems, evidence and research for mental health. (WHO, 2016, para. 3)

These objectives are based on the understanding that mental health services in many parts of the world are not only of poor quality, but may actually thwart the recovery process. For example, it is not uncommon for people to be chained to their beds or locked up with no human contact. Such human rights violations, however, are not limited to residential inpatient facilities; many people in outpatient and community care also face restrictions on their basic human rights (WHO, 2016).

The Sustainable Development Goals and the WHO's efforts to increase focus on mental health and well-being worldwide open up many possibilities for creative planning and participation in international human rights projects. However, in order to contribute to effective program development and implementation, a basic understanding of global movements is essential.

Effective Leadership and Governance

In order to strengthen leadership and governance for worldwide mental health programs, a sustained effort must be made to include global perspectives in the training of psychologists. This is particularly important as the majority of psychologists are trained in Western countries, such as the United States. As the U.S. is home to a multicultural population, we are often required to attend to the needs of people from different backgrounds on a regular basis. Although this has inspired the inclusion of multicultural viewpoints in educational endeavors, these perspectives are often seen as adjacent to Western norms which continue to dominate the discipline. Internationalizing psychology thus requires us to critically assess our assumptions of "normal." What fits in a North American or Western context may not fit in others (Bullock, 2014), but if we continue to base our curriculum and practice on research that has been conducted with American college students as the population of choice, we are doing a disservice to the psychologists we train.

When I (Lutz) was given the task to develop a course on Global Mental Health and Human Rights for one of The Chicago School of Professional Psychology's (TCS) international psychology programs, I felt excited and honored to play a part in educating students on what I consider to be one of the most important topics today. As a German, I feel a personal connection to the history of the international human rights movement. After the Holocaust, my parents' generation was confronted with its own parents' role in creating the need for a global morality to prevent the possibility of future atrocities.

As immigrants to the U.S. and proponents of international psychology, my co-author and I tend to look at psychological concepts from an international perspective rather than an explicitly Anglo-western view. For example, in my work with immigrants from culturally-diverse backgrounds, at times I find that I am expected to take on the role of a leader rather than a partner on the path to wellness. Understanding this expectation helps me be more transparent and supportive in my therapeutic approach without compromising the person's trust. My co-author brings similar perspectives to her work as an educator and researcher specializing in international and culturally-diverse populations. While working in the Middle East, for example, she was continually evaluating content and teaching methods rooted in Western norms to determine their efficacy with her Gulf Arab students. The reflective thinking that we both learned from our international psychology studies helps us to do better in our respective fields.

Teaching Global Mental Health

Building a curriculum generally begins with institutional learning goals and proceeds in a systematic manner to structure in program competencies, program learning outcomes, course learning outcomes, and possibly even module learning outcomes. Setting institutional goals first can streamline the process of designing a meaningful course; however it should not take away from creating learning experiences that inspire curiosity, engagement, and commitment to the topic.

When I was a child, my father, a physiologist, once took my brothers and me to one of his lectures at the local university. I remember vividly how this event influenced my thinking about teaching. We sat excitedly in the highest ranks of the auditorium, seeing our dad in a white coat near a chalkboard far away in the front. As children between 5 and 7 years of age, we drew some attention from the "grown-up" students, which was fun. While I anticipated not understanding what my dad would be talking about, I still expected to be impressed by his brilliant performance. However, together with the rest of the "real" students, I was soon bored to death, staring at the little white figure in the front reading off his notes. Unable to hide my disappointment, I later came to understand that this was considered academic teaching.

Unfortunately, this "sage-on-stage" lecture style of imparting knowledge continues to be used in higher education classrooms. In some cases, it represents the dominant instructional strategy (Smith & Valentine, 2012). Having worked in education for many years, my co-author has witnessed this first-hand in classrooms in the U.S. and overseas. However, in teaching about psychological well-being based on human rights, a purely academic lecture style seems counterproductive. After all, we are talking about a global movement that seeks to convince, engage, create commitment, and change how we as human beings treat each other and our world.

The institutional learning outcomes of courses offered at TCS address scholarship, diversity, and professional behavior and practice (TCS, 2016). The successful translation of such learning goals into a vibrant and effective learning environment depends on the correct balance between theories and practical approaches, as well as on incorporating lived experiences and current events. The learning outcomes for "diversity" in the global mental health and human rights course, for example, ended up covering a wide range of relevant topics including global citizenship, Western and non-Western approaches to human rights, political and economic globalization, colonialism and contemporary systems of privilege, cultural competence, international humanitarianism, and the protection of vulnerable and oppressed populations (TCS, 2013).

Juxtaposing theoretical discussions with relevant current events can help students see the application of theories to real world situations. In 2015, when the American Psychological Association (APA) set up the vote to base their ethical principles on human rights and eliminate their members' participation in military interrogations, my class viewed the movie "Doctors of the Dark Side" (Davis, 2011), which addressed the role of psychologists in the torture of detainees at Guantanamo Bay. The week of the vote we exchanged our expectations and predictions regarding the outcome. While all students agreed that in general, torture is a human rights violation and in opposition to the Hippocratic Oath's central tenet to "do no harm," many thought that psychologists working for the military needed to follow orders, rather than refuse involvement by referencing human rights. We discussed national security demands, the experience of military personnel, the (in)effectiveness of torture, the Stanford Prison Experiment, and the consequences of a clear "no" to psychologists' engagement in interrogations. The class was divided between those convinced of military necessity and those who advocated for social justice. Essentially our discussion forum became a microcosm of the arguments of the APA at large.

Even as I found myself clearly on the side of the social activists, it was very rewarding to create a safe space for differing opinions, thus encouraging such a rich discussion to take place. On August 7, 2015, when the news broke regarding the APA's decision to base their ethics on human rights and disengage from military interrogations, I felt a tremendous sense of hope and relief. However, I still needed to keep the discussion space open for both supporters and opponents of the resolution. While admittedly, the decision posed a dilemma for military psychologists, we also explored how the dissident psychologists had engaged in a 13-year struggle to get to this rights-based victory which began in 2006 when the torture scandal became public. Topics of discussion included the willingness to be considered a defiant outsider, the sacrifices and dedication of a prolonged legal struggle, and the tenacity to hold up higher moral standards against powerful opponents.

Contributing to egalitarian and rights-based dialogue, however, requires continuous effort to encourage and engage in difficult conversations. In another class, my students watched the film "The Color of Fear" (Mun Wah, 1997), which provides an important message about diversity, racism, privilege, and colorblindness by the dominant culture. When the class debated what meaningful prevention and action in the face of intercultural conflict could look like, a Jewish student brought up that her grandmother had survived the Holocaust. I decided to apologize to her as a German. Although I was not alive during the Second World War, I am part of the culture that was responsible for the systematic large-scale crimes against humanity. The giving and receiving of this gesture became a beautiful experience of the power of apology for the student, who had never heard someone take personal responsibility for the Holocaust before. For me, the event was profound as well, since I personally felt the impact of this small gesture, even generations after.

Globalization and Justice

When examining psychological well-being worldwide it is important to look at globalization as the basis of current international interaction. The past director of the WHO's psychiatric research center in Honolulu, psychologist Anthony Marsella (2012), defines globalization in the following manner:

> Globalization is both a process and product (as a set of processes globalization refers to historical and contemporary economic, political, cultural, geographic, and technical events, forces, and changes that alter our individual and collective lives by virtue of their immediate and/or future global proportion and consequences for interdependency [p. 461]; ... as an outcome, globalization refers to the negative and/or positive economic, political, cultural, geographic, technical, psychosocial, and health consequences of globalization processes [p. 462]); the globalization process and product are reciprocally determined; the primary drivers of globalization are all events, forces, and changes that are transnational, transcultural, and transborder, especially: capital flow, ownership, trade, telecommunications, transportation, political and military alliances, and international agencies. (p. 460-461)

This definition highlights the complexity, the motivations behind, and the political nature of what we know mainly as an abstract term. For most students, globalization means finding chains like Starbucks all over the world, and that international business is looking for the cheapest possible labor market. Although globalization is based on economic interests and principles, it also has social and political implications based on continuing competition for alliances between sovereign nation-states and the growing network of individuals and corporations that comprise a global marketplace (Marsella, 2012).

We often have a limited understanding of the economic base and far-reaching consequences of globalization for social justice. It is therefore important to educate ourselves on a global approach to psychology, which takes into consideration the markets with their possibilities and deficiencies. The economist and psychologist Per Espen Stoknes (personal communication, April 23, 2016) suggests a creative exercise that involves seeing the market as a psychotherapy client. Rather than judging or condemning it, he recommends approaching it with curiosity and compassion for its deficiencies. Stoknes (2009) relates the nature of markets to that of the Greek god Hermes, who as a young child lied about stealing Apollo's cattle. When caught and brought before Zeus for justice, Hermes was able to "sweet-talk" his way out of punishment. He then proceeded to negotiate a deal with the owner of the cattle, which benefitted them both. Such relationships define the essence of markets. If we can begin to view markets as "conversations, the important question then becomes: What characterizes markets that also strengthens social relationships and doesn't destroy nature?" (Espen Stoknes, 2009, p. 116)

Using mythology to understand the complexity of modern relationships can be a powerful way of engaging students and inspiring creative thought. Students not only re-discover the power of fair trade, but some have diagnosed the market with narcissism, anti-social personality disorder, or manic episodes. When exploring how Hermes' potential might be used for social justice and sustainable living, Stoknes (2009) reminds us of the Greek god's willingness for sacrifice and his exemplary conflict-resolution skills. A global community psychology could develop a strengths-based approach around such topics. Thus, thinking of economic forces as patients on a therapy couch or as a Greek messenger god with winged heels can limit a bipolar or judgmental view about globalization.

Emphasizing social justice is of utmost importance in current market-based conversations. Marsella (2006) describes our era as:

> ...times that are confronting us with an endless stream of abuses to human dignity and welfare, and times that are presenting serious threats to the source, distribution, and restoration of justice! ... Times that require reflection on the roots of justice that reside in our human nature. (p. 121)

The need to stay creative and strategic in the face of our complex and often overwhelming analysis of the factors that influence psychological well-being in the face of globalization can be facilitated by another excursion into the realm of mythology. According to the ancient Egyptians:

> Every day a golden vessel floats across the skies for 12 hours. One of the passengers is Re, the god of the sun and lord of flames. During the following 12 hours of night, he and the other divine passengers of the sun ship cross the realm of the dead. There the snake god Apophis is trying to destroy the golden vessel, so that there would be eternal night. But the divine passengers are strong: Isis, rich with cleverness, Heka, the god of magic, and Maat, the goddess of justice and order, are three of them. ... With their joint resourcefulness, magic and strength they overcome the dark powers and the vessel re-emerges shining on the eastern sky each morning. (Lehmann, 2011)

This myth emphasizes the balance between night and day and light and shadow, but also emphasizes the re-occurring struggle to establish justice and order against contrary forces that need to be reckoned with by using all of our skills. Transferring the myth to human behavior, it can also illustrate the interplay between two opposing positions: one that emulates a reckless "survival of the fittest" mentality versus one that imbues our ancient relationship to justice. As Marsella (2006) points out, human beings are capable of both destruction and nurturing. Recognizing this, we must actively create contexts that nurture the life-affirming side of human nature and limit the damaging characteristics.

Recognizing and owning the potential for violence, ignorance, and destruction as well as the potential for social engagement and compassion at macro and micro levels is a critical aspect of learning to promote psychological well-being in the global context. After exploring the positive and negative impact of globalization and the hopeful fact that we are not by nature condemned to just exploit, fight wars, and destroy our planet, the evolution of our sense of justice toward the Universal Declaration of Human Rights (UDHR) follows as a necessary next step in human ethical and moral development. Marsella (2006) defines justice in the following way: "Justice exists when individual welfare and well-being is extended to the collective, thus, expanding our identity, consciousness, and potential for contributing to life" (p. 127). He points to the United Nations Development Report 1999 as a guide to achieving globalization within the framework of social justice. This entails consideration of the following:

1. Ethics–Less violation of human rights;
2. Equity–Less disparity among nations;
3. Inclusion–Less marginalization of people and countries;
4. Human Security–Less political and economic instability and vulnerability;
5. Sustainability–Less environmental destruction; and
6. Development–Less poverty and deprivation. (Marsella, 2012, p. 469)

Fair trade that prioritizes the common good over corporate financial interests seems to be the path less travelled. However, criticism to partnerships such as the North American Free Trade Agreement (NAFTA) and the Trans-Pacific Partnership (TPP) is re-emerging in the current presidential election debates on the Democratic as well as Republican side, and makes a fair trade solution more plausible (Goodman, 2016).

Understanding Historical Injustice and Cultural Diversity

In our experience, students get discouraged and angry when confronted with the understanding of how little they know about the powers that rule our world. Some cling to the positive effects of globalization and how at least there are medical and social achievements that have made the world a better place. Others want to go out and act against those who they believe are the modern-day villains. However, psychological actors on a global level must learn how to tolerate and process the discomfort of being beneficiaries of what has damaged and violated others and their environment.

For years, the California psychotherapist, Gina Swan, has emphasized the need for cultural attunement of people in the helping professions. She has designed and provided cultural competency trainings. Gina Swan also introduced diversity workshops based on the film "The Color of Fear" (Mun Wah, 1994) to mental health institutions. Swan and I have noticed over the years how little the mental health community knows about historical oppression in the U.S. For example, many therapists are unaware of the internment of people of Japanese descent in camps from 1942 to 1946 (ushistory.org, 2016) or the structural racism documented in American laws. For example, disallowing property ownership based on race was declared unconstitutional in 1948 (Silva, 2009), but can be found in property titles to this day. Interracial marriage state laws became unconstitutional in 1967, but existed in Alabama until the year 2000 (About, 2016).

Since planners and providers of training in global psychological well-being must be aware of the causes of inequality and conflict on the micro and macro levels, Swan (personal communication, August 25, 2016) suggests adding coursework about the historical traumatization of specific populations in the U.S. to the curriculum for the mental health professions. This is essential to understanding how social injustice is not just a problem "somewhere else" in the world, but rather one that continues to affect communities in our own country. We recommend addressing the context of discrimination on a national level in order to sensitize the actors of psychological well-being worldwide to the concept of privilege in our own backyards. In order to be effective, trust and safety must be established in the learning environment approaching this theme.

As a German, I will never forget how I learned in school about the Holocaust. It started in 3rd grade during religious studies and history as part of the de-Nazification education of the German population in the 1960s. We watched documentary footage of the death camps and were taught that our grandparents created this horror. I remember running home from school and asking my mother what she knew. My mother replied she had been a child too young to understand what happened. There were lots of silences and awkward excuses when I went on to ask my grandmother whether she had known about the Holocaust. She replied she mainly remembered the creation of the "autobahn," the freeway system established during the war. During another visit to my grandparents' home, my cousin found my grandfather's Second World War uniform in the attic. He was punished and told to put it away and to never bring up the subject again. A sense of fear and silence shrouded the topic, but as children, we were relentless in our quest for understanding what we were told by the different parties.

We believed the messages from school and church that it was our responsibility to never let a Holocaust happen again, even if it meant sacrificing our lives. My little brother and I discussed at night what we should do if our older brother turned out to be another Hitler. Later, in our teens, we argued with our grandparents and those of their generation. Particularly during international travels, we felt a sense of shame, trans-generational guilt, and a profound responsibility regarding the German role in the Holocaust.

The early sensitization and education about the guilt of the German people in crimes against humanity is an example of how generations can be taught to be wary of authoritarian power structures, nationalism, and the use of other cultures as source of all evil. While my generation in Germany was confronted with understanding and admitting historical guilt in a very direct and painful way, a dialogue-based encounter with historical and current injustice still seems very necessary in forming our cultural identities as we become global promoters of mental health. Colonialism and its consequences for indigenous peoples, recent wars and their justifications, slavery, environmental destruction and exploitation of resources that leave only devastation are just a few examples of areas in which we need to take responsibility, if only for the benefits we have received. The American writer, Martin Amis, confirms:

> It is the rule that your parents are a bit more racist than you, and your children will be less racist than you. The degree can be changed gradually, and old habits can be fought with extensive national efforts. … I respect Germany in this aspect. It is incredible what the Germans did to process the Holocaust. Young people want to talk about it. This is a great success! (Amis & Kuemmel, 2016)

However, just as the golden vessel of the sun, with justice as its passenger, is descending into the night of struggle, the current upswing of hostility against refugees, immigrants, or different ethnicities in many parts of our world must challenge us. We have to use our sense of justice, courage, wit, and wonder to find a way through rekindled and ancient racism into another day of shared humanity. This is not an easy endeavor.

Introducing the Universal Declaration of Human Rights

The Universal Declaration of Human Rights and the U.N. Refugee Convention are as timely today as they were when created in response to World War II and its aftermath. According to Wasserstein (2011), by 1950, 11.5 million Germans alone (not counting Jews, Poles, Ukrainians, Belorussians, Ukrainians, Estonians, Latvians, Lithuanians, Croats, and others) had fled expulsion or left Eastern Europe voluntarily to resettle in the west ("Further Expulsions," para. 3). These documents guaranteed the right to asylum in countries away from persecution and prohibited the forcible return of refugees.

Sixty-seven years later, by the end of 2015, as a result of the humanitarian need created by the wars in the Middle East, 800,000 refugees arrived in Germany (Healy, 2016, p. 18). The German chancellor, Angela Merkel, became the "2015 Person of the Year" in Time Magazine by adopting a large-scale humanitarian policy for refugees (Hoffman, 2016). She has since stumbled into a crisis which has reintroduced border controls and prompted accusations of importing terrorism into the country. Additionally, the root causes of the refugee situation have not been addressed. "There are no prospects for peace in sight in Syria, Libya remains a failed state and Iraq is, despite some territorial gains against Islamic State, still far from establishing peace" (Hoffman, 2016).

Racism and fear of immigrants is very much alive in the U.S. as well. As a Muslim American, my co-author has been struggling with the increasing voices of Islamophobia that have become louder through the rhetoric of the 2016 presidential campaign. Students of global mental health must have an understanding of the historic dimensions of the refugee crisis and the inevitability that more regions of our planet may become uninhabitable due to war or environmental disasters, thus triggering the continued displacement of inhabitants in the future. I have found it helpful to let students evaluate what is being done to support refugees or internally displaced people in existing organizations in their country and around the world. This way, they can examine the policies being implemented and use principles of community psychology to evaluate the levels of compassion, collaboration, social justice, and accountability (Nelson & Prilleltensky, 2006) of current practices.

However, looking critically at the language and approach of the human rights movement itself is necessary in order to understand the complexity of true partnership and inclusion on a worldwide level. While I have seen students gain a sense of hope and direction for their involvement to support global well-being when learning about the Universal Declaration of Human Rights, it is often hard for them to afford a critical orientation toward this approach. For example, when facing the dilemma of specific cultural practices such as female genital mutilation, it becomes complicated to negotiate a culturally appropriate but also rights-based perspective. The lack of binding provisions for human rights on national and international levels, the finger-pointing at non-Western nations while ignoring our own affronts to human rights laws such as the death penalty in the U.S., and the individualist orientation of the human rights movement are all important themes for discussing the enormous task of formulating universal policies of social justice. Inviting critical dialogue into the classroom has been a powerful experience to address the ethical and practical challenges of global mental health.

As Western students and teachers of worldwide psychological well-being, we often struggle with integrating approaches based on other worldviews. As an emerging paradigm, International Psychology embraces the importance of micro-cultures in the macro-culture of global interdependence by considering indigenous approaches within the methodological framework of social science (Larsen et al., 2011). A comparison of the structure and focus of the Universal Declaration of Human Rights with that of the Universal Declaration of the Rights of Mother Earth (Eastaugh & Sternal-Johnson, 2010), which originated in Bolivia in 2010, can make the possibilities and necessity of such thinking visible. The Rights of Mother Earth achieves a holistic approach to the interdependence of life on our planet while addressing the roots of individual suffering on a macroscopic level, thus providing an excellent example of the importance of indigenous and collective wisdom in current times:

Article 1. Mother Earth

1. Mother Earth is a living being.
2. Mother Earth is a unique, indivisible, self-regulating community of interrelated beings that sustains, contains and reproduces all beings.
3. Each being is defined by its relationships as an integral part of Mother Earth.
4. The inherent rights of Mother Earth are inalienable in that they arise from the same source as existence. (Eastaugh & Sternal-Johnson, 2010)

Such a holistic approach to the refugee crisis may seem utopian to the Western mind. However, it can help us focus on the collective task of preserving the planet as part and parcel of mental and physical well-being.

Global Mental Health

Internationalizing the historical context of mental health is an important facet of the curriculum in order to move away from a culturally egocentric approach to psychological well-being. Students and faculty alike are seldom aware that the earliest approaches to alleviating suffering stem from ancient India, China, and Greece. Patel, Minas, Cohen, and Prince (2014) describe the international similarities in treatment of mental health conditions in the ancient world as "herbal potions and acupuncture, ... massage and Yoga, ... baths, balanced diet, and exercise" (p. 3-4). According to Patel et al., there was communication between the physicians of those regions, and a common theory of illness was based on "imbalances in life forces" (p. 3). Similarly, it often comes as a surprise to Western students that some of the first institutions for the treatment of mental illness were Islamic hospitals, "established early in the eighth century in Fez and Bagdad" (p. 4), and that the first psychiatric hospital in the Western hemisphere opened in Mexico in 1567. Additionally, in "the Aztec, Mayan, and Incan empires ... trephination was practiced ... [and] the utilization of psychotropic and hallucinogens was apparently widespread, as were religious practices, baths, bloodletting, and fasting" (p. 6).

Patel et al. fault colonialism for the systematic destruction of knowledge about indigenous approaches. To illustrate the existence of extensive knowledge about health in the time before colonialization, we suggest introducing the voice of the Indigenous Peruvian Felipe Guaman Poma de Ayala, who chronicled the Andean life during colonization by the Spaniards in 1613. Guaman Poma tried to convince the Spanish that the Indigenous culture in Peru was advanced and not inferior to that of the colonizers. He explained that:

> ...the Indian surgeons, barbers, and licentiates who heal and bleed, and who know and understand about medicines, illnesses, sores, the herbs that are used to heal, and the medicines and purges ... are as good at healing as any doctor or licentiate of [the colonizer's] medicine. (De Ayala, 2006, p. 280)

This appeal is still important today in order to remind international actors in mental health to understand existing local health systems and resources, rather than focusing solely on exporting Western approaches.

While the first model for Western community psychology dates back as far as the 14th century, the approach was only briefly considered an alternative for hospitalization of the mentally ill in the 1800's when asylums became costly and overcrowded (Patel et. al, 2014). Conversely, colonial psychiatry, with its emphasis on institutionalization, spread around the world and continues to be practiced in the former colonies that have now turned into "low-income countries" (p.7).

Since the 1960s, mental health experts in Western Europe and North America have re-recognized the value of community-based mental health care and have found that it is more efficient than institutionalization. They have acknowledged the harmful effects of lengthy stays in asylums and increasingly appreciate "the civil and human rights of persons with mental disorders" (Patel et. al, 2014, p. 8). However, according to Paul Farmer, the Chair of Harvard University's Department for Global Health, the urgency for addressing global mental health problems is great, with studies showing that 12 to15 percent of global diseases are attributed to neuropsychiatric disorders, a greater percentage than what is attributed to infectious diseases (Farmer, Yong Kim, Kleinman, & Basilico, 2013, p. 215).

Looking back at the history of mental health care, global mental health actors can find inspiration for the integration of ancient and indigenous ideas into modern approaches. Students often equalize traditional healing practices with harmful techniques (e.g., female genital mutilation) or practices preventing effective medical care (e.g., South Africa's past health policy to treat AIDS with anti-poverty initiatives only (Boseley, 2008), which led to an increased spread of the epidemic). However, some new pathways in mental health seem to focus on integration and collaboration rather than on competition. For example, training and paying lay people for foster care of the mentally ill might be re-examined as a community-based option.

We cannot over-emphasize the need for teaching an integrative and open approach to psychological well-being for global actors in order to decolonize mental health practices and create partnerships with local communities.

Mental Health, Culture, and Human Rights

An important part of the curriculum for psychological well-being worldwide based on human rights is exploring what it means to be culture-bound, and how to recognize culture-bound phenomena to prevent misinterpretations and conflicts. One critic of exporting Western mental health treatment across the globe is Ethan Watters (2010) who published case studies of the mistakes by well-meaning providers. He concluded that providers focusing on psychological trauma often came into affected communities convinced that trauma had a universal effect on people and that they knew how best to treat it. In many incidents, Western mental health providers neither assessed nor involved the local communities in discussing the support they needed or wanted. In fact, providers who focused on issues other than mental health did a better job of including community perspectives (Watters, 2010, p. 79). Such culturally inappropriate measures have appeared in many of my students' papers, even after a whole course of sensitizing information!

In the module on cultural rights by the International Human Rights Internship Program (IHRIP, 2000) at the University of Minnesota Human Rights Resource Center, Ann Blyberg discusses the complexity of this issue in depth. While "the right to freely participate in the cultural life of the community" is anchored in the UDHR's Article 27 (U.N., 1948), definitions of culture remain general and cultural values have been hard to specify. The concept of self-determination within countries can be particularly controversial as cultural inclusion might be considered important on the one hand, but on the other, it may not be accepted by some people from the indigenous culture. Blyberg (in IHRIP, 2000) uses the example of improving education on a Navajo reservation that had very low academic outcomes. Stronger cultural identification with the Navajo cultural roots led to better outcomes than did identification with the dominant Anglo-

European model of instruction. This led to the implementation of bilingual education in Navajo and English, as well as training for teachers to promote the development of a culture and language-based curriculum. Blyberg cautions that education

> ...is never value-free, and formal, state-sponsored education is designed to convey the content and perpetuate the values that are important to the state. That content and those values may be at variance with the values that a minority culture seeks to perpetuate for itself. (Blyberg, IHRIP, 2000, "Economic and Social Rights," para. 1)

This may be particularly difficult to address when the educational content explicitly or implicitly espouses the superiority of the dominant culture.

Where social and mental health are concerned, it is important to realize that a person's culture is essential to his/her identity and if that culture is at risk, then the well-being of that person is also at risk. It is therefore imperative that we examine the sociopolitical context in order to understand how institutionalized forms of culture affect communities, both positively and negatively (Blyberg in IHRIP, 2000). The right to culture in itself presents a collective theme in the discussion of individual human rights. Self-development and creativity do not exist in a vacuum. When indigenous and Western cultures clash, the challenge is to integrate endogenous sources of knowledge in creative ways. While technology, medical practices, and individual rights might be adapted by an indigenous population, a Western culture can benefit from learning how to re-emphasize community mental health and support for people who may be disconnected or at-risk within the individualistic mainstream culture.

I have found that this bi-directionality of cultural influence is often hard for Western students to understand. They can easily get overwhelmed and confused when realizing that there are no easy answers for the complex dilemma between individual and cultural rights.

"How do I know whose cultural right are more important?"

"What's the point of focusing on culture anyway?"

Such questions reveal the extent of students' frustration. However, once students are able to accept the discomfort of letting go of the dualistic nature of right and wrong, these discussions can develop creative problem-solving and critical thinking skills. Students can begin to recognize the importance of context, as well as the shortage of culturally-attuned solutions. This opens up a wealth of opportunities to contribute to a decolonizing agenda.

Decolonizing Research Practices

Although research is an integral part of developing both training programs and interventions to improve well-being, evidence-based practices continue to be based on the results of research conducted in Western societies. The acronym WEIRD was coined by Heinrich, Heine, and Norenzayan (2010) to represent the majority of researchers and research participants in the extant literature: Western, Educated, Industrialized, Rich, and Democratic. The term is particularly relevant as the culture of the mainly European-American college population that makes up the WEIRD community is, in fact, unusual compared to other cultures around the world. In a study of top psychology journals, Arnett (2008) found that 96% of research participants come from Western industrialized nations, yet these countries only represent about 12% of the world's population (p. 602-603). Thus, by using a WEIRD group of people to describe the "normal" or "desirable" characteristics of human experience, research practices continue the colonization of non-Western and indigenous communities whose traditional knowledge systems and worldviews are made to fit within the confines of Western research methods.

To overcome this challenge, researchers have begun to focus on collaborating with local communities. However, effective collaboration is dependent on the level of trust and rapport that researchers can develop with members of the local communities. Unfortunately, these are often undermined by the widely-held assumption that Western methods are the only ways that can deliver scientifically rigorous results. Traditional research methods place the investigators in a position of power. We define the area of enquiry, the research questions, and the hypotheses. We collect data from respondents who are the subjects or perhaps more aptly, the objects of our research. We then interpret our results based on the existing literature and our understanding of the phenomena. Although qualitative methods do require researchers to reflect on the subjectivity of personal worldviews when interpreting data, the crux of the responsibility for understanding the data lies with the research team. Thus, traditional models are often interpreted by indigenous populations as disempowering to their communities, perpetuating stereotypes, and benefiting only the careers of investigators, with little to no benefit being brought to the local communities (Simonds & Christopher, 2013). It is not surprising, then, that non-Western and indigenous communities may be hesitant to engage in academic research.

Decolonizing research requires investigators to go beyond collaboration using pre-determined Western methodologies; instead, it presupposes a system of research that places indigenous values and protocols at the center. This does not mean that existing methods and theories should be rejected, but rather that they should be framed as flexible assumptions that can be adapted to the needs and ways of knowing that are most representative of local worldviews (Simonds & Christopher, 2013).

Community-based participatory research (CBPR) is the umbrella term for a variety of methods, such as participatory action research and mutual inquiry, that are being used to facilitate the integration of non-Western ways of knowing into the research process. CBPR has gained popularity as an orientation to research that veers away from investigator-driven methods to focus on scientific enquiry that emerges from the needs of local communities. In CBPR, community members play key roles throughout the process, from identifying the research problem to the collection, analysis, and interpretation of data, as well as the application of knowledge to inform educational and policy decisions (Minkler & Wallerstein, 2008). Thus, community members are not only research participants or gatekeepers to information, but rather integral members of the research team. By centering the values and traditions of local communities in the process, research practices can begin to change the balance of power between investigators and participants, allowing for the creation and dissemination of more relevant and valid information regarding non-Western communities.

Such a partnership would be of particular significance to local communities where English is not the primary or even secondary mode of communication. Lincoln and Gonzales y Gonzales (2008) note that one of the ways in which scholars can begin to decolonize research practices is by working with bilingual or multilingual data. As English is the dominant language for the dissemination of academic research, the voices of non-English speakers are often unavailable to Western scholars, who are also predominantly English speakers.

> This global status of English alongside the documented growth in English-medium publications means that scholars from around the world are under considerable pressure to publish in English. While such pressure is keenly experienced by scholars writing out of non-Anglophone contexts who have to make difficult decisions about which writing to do in which languages, Anglophone scholars often seem unaware of the privileged position they (we) hold, or the invisible benefits that such a position ensures. (Lillis & Curry, 2010, p. 1)

The privileged status of English in academic circles (and within academic publishing in particular) has the effect of essentially silencing the perspectives of many non-English speaking communities. Thus, a partnership between researchers and local communities would allow non-English speakers to have a voice in mainstream literature.

In an upcoming anthology of personal narratives on veiling, for example, my co-author consciously reached out to non-native English speakers to include their perspectives on the topic. In order to do this, she and her co-editor worked with contributors from a variety of cultural and linguistic backgrounds. Given the relationship between veiling, head-cover, and the perception of foreignness in Western, non-Muslim societies (Ruby, 2006), they felt that it was important to look at the various ways in which veiling is perceived in different parts of the world and in different contexts.

What is an oppressive practice in one context, for example, may be a symbol of female empowerment in another (Read & Bartkowski, 2000), and so a decolonizing approach using personal narratives was chosen to explore this phenomenon.

A great deal of collaboration and discussion went into the writing of each narrative to maintain the authenticity of those voices while adhering to the structural and communicative aspects of the English language. Colloquial terms as well as the fluidity of language were particularly challenging – especially as the editors are South Asian Americans and the publisher is based out of the U.K. Phrases and cultural contexts that were understood by some parties were incomprehensible to others!

As the contributors were ultimately responsible for their message, it was important to reflect on both their words and their intentions. Thus, the essays were drafted and re-drafted a number of times to ensure readability for international audiences. In many cases, foreign words and phrases were kept intact in the essays in order to allow for the nuances of the heritage language and culture to be communicated to bilingual readers – a strategy espoused by Lincoln and Gonzales y Gonzales (2008). As such, the veiling anthology is an effort to decolonize research by examining a controversial practice such as veiling from an approach that allows authentic experiences to be shared with an international audience.

Trauma and Mental Illness

When focusing on psychological well-being worldwide, it is imperative to understand the obstacles to global mental health and human rights. The Substance Abuse and Mental Health Services Administration (SAMHSA) published a treatment improvement protocol that establishes trauma as a major contributor to mental health disorders nationwide (SAMHSA, 2014). Additionally, the former United Nations official and Senior Advisor to the Nonviolent Peaceforce, Rolf Carriere (2014), emphasized the need to place effective trauma treatment at the forefront of worldwide efforts to increase psychological well-being. He suggests that we decipher the various forms of violence around the world in order to understand the magnitude of the problem. For example, natural violence such as flooding and droughts has increased with climate change and is estimated to be affecting 268 million people worldwide. Direct violence includes the intent to harm, which affects approximately 1.5 billion people who are living in war zones or other violent places. Structural violence, such as extreme poverty, affected 1.2 billion people in 2014 and cultural violence is often rooted in direct and structural violence which is manifested in beliefs and attitudes about power and the "need" for violence (Carriere, 2014, p. 188-189).

The growing trend to prioritize the impact of trauma and trauma education therefore needs to be addressed within the curriculum for mental health actors worldwide. The principles of this focus provide an important opportunity for international organizations to realize the prevalence of trauma, recognize its effect on all individuals involved (including their own workforce), and respond by using knowledge to inform their practices (SAMHSA, 2012). The implementation guidelines further highlight the need for physical and emotional safety by improving cultural and factual competence. Often students in international psychology or community psychology programs lack a clinical background that prepares them for the work with, or planning of mental health services for, traumatized populations. Some switch from areas like business or management in order to find a more meaningful way to help those in need. In order to alert them to the importance as well as the opportunities in addressing trauma worldwide, it is helpful to integrate the topic of trauma into the curriculum.

The "window of tolerance" model (Corrigan, Fisher, & Nutt, 2011) is an easy way to illustrate the impact of traumatic stress on the human system. According to this model, our day-to-day experiences can be adaptively integrated when they fall within a spectrum that we have learned to tolerate. A trauma response occurs when the amount of traumatic stress we can handle has been exceeded and we have to resort to survival mechanisms such as fight, flight, or physical immobility in order to regulate our emotions. Once the level of arousal has become bearable again, we revert to thinking creatively and strategically. However, if we are unable to integrate the memories of a traumatic event, they can re-emerge in involuntary flashbacks, nightmares, physical symptoms, and other responses that interfere with daily life (Corrigan, Fisher & Nutt, 2011). Fairytales can be used to illustrate this mechanism. For example, in Grimm's Hansel and Gretel (2015), the children lost in the woods use strategic thinking and creativity to overcome the witch. They demonstrate resiliency in the face of hardship by tricking the witch on several occasions. In contrast, Sleeping Beauty (Grimm, 2014) leaves her window of tolerance and spends years in a hypo-aroused state. She only returns to active living by means of a loving connection.

Folk tales from indigenous cultures address the universal phenomenon of healing through a different lens. An indigenous tale from Guyana (Gahbler, Becker, Simon, & Stosberg-Lindert, 2016), for example, tells the story of the courtship between a lone human survivor of a war and the daughter of the vulture king. Grief-stricken, the human survivor first lies down next to the dead in the hopes of joining them. When he doesn't die, he clings to the next living creature in his reach: the daughter of the vulture king who is able to transform into a woman at will. After living with him on earth for a while, she wants to return to her family, so he joins her in the sky. There, he finds himself an outsider, forced to undergo many trials to keep his relationship with the vulture king's daughter. With the support of helpers from the natural world, he is able to complete the challenges set by her disapproving father until eventually he chooses to return to the human realm without her. He brings back a kernel of corn to begin life again on earth.

This story illustrates how trauma can take people to a different reality, away from the life they know. Little by little, they can begin to trust the world again. When they choose to return to their community, they need the necessary skills to thrive again amongst their own. Thus, the folktale highlights an indigenous approach to healing from trauma that involves re-establishing a positive relationship with the community, the environment, and the self.

Collaborations and Experiential Learning

The United Nations Department of Economic and Social Affairs (2015) authored the sustainable development goals for all participating countries, and Carriere (2014) and SAMHSA (2012) emphasized the need to understand and treat trauma collectively. After assessing, sharing, and learning about feasible projects, the implementation of initiatives is the next logical step. However, this is highly dependent on the capacity for collaboration among various partners. Experiential learning programs focusing on human rights can open up avenues for sustainable collaboration by connecting students with human rights organizations to investigate violations, participate in advocacy initiatives, and engage in human rights campaigns. Currently, such programs are mainly offered through law clinics like Harvard (The Human Rights Program, 2016) and the University of Texas at Austin (2016).

Renowned health and human rights scholar Alicia Ely Yamin emphasizes that there is no single approach to human rights in the field of global health, but human rights-based approaches aid accountability by upholding the responsibility of the state to its citizens. According to Yamin, this is the defining feature that differentiates human rights approaches from needs-based ones (Webb, 2016). In my classroom, I have observed that when assigned the task of evaluating and designing a non-profit agency, many students forget to familiarize themselves with the local context and culture. They want to "bring their knowledge," "educate the ignorant locals about the ineffectiveness of shamanism," "innovate," "change," and "bring up-to-date those ineffective local agencies." Only very few students remember values such as "self-determination," "respect to diversity," "participation and collaboration," or "support for community structures" (Nelson & Prilleltensky, 2006). To provide experiential learning opportunities in a culturally competent and rights-based approach, we recommend modeling global collaboration by including international speakers. Presenters who have worked with human rights projects worldwide can provide a practical link for the application of culturally-attuned methods in research and project development. During a recent guest lecture in my Global Mental Health and Human Rights course at TCS, Rolf Carriere discussed some ideas on how to become active global collaborators. The talk brought to life the suggestions he espoused in his article, "Scaling up What Works" (2014):

- Systematically map all significant stakeholder organizations, including pertinent UN agencies (UNHCR, Red Cross, UNICEF).
- Design a grand partnership strategy for (and with) each of them,
- Plan the first global conference on trauma therapy bringing together principal stakeholder representatives.
- Organize strategic planning meetings at national, regional, and global levels.
- Identify and approach potential champions, goodwill ambassadors, and celebrities of national and global appeal for policy advocacy and to support the cause.
- Begin work on an authoritative annual State of the World's Trauma Report.
- Produce a powerful advocacy film on EMDR and other trauma therapies (Carriere, 2014, p. 193-4).

He also invited students and readers alike to support the Global Initiative for Trauma Treatment (GIST-T), which "intends to help expand current efforts to scale up trauma treatment for peace operations personnel and humanitarian staff of international organizations, and for the traumatized populations they serve" (Carriere, personal communication, August 28, 2016). Carriere, who serves as the Senior Advisor for GIST-T, can be contacted at rolfcarriere@gmail.com for lectures or consultations and will use the proceeds to further GIST-T.

During our doctoral studies, my co-author and I found the international field experiences to be the most powerful part of our education. Visiting the organization "Community Action for a Safer Environment" (CASE) in a poverty and crime-ridden former township of Cape Town, South Africa, for example, allowed our cohort to experience hands-on how community work can be organized by the affected community members themselves. Similarly, engaging with the community-based Maori mental health programs in New Zealand left an indelible mark on our understanding of the long-term effects of colonization on the disenfranchisement of indigenous people. Our experiential learning opportunities provided us with insights that could not be gained solely through classroom activities.

Final Thoughts

As we have discussed in this chapter, the international focus on mental health taking shape with the U.N.'s Sustainable Development Agenda is an opportunity to teach awareness about global mental health and human rights. Our suggestions for an engaging, comprehensive curriculum included emphasis on the following topics:

- Effective leadership skills sensitive to non-western perspectives,
- Ethical decision making on current world events in a safe learning environment
- Social justice in the age of globalization
- Responsibility tied in with the human potential for violence and for justice
- The micro and macro levels of social injustice in our own backyard
- Individual human rights in conjunction with collective cultures
- Indigenous holistic views such as the rights of the earth
- An international perspective on mental health
- Cultural exchange and bi-directional learning
- Decolonizing research practices through collaboration with local communities based on local values
- Becoming trauma-informed
- Collaborations and experiential learning with experienced practitioners across the world.

We believe that connecting the personal and the global is necessary to stimulate out-of-the-box thinking about the complex themes in the area of global mental health and human rights. It is our hope to generate engagement and bring up-to-date information to the training of key stakeholders in psychological well-being worldwide.

References

About, Inc. (Ed.). (2016). *Interracial marriage laws.* Retrieved from http://civilliberty.about.com/od/gendersexuality/tp/Marriage-Rights-History-Timeline.htm

Amis, M., & Kuemmel, P. (2016, August 7). In Zeitonline (Ed.), *Was bedeutet dieser Irrsinn, Martin Amis?* Retrieved from http://www.zeit.de/2016/31/usa-donald-trump-terrorismus-martin-amis/komplettansicht (translated by Lutz)

APA. (Ed.). (2015, August). *APA Council Policy Manual.* Retrieved from http://www.apa.org/about/policy/

Arnett, J. (2008). The neglected 95%: why American psychology needs to become less American. *American Psychologist, 63*(7), 602–614.

Boseley, S. (2008, November 6). *Mbeki Aids denial caused 300,000 deaths.* Retrieved from https://www.theguardian.com/world/2008/nov/26/aids-south-africa

Bullock, M. (2014). Internationalization in psychology and in APA: A process, not an outcome. *Psychology International.* Retrieved from http://www.apa.org/international/pi/2014/03/column.aspx

Blyberg, A., IHRIP, (2000). *Module 17: cultural rights.* Retrieved from http://hrlibrary.umn.edu/edumat/IHRIP/circle/modules/module17b.htm

Carriere, R. (2014). Scaling up what works: using EMDR to help confront the world's burden of traumatic stress. *Journal of EMDR Practice and Research, 8*(4), 187-195.

The Chicago School of Professional Psychology. (2013). *Syllabus.* Chicago, IL: Author.

The Chicago School of Professional Psychology. (2016). *2014-2015 Academic catalog and student handbook.* Retrieved from http://catalog.thechicagoschool.edu/content.php?catoid=42&navoid=2001#Statement_of_Values_

Corrigan, F. M., Fisher, J. J., & Nutt, D. J. (2011). Autonomic dysregulation and the Window of Tolerance model of the effects of complex emotional trauma. *Journal of Psychopharmacology, 25*, 17-25.

Davis, M. (Director). (2011). *Doctors of the dark side* [Motion picture]. United States.: Shelter Island of TDC Entertainments.

De Ayala, G. P. F. (2006). *The first new chronicle and good government abridged* (D. Frye, Trans.). Indianapolis, IN: Hackett Publishing Company.

Espen Stoknes, P. (2009). *Money & soul.* Foxhole, United Kingdom: green books.

Farmer, P., Yong Kim, J., Kleinman, A., & Basilico, M. (2013). *Reimagining global health.* Berkeley, Los Angeles: University of California Pres.

Gahbler, W., Becker, F., Simon, R., & Stosberg-Lindert, U. (Eds.). (2016, August 13). *Der Besuch im Himmel.* Retrieved from Gemeinschaftspraxis fuer Anaesthesie und Schmerztherapie Web site: http://www.schmerzkreis.net/liste-der-maerchen.html

Goodman, A. (Ed.). (2016, August 9). *Matt Taibbi: Trump's all white male economic team includes 'financial crisis villain' John Paulson.* Retrieved from http://www.democracynow.org/2016/8/9/matt_taibbi_trumps_all_white_male

Galtung, J. (2008). *50 Years: 25 Intellectual landscapes explored.* Bergen, Norway: Transcend University Press.

Grimm. (2014). In R. Godwin-Jones (Ed.), *Sleeping Beauty.* Retrieved from http://germanstories.vcu.edu/grimm/dorneng.html

Grimm. (2015). In eastoftheweb shortstories (Ed.), *Brothers Grimm Hansel and Gretel.* Retrieved from http://www.eastoftheweb.com/short-stories/UBooks/HanGre.shtml

Healy, H. (2016). Fight for the heart of Europe. *New Internationalist, 489*, p.12-18.

Henrich, J., Heine, S.J., & Norenzayan, A. (2010). The weirdest people in the world? *Behavior and Brain Sciences, 33*, 61-83.

Hoffman, C. (2016). *Merkel's humane refugee policies have failed.* Retrieved from http://www.spiegel.de/international/europe/the-limits-of-humanity-merkel-refugee-policies-have-failed-a-1079455.html

The Human Rights Program. (Ed.). (2016). *Human Rights@Harvard Law: Experiential Learning.* Retrieved from udents/ad-hoc-experiential-learning-opportunities/

Incayawar, M., Wintrob, R., Bouchard, L., & Bartocci, G. (Eds.). (2009). *Psychiatrists and traditional healers: unwitting partners in global mental health.* Hoboken, NJ: Wiley & Sons.

Lehmann, M. (2011). *Maat.* Retrieved from www.oldegypt.com, (translated by Lutz)

Lillis, T. M., & Curry, M. J. (2010). *Academic writing in global context.* London: Routledge.

Lincoln, Y. S., & Gonzalez y González, E. M. G. (2008). The Search for Emerging Decolonizing Methodologies in Qualitative Research Further Strategies for Liberatory and Democratic Inquiry. *Qualitative Inquiry, 14*(5), 784-805.

Marsella, A. (2006). Justice in a global age: Becoming counselors to the world. *Counselling Psychology Quarterly, 19*, 121-132.

Marsella, A. (2012). Psychology and globalization: understanding a complex relationship. *Journal of Social Issues, 68*, 454-472.

Marsella, A. J. (1997). "Globalization and psychosocial health and well being." Honolulu, HI: Public Lecture, Globalization Lecture Series, Matsunaga Peace Institute, University of Hawaii.

Marsella, A. J. (2001). "Globalization and psychology." Invited Address. Los Angeles, CA: American Psychological Association Annual Convention.

Minkler, M., & Wallerstein, N. (Eds.). (2008). *Community-based participatory research for health: From process to outcomes.* San Francisco, CA: John Wiley & Sons.

Moodley, R., & West, W. (Eds.). (2005). *Integrating traditional healing practices into counseling and psychotherapy.* Thousand Oaks, CA: Sage.

Mun Wah, L. (Director). (1994). *The color of fear* [Motion picture]. United States: Veremos Productions LLC.

Nelson, G., & Prilleltensky, I. (2006). *Community Psychology: in pursuit of liberation and well-being.* New York: Palgrave-MacMillan.

Patel, V., Minas, H., Cohen, A., & Prince, M. J. (Eds.). (2014). *Global mental health: Principles and practice.* New York: Oxford University Press.

Read, J. N. G., & Bartkowski, J. P. (2000). To veil or not to veil? A case study of identity negotiation among Muslim women in Austin, Texas. *Gender & Society, 14*(3), 395-417.

Ruby, T. F. (2006, February). Listening to the voices of hijab. *Women's Studies International Forum, 29*(1), 54-66.

Silva, C. (2009). In Seattle Civil Rights & Labor History Project (Eds.), *Racial restrictive covenants: enforcing neighborhood segregation in Seattle.* Retrieved from http://depts.washington.edu/civilr/covenants_report.htm

Simonds, V. W., & Christopher, S. (2013). Adapting western research methods to indigenous ways of knowing. *American Journal of Public Health, 103*(12), 2185–2192.

Smith, D. J. and Valentine, T. (2012). The use and perceived effectiveness of instructional practices in two-year technical colleges. *Journal on Excellence in College Teaching, 23*(1), 133-161.

Substance Abuse and Mental Health Services Administration. (2012). SAMHSA's working definition of trauma and principles and guidance for a trauma-informed approach [Draft].Rockville, MD: Substance Abuse and Mental Health Services Administration.

Substance Abuse and Mental Health Services Administration. (2014) *Trauma-informed care in behavioral health services: Treatment improvement protocol (TIP) Series 57.* HHS Publication No. (SMA) 13-4801. Rockville, MD: Substance Abuse and Mental Health Services Administration.

United Nations. (1948, December 10). *The Universal Declaration of Human Rights.* Retrieved from http://www.un.org/en/documents/udhr/

United Nations Department of Economic, & Social Affairs. (Eds.). (2015, September). *Sustainable Development Knowledge Platform.* Retrieved from https://sustainabledevelopment.un.org/#

The University of Texas at Austin. (Ed.). (2016). *Learn more about the human rights clinic.* Retrieved from https://law.utexas.edu/clinics/human-rights/course-info/about/

UShistory.org. (Ed.). (2016). *America in the Second World War: 51e. Japanese-American Internment.* Retrieved from http://www.ushistory.org/us/51e.asp

Wasserstein, B. (2011, February 17). *European refugee movements after World War Two.* Retrieved from http://www.bbc.co.uk/history/worldwars/wwtwo/refugees_01.shtml

Watters, E. (2010). *Crazy like us.* New York: The Free Press.

Webb, A. (2016, September 7). *Health, equity and human rights.* Retrieved from http://humanrights.uconn.edu/2016/09/07/health-equity-and-human-rights-whats-the-added-value-of-a-rights-based-approach/

World Health Organization. (Ed.). (2016). *Comprehensive mental health action plan 2013-220.* Retrieved from http://www.who.int/mental_health/action_plan_2013/en/

CHAPTER 18

The Role of Mental Health in Peacebuilding Interventions: A 3B's Analysis Approach

Tristan Hansell, Lisa M. Brown, and Robert Groelsema

This chapter argues that when trauma interventions are informed by culture and context, we are able to come to a deeper understanding of factors that foster resilience in communities and contribute to more effective ways of healing and peacebuilding. Several studies have emerged indicating that using Western approaches to treat mental illness in non-Western cultures could, in some instances, result in detrimental effects such as increasing traumatic stress or complicating the recovery process (Sijbrandij, Olff, Reitsma, Carlier, & Gersons, 2006). The understandably high estimates of mental health disorders in post-conflict and conflict societies make analyzing the role of mental health within peacebuilding interventions imperative. Interventions that address mental health from culturally sensitive, psychosocial perspectives not only contribute to the well-being of individuals and societies, but also have the potential to strengthen peacebuilding initiatives and reduce conflict recidivism.

Applying a mental health perspective to peacebuilding aids in understanding the high resurgence of conflict in fragile states and can inform development or implementation of alternative approaches to solving complex issues in low resource environments (Pham, Weinstein, & Longman, 2004; Vinck, Pham, Stover, & Weinstein, 2007). The mental health of those living in conflict and transitional societies, particularly those who are displaced, is complicated by contextual factors. Psychological health is influenced by pre-existing disorders, traumatic experiences during conflict, and post-conflict psychosocial stressors and resource insufficiency.

392

In this chapter, psychosocial interventions are defined as interventions developed to positively influence both relationships within communities and individual thought and behavior, not to the exclusion of biopsychological interventions. Though the exclusion of biopsychological interventions often forms the distinction between medical and psychosocial interventions, researchers in this field have become increasingly aware of the need for combining biological, psychological, and social approaches (Williamson & Robinson, 2006). This combination leads to the development of integrated care for patients. Integration of care is important in cases of trauma when expressions of distress can often be somatic, stigmatizing, and variable in different cultures and contexts.

To illustrate the effectiveness of psychosocial interventions and peacebuilding interventions on global mental health, we will consider a *binding, bonding, and bridging* (3B's) perspective. The 3B's model was developed by Catholic Relief Services (CRS) as a community peacebuilding strategy to strengthen social cohesion in deeply divided, conflict-affected societies (CRS, 20106). To the bonding and bridging of social capital theory, the 3Bs methodology adds binding, which is the space for mental and emotional healing and transformation that occurs within an individual. Binding at an individual level is intended to facilitate effective relationship building within single-identity groups (bonding), and for resolving intergroup grievances and reconnecting estranged and adversarial groups across social divides (bridging) (CRS, 2016). We will refer to these concepts throughout the chapter to highlight aspects of psychosocial peacebuilding interventions.

This chapter draws on four main strands of literature: global health, political science, sociology, and psychology. It utilizes case studies from Africa, the Middle East, and South America to illustrate how culture and context relate to conflict, peacebuilding and mental health. To highlight key components of psychosocial peacebuilding, we divide our discussion into four parts. First, we examine the "psych" of psychosocial, second, we look at the "social' within psychosocial, third, we describe the impact of conflict and trauma on youth, and fourth, we emphasize the importance of mental health to peacebuilding and to preventing conflict recidivism.

The Psych in Psychosocial

Culturally informed practices help mitigate the stigma surrounding mental health in many countries. Trauma, shame, guilt, grief, anxiety, and depression typify conflict and post-conflict societies. Acknowledging these aspects and embedding mental health interventions in tandem with other health programming such as maternal-child care, nutrition, and infectious disease prevention reduces stigma, facilitates access to health care, and provides much needed conjunctive care (Jegannathan, Kullgren, & Deva,

2015). Eisenman et al. (2006) observed how primary care providers in post-conflict societies focused on recognition of trauma symptoms and effectively managed mental health disorders, which in turn increased access to care for patients. By focusing on somatization symptoms and applying culturally-informed diagnoses and treatments, Eisenman and colleagues contend that developmental health programs can help destigmatize mental health, reduce misdiagnoses, and adapt Western approaches to treat mental health in post-conflict societies more effectively.

Women are particularly vulnerable to abuse and stigmatization during violent conflicts (Gizelis, 2011). They also cope with domestic abuse, and in theocracies, high levels of discrimination and marginalization (Hajjar, 2014). Because of rape and sexual and physical assault, women contract sexually transmitted diseases and have unwanted pregnancies that lead to rejection by their families and communities. Strategies to counter stigma and shame include building resilience, acknowledging personal strengths, and putting value on physical and social assets. Treatment provided in Sierra Leone illustrates the value of contextual mental health programming that specifically focuses on destigmatizing women's mental health in a post-conflict society (Betancourt et al., 2010).

Sierra Leone

From 1991 to 2002, Sierra Leone experienced a brutal civil war between the ruling regime and the Revolutionary United Front (RUF). Fueled by blood diamonds, the decade-long war resulted in thousands of deaths and the displacement of hundreds of thousands more (de Jong, Mulhern, Ford, van der Kam, & Kleber, 2000, p. 2068). Questionnaires collected from Sierra Leone residents in 1999 documented that 41% of respondents witnessed the murder of a loved one and 99% suffered from a trauma disturbance (de Jong et al., 2000, p. 2067). Civilians caught in the violence were raped, tortured, and killed by perpetrators from both sides of the conflict (Amowitz et al., 2002).

The conflict left an entire population either directly or indirectly traumatized. Tens of thousands became disabled through torture and the amputation of limbs (Berghs, 2011, p.1402). Amputees became unwanted reminders of the past and were stigmatized and shunned by society, resulting in their inability to provide for themselves and their families (Amowitz et al., 2002). Humanitarian programs designed to address their mental and physical needs and to decrease stigma had some success (Conteh & Berghs, 2014). One intervention relied upon traditional proverbs to lessen stigma and to encourage acceptance, forgivenesss, and reconciliation by developing a "there's no bad bush" campaign (Stovel, 2008). Another program established soccer leagues for the disabled to reconnect amputees to their home communities and to encourage resilience

(Wessells, 2008). Other forms of financial and social support came from the national government, non-governmental organizations (NGOs), and the international community and assisted war victims with transportation, crutches, and jobs. However, the humanitarian assistance eventually shifted towards programs focused on poverty reduction and mainstream national health, thereby leaving the needs of many amputees inadequately addressed (Conteh and Berghs, 2014).

Stigma also affected women abductees. Although male and female returnees were stereotyped as violent – and were therefore avoided and isolated – female returnees were also considered damaged property and were ostracized. As such, they were unable to marry and prosper (Betancourt et al., 2008). One of the most effective methods to counter stigma was to encourage family and the community to help returning female child soldiers reintegrate into society (Theresa Stichick Betancourt et al., 2010). Families and communities applied traditional healing practices that spiritually cleansed females, making them culturally acceptable (Stark, 2006). For male soldiers, community-based interventions that encouraged dialog and truth telling were found to be effective. For both males and females, interventions that combined traditional healing techniques, such as dance and use of proverbs, increased empathy between members from all groups of society (Wessells, 2008).

In contrast to grassroots approaches, the highly visible national Truth and Reconciliation Commission (TRC) processes mostly failed to achieve "reparations and reform" (Graybill, 2011). Instead of connecting victims to family and community support systems, the TRC tried to offer a gender sensitive stage in which victims' voices could be heard. From a mental health perspective, rehabilitation efforts could have been more successful if they had addressed issues that the women cared about most, such as providing for their children and restoring relationships with friends and family (Graybill, 2011).

Similarly, Medeiros (2007) found that many of the street children in Sierra Leone were former child soldiers who had been stigmatized and shunned by their family and community. The loss of social support from their soldier and home communities rendered this population especially vulnerable to negative mental health outcomes. However, without adequate interventions to increase individual, group, and community trauma awareness and resilience, ex-child soldiers turned to street gangs for acceptance – a lost opportunity for healing. Traumatized Sierra Leonean children, youth, and their support communities inflicted long-term social costs on the country to the detriment of reconstituting scarce social capital, rebuilding critical social cohesion, and avoiding conflict recidivism.

On a more positive note, since 2002, Sierra Leone has held non-United Nations-supervised elections and witnessed a peaceful transfer of power at the ballot box. The country has also overcome a major Ebola public health crisis. Continued incorporation of mental health into public health settings and utilization of gender-neutral assessments and treatments has aided in destigmatizing mental health treatment in Sierra Leone (Betancourt et al., 2008; Medeiros, 2007).

Refugees and Internally Displaced Persons (IDPs)

Impacts on refugees and internally displaced persons (IDPs) are essential considerations in peacebuilding outcomes, both in regards to the void created in their home communities and for the challenges faced when reintegrating and coexisting with host communities. Many victims of violence and conflict seek refuge in camps in neighboring countries sometimes for days or weeks, and often for years. It is common for refugees to be stereotyped as violent and mistaken for ex-soldiers. Consequently, refugees experience maladaptive psychosocial adjustment, much like many Liberian refugees who fled to Sierra Leone did (Abdullah, 1998). Refugees also suffer discrimination and victim-blaming. They often are dismissed as poor, lazy, violent, or gangster-like (Loescher, 2002). Refugees with temporary resident status were found to have poorer mental health outcomes, and fears resulting from past trauma experiences have been linked to resistance to repatriate (Steel et al., 2006). Given the sizeable numbers of refugees worldwide, it seems logical to focus greater attention on their long-term psychosocial needs. Such interventions could advance social cohesion, peacebuilding, and development.

Refugee psychology has become a field of its own. It encompasses trauma due to separation from loved ones, loss of occupation and home, and estrangement from familiar surroundings. In practice, mental health therapy, psychological assessment, and social support services typically receive limited attention in resettlement communities. Deeper psychosocial capacity building, which is vital for successful co-existence with host communities and for resettlement, is often missing. Cultural orientation and language trainings are important, but orienting refugees to the host communities' political, economic, and social services systems and introducing them to social norms and outlets within the refugee and host communities allows for economic and social capital acquisition. As CRS' experience in northwest Central African Republic and Cameroon shows, binding, bonding, and bridging exercises conducted with IDPs, refugees, and refugee-impacted communities can be highly effective in facilitating the return of IDPs and refugees to their homes (Talla, 2016).

Mental health initiatives for refugees and IDPs must take into account the cultural underpinnings from the person's past and must consider the effects of resettlement processes. The lack of self-determination within resettlement has been associated with negative outcomes, including poor mental health and violence (Simich, 2003). Refugees should be empowered and assisted to seek out extended family for better resettlement outcomes (Simich, 2003). Experience shows that when refugees going through resettlement are guided by individual volunteers, stress is reduced, academic achievement is higher, and employment prospects improve (Mcspadden, 1987). Building social capital within resettlement communities starts with trauma interventions, and effective strategies for strong social cohesion are needed on individual, societal, and political levels (Elliott, & Yusuf, 2014).

The Social in Psychosocial

Mental health is connected to intragroup bonding and intergroup bridging in conflict zones. Putting an end to fighting, protecting civilians, creating safe spaces, and holding intra- and inter-group meetings are vital to peacebuilding (Korir, 2009). In addition, individual transformative peacebuilding can empower other individuals in groups and can develop social capacity for political change (Plonski, 2005).

The symbiotic relationship between psychological and social interventions eliminates the need to focus exclusively on one approach. When a person is able to process their own trauma, they become emotionally available to empathize with opposition groups; similarly, this ability to empathize increases protective factors against mental health disorders (Weder, García-Nieto, & Canneti-Nisim, 2011). Bosnia and Herzegovina are good examples of bottom-up peacebuilding endeavors in which an emphasis was placed on developing shared understanding and relationships that promote social cohesion and peacebuilding, with examples of both bonding and bridging interventions (Phillips, Hemmer, Garb, & Graham, 2006). Interventions aimed at increasing horizontal social capital in the Israel-Palestine conflict and in Bosnia and Herzegovina will be explored next. Comparative outcomes stress the importance of mental health, culture, and context in promoting the development of social cohesion.

Israel-Palestine Conflict

The Israeli-Palestinian conflict is historically deep-rooted and long-lasting, and it has been devastatingly traumatic for both sides. Disputes began in the late 1800's over sovereignty during the Zionist movement and became an inter-state conflict with the establishment of Israel in 1948 (Shafir, 1989). There have been multiple attempts to build peace, the most recent of which involved two-party state solution (Breslau, 2010). Since this conflict is deeply rooted in history, the issues dividing the principal actors are embedded within generational culture. In contexts like this, psychosocial interventions must base their efforts in both psychological and sociological principles aimed at reducing intergroup bias. At the same time, they must give recognition to individual suffering and points of view. Horizontal social capacity building across ethnic groups allows for recognition of in-group experiences. Concurrently, it recognizes similar experiences in outgroups and attempts to eliminate in-group bias through both bonding and bridging (Handelman, 2016).

Several programs in Palestine have attempted to bridge the divide between Israelis and Palestinians. *Beyond Bullets and Bombs: Grassroots Peacebuilding between Israelis and Palestinians* (Kuriansky, 2007) provides illustrations of such initiatives. To stand a better chance of obtaining peaceful conflict outcomes, Kuriansky highlights the need for developing and sharing trauma narratives within and between adversarial groups by combining elements of bonding and bridging (see also Ross, 2004). Socialization of the population within institutional settings like schools, associations, clubs, and places of worship also offers promising avenues to reshape entrenched attitudes and behavior (Paffenholz, 2010). Wallach and Wallach (2000) found that bringing schoolchildren to neutral places to develop relationships humanizes "the other" and reduces the tendency to label and stereotype. Furthermore, acknowledgment of past suffering and traumatic experiences can aid in the process of rehabilitation and reconciliation when implementing programs (Becker, 2015). Above all, it may be argued that although difficult and time consuming, grassroots, person-to-person interventions are the most realistic approach for enabling change within the holy land because of the deep-rooted, long-repeated narrative from both sides that impedes progress in social and political reform (Weder et al., 2011).

Bosnia and Herzegovina

The Bosnian War (1992-1995) witnessed fighting among Muslim Bosnians, Orthodox Serbs, and Catholic Croats in a bid for sovereignty following the dissolution of the former Yugoslav territory (Belloni, 2009). At least 20,000 persons were raped, 100,000 people died, and more than two million were displaced (Momartin, Silove, Manicavasagar, & Steel, 2004, p. 232). The war ended with intervention from North Atlantic Treaty Organization (NATO) forces (Daalder, 1998) and the signing of the Dayton peace agreement in 1995 (Belloni, 2009).

Although the Dayton Accords brought an end to overt conflict, the agreement encouraged ethno-national politics in Bosnia and Herzegovina (Pinkerton, 2016). As a result, the belligerents erected post-war barriers between ethnic groups while vying for power in what they viewed as a zero-sum game. Given the situation, post-war psychosocial programs were developed to address both trauma and social cohesion by reducing inter-ethnic barriers (Derrida, 1997) and by eliminating systemic intergroup bias and favoritism on societal and political levels (Keil & Perry, 2015).

Among the daunting psychosocial challenges facing the new country was the prevalence of Post-Traumatic Stress Disorder (PTSD) in children. Although depression and anxiety disorders were found to be within normal clinical limits after the war, the rate of PTSD in children was estimated to be 74% (Smith, Perrin, Yule, Hacam, & Stuvland, 2002, p. 147). Similarly, a decrease in perceived power and self-esteem, associated with depressive symptoms, was noted in the general population (Carballo et al., 2004). This decrease has been linked to the continuing political ethnic divisions in the country that foster interethnic competition and discrimination. These divisions prevent citizens from forming interethnic associations and coalitions that could otherwise aggregate social, economic, and political needs across groups and constructively engage with and hold the government accountable to the will of people for the common good (see Carballo et al., 2004).

One means of treating PTSD and raising self-esteem in Bosnia and Herzegovina was addressing stigma. Researchers have found that simply replacing the phrase "mental illness" with "mental health" allowed people who would benefit from treatment to accept help (Hasanović, Sinanović, Pajević, Avdibegović, & Sutović, 2006). In other instances, researchers observed that using music and art therapy trauma reduced symptoms in children (Heidenreich, 2005; Kollontai, 2010; Hasanovic et al., 2009). If interventions aimed at addressing trauma have failed, it is largely because they did not recognize that the comorbidity with mood disorders was also related to continued divisions between families, soaring unemployment, lack of resources, and displacement (Carballo et al., 2004).

Above all, the goal of social cohesion interventions was to bring people together to develop empathy, compassion, trust, and communication. Similar to the soccer leagues for the disabled in Sierra Leone, youth football leagues restored families and communities and built inter-ethnic relationships in Bosnia and Herzegovina; however, some sports programs in active conflict zones fostered intergroup bias (Gasser & Levinsen, 2004). Further, instead of bridging social and ethnic divides, the distribution of foreign aid and government institutions within the country have reinforced ethnic boundaries, thereby perpetuating the conflict (Carballo et al., 2004).

In sum, post-war Bosnia and Herzegovina faced significant developmental challenges that were more formidable and difficult to address because of interethnic barriers and untreated trauma. 41% of the population had acquaintances only from their own ethnic group (O'Loughlin, 2010, p. 47). The minimal social trust among adult populations (Hoogenboom & Vieille, 2010) and the high levels of PTSD in children could benefit from a more holistic psychosocial approach along the lines of the 3Bs. Moreover, greater attention to the vertical axis of social cohesion could alleviate the structural discrimination perpetuated by the state.

Nearly half of the population of Bosnia and Herzegovina wanted to develop friendships with other nationalities (O'Loughlin, 2010, p. 47). If this interest could be coupled with an emerging awareness of the critical role that caregivers play in mental health and peacebuilding, the country would have more effective programming focused on psychosocial family interventions that promote development of coping skills, knowledge of child development, communication skills, and normalizing of experiences through group work (Dybdahl, 2001).

The Challenge of Youth

South Africa is often praised for its peaceful post-apartheid transition. Citizens hoped they would find forgiveness and justice through the Truth and Reconciliation Commission (TRC), but two decades later, South Africans express discontent regarding the lack of justice and progress in equal economic opportunities and land redistribution. Globally, South Africa ranks in the top ten for the highest crime rates (Breetzke, 2016, p. 277), has the fourth-highest prevalence of HIV/AIDS (CIA, 2014, People and Society subsection, para. 25), and has the world's second-highest inequality in wealth distribution as measured by the Gini Index (.63) (CIA, 2014, People and Society subsection, Country Comparison-Gini Index Table).

According to the CIA, South Africa typifies the developing world's youth bulge and high population growth rate. South Africa has 54.3 million (para. 1) people with an annual population growth rate of .99% (para. 10) (CIA, 2014, People and Society subsection). Fifty-four per cent of South Africans are younger than 24 years of age (CIA, 2014, People and Society subsection, para. 7). As with Sierra Leonean youth, South African youths have experienced devastating losses. In South Africa, these losses include the deaths of family members and friends from acquired immune deficiency syndrome (AIDS). Furthermore, youth have been exposed to crime and urban violence and face dismal job prospects. Approximately 22% of the population has had no schooling, and only 12% has had access to higher education (Rensburg & Botha, 2014, p.145). Reducing crime rates, preventing gang violence, and strengthening social cohesion over the long term will depend on effective psychosocial interventions and youth programs (Chase et al., 2007). Internationally, the growing number of children being forced to participate in conflict as perpetrators has led to severe damaging effects on an individual and societal level (Chase et al., 2007). Psychosocial interventions designed specifically for former child soldiers in northern Uganda and Mozambique might serve as models for other countries where psychosocial interventions for youth are in short supply.

Mozambique

The Mozambique Civil War began in 1977 and lasted until 1992. Fighting between the ruling party, the Front for Liberalization of Mozambique (FRELIMO), and the Mozambique Resistance Movement (RENAMO), claimed almost one million lives and displaced more than five million more (Andersson, 2016, p. 28). Both sides committed atrocities, engaged in forced enlistment, forcibly relocated civilians to cramped camps and villages, and took away their livelihoods (Englund, 2002). Actions by both RENAMO and FRELIMO led to massive starvation of civilians, resulting in hundreds of thousands of deaths (Andersson, 2016, p. 29).

In 1992, following the Rome Peace Accords, United Nations (U.N.) peacekeeping forces entered the country and oversaw a two-year transition culminating in national elections (Fearon, Humphreys, & Weinstein, 2009). Traditional healers in village and town ceremonies conducted one of the more effective programs. Local leaders brought child soldiers back into their home communities to cleanse them of the "war pollution" they had acquired in battle (Pouligny, 2005). Elders and spiritual leaders led symbolic ceremonies in which victims/perpetrators of war could shed the evil that came from being in war and be forgiven and welcomed back into the community (Stark, 2006). In contrast, in a Western therapeutic intervention, Mozambique youth verbally acknowledged their trauma instead of processing it through spiritual experiences or community practices. This resulted in negative effects leading to increased symptomatology (Honwana, 1997).

Despite the relative success of psychosocial programs in Mozambique, fresh fighting between RENAMO and the highly centrist and autocratic FRELIMO-led government broke out in 2013 (Reisinger, 2009). A number of factors accounted for this relapse into violence. They included the politicization of international aid, corrupt resource management (Reppell, Rozen, & de Carvalho, 2016), failure to decentralize the government, and lack of collaboration among peacekeeping and peacebuilding organizations (Reppell, Rozen, & de Carvalho, 2016). In addition, the United Nations Development Program (UNDP) short-term peace building focused on disarmament, demobilization, and reintegration (DDR), rather than on conflict resolution, mental health services, and social cohesion (LeFranc, 2011). As absorptive, adaptive, and transformative capacities of youthful individuals and communities expand, they will improve their resilience to endogenous and exogenous shocks, and they will be better positioned in the future to demand democratic decentralization and accountability for transparent, inclusive government services (Usaid, 2012).

Uganda

Uganda has experienced protracted periods of violent conflict from the Idi Amin dictatorship of the 1970s to the armed rebellion and ascendency to power of Yoweri Museveni in 1986. From 1987 to 2010, self-proclaimed prophet, Joseph Kony, led a movement called the Lord's Resistance Army (LRA), which staged attacks on government forces, but also forcibly recruited child soldiers, kidnapped and enslaved girls, committed atrocities against civilians, and generally terrorized the Acholi people of northeastern Uganda (Vinck et al., 2007). Citizens were caught between the LRA and Museveni's troops in a catch-22 of assumed guilt from both sides (Roberts, Ocaka, Browne, Oyok, & Sondorp, 2008). Some two million IDPs were moved into confined areas resembling concentration camps, which the LRA could easily attack (Branch, 2007, p. 181).

In 2006, a ceasefire was reached between Museveni's Ugandan People's Defense Force (UPDF) and the LRA that pushed the remaining LRA forces into neighboring territories. The peacebuilding process that followed was contentious. The involvement of the International Criminal Court (ICC) pitted proponents of retributive justice against advocates for restorative justice and traditional reconciliation. Moreover, the blurred lines between perpetrators and victims complicated the peacebuilding process. Over the course of the war, the LRA recruited more than 25,000 children and forced them to fight and commit atrocities (Chatlani, 2006, p. 278). Although reaching peace was the main goal of Ugandan citizens, prosecuting only LRA and not UPDF combatants was perceived as a double standard (Chatlani, 2006).

Often described as a war on children, the LRA-UPDF conflict provided insights for evaluating peacebuilding interventions targeted at youth. First, researchers found that citizens living with PTSD or depression in Uganda were more likely to prefer violent over peaceful means for ending the conflict (Vinck et al., 2007). Second, the way traumatic events were processed was found to dramatically affect mental health outcomes, especially for children (Betancourt & Khan, 2008). Third, "meaning making" after traumatic events was found to reduce or prevent the development of PTSD (Betancourt, Meyers-Ohki, Charrow, & Tol, 2013). Following exposure to life-altering traumatic events, child soldiers, IDPs, and refugees reported that their whole world changed. Often, the people essential in processing the events were no longer part of a child's life. Child soldiers were subjected to forced violence, substance abuse, sexual assault, and physical and psychological torture. The extent of suffering, the fragmentation of society, and the absence of individual social support created the need for in-depth, widespread, and extended rehabilitation programs (Roberts et al., 2008).

Individual therapeutic interventions have been shown to be effective in youth populations in Uganda, and even though it is not feasible to deliver these interventions to a large majority of the population, they should not be undervalued because of the extent of trauma within this population. By using local trainees as therapists and conducting sessions within community home settings, narrative exposure therapy has shown to be effective at reducing PTSD symptoms in former child soldiers in Uganda (Ertl et al., 2010). Interpersonal therapy was also found effective in adolescent girls (but not boys) in reducing depression and PTSD symptoms (Bolton et al., 2007). Research has focused on interventions with the specific aim of reducing trauma, but a deeper understanding of factors of resilience within the child soldier subgroup of the population is needed (Betancourt & Khan, 2008).

Societal level interventions to address trauma in Uganda have been designed mainly through the lens of resilience by focusing on social support, meaning making, and attachment (Betancourt & Khan, 2008). Meaning making following a traumatic event is the way in which one is able to understand and make sense of events and is a significant contributor to mental health outcomes in individuals. The separation from family and loved ones following traumatic events disrupted attachment patterns and altered meaning making in youth. This contributed to poor mental health outcomes and the determent of resilience.

Psychosocial interventions focusing on resilience and developmental goals that were conducted in school-based settings were found ineffective across four countries in the region (Ertl & Neuner, 2014). Studies like these underscore the importance of culture and context, individual experience, reaction, and meaning making during war (Kalksma-Van Lith, 2007). Scholarly research also showed that the role and experience of females in conflict must be given distinct attention. There is a need for gender-sensitive health programs as well as programs designed to decrease stigmatization and increase recognition of traumatic experiences for women during war (Liebling-Kalifani et al., 2008).

Mental Health and Recidivism

According to the International Federation of Red Cross and Red Crescent Societies (IFRC), psychosocial interventions promote the restoration of social cohesion. In turn, social cohesion fosters a decreased chance for recidivism of violence by striving to restore fundamental aspects of a community like trust and resilience. Although it is often argued that economic factors are the main determinants of conflict recidivism (P. Collier, Hoeffler, & Soderbom, 2008), one report found that World Bank spending had "no systematic effect on either conflict recurrence or economic recovery" (Flores & Nooruddin, 2009, p. 1). Recidivism, instead, was linked to anti-social personality traits, lack of education, and weak social support in former soldiers (Kaplan & Nussio, 2016).

To understand the link between mental health and conflict recidivism, it is helpful to compare and contrast experiences from post-conflict societies that have succeeded in maintaining the peace with those of societies that have slid back into conflict. In this respect, we will single out the role of social cohesion strengthening related to mental health in conflict and post-conflict societies. Research shows that 20-50% of countries that have experienced violent conflict return to civil war within a five year period (Suhrke & Samset, 2007, p. 195).

Columbia

Columbia experienced one of the longest violent conflicts. It concluded in 2016 with a peace agreement between the government and the rebel forces, the Revolutionary Armed Forces of Colombia (FARC). The conflict was known as the "forever war" because violence raged for more than fifty years, making the conflict the longest civil war in world history (Johnson & Jonsson, 2013). The FARC claimed to represent the economically disadvantaged and rapidly gained support from other military and rebel groups that shared their goal to restore government to the people (Gill, 2008). Hundreds of thousands died, millions were displaced, and millions more suffered human rights violations committed by both sides of the conflict (Gill, 2008, p. 136). In 2012, peace negotiations began but were bogged down over the issue of amnesty for FARC fighters (Johnson & Jonsson, 2013). Most Columbians were in favor of punitive justice, which made it virtually impossible to reunite former combatants with their families and reintegrate into their communities (Kaplan & Nussio, 2016).

Poor mental health outcomes are often associated with increased recidivism in post-conflict societies. Indeed, some studies have identified appetitive aggression as a protective factor against the development of PTSD (Meyer-Parlapanis et al., 2016). Appetitive aggression is the positive regard towards violent and aggressive acts. In Colombia, those who willingly gave up fighting and had low appetitive aggression, in contrast to those who were forced to disarm collectively, were more likely to develop PTSD and therefore to be more predisposed to violence (Weierstall, Castellanos, Neuner, & Elbert, 2013). This is an important point within the context of peacebuilding and elimination of potential recurring violence. Although former soldiers suffering from PTSD might receive more interventions and aid, those showing resilience were more likely to return to violence because of appetitive aggressive tendencies.

Evaluating individual-level reactions and meaning making after conflict is essential to appropriately applying interventions to decrease recidivism rates. The involvement of IDPs in the peacebuilding process and in determining funding and reconciliation measures has been noted in research conducted in Colombia and has been a deterrent in other state's progress to peace (as noted previously) (Ferris, 2009). In Colombia, mental health has been found to be most directly correlated to income, rather than to negative social capital (Harpham, Grant, & Rodriguez, 2004). Being a woman and lacking education were the two factors that contribute most to poor mental health. This illustrates the need for both bottom-up and top-down peacebuilding processes as a means to stop recidivism. In Colombia, traumatic experiences and social fabric were not found to be as influential on mental health outcomes relative to economic and educational opportunities (Harpham et al., 2004).

Central African Republic

Since independence in 1960, the Central African Republic (CAR) has experienced cycles of violent conflict and coup d'états (Kane, 2014). CAR sits at the epicenter of an unstable region, which includes Darfur, Sudan, South Sudan, and northeast Democratic Republic of the Congo (DRC). The LRA continues to terrorize villagers in northeast DRC, South Sudan, and southeast CAR. The Seleka rebellion began in December 2012 when a coalition of fighters from the north swept across the country, eventually seizing Bangui on March 24, 2013 (Groelsema & Talla, 2016). Many youth, facing bleak employment prospects, joined armed groups. Violence, lawlessness, and destruction of property ensued, targeting civilians. Anti-Balaka militias sprang up to counter Seleka, ultimately forcing many indigenous and *Mbororo* (Peuhl herders) Muslims to flee the northwest. In 2014, a transitional government was established, and in late 2015 and early 2016, Faustin Archange Touadera was elected president in national elections.

Although the recent conflict is rooted in poor governance and inequality, conflict actors seized upon differences in faith to divide communities. The resulting inter-religious dynamic polarized CAR and instilled fear, mistrust, and hatred between Muslims and Christians. The horrific atrocities were considered by some to be genocide (Vinck & Pham, 2010). To address social disintegration, the interim government requested CRS to train its leaders and civil servants in social cohesion. Some 1,000 officials from the Ministry of Reconciliation and other government agencies, in addition to civil society leaders, participated in CRS' social cohesion strengthening workshops during 2014-2015 (Groelsema & Talla, 2016, p. 2, "How we do it" subsection).

Much of the recent violence occurred within IDP camps, where displaced individuals and families sought protection and food. Observers estimated that the majority of Central Africans witnessed violence directly and that more than half of the adult population qualified as depressed or suffering from anxiety (Vinck & Pham, 2010, p. 544). Deep divisions along sectarian lines made it imperative that bonding and bridging activities continued in the post-conflict period. However, in late 2016, large Muslim populations were still residing across the border in Chad and Cameroon (Kane, 2014). To initiate bonding and bridging, CRS led social cohesion workshops in northeast Cameroon with Mbororo Muslim refugees and their host communities and with Christian residents of home communities where Muslims had fled. These activities were vital for preparing refugees and IDPs to return to home communities and increased the chances for success of DDR programs.

Efforts to establish peace and stability were long-term in CAR. In collaboration with USAID and the Gerald and Henrietta Rauenhorst (GHR) Foundation, CRS began leading a Global Development Alliance (GDA) consortium in 2015, which supported an Inter-Religious Platform (IRP) in implementing horizontal and vertical social cohesion strengthening, livelihoods development, and peace education nationally within CAR. The social cohesion component utilized the 3Bs model to which elements of Appreciate Inquiry (AI) were added (CRS, 2016). The GDA consortium enlisted Palo Alto University, an institution focused on psychological research and clinical training, to evaluate and inform psychosocial practices. The intent was that collaboration among government, local and international NGOs, civil society, and researchers would result in more informed and effective mental health practices forming an integral part of peacebuilding processes.

Conclusion

This chapter reviewed the significance of culture and context in informing trauma and highlighted differences in coping, symptoms, meaning making, and factors of resilience. The case of Israel and Palestine can be used to illustrate the role of mental health within binding, bonding, and bridging (referred to as the 3Bs framework) of peacebuilding. People who experienced war or structural violence needed binding for personal transformation; they needed bonding with members of their identity group to reach agreement on their historical grievances, present demands, and view of the "other"; they needed bridging to engage traditional adversaries in non-violent, productive ways that acknowledged the right of the other to exist, to mutually prosper, and to live harmoniously with each other. Although the mix and sequencing of binding, bonding, and bridging activities will vary according to context, post-conflict and conflict-prone countries like Sierra Leone, Columbia, and CAR can advance peacebuilding and avoid conflict recidivism through a more intentional and informed combination of psychosocial and broader peacebuilding activities for traumatized civilian populations.

The integrative model, developed by Miller and Rasmussen (2010), applied a sequenced approach to mental health intervention first by addressing daily stressors and then by providing essential mental health services for people who were still struggling after their daily stressors had been reduced or better managed. Nonetheless, many of the necessary coping skills needed for addressing and eliminating daily stressors were often attained via mental health treatment. In highly conflicted environments like Colombia, providing opportunities to overcome daily stressors should not be stigmatized or considered detrimental. In contexts of war and mass violence, in which trauma and social fracturing are the main contributors to poor mental health, psychosocial peacebuilding can enhance mental health while contributing to more productive and sustainable social, political, and economic outcomes.

This review is not meant to denigrate Western mental health practices. Rather, it highlights the additional benefits of socio-cultural approaches, which together accentuate the benefits of citizen involvement in decision-making. Acknowledging the intertwining nature of mental health, social cohesion, and peacebuilding paves the way for reconciliation on multiple levels. A vibrant social fabric is a key contributor to resilience. Developing social cohesion, through horizontal bonding and bridging and vertical social capitalization, aids in protecting against recidivism and negative mental health outcomes.

Interventions that address mental health in conflict or post-conflict societies are increasing internationally and have the goal of destigmatizing access and use of mental health treatment. The role mental health plays within peace-building processes is increasingly acknowledged, and this allows for the development of culturally appropriate assessments and treatments. Research should first establish the relevance and appropriate approach within a particular population and then continue to expand on developing and evaluating the effectiveness of culturally adapted mental health interventions.

References

Amowitz, L. L., Reis, C., Lyons, K. H., Vann, B., Mansaray, B., Akinsulure-Smith, A. M., … Iacopino, V. (2002). Prevalence of war-related sexual violence and other human rights abuses among internally displaced persons in Sierra Leone. *Journal of the American Medical Association, 287*(4), 513–521. http://doi.org/10.1001/jama.287.4.513

Belloni, R. (2009). Bosnia: Dayton is dead! Long live Dayton! *Nationalism and Ethnic Politics, 15*(3), 355–375. http://doi.org/10.1080/13537110903372367

Berghs, M. (2011). Embodiment and Emotion in Sierra Leone. *Third World Quarterly, 32*(8), 1399–1417. http://doi.org/10.1080/01436597.2011.604515

Betancourt, T. S., Borisova, I. I., Williams, T. P., Brennan, R. T., Whitfield, T. H., de la Soudiere, M., … Gilman, S. E. (2010). Sierra leone's former child soldiers: A follow-up study of psychosocial adjustment and community reintegration. *Child Development, 81*(4), 1077–1095. http://doi.org/10.1111/j.1467-8624.2010.01455.x

Betancourt, T. S., & Khan, K. T. (2008). The mental health of children affected by armed conflict: protective processes and pathways to resilience. *International Review of Psychiatry (Abingdon, England), 20*(3), 317–28. http://doi.org/10.1080/09540260802090363

Betancourt, T. S., Meyers-Ohki, S. E., Charrow, A. P., & Tol, W. A. (2013). Interventions for children affected by war: an ecological perspective on psychosocial support and mental health care. *Harvard Review of Psychiatry, 21*(2), 70–91. http://doi.org/10.1097/HRP.0b013e318283bf8f

Betancourt, T. S., Simmons, S., Borisova, I., Brewer, S. E., Iweala, U., & de la Soudière, M. (2008). High hopes, grim reality: Reintegration and the education of former child soldiers in Sierra Leone. *Comparative Education Review, 52*(4), 565–587. http://doi.org/10.1086/591298

Bolton, P., Bass, J., Betancourt, T., Speelman, L., Onyango, G., Clougherty, K. F., … Verdeli, H. (2007). Interventions for depression symptoms among adolescent survivors of war and displacement in northern Uganda: a randomized controlled trial. *JAMA : The Journal of the American Medical Association, 298*(5), 519–527. http://doi.org/10.1001/jama.298.5.519

Branch, A. (2007). Uganda's civil war and the politics of ICC intervention. *Ethics & International Affairs, 21*(2), 179–198. http://doi.org/10.1111/j.1747-7093.2007.00069.x

Breetzke, G. D. (2016). Examining the spatial periodicity of crime in South Africa using Fourier analysis. *South African Geographical Journal, 98*(2), 275-288.

Breslau, D. (2010). Review: One state, two states: Resolving the Israel/Palestine conflict. *Contemporary Sociology, 39*(1), 68–69. http://doi.org/10.1177/0094306109356659kk

Carballo, M., Smajkic, A., Zeric, D., Dzidowska, M., Gebre-Medhin, J., & Van Halem, J. (2004). Mental health and coping in a war situation: The case of Bosnia and Herzegovina. *Journal of Biosocial Science, 36*(4), 463–477. http://doi.org/10.1017/S0021932004006753

Chase, R., Doney, A., Sivayogan, S., Ariyaratne, V., Satkunanayagam, P., & Swaminathan, A. (2007). Mental health initiatives as peace initiatives in Sri Lankan schoolchildren affected by armed conflict. *Medicine, Conflict, and Survival, 15*(4), 379-90–3. http://doi.org/10.1080/13623699908409479

CIA. (2014). The World Factbook 2013-14. Retrieved from https://www.cia.gov/library/publications/the-world-factbook/index.html

Collier, P., Hoeffler, a., & Soderbom, M. (2008). Post-conflict risks. *Journal of Peace Research, 45*(4), 461–478. http://doi.org/10.1177/0022343308091356

Collier, P., & Sambanis, N. (2002). Understanding civil war. *Journal of Conflict Resolution, 46*(1), 3–12. http://doi.org/10.1177/0022002702046001001

Daalder, I. H. (1998). Decision to intervene: How the war in Bosnia ended. *Foreign Service Journal, 75*(12), 24 ff. Retrieved from http://www.brookings.edu/research/articles/1998/12/balkans-daalder

de Jong, K., Mulhern, M., Ford, N., van der Kam, S., & Kleber, R. (2000). The trauma of war in Sierra Leone. *Lancet, 355*(9220), 2067. http://doi.org/10.1016/S0140-6736(00)02364-3

Dybdahl, R. (2001). A psychosocial support programme for children and mothers in war. *Clinical Child Psychology and Psychiatry, 6*(3), 425–436. http://doi.org/http://dx.doi.org/10.1177/1359104501006003010

Englund, H. (2002). From war to peace on the Mozambique-Malawi borderland. Edinburgh University Press, Vol. 26.

Ertl, V., & Neuner, F. (2014). Are school-based mental health interventions for war-affected children effective and harmless? *BMC Medicine, 12*(1), 84. http://doi.org/10.1186/1741-7015-12-84

Ertl, V., Pfeiffer, A., Saile, R., Schauer, E., Elbert, T., & Neuner, F. (2010). Validation of a mental health assessment in an African conflict population. *Psychological Assessment, 22*(2), 318–324. http://doi.org/10.1037/a0018810

Fearon, J. D., Humphreys, M., & Weinstein, J. M. (2009). Can development aid contribute to social cohesion after civil war? Evidence from a field experiment in post-conflict Liberia. In *American Economic Review* (Vol. 99, pp. 287–291). http://doi.org/10.1257/aer.99.2.287

Ferris, E. (2009). Internal displacement and peacebuilding in Colombia. *Brookings-Bern Project on Internal Displacement*, 71.

Flores, T. E., & Nooruddin, I. (2009). Financing the peace: Evaluating World Bank post-conflict assistance programs. *Review of International Organizations*, *4*(1), 1–27. http://doi.org/10.1007/s11558-008-9039-0

Gizelis, T.-I. (2011). A country of their own: Women and peacebuilding. *Conflict Management and Peace Science*, *28*(5), 522–542. http://doi.org/10.1177/0738894211418412

Groelsema, R. & Talla, J. "Secured, Empowered and Connected Communities (SECC) Strategic Objective 4 Learning Exercise." CRS, Baltimore, MD, September, 2016.

Hajjar, L. (2014). Religion, state power, and domestic violence in Muslim societies: A framework for comparative analysis. *Law & Social Inquiry*, *29*(1), 1–38. http://doi.org/10.1111/j.1747-4469.2004.tb00329.x

Harpham, T., Grant, E., & Rodriguez, C. (2004). Mental health and social capital in Cali, Colombia. *Social Science & Medicine*, *58*(11), 2267–2277. http://doi.org/10.1016/j.socscimed.2003.08.013

Hasanović, M., Sinanović, O., Pajević, I., Avdibegović, E., & Sutović, A. (2006). Post-war mental health promotion in Bosnia-Herzegovina. *Psychiatria Danubina*, *18*(1–2), 74–78.

Hasanovic, M., Srabovic, S., Rasidovic, M., Sehovic, M., Hasanbasic, E., Husanovic, J., & Hodzic, R. (2009). Psychosocial assistance to students with posttraumatic stress disorder in primary and secondary schools in post-war Bosnia Herzegovina. *Psychiatr Danub*, *21*(4), 463–473.

Honwana, A. M. (1997). Healing for peace: Traditional healers and post-war reconstruction in southern Mozambique. *Peace and Conflict: Journal of Peace Psychology*, *3*(3), 293–305. http://doi.org/10.1207/s15327949pac0303_6

Hoogenboom, D. A., & Vieille, S. (2010). Rebuilding social fabric in failed states: Examining transitional justice in Bosnia. *Human Rights Review*, *11*(2), 183–198. http://doi.org/10.1007/s12142-009-0129-z

Jegannathan, B., Kullgren, G., & Deva, P. (2015). Mental health services in Cambodia, challenges and opportunities in a post-conflict setting. *Asian Journal of Psychiatry*, *13*, 75–80. http://doi.org/10.1016/j.ajp.2014.12.006

Johnson, K., & Jonsson, M. (2013). Colombia: Ending the forever war? *Survival*, *55*(1), 67–86. http://doi.org/10.1080/00396338.2013.767407

Kane, M. (2014). Interreligious violence in the Central African Republic. *African Security Review*, *23*(3), 312–317. http://doi.org/10.1080/10246029.2014.931625

Kaplan, O., & Nussio, E. (2016). Explaining recidivism of ex-combatants in Colombia. *Journal of Conflict Resolution*, 1–30. http://doi.org/10.1177/0022002716644326

Kollontai, P. (2010). Healing the heart in {Bosnia}-{Herzegovina}: art, children and peacemaking. *INTERNATIONAL JOURNAL OF CHILDRENS SPIRITUALITY*, *15*(3, SI), 261–271. http://doi.org/10.1080/1364436X.2010.523073

Kuriansky, J. (2007). Beyond bullets and bombs : grassroots peacebuilding between Israelis and Palestinians. *Contemporary Psychology*, xxvi, 382 .

Liebling-Kalifani, H., Ojiambo-Ochieng, R., Marshall, a., Were-Oguttu, J., Musisi, S., & Kinyanda, E. (2008). Violence against women in Northern Uganda: The neglected health consequences of war. *Journal of International Women's Studies*, *9*(3), 174–193.

Mcspadden, L. a. (1987). Ethiopian refugee resettlement in the Western United States: social context and psychological well-being. *The International Migration Review*, *21*(3), 796–819. http://doi.org/12314906

Meyer-Parlapanis, D., Weierstall, R., Nandi, C., Bambonyé, M., Elbert, T., & Crombach, A. (2016). Appetitive aggression in women: Comparing male and female war combatants. *Frontiers in Psychology, 6*(JAN). http://doi.org/10.3389/fpsyg.2015.01972

Miller, K. E., & Rasmussen, A. (2010). War exposure, daily stressors, and mental health in conflict and post-conflict settings: Bridging the divide between trauma-focused and psychosocial frameworks. *Social Science and Medicine, 70*(1), 7–16. http://doi.org/10.1016/j.socscimed.2009.09.029

Momartin, S., Silove, D., Manicavasagar, V., & Steel, Z. (2004). Comorbidity of PTSD and depression: Associations with trauma exposure, symptom severity and functional impairment in Bosnian refugees resettled in Australia. *Journal of Affective Disorders, 80*(2–3), 231–238. http://doi.org/10.1016/S0165-0327(03)00131-9

O'Loughlin, J. (2010). Inter-ethnic friendships in post-war Bosnia-Herzegovina: Sociodemographic and place influences. *Ethnicities, 10*(1), 26–53. http://doi.org/10.1177/1468796809354153

Paffenholz, T. (2010). *Civil Society and Peacebuilding. Civil Society and Peacebuilding A Critical Assessment.* Retrieved from http://www.mendeley.com/research-papers/search/?query=peacebuilding+mechanisms+

Pham, P. N., Weinstein, H. M., & Longman, T. (2004). Trauma and PTSD symptoms in Rwanda: implications for attitudes toward justice and reconciliation. *JAMA : The Journal of the American Medical Association, 292*(5), 602–612. http://doi.org/10.1001/jama.292.5.602

Phillips, M., Hemmer, B., Garb, P., & Graham, J. (2006). Putting the "up" in bottom-up peacebuilding: Broadening the concept of peace negotiations. *International Negotiation, 11*, 129–162. http://doi.org/10.1163/157180606777835739

Plonski, S. (2005). Developing agency through peacebuilding in the midst of intractable conflict: The case of Israel and Palestine. *Compare: A Journal of Comparative and International Education, 35*(January 2015), 393–409. http://doi.org/10.1080/03057920500331454

Pouligny, B. (2005). Civil society and post-conflict peacebuilding: Ambiguities of international   programmes aimed at building "new" societies. *Security Dialogue, 36*(4), 495–510. http://doi.org/10.1177/0967010605060448

Reisinger, C. (2009). A framework for the analysis of post-conflict situations: Liberia and Mozambique reconsidered. *International Peacekeeping*, (March 2013), 37–41. http://doi.org/10.1080/13533310903184689

Rensburg, R., & Botha, E. (2014). Is Integrated Reporting the silver bullet of financial communication? A stakeholder perspective from South Africa. *Public Relations Review, 40*(2), 144-152.

Roberts, B., Ocaka, K. F., Browne, J., Oyok, T., & Sondorp, E. (2008). Factors associated with post-traumatic stress disorder and depression amongst internally displaced persons in northern Uganda. *BMC Psychiatry, 8*, 38. http://doi.org/10.1186/1471-244X-8-38

Ross, G. (2004). Guide: Media guidelines: From the "Trauma Vortex" to the "Healing Vortex". [References]. *Journal of Aggression, Maltreatment & Trauma, 9*(3–4), 394. http://doi.org/10.1300/J146v09n03_09

Shafir, G. (1989). *Land, labor, and the origins of the Israeli-Palestinian conflict, 1882-1914.* Univ of California Press; 1996 Aug 19

Sijbrandij, M., Olff, M., Reitsma, J. B., Carlier, I. V. E., & Gersons, B. P. R. (2006). Emotional or educational debriefing after psychological trauma: Randomised controlled trial. In *British Journal of Psychiatry* (Vol. 189, pp. 150–155). http://doi.org/10.1192/bjp.bp.105.021121

Simich, L. (2003). Negotiating boundaries of refugee resettlement: A study of settlement patterns and social support. *Canadian Review of Sociology/Revue canadienne de sociologie, 40*(5), 575-591.

Smith, P., Perrin, S., Yule, W., Hacam, B., & Stuvland, R. (2002). War exposure among children from Bosnia-Hercegovina: Psychological adjustment in a community sample. *Journal of Traumatic Stress, 15*(2), 147–156. http://doi.org/10.1023/A:1014812209051

Stark, L. (2006). Cleansing the wounds of war: An examination of traditional healing, psychosocial health and reintegration in Sierra Leone. *International Journal of Mental Health, Psychosocial Work & Counselling in Areas of Armed Conflict, 4*(3), 206–218. http://doi.org/10.1097/WTF.0b013e328011a7d2

Steel, Z., Silove, D., Brooks, R., Momartin, S., Alzuhairi, B., & Susljik, I. (2006). Impact of immigration detention and temporary protection on the mental health of refugees. *British Journal of Psychiatry, 188*(JAN.), 58–64. http://doi.org/10.1192/bjp.bp.104.007864

Stovel, L. (2008). "There"s no bad bush to throw away a bad child': "tradition"-inspired reintegration in post-war Sierra Leone. *The Journal of Modern African Studies, 46*(2), 305–324. http://doi.org/10.1017/S0022278X08003248

Suhrke, A., & Samset, I. (2007). What's in a figure? Estimating recurrence of civil war. *International Peacekeeping, 14*(2), 195–203. http://doi.org/10.1080/13533310601150776

Usaid. (2012). Building resilience to recurrent crisis - USAID policy and program guidance. *Zhurnal Eksperimental'noi I Teoreticheskoi Fiziki, 32*. http://doi.org/10.1007/s13398-014-0173-7.2

Vinck, P., & Pham, P. N. (2010). Association of exposure to violence and potential traumatic events with self-reported physical and mental health status in the Central African Republic. *JAMA, 304*(5), 544–552. http://doi.org/10.1001/jama.2010.1065

Vinck, P., Pham, P. N., Stover, E., & Weinstein, H. M. (2007). Exposure to war crimes and implications for peace building in northern Uganda. *JAMA : The Journal of the American Medical Association, 298*(5), 543–554. http://doi.org/10.1001/jama.298.5.543

Weder, N., García-Nieto, R., & Canneti-Nisim, D. (2011). Peace, reconciliation and tolerance in the Middle East. *International Journal of Mental Health, 39*(4), 59–81. http://doi.org/10.2753/IMH0020-7411390404

Weierstall, R., Castellanos, C. P. B., Neuner, F., & Elbert, T. (2013). Relations among appetitive aggression, post-traumatic stress and motives for demobilization: a study in former Colombian combatants. *Conflict and Health, 7*(1), 9. http://doi.org/10.1186/1752-1505-7-9

Williamson, J., & Robinson, M. (2006). Psychosocial interventions , or integrated programming for. *Intervention: The International Journal of Mental Health, Psychosocial Work and Counselling in Areas of Armed Conflict., 4*(1), 4–25.

CHAPTER 19

Project 1948: Establishing an NGO in Global Health

Aaron Hermann, Jenifer L. White, and Klara Lubej

One does not simply establish a non-governmental organisation (NGO) in global health... There are numerous steps and perils on the path to success. How sustainable and successful a company becomes is very much impacted by the planning, preparation, initial knowledge and skills of staff, and experiences of staff at the origins of the organisation. One would be hard-pressed to find any company in the world that could honestly say that the steps involved in its establishment were easy and without great obstacles. The reality of doing business in a global context with varying cultural norms and values is that complexities will always arise. How an organisation confronts and solves these complexities is dependent on understanding the global situation and local market situations in its host country. Finances alone are not sufficient to guarantee success – a lesson hard-learnt by all too many organisations throughout history. Solid business plans, systems, practices, knowledge, goals, and missions are a must for a company looking to operate globally.

Establishing an NGO in global health presents extensive challenges, including time, budget, and political constraints (Stevens, 2012). The realities of the global situation are perhaps most pertinent to a global health organisation, mainly due to the nature of its industry. The health industry is one with high levels of personal contact, and as such, organisations in it are people-oriented ventures. In many ways, NGOs are not altogether different from a traditional global company. For example, they may provide goods and/or services, their customers are the core of their operations, and without knowledge of their customers' behaviours, preferences, and situations, the organisation cannot flourish. This does not mean that one should apply the same practices to both NGOs and traditional global companies without careful consideration, but it does mean that certain global factors of business will impact both types of entities. Overall, comprehensive scanning of the industry is vital for a global health NGO, just as it would be for any multinational company. Scanning is used to identify numerous factors such as Strengths, Weaknesses, Opportunities, and Threats (SWOT) of an organisation and the market around it. Through this, an organisation is able to better prepare for the global market.

International Business Risks

In this globalized world, an increasing number of businesses are choosing to expand their operations overseas. Some, like born global firms, begin their lifecycle in the global arena but must still be aware of the factors influencing global business. In either case, accompanying these decisions are a series of risks threatening to end operations before they have even begun. This is true for every industry, not just health. In any international endeavour, organisations will need to recognise and face the risks associated with undertaking global ventures. Of course, these risks will differ from country to country, industry to industry, and organisation to organisation; however, be the organisation for-profit or non-for-profit, they must be aware of and prepare for any number of factors which may come into play in the global arena.

Generally speaking, there are four main categories of international business risk associated with a decision to operate globally or extraterritorially. The level and extent to which these affect an organisation will differ due to a number of factors (i.e., operating industry, size, employee specifics, product or service offerings, country of expansion/operation, etc.). These four categories are 1) Cross-Cultural Risk, 2) Country Risk, 3) Financial Risk, and 4) Commercial Risk. In the case of a global health venture, each of these risks can play a role in decision making, expansion, and business operations, and as such, companies must take care to identify, prevent, and address these risks.

Of all of these four categories of risks, two play a particular role in the operations of global health NGOs (and more generally, in culture/health-rich industries): Cross-Cultural Risk and Country Risk. Both are perhaps the most difficult to account for, quantify, and monitor, yet they are vital for successful operations in a foreign nation. First and foremost, one must be careful and observant of Cross-Cultural Risks when engaging in a highly people-orientated venture, such as is the case in the health industry. The personal interaction between business and customers, particularly the close and personal nature of the contact, means that there is considerable potential for cross-cultural misunderstanding and faux-pas.

Cross-Cultural Risks

Cross-Cultural Risk can be defined as the consequences and effects caused by differences in culture which place human matters of value in jeopardy. Culture refers to more than just language and values – it also incorporates behaviour, norms, ethics, etc. Cultural manifestations can be grouped into two categories: tangible (e.g., dress, dance, religion, music, etc.) and intangible (e.g., locus of control, gender roles, Power Distance, concept of self, etc.). Culture is a major factor in the success or failure of an international venture. The clash of cultures or failure to incorporate differences in culture (either within an organisation or in its sphere of influence) can result in major detrimental effects, as has been demonstrated by some of the world's largest and most successful companies in history, companies such as Swissair (Hermann & Rammal, 2010) and Chrysler Group LLC.

There are numerous avenues for issues to occur when discussing culture and Cross-Cultural Risk. Perhaps one of the most obvious of these is that of language. Despite the fact that in the last 70 years, English has become one of the most widely used languages for businesses in the world, it is not the only business language. Whilst some of the world's most influential companies, like Red Bull GmbH, are using English as their main operating language, there are still many global firms (primarily French, German, and Japanese) which chose to retain their native language as the operating language. Similarly, communications with customers and stakeholders are not always possible in English. There are a number of nations where the traditional "global languages," (English, French, German, or Spanish) are not widely used, and as such, communication only in these languages can create a plethora of problems for a firm. This can be seen in nations in the southern Balkans, where, even among the younger generations, English, French, German, and Spanish are not widely spoken. In global health, an example of the risks language barriers pose can be seen in an organisation such as *Médecins sans Frontiers*. Imagine if the doctors or nurses could not speak the local language – communication with patients would be next to impossible. In any case, it is always a good idea for a firm operating in a foreign nation to be able to communicate in the native language. This practice helps to eliminate potential misunderstandings and facilitates improved relations between the organisation and its stakeholders.

Hofstede's Dimensions

On a more intangible level, Hofstede (1980) outlines six components of culture, which include: 1) Individualism vs. Collectivism, 2) Power Distance, 3) Uncertainty Avoidance, 4) Masculinity vs. Femininity, 5) Long-Term Outlook vs. Short-Term Outlook (sometimes also known as the Confucius Dynamism), and 6) Indulgence vs. Restraint. Each of these elements plays a role in business operations, stakeholder interactions, and employee relations. Overall, they can contribute to the success or failure of a firm.

Individualism vs. Collectivism

This concept relates to one's view of one's primary function in society, be this to oneself or to the collective (i.e., greater society). To elaborate, individualism refers to a person's emphasis being placed on him/herself and his/her immediate family. This impacts how people behave, their motivations, competitive nature, etc. Collectivism, on the other hand, can be defined as a person's belief in the needs of the community, the ties between individuals, and the cooperative nature of his/her existence. As such, the impact of individualism/collectivism in a global health NGO may not be limited to the preferences of their customers, but this factor can also influence employment elements such as staff recruitment, employee interactions, etc.

Power Distance

Power Distance refers to the gaps of power which exist in societies, and how societies deal with those perceived inequalities. This element has particular impact on employee relations. Companies which hire employees from cultures differing significantly from their own may more frequently come across issues relating to reporting, decision making, etc. High Power Distance cultures tend to exhibit more autocratic business structures and provide less autonomy to lower-level employees. Employees from these cultures are less likely to question decisions from top level management, even in situations where they are aware that an alternative would result in improved outcomes. Low Power Distance cultures tend to exhibit the opposite. Organisations tend to be flatter, with fewer differences between top-level managers and lower-level managers. This in turn creates situations where employees may be more willing to approach high-level managers and are more comfortable asking questions of their managers; however, this may create greater feelings of inequality in situations where large disparities exist in pay or reward systems.

Uncertainty Avoidance

Uncertainty Avoidance can be defined as the willingness of individuals in a society to take risks. High Uncertainty Avoidance cultures are less likely to take risks, especially when the situation is unclear or when the process involves dangerous or uncertain outcomes. Low Uncertainty Avoidance cultures are, on the other hand, more willing to undertake risks even in unclear situations. This is of particular importance particularly when it comes to aspects such as decision making or undertaking of new ventures.

New medical practices or services are more likely to be readily accepted and embraced in nations where there is Low Uncertainty Avoidance.

Masculinity vs. Femininity

Masculinity vs. Femininity refers to the nature of a culture's orientation and tendencies to embrace and exhibit traditional male and female roles. In masculine cultures, individuals value ambition, competitiveness, assertiveness, etc. In feminine cultures, emphasis is placed on interdependence among people, caring for the less-fortunate, nurturing roles, etc. One should be aware that both males and females in each of these cultures can exhibit these characteristics; they are not gender specific. These factors play a role in workplace motivation and reward systems. People from masculine cultures tend to respond better to material rewards, pay, etc. Individuals from feminine cultures, on the other hand, tend to respond better to rewards which enhance relationships. This affects the global health industry. Feminine-based cultures tend to place more emphasis on health, and greater investment in health accompanies this focus. As such, an NGO in global health may find it beneficial to headquarter operations in feminine-based nations.

Long -Term Outlook vs. Short-Term Outlook

This concept is a culture's orientation towards long-term versus short-term goals, or how far into the future a nation plans. Moreover, it refers to the extent to which a culture derives satisfaction from short- or long-term outcomes. As such, Long-Term Outlook cultures place more emphasis on matters such as planning and living; outlook extends decades into the future. A Short-Term Outlook culture focuses more on the here and now; outlook rarely extends beyond five to ten years into the future. Anglo societies are short-term oriented, whereas Asian nations are long-term oriented. A nation's support of a venture is oftentimes affected by the extent to which the nation's culture is long-term oriented. Simply put, a nation can either view a global health operation as something needing long-term support in order to eventually see benefits, or as something from which it can expect immediate outcomes.

Indulgence vs. Restraint

This concept describes a culture's view of basic and natural human drives and gratification, particularly those related to life's enjoyment. Cultures with greater levels of indulgence are more likely to seek out enjoyable activities. This has an impact on the services and products offered in a country as consumer preference and behaviour will play a major role in consumer purchasing habits. Similarly, cultures with higher levels of indulgence will have different motivating factors. As such, reward systems and human resource (HR) policies will need to be adapted to account for these differences. For example, a culture with high levels of indulgence may not find recognition-based rewards systems (such as employee of the month awards) particularly motivating; financial rewards may be more motivating to such individuals.

These are but a few of the elements of culture affecting international business operations. There are a plethora of other elements which impact how a firm does business in a foreign nation. Some of these include: 1) Concepts of time (e.g., relating to punctuality), 2) Work ethic, 3) Concepts of autonomy, 4) Length of employment (lifelong or temporary), 5) Teamwork orientation, and of course 6) Etiquette and customs. An additional point of particular importance in the global health industry is the different cultural norms and beliefs relating to the interactions between females and males. An example of this can be seen in the traditional culture of the Aboriginal Australian. The segregation of roles in traditional Aboriginal culture, as well as Aboriginal avoidance practices, are such that certain roles/events can only be observed by one of the two genders; there must be no mixing. On the other hand, in many "Western" cultures, a female visiting a male doctor or vice versa is considered perfectly acceptable. This is not the case in all cultures. There are some societies that believe that it is necessary for female patients to visit female doctors and male patients to visit male doctors. As such, a firm looking to operate in a foreign nation, particularly in one with a very different culture, must be aware of the norms relating to female/male interactions. This is vital in order to prevent any offence or negative business consequences.

Country Risks

Country Risk refers to potential losses or other adverse effects as a result of changes and developments in a nation's legal or political environment. These risks include government takeover of business assets, embargos and sanctions, legislative changes, bureaucratic red tape, inadequacy of the legal system, and corruption/economic mismanagement.

Government Takeovers

Government takeovers can vary from country to country. Generally, there are two categories of government seizures: 1) confiscation, which is seizure without compensation, and 2) expropriation, which is seizure with compensation (Wild, Wild, Han & Rammal, 2007). One example is the petrochemical industry in Venezuela. The Venezuelan government's decision to change the ownership of national oil reserves to state-owned had a significant impact on the international firms operating in the Venezuelan market.

Embargoes and Sanctions

Embargoes and sanctions can take numerous forms but include actions such as trade restrictions (either complete or concerning a certain good/service) or prohibiting transactions with a particular country. Embargoes are generally considered to be complete restrictions on trade and dealings with a country (with few exceptions, like humanitarian aid). An example of this was the United States' embargoes on Cuba. Sanctions, on the other hand, are less overarching. Sanctions are generally limited to specific goods or items or to a particular industry. An example of this is the United Nations' (U.N.) sanctions on North Korea. This is important for a global health company to know because it may limit what supplies or raw materials (e.g., chemicals, drugs, etc.) they can import or export from the nation in question.

Legislative Changes

Legislative changes that can affect a company include changes in marketing law, foreign ownership laws, environmental laws, contract laws, medical registration laws, etc. These changes may or may not be tied to a government change. Because of this, many international businesses will assess the likelihood if, in a given election, a change in the leading political party will occur. It should, however, be noted that legislative changes are not only a consequence of political change. Political parties may change their perspective on a particular point during their term in office for political, economic, or military reasons, and as a result, legislative change may occur. Likewise, simply because there is a change in government does not necessarily mean that there will be a change in legislation. This complexity is part of the ambiguity and difficulty associated with Country Risks. It also demonstrates the need for environmental scanning and preparation.

Bureaucratic "Red Tape"

Bureaucratic red tape includes an assortment of formal government regulations which may result in inefficiencies or a hindrance of company operations. A few examples of bureaucratic requirements are taxes, permit and licensing requirements (such as the registration of doctors or nurses), procedures or requirements for setting up a company, etc. It has been argued that bureaucratic red tape is linked to the Gert Hofstede's Uncertainty Avoidance. This is to say, the more a culture is prone to fear the uncertain, the more bureaucratic processes are put in place to protect against this fear (Hofstede, 1980). These regulations and requirements are sometimes used as a means to protect national firms and/or limit the potential of international firm operations and market share in a country.

Inadequacy of the Legal System

This refers to the extent to which a county's legal system is able to cope with the necessities of international business and the demands of global corporations. These demands include issues related to contracts, negligence claims, dispute resolution, etc. Issues may arise when foreign companies have difficulties with domestic companies or even other third nation corporations.

Corruption or Economic Mismanagement

As the name would suggest, corruption or economic mismanagement refers to the level of impact businesses may experience due to issues of corruption or mismanagement of national economic situations. To prepare for these issues, companies have an assortment of tools at their disposal to research and learn before entering a new market. A global NGO, Transparency International, provides a series of resources which companies can use to help make market-entry decisions. These include the Corruption Perception Index (Transparency International, 2015) and country-specific information relating to corruption levels.

A company seeking to expand business must ensure appropriate research and scanning is conducted before market entry occurs. Likewise, they must ensure strict adherence to local laws and may consider alliances with local partners to ensure minimisation of risk. The list of possible methods to minimise Country Risks are extensive; however, one fact remains clear: in order to succeed, companies must consider these risks seriously.

Recruitment and Staffing

There are a number of options for international organisations concerning recruitment. Regarding overarching staffing approaches, there are generally considered to be four primary approaches: ethnocentric, polycentric, geocentric, and regiocentric. Each has pros and cons, and one may find that different firms derive different benefits from each approach.

The ethnocentric approach is one in which an organisation fills positions (particularly management positions) with nationals from the home nation. This approach is often utilized by organisations which employ quality management strategies such as Total Quality Control and Just-in-Time. Historically, companies like BMW have employed such staffing approaches. Two benefits that generally accompany this approach include a more uniform organisational culture and the fact that systems and processes used in the home country do not need to be altered. One of the key drawbacks of this system is that the organisation runs the risk of stagnant organisational cultures; this in turn creates subsequent issues related to engaging in new ventures. Perhaps more importantly, this approach does not make the transfer of local knowledge and experience particularly easy.

The polycentric approach is the opposite of the ethnocentric approach. This approach is one in which organisations fill positions with nationals from the host country. As with the ethnocentric approach, there are possible drawbacks that accompany the benefits. Firstly, organisations run the risk of culture clash. In other words, a blend of two different corporate (or national) cultures may create difficulties with daily processes or business systems. Similarly, it has been argued that the hiring of host-nation nationals creates added costs of training for the employees. On the other hand, the benefits include a more diversified workplace, new ideas, and a more diversified HR base. Colgate Palmolive is an example of a major international company that employs this staffing approach.

The geocentric approach can be defined as a "best fit" approach. Positions are filled by those considered to be the best for the position, regardless their origin. These staff members may be home country nationals, host country nationals, or third-country nationals. Two benefits of this approach include a decrease in resentment among other staff (since favouritism is not shown) and the fact that selected staff usually already have significant international experience; this experience can then be more readily passed on to the other staff through training and development programs. Some disadvantages are that the HR recruiting process may be longer, more complex, and requires more scrutiny. Furthermore, there can be additional costs associated with relocation of staff, and compensation for such employees is often higher. Many global universities follow the geocentric approach, hiring academics from all over the world. Volkswagen also employs the geocentric approach for its global operations.

The final approach is that of regiocentric staffing. This approach is, in many ways, a hybrid of the geocentric and either the polycentric or ethnocentric approach. This approach is one in which organisations hire the most qualified person for the position, not from a global perspective but from a regional perspective. For example, a Finnish organisation decided to open operations in Singapore, but instead of hiring local Singaporean employees or Finnish employees, the recruitment drive is expanded to include other surrounding countries in the region of Southeast Asia. As such, employees may come from Hong Kong, Malaysia, Thailand, the Philippines, etc. A company might choose this approach if it plans to do business with other countries in the region or if there are particular intricacies of the region which must be considered in order to successfully operate a company in the host country. The benefits of the regiocentric approach are similar to that of the geocentric approach. It usually accompanies an increase in diversity which benefits the organisational culture and decision making. Drawbacks are also similar. These include possible clashes between differences in organisational or national culture. Moreover, a company must be careful because any regional issues between countries (such as trade disputes or historical grievances) may be brought in with new staff.

Overall, these risks may be experienced by any organisation or company. Whilst these factors are, in theory, always present, the realities of how these elements will effect an organisation will differ from one organisation to another. As such, it seems prudent to now provide a specific case study of a global health NGO that showcases these factors.

Project 1948: A Case Study

Project 1948 is a U.S.-based, global health NGO with an international focus in Bosnia and Herzegovina. The primary focus of Project 1948 is convergence between mental health and social change. The organisational objective is to create awareness and encourage change in the international community by 1) promoting intercultural dialogue, 2) collectively empowering young adults through photography to begin a conversation with policymakers, and 3) inform the global community of the plight of youth in Bosnia and Herzegovina. This approach encourages freedom of expression and helps to promote a sense of well-being, confidence, self-esteem, and good mental health of the participants.

Project 1948 connects history, participants, society, and culture. Through intercultural and interethnic dialogue, participants elicit conversation and understanding. It was felt that the global community needed to understand human rights abuses under political deadlock and how to get involved (Ishay, 2008). Project 1948 objectives are furthered by bringing people together, building relationships, and sharing resources. The organisation presents the perspectives of marginalized groups to provide direct insight into restructuring and implementing national and international policies and procedures. Through sharing, the staff of Project 1948 have facilitated in building bridges with decision-makers and creating partnerships for community change.

Photo-Voice as the Project's Core

Project 1948's primary avenue for the promotion of mental health and social change is the "Photo-Voice" initiative. Participants are given photography equipment for three weeks to document their daily lives. From this, they can choose to demonstrate challenges, social connections, or any aspect of their lives that they value or feel warrants documentation. In particular, participants are asked to photograph aspects of the world around them that they see as restricting their personal freedoms, rights, or health. The participants then sit down with Project 1948 staff to discuss their photos, why they chose them, what significance they play and how they interact with their world. They also answer a series of semi-structured questions relating to their perceptions and desires. The photo-voice method was selected due to the power of visual media in the modern world. Ample research has demonstrated the positive impacts visual media can have on a person's life and on the lives of those around them (Rose, 2012).

Following the interviews, the results are compiled as reports and presented to various authorities and government bodies throughout Bosnia and Herzegovina and to global organisations such as the U.N. This information is presented with the hope of eliciting change and creating awareness for the plight of young Bosnian and Herzegovinians. As participants engage in critical reflection, they may advocate for change in their communities by using the power of their images and stories to communicate. The hope is that this communication, coupled with the results of the interviews, will effect change by showing politicians in Bosnia and Herzegovina that the younger population is unhappy with the current state of affairs. Later, the images are placed on public display and published through various media outlets both in print and online. Through the data collected during this process, Project 1948 highlights policies and issues that impact participants, thereby directing policy-change efforts toward those that would be most meaningful (Wang & Burris, 1997).

The Photo-Voice initiative allows Project 1948 to involve a participatory-action research strategy based on the understanding that people are experts on their own lives (Butler-Kisber, 2010). Project 1948 employs a two-part model: 1) displaying the visual language of photography while highlighting community concerns and 2) catalysing policy change through youth capacity building. The organisation takes an innovative approach to achieving sustainable peace and empowers young adults to begin an international dialogue to hold officials and institutions accountable at all levels of government. Photography and the Photo-Voice project can provide a voice to the most marginalised of society. It provides young adults with hands-on photography experience and the opportunity to make a difference in their community. The project also aims to cultivate collective identity and inter-ethnic cooperation and friendship among Bosnians, Croatians, Serbians, and Herzegovinians. Social inclusion is the cornerstone of this NGO's approach. Engagement with the arts can propel young adults to become community leaders, effectuate change, and strengthen their institutional representation. The aim of this initiative is to help participants develop an interest in activism in order to benefit their community. This newly-founded interest increases engagement in humanitarian affairs or lead charity initiatives (Wang, 1999). The power of photography gives direct insight into the everyday lives of the people of Bosnia and Herzegovina, and through this, the project is helping to create a future for the youth of the nation. The combination of these powerful tools and a person's drive can truly make changes for the young people of Bosnia and Herzegovina.

It is anticipated that one of the most powerful outcomes of Project 1948 will be the long-term relationships built among international governments, the U.N., the government of Bosnia and Herzegovina, and our diverse participants, who have shared a memorable community experience that influences policy-change. Project 1948's vision is to give a camera. Its mission is to give a voice. Furthermore, the Photo-Voice initiative allows the youth of Bosnia and Herzegovina to express their own concerns about growing up as a post-Dayton generation.

The Case of Bosnia and Herzegovina

For centuries, the protection of human rights has been a worrisome issue in Bosnia and Herzegovina. Moroever, the struggle to uphold the principles of the Universal Declaration of Human Rights (UDHR) has simmilarly been difficult, not only for the people of Bosnia and Herzegovina, but also for the global community. Bosnia and Herzegovina has a long history of human rights violations, dating back long before the tragedies of the 1990s. One can trace the history of human rights violations in region of modern day Bosnia and Herzegovina as far back as the Roman period, during the times of the Illyrian Wars, and perhaps even further. In many ways, Bosnia and Herzegovina is under political deadlock as a result of the constitution that developed from the Dayton Peace Accords (1995). The Dayton Peace Agreement was an international effort to implement peace in November 1995 (and end the Bosnian War in the southern Balkans) between the Bosniaks, Croats, and Serbs in order to further protect human rights among the ethnic divisions (Cousens & Cater, 2001). The youth sections of society are amongst the most marginalised and vulnerable in Bosnia and Herzegovina. The Bosnian government, with its tripartite presidency, is often denounced for its failure to recognize the importance of listening to the voices of younger people (Magil & Hamber, 2011). Moreover, freedom of the press is severely limited in Bosnia and Herzegovina. As a society, Bosnia and Herzegovina is often subject to human rights abuses and discrimination in employment, education, and official representation. As such, violence and discrimination against these vulnerable groups need to be addressed. Generations raised in the former Yugoslavia were exposed to distinctive cultural and societal norms. Socialist society, culture, and government were intertwined with the lives of the populace. This brought a number of issues which eventually led to the Bosnian War. The end of the war brought major changes in Bosnia and Herzegovina – a new way of living. With this new life came new challenges, including some that the older generations simply had not been exposed to in their time on the planet. These challenges have severely impacted the mental health of the youth in Bosnia and Herzegovina, particularly amongst minorities like the Roma and Jewish populations. Project 1948 found itself in a unique situation with risks relating to international business in all arenas of the venture. Of course, one of the key barriers was language. Given that Bosnia and Herzegovina has limited use of the more common global languages, initial communication and research was quite a difficult task. The necessities to just enter the Bosnian and Herzegovinian market were not clear. As such, it was vital to engage the services of a native speaker, translator, and/or interpreter in order to navigate the troubled waters of initial market entry. Serbo-Croatian was, for a time, widely used across the country, but the oldest and youngest generations were not taught it. Related difficulties extend further into Project 1948's business tasks. Whilst English is spoken amongst the younger generation, it is still not common, and as such, using it caused misunderstandings. It is therefore suggested that companies use the native languages of the regions of Bosnia and Herzegovina in order to ensure more efficient and effective communication with customers and stakeholders.

Concepts and norms of time were likewise an issue; operating with a Western approach meant that many employees from Western countries felt as though the Bosnian and Herzegovinian approach to work is considerably more relaxed. This affected the working relationships between Bosnian and Herzegovinian stakeholders and Western stakeholders. Moreover, these cultural differences affected meeting arrangements, the processing of paperwork, and requests made through official channels. Generally speaking, these processes were lengthy, and as such, considerable preparation was required in order to have tasks completed at the desired time. At times, it was recommended to begin making necessary arrangements at least one year in advance in order to ensure deadlines did not expire.

Likewise, religion and regional variations were a major factor impacting operations in Bosnia and Herzegovina. Bosnia and Herzegovina is a unique country with a unique governmental structure and ethnic arrangement. The nation is split into three main regions which differ not only in religious majorities and languages but also have distinct administrative systems. At times, these regions (Republika Srpska, Federation of Bosnia and Herzegovina, the Brčko District) have very little interaction; therefore, communication between the regions can be tense. One should also point out the somewhat separate Herzegovinian region, which is known unofficially as the "Trebinje Region" and consists of a mixture of the cultures of Bosnia and Herzegovina. Despite this, there is still a percentage of the population in this region that identifies as Herzegovinian.

The varying dominant religions and ethnic groups in each area also play a role in how an organisation conducts operations. The population of the

Republika Srpska, which is predominately Serbian Orthodox, has very different expectations and social norms from the mainly Muslim population in the Federation of Bosnia and Herzegovina. These norms and values come to the forefront, particularly in regards to personal matters such as opinions, beliefs, and feelings. Finally, the Brčko District has a predominantly Croatian and Catholic populace. These three (some argue four) regions create further complexity for global companies operating in Bosnia and Herzegovina.

Similarly, with regards to Country Risk, Bosnia and Herzegovina presented some challenges to operations and successful completion of the venture. The aforementioned administrative and regional complexity of Bosnia and Herzegovina is one of the first difficulties a company will confront. Each region retains autonomy over education, administration, laws, policies, etc., and this creates a great deal of complexity regarding nationwide access for an NGO. These difficulties are not confined to the political and bureaucratic barriers and obstacles (which can create considerable hurdles) but also extend into interactions between the populace in respective regions, transport, communications, infrastructure, access to materials and resources, etc. One Country Risk that could affect NGOs is the possible referendums in the region of Republika Srpska. There is considerable debate as to whether a referendum should be held to determine if the region should return to the Republic of Serbia or remain part of Bosnia and Herzegovina. If such a referendum occurs and results in the former, then an organisation based in the largest city of Republika Srpska, Banja Luka, may find itself in an altogether new market and country – one for which it perhaps did not prepare. There is a third option, though less likely: the region may seek complete succession. Similar debates are taking place in the Brčko District with the Croatian populace, though with less enthusiasm and a more complex arrangement if it were to occur. There are some attempts of the same sort in the Trebinje Region, but again, to a much smaller degree. In such cases, there are obvious, far-reaching consequences for an NGO than surpass just country access. New laws, customer behaviour/preferences, taxes, regulations, etc. could easily impact organisational operations. All in all, despite the fact that Bosnia and Herzegovina is a single nation, organisations and individuals from Western countries may find the administrative and district systems in place to be confusing, as if there are three separate nations as opposed to just one. Bosnia and Herzegovina is a unique nation, and each region should be treated with respect and acknowledgement of their differences. Thus, operations must incorporate these realities in order to operate successfully in this complex market. Continuous monitoring and evaluation of the situation in Bosnia and Herzegovina is needed to ensure the sustainability of the operations.

Financing and Staffing the Project

The task of founding the NGO included facilitating a global team of photographers, writers, human rights enthusiasts, and policy specialists. As such, establishing Project 1948 was a complex process, not only due to reasons of logistics and human resources, but also due to constant barriers like time, budget, and political constraints.

Regarding financing Project 1948, it was necessary to turn to alternative sources of sponsorship and funding. The normal sources often include international organisations, research groups, non-for-profit groups, and nation states. However, these sources of funding are extremely competitive, and a small start-up without a track history and with new and unique approaches to operations is not likely to be awarded any such funds. Similarly, whilst Bosnia and Herzegovina has indeed made advancements in the past 20 years, economically, it is still one of the poorest European nations. This creates problems for local sourcing of funds as many Bosnia and Herzegovinian companies simply cannot afford to invest in programs directed towards corporate social responsibility. As such, alternatives were both needed and desirable. Naturally, these sources depend on the specific product or service, but there are general categories one can refer to for these alternative sources.

One alternative source is private companies that provide useful product offerings to your company. For example, cameras are vital to the work of Project 1948, so approaching camera companies could be beneficial. In other words, funding need not be in the form of financial offering, but can also be in the form of logistic support, products, food, or supplies.

Another alternative source is in the organisational goals. Project 1948's goals include the protection of women's rights and ethnic rights and equalities. As such, it was beneficial to approach other organisations and entities with the same goals. Women's rights groups often have funding or research opportunities available. Similarly, ethnic and religious rights organisations provide many funding possibilities. These include organisations for the protection of migrants, religious freedom groups, groups fighting anti-Semitism, and of course, human rights groups.

Recruitment likewise requires a bit of lateral thinking. Traditional sources of recruitment, whilst still an option, have a number of drawbacks for an NGO. The main drawback of traditional recruitment is the cost associated with hiring traditional recruitment agencies. These costs can be excessive, and a non-for-profit organisation must ensure that their resources are being used in the most efficient and effective manner possible. As such, alternative avenues for finding staff are ideal. Generally speaking, volunteers are the backbone of NGOs. Without the services of volunteers, many of the NGO activities would simply not be possible. In the case of Project 1948, one of the most effective tools for recruitment is the United Nations Volunteer program. This takes many forms, from online volunteering to the more traditional in-person forms. With much less outlay than traditional recruitment platforms, this platform provides avenues for the global sourcing of human resources and affords the opportunity to hire the skills of highly experienced personnel,

Similarly, Project 1948 was able to work in unison with other global and local NGOs. These partnerships included organisations such as Photographers Without Borders, The Global Goals, OnGood (the .NGO domain), United Nations Department of Economic and Social Affairs, United Nations Volunteers. These partnerships provided opportunities to source highly-skilled and experienced personnel. Of particular benefit was the fact that many of these people had prior experience not only working in the international arena of human rights, women's rights, ethnic and minority rights, and/or migration issues. These partnerships provided opportunities for creating awareness of Project 1948 through use of online platforms and magazines.

Spreading the Word: Project 1948's Marketing

As is the case for for-profit companies, marketing in an NGO is an important part of operations and vital for the success and sustainability of the company. This is particularly true for Project 1948. Before all else, the organisation needs to promote awareness of its endeavours and goals.

Whilst traditional avenues for publicity (television, radio, etc.) are viable options, they are expensive. Given resource limitation, the awareness campaign needed to take a different form, at least at the beginning. Some useful avenues were online blogs, magazines, and social media. Of particular importance to a fledgling NGO are publications with large, diverse readerships, including social media platforms like Facebook, Instagram, Twitter, and human rights blogs. Whilst publication in journals is a possible marketing opportunity, it is quite time-consuming to produce articles for them, they have specific requirements which are often in conflict with NGO goals, their review times are lengthy, and they have limited readership.

Another source of publicity is media channels – not typical, paid advertisements, but rather public relations (PR) campaigns. There are two types of PR campaigns available for organisations: proactive and reactive. An organisation should focus on proactive PR and only use reactive PR if necessary. Proactive PR is designed to create buzz about a new product or service that offers something unique and interesting. Reactive PR is only initiated after a problem occurs and is often used to repair damage. Project 1948 was in a position to use proactive PR because of the novel nature of its work. Proactive PR can take many different forms; however, public releases and executive statement releases are of the greatest benefit to

NGOs. The goal of this approach is to win free, positive press coverage. There are a number of benefits to this kind of publicity, including: 1) low cost, 2) positive image building, and 3) higher credibility (because it is perceived as not being paid-for publicity).

Localization

When establishing a global company, localization is an important factor for daily operations and marketing purposes. Global companies must be aware that a successful business strategy in the company's local market might not have the same results in a foreign market and therefore must be localized. Localization can be defined as a process of "taking a product and making it linguistically and culturally appropriate to the target locale (country, region and language) where it will be used" (Esselink, Vries & Shiera, 2000, p. 3). This can be applied to products, services, and operations in foreign business environments.

Moreover, localization encompasses adaptations of a company's products/services to the culture, taste, needs, propriety, and history of the target market in order to best satisfy customers' preferences. This can include adaptation of languages, symbols, colors, date and time systems, currencies, page layouts, voltages, keyboards, and approaches to staff recruitment. In Chinese culture, for example, red and yellow are considered lucky colors and are therefore widely used. Yellow is associated with royalty and power of the throne, and red is associated with happiness, success, and good fortune. On the other hand, white is associated with mourning in Chinese culture, so companies should be careful when using it. Another example is website layout. Research has demonstrated that people tend to read in an F-shaped pattern, which means they read from left to right (Nielsen, 2006). Consequently, the main piece of information should be on the left side. But that is only true for some countries, including those traditionally classified as Western. People in Arabic countries, however, read from right to left. Hence, websites intended for the Arabic market should position their information differently.

A simple example of localization is a translation of the company's webpage into the language of the target market so customers can access the information in their mother tongue, which is, according to the Common Sense Advisory's research (2006), more important than price for 56.2% of customers (p. 2). Moreover, various studies and surveys show that users prefer websites to be in their mother tongue (European Commission, 2011; Common Sense Advisory, 2006). Web users tend to stay on a website two times longer if it is in their native language (Forrester Research, 2009, p. 1). Furthermore, the likelihood of the purchase increases three times if a website is localized (Forrester Research, 2009, p. 1). In situations where companies provide customer service centres, the associated costs are cut in half if the instructions are translated into the language of the local market. This is not only because of the reduced time and costs involved in training, but also because of factors such as a reduced likelihood of errors and employee mistakes (Forrester Research 2009, p. 1).

Sometimes a failure to localize and adapt products/services to the local market can lead to serious consequences for business, harm a company's reputation, and result in lower revenues. Some of the world's largest companies, including Pepsi, Electrolux, Nike, and McDonald's, have experienced these consequences. For example, Proctor and Gamble introduced a product called Vicks Cough Drops to the German market. Unfortunately, they were not aware that the German pronunciation of the letter "v" is "f," which made "Vicks" sound like a German term for sexual penetration. Consequently, the company decided to change the name into Wicks, which in German is pronounced the way the company originally intended.

Gerber, as with Procter and Gamble, experienced the negative consequences of poor (or no) localization techniques. The company started selling their baby food in the African market and decided to use the same packaging as in their local market, which had an image of a baby on it. This is a normal marketing technique in many Western markets, but the company failed to research local norms and marketing habits. Due to high illiteracy rates, many local companies print images of the content of the product on the label. Because of this, local consumers actually thought the Gerber baby food contained babies. The importance of cultural sensitivity is obvious; a global company needs knowledge and understanding of local norms and must show respect for the local culture when entering foreign markets.

In the case of Project 1948, only minor adaptations, such as a translation of the surveys and documents into Bosnian language, could make a huge difference in acquired results. This is due to the fact that many citizens are not as comfortable with English as they are with their mother tongue. Even a person is reasonably fluent in English, the psychological standpoint from which they derive their expressions of feelings and deep emotions will differ to that which is derived from their native language. If forced to speak in English, participants may not answer the questions with the same depth or accuracy as they would in their native language. Additionally, it is important to educate home country employees (that deal with the host country nationals) about the Bosnian market before entering it because misunderstandings of the the complex political, cultural, and linguistic situation in Bosnia and Herzegovina could easily lead to gaffes. To some, a seemingly-easy task like translation might not seem problematic or even necessary, but in the case of Bosnia and Herzegovina, there are three official languages used in different parts of the country: Bosnian, Croatian and Serbian. These intricacies need to be taken into account when preparing a business strategy and international venture.

Conclusion

The complexities of creating an international, health-based NGO are varied and numerous. What may appear to be a simple process from the outset is actually a very difficult endeavour. However, the rights of the participants and the future of the nation are worth the effort. The complexities of cultures and countries around the world make such endeavours difficult but also so worthwhile, and in many ways, so much more interesting. The realities of the Bosnian War and the long history of Yugoslavia and Bosnia and Herzegovina make Project 1948's efforts difficult. Yet, if in the future, the Project truly does create changes for the betterment of human rights and policy in Bosnia and Herzegovina, then the risks and barriers to the international venture were worth all the hardship.

Questions

1. You are in charge of the global operations of a U.S.-based health NGO seeking to expand internationally. Your company has decided to expand into Asia, in particular into Bangladesh and Nepal. Answer the following questions, keeping in mind the lessons of the chapter:
    a. Can your organisation apply the same systems and processes for both countries? Explain why, why not, and give pros and cons of each approach.
    b. Research Hofstede's findings on both countries and discuss what each element means for your organisation.
    c. For each country, list the possible risks and challenges your organisation may face while establishing your operations in each of the foreign nations.
2. As head of the marketing department for a Swiss pharmaceutical firm, you are responsible for the expansion of your firm's corporate social responsibility programs into Slovenia. Make recommendations for a marketing campaign for your firm using the corporate social responsibility programs of a well-known pharmaceutical company. Make sure to apply and discuss the Cultural and Country Risks associated with the Slovenian market.
3. You are working as a HR officer for a newly established global NGO in health. You have been informed by your manager that the NGO needs new staff because of recent expansion of operations. It is therefore your responsibility to undertake two tasks:
    a. Investigate possible avenues for recruitment and explain why you have selected your choices.

      b. Make recommendations for staffing and recruitment practices and give reasons for your answers.

4. Research the current situation in Bosnia and Herzegovina.

      a. Explain the issues a Bosnia and Herzegovinian health NGO might face when trying to operate in the global market.

      b. Which cultural and country elements may create issues for the NGO when attempting to operate in Sudan?

      c. In what ways can the Bosnia and Herzegovinian NGO address the risks associated with its global operations? Make use of theories and concepts covered in the chapter.

5. Having recently graduated from your doctorate, you have decided to apply what you have learnt to help less-fortunate people around the world. You have decided to open an NGO in the area of Human and Ethnic Rights. You are an Austrian-registered NGO, and you have decided to focus initially on the European region. Answer the following questions:

      a. Which parts of Europe will you begin to focus on? Why?

      b. Create a draft plan for the steps you will take to establish your NGO. Include elements of financing, marketing, recruitment, and any other elements you feel are important to the setup of your NGO.

      c. Using the lessons you have learned in this chapter, explain what barriers you may face in the countries you selected in part A of this question. Provide details on what you will do in order to minimise or prevent these risks.

References

Butler-Kisber, L. (2010). *Qualitative inquiry: Thematic, narrative and arts-informed perspectives.* London: Sage Publications.

Common Sense Advisory. (2006). Can't read, won't buy: Why language matters on global websites. Retreived from http://www.commonsenseadvisory.com/AbstractView/tabid/74/ArticleID/957/Title/CantReadWontBuyWhyLanguageMattersonGlobalWebsites/Default.aspx

Cousens, E., & Cater, C. (2001). *Toward peace in Bosnia: Implementing the Dayton accords.* Boulder: Lynne Rienner Publishers.

Esselink, B., Vries, A., & Shiera, O. (2000). *Practical guide to localization.* Philadelphia: John Benjamins Publishing Company.

European Commission. (2011). User language preferences online: Analytical report. Retreived from http://ec.europa.eu/public_opinion/flash/fl_313_en.pdf

Forrester Research. (2009). Translation and localization of retail web sites: Maximizing the international experience through tailored offerings. Retrieved from https://www.forrester.com/report/Translation+And+Localization+Of+Retail+Web+Sites/-/E-RES54629

Hermann, A., & Rammal, H.G. (2010). The grounding of the "flying bank". *Management Decision, 48*(7): 1048 – 1062.

Hofstede, G. (1980). *Culture's consequences: International differences in work-related values.* Beverly Hills, Sage Publications.

Ishay, M. (2008). *The history of human rights: From ancient times to the globalization era.* Los Angeles: University of California Press.

Magil, C., & Hamber, (2011), "If They Don't Start Listening to Us, the Future Is Going to Look the Same as the Past": Young People and Reconciliation in Northern Ireland and Bosnia and Herzegovina, *Youth Society*, 43 (2): 509-527

Nielsen, J. (2006). F-shaped pattern for reading web content. Nielsen Norman Group. Retreived from https://www.nngroup.com/articles/f-shaped-pattern-reading-web-content/

Rose, G. (2011). *Visual methodologies: An introduction to researching with visual materials.* Thousand Oaks, CA: Sage.

Ryan, L., and Mackinnon, S. (2016). Photovoice: Using pictures to tell a story. Ed. A. Crowe, in A. R. Vollman (Ed.), Canadian Community as Partner: Theory and Multidisciplinary Practice. 4th ed. Philadelphia, PA: Lippincott Williams & Wilkins.

Stevens, M., & Gielen, U. (2012). *Toward a global psychology: Theory, research, intervention, and pedagogy.* Hove: Psychology Press.

Transparency International. (2015). Corruption perception index 2015. Retrieved from http://www.transparency.org/cpi2015

US Department of State. (1995). Dayton accords. Retrieved from http://www.state.gov/p/eur/rls/or/dayton/

Wang, C. (1999). Photovoice: A participatory action research strategy applied to women's health. *Journal of Women's Health, 8*(2): 185-92.

Wang, C., & Burris, M. (1997). Photovoice: Concept, methodology, and use for participatory needs assessment. *Health Education and Behavior, 24*(3), 369-387.

Wild, J., Wild, K., Han, J., & Rammal, H., (2007) *International business: the challenges of globalisation,* Frenchs Forrest, Pearson Education Australia.

CHAPTER 20

Establishing a Virtual Academy for Overcoming Global
Poverty: Taking Knowledge into Action

Marlene J. Cohen and Joseph Martin Stevenson

Introduction

> *"Our greatness lies not so much in being able to remake the world...as in being able to remake ourselves."*
> — *Mahatma Gandhi (Rothenberg, 2007, p. 729)*

This chapter details the development of a technological infrastructure, Virtual Academy for Overcoming Global Poverty (VAOGP), that allows undergraduate and graduate students and faculty to examine global poverty online, onsite, and in class. The area of poverty is central to the new charter of the United Nations (U.N.). This infrastructure would facilitate online discussions between students from various countries and allow them to conduct research and to examine methods and means to mitigate poverty. Students in Europe, Africa, Latin America, and Canada could correspond with students in the United States and throughout the world on common topics.

Poverty is everywhere and does not discriminate based on venue. VAOGP is committed to taking current knowledge into action to address poverty in all its forms in a sustainable manner. VAOGP fulfills this mission by: conducting and encouraging research to identify causes and effects of global poverty; assisting corporate sectors with global strategies and economic development directed at alleviating poverty; employing the international resources of The Chicago School of Professional Psychology

433

(TCSPP) to identify local and global partners for research projects and activities designed to prevent and combat poverty; acknowledging the powerful link between mental health and economic security by including existing TCSPP Global programs and incorporating multidisciplinary issues and solutions surrounding poverty into online; understanding and activating the potential of technology to advance diagnosis/treatment of mental health (and therefore economic security) in the global community; and addressing economic and technological inequities (including access to the internet and digital technologies) that contribute to and perpetuate poor health, dislocation of individuals/families, and high rates of poverty.

The issues surrounding global poverty are complex and are not likely to be resolved by one field of study, one location, or one institution. Creating a space for ongoing and dynamic open discussion about effective, efficient, and sustainable interventions will allow for greater hope in addressing this critical, societal challenge for the voiceless and marginalized around the world. The virtual collaborative work from this new VAOGP will not only contribute to transdisciplinary global conversations about growing poverty throughout the world, but will also help to fill gaps in the literature and address voids in the research. This could have impact, influence, and implication for public policy on a global scale with vast returns on intellectual investment from a bold new global academy using the internet for altruistic and academic rationale versus financial and commercial reasons.

The Development of the Concept

> *"Others have seen what is and asked why. I have seen what could be and asked why not."*
> — *Pablo Picasso (Picasso, 2000, p. 1)*

In our optically advancing and digitally accelerating age, how can we bring students and faculty together – from a distance – to study global poverty from around the world through cyberspace technology?

The concept covered in this chapter calls for the development of a technological infrastructure (Virtual Academy) that allows undergraduate students and faculty to examine global poverty with an academic focus. This foundation would facilitate scholastic dialogue between students and faculty on a global level and allow them to initiate research and to examine interventions that will eliminate poverty. Poverty affects us nationally and internationally. The issues related to poverty could easily figure into a student's continuing education and allow students and academic advisors to explore potential solutions to this meaningful area of study.

Higher education must continue to be committed to providing its students, faculty, staff, and surrounding community with meaningful educational experiences that focus on a global perspective – experiences that foster the diversity of international cultures, the need for a productive process of intercultural synergy, and the acquisition and international understanding of an increasingly interdependent global economy.

As both academic and economic sectors become increasingly interdependent, the opportunities to build synergy for mutually beneficial success will grow. This is particularly paramount as the United Nations Educational, Scientific and Cultural Organization (UNESCO, 1995) suggested post-secondary institution diversification. Program diversification is a welcome development as we redesign higher education, its curriculum, co-curricular cognates, and extra-curricular activities. These changes will be beneficial to learners and teachers who are preparing for the challenges of the next global millennium.

To carry out this commitment, a technological infrastructure for a growing international academy within a global economy is necessary and its core focus should be poverty. An online global academy could focus on the following primary goals: (1) to provide an internationally-focused model curriculum for students, faculty, and staff to study poverty, (2) to assist the corporate sectors with global strategy and economic development regarding poverty, (3) to provide corporate and college clients and constituencies with training in economics, culture, language, and social welfare issues, (4) to facilitate an international network of data bases on poverty and the global economy for academic, corporate, and governmental communities, and (5) to engage both students and faculty in critical thinking, character building, service learning and global citizenship.

In *The Future of State Universities*, Roskens (1985) warned that, "Americans [would] become increasingly aware of and influenced by the fact that they live in an emerging world community and economy" (p. 27). Magrath and Borgestad (1985) add that as the global community shrinks and countries become more intertwined economically, politically, and for security, there is an increased demand for international awareness, cooperation, and competence. Meeting such demands is a fundamental responsibility of any nation's educational system.

In *The International Dimension in U.S. Higher Education*, Spalding (1989), for the Association of American Colleges, recognizes that, "We live in an era in which America's international competitiveness has become key to national well-being, if not economic survival" (p. 2). As far back as 1816, Thomas Jefferson noted, "An educated citizenry is a vital requisite for our survival as a free people" (Wagoner, 2004, p. 113). Today, we live in a global economy, and education must therefore include commitment to the knowledge that will yield success.

The nexus of academic discussions about emerging global challenges could center on the following changes, conditions, circumstances, and consequences (Stevenson, 2013):

- Locally, regionally, and globally expanding and enhancing multiculturalism and convergences within and across nations to enhance technology and cultural change;
- Eliminating disparity in the divide between the less and more fortunate, resulting in human equity and justice;
- Increasing collaboration from privately and publicly funded schools about the definition of an educated person;
- Finding solutions for income related hardships, economic crises, increased unemployment rates, and national disasters resulting in growing concern for future generations;
- Altering morals to ensure the development of a societal continuum that ranges from highly conservative voices to highly liberal voices with beliefs that promote common respect and acceptance and tolerance;
- Demystifying historical opinions about race and discrimination complicated by biased attitudes on campus and the community about the status quo;
- Eliminating concerns about self-preservation, territorialism, individualism, territorialism, and religious disagreement amid unpreparedness for expanding globalization;
- Reducing citizen powerlessness related to impacting governmental, educational, and corporate decisions;
- Increasing voice, contribution, and influence of women and ethnic minorities;
- Eliminating conflict-ridden discourse about entitlements, rights, and privileges resulting in intolerance and restriction of human rights;
- Addressing waning respect for freedom of expression and disregard for human dignity creating ambiguity about the principle of higher education for the greater good;
- Changing habits of human behavior concerning perceptions, and opinions based on heightened emotionalism versus facts, objective analysis and data driven decision making;
- Addressing resentment and opposition to socio-progressive change made more complex by changing technology, resulting in high tech versus high touch;
- Unearthing repressed human feelings of those living in the south related to human rights issues of the Old Deep South (Post Civil War) and New Deep South (Post Civil Rights);

· Tackling the waning confidence in the possibility of the American Dream and increasing incidents of behavior based on over-sensationalized reactions to current events;

· Addressing fear of losing perceived freedoms, rights and liberties, losing position in society, losing historical individuality, losing freedom of choice, and fear of the unknown.

This concept of a virtual academy calls for the transnational development of a technological infrastructure that facilitates academic opportunities for students and faculty to conduct research and scholarship online and in-class in areas that impact and implicate global urban poverty.

As a working conceptual document, the next section will review urban poverty conditions – both nationally and globally – emerging technologies, higher education trends, public service development, and systemic issues. It will conclude with recommendations for further development.

Historical Context

"Extreme poverty anywhere is a threat to human security everywhere."
— *Kofi Annan, Seventh Secretary-General of the United Nations (2002, p. 1)*

Over four decades ago, Fantini and Weinstein (1968), in *The Disadvantaged: Challenge to Education*, cited a colleague who commented: ". . . historians may write of this cycle as the opening phase of an educational revolution...powerful, purposeful, reshaping of our educational institutions" (p. 418). Earlier in the same work, they advocated that, ". . . education is called upon to solve such problems as social mobility, work force, and employment, poverty, social injustice and segregation" (p. 56). That same year, Featherstone (1968) of Michigan State University cited a colleague as projecting in *Urban Schooling* that, ". . . by 1999, our urban population will reach nearly 250 million; urban wealth will increase fourfold, and the average family income will be much higher, even in today's purchasing power, to build that growth . . ." (p. 286). He later cites another colleague as concluding, ". . . the university comes closest to being able to identify itself with the whole of the urban scene...(p. 213) Respective disciplines can touch every aspect of circumstances of the nation's poor. This inspired both Presidents John F. Kennedy and Lyndon B. Johnson (Johnson, 1964) as they declared (in 1963 and 1964, respectively) the historic "War on Poverty." As reflected later by Church (1976): ". . . children of poverty came to school nutritionally deprived, in poor health, and with aspirations already circumscribed" (p. 432).

In 1990, the Business-Higher Education Forum of the American Council on Education (ACE) provided a synopsis of the above present conditions of urban life in the preface of their widely disseminated publication, *Three Realities: Minority Life in the United States*. The Business-Higher Education Forum report warns, ". . . severe minority poverty in U.S. remains a paradox in a just and compassionate society" (p. 213). The report culminates with recommendations relative to out-of-wedlock births, public education employment, and public assistance reform. Nationally, Jargowsky (1997) speculates:

> . . . between 1970 and 1990, neighborhood poverty in U.S. metro areas, considered collectively, grew along virtually every dimension. Ghettos, barrios, and other slum neighborhoods expanded in size, number of residents, number of poor residents, and the proportion of the metro population within them. (p. 29)

One could speculate that the recommendations, primarily developed by ACE for higher education and corporate audiences, probably did not reach readers of professional business journals or other academic publications commonly circulated among many international groups. Moreover, frequently, reports prepared by academicians and corporate leaders lack real life, "theory into practice" application with action plans for designating resources, responsibility, time frames, and anticipated outcomes and methods for assessing expected results. This could frustrate practitioners in the workplace, activists in the field, and both students and faculty in the modern college classroom.

The ACE recommendations were proposed on the birth of a new decade, when according to Davis and McCaul (1990) in *At-Risk Children and Youth*:

- 1 million students do not complete their secondary education (p. 4)
- 1.5 million teens become expectant with child (p. 4)
- At least 100,000 children are homeless each night (p. 4)
- Over 5,000 young people commit suicide each year (p. 4)
- A reported 2.2 million cases of child abuse and neglect occurred in 1987 (p. 4)
- 15% of urban high school graduates are able to read at less than a 6th grade level (p. 4)
- About 10 million children are without regular medical care (p. 4)
- Almost 20 million children under 17 years of age have never visited a dentist (p. 4)
- Approximately 3 million children have a serious problem with alcohol abuse (p. 4)

More specific to poverty, the authors warned that:

- Children represent 40% of the country's poor even though they make up 25% of the U.S. population (p. 20)

- Overall, about 1/5 of all U.S. children live in households below the poverty line (p. 20)
- 46% of black children exist below the poverty line (p. 20)
- 40% of Hispanic children exist below the poverty line (p. 20)
- 16% of white children exist below the poverty line (p. 20)
- Of the 3 million newly classified as poor, 2 million are Caucasian (p. 20)
- 54% of the poorest children live with single mothers (p. 20)
- In the U. S., every 53 seconds a child dies of poverty (p. 20)

In their subsequent report, Davis and McCaul (1991) concluded that:

. . . children represent the largest and fastest growing group of poor in U.S, forty percent of the poor in U.S. are children...more Americans are poor today than before the war on poverty was initiated in 1964. . . .nearly 40,000,000 people of all ages live in the families below the official poverty line...the younger a child is today in this country, the greater are his/her chances of being poor. (p. 35)

More recent research communicates similar conditions. The Editors of the Chronicle of Higher Education's Almanac (1994) reported a national poverty rate of 18.3% for youth under the age of eighteen (p. 3). These characteristics provide a compelling foundation for all of us in global higher education to conduct applied research, compare and contrast experiences, and develop a "virtual" forum to discuss interventions.

Every year from 1990 to 2014, the status dropout rate was lower for White youth than for Black youth, and the rates for both White and Black youth were lower than the rate for Hispanic youth. During this period, the status dropout rate declined from 9.0 to 5.2 percent for White youth; from 13.2 to 7.4 percent for Black youth; and from 32.4 to 10.6 percent for Hispanic youth. As a result, the gap between White and Hispanic youth narrowed from 23.4 percentage points in 1990 to 5.3 percentage points in 2014. Most of this gap narrowed between 2000 and 2014, when the gap between White and Hispanic youth decreased from 20.9 to 5.3 percentage points. Although the rates for both White and Black youth declined from 1990 to 2014, the gap between the rates in 2014 did not measurably differ from the gap between the rates in 1990. However, the White-Black gap narrowed from 6.2 percentage points in 2000 to 2.2 percentage points in 2014 (Institute of Education Sciences, 2016, p. 1).

The U.S. Department of Health and Human Services stated, "In 2014, there were 24.2 births for every 1,000 adolescent females ages 15-19, or 249,078 babies born to females in this age group. Nearly 89 percent of these births occurred outside of marriage" (U.S. Department of Health and Human Services, 2016, p. 4). According to the authors' calculations, this is a decrease of over 66% since 1990.

However, homelessness among children has significantly increased since 1990. "A staggering 2.5 million children are now homeless each year in America. This historic high represents one in every 30 children in the United States" (National Center on Family Homelessness, 2016, p. 1).

In a study conducted by Graham and Teague (2011), the reading levels of students in suburban, urban, and rural school students were compared. While reading levels of urban and rural third grade students lagged behind suburban students, they found that socioeconomic status was more strongly correlated to lower reading levels than the location of the student.

According to global data in 2007, 9.2 million children die before they reach age 5 (UNICEF, 2009, p. 30). Many of these children die from causes that could have been prevented through proper health care and living conditions.

Poverty has harmful effects on individuals in society, which in turn negatively impact human potential. Research has supported this premise for many years. In 2002, the International Union for the Conservation of Nature reported that the disparity between rich and poor countries continues to grow, both within each country and between them. Research has found a consistent relationship between educational and economic outcomes (Van der Berg, 2008), indicating that strengthening the educational experience may improve economic results.

While better educational outcomes may combat poverty, parents in low-income families may not have the experience necessary to provide the same level of intellectual stimulation as parents in higher-income families (Engle & Black, 2009). Parents in low-income families also tend to read less often to their children, which decreases phonemic awareness and comprehension skills. Furthermore, poverty also has a negative impact on educational development due to lack of resources (Lacour & Tissington, 2011).

These issues extend across the globe and are not specific to any one country or culture. For example, Van der Berg (2011) reports that poverty has had a negative impact on length of education in South Africa, and this has affected skill shortages in the labor market. Here in the U.S., the combination of minority status and income has had a significant effect on educational outcomes (National Student Clearinghouse, 2015). Additional research in the U.S. indicates a substantial achievement gap attribute to low-income status (Harvey, 2015).

Even more disturbing is the relationship between low-income children's educational outcomes and later incarceration in the criminal justice system (Adamu & Hogan, 2013). "The term 'school-to-prison pipeline' has become a powerful metaphor to capture the processes by which children – typically low-income children of color – are pushed out of school and into the criminal justice system" (Adamu & Hogan, 2013, p. 1).

The many, unrealized talents of these individuals equate to tragic waste of human potential.

Coley & Baker (2013) point to improved educational experiences for low-income children as a potential resolution. Stevenson (2003) adds to this solution by suggesting that technology be used to improve educational outcomes for low-income children and adults. We are no longer limited to the location of educational resources as access to the internet can provide much-needed educational expertise wherever the infrastructure for internet access exists.

More recently, the Center for Law and Social Policy (CLASP) (2016) reported a 1.3% decrease in poverty between 2014 and 2015, with approximately 1 million less children living in poverty (p. 3). They point to changes in public policy, including the Affordable Care Act, as the impetus for this improvement. With the upcoming presidential election in the near future, CLASP calls for us to keep poverty as a focus.

Based on this historic data, it is clear that poverty remains a serious global problem. This problem will most likely not be solved by any one discipline or organization. With this in mind, the concept of a virtual academy that is comprised of the interdisciplinary efforts of faculty and students in higher education across multiple fields of study and in conjunction with private and public entities with a focus on elimination of poverty could provide a more thorough and comprehensive vehicle for tackling the issues of poverty.

Developing the Vision

"The world is a dangerous place, not because of those who do evil, but because of those who look on and do nothing."
— *Albert Einstein, theoretical physicist*
(Crowley, 2016, p. 3)

In September 2015, we (the present authors) initiated the process of developing a virtual academy devoted to overcoming global poverty at TCSPP. This process began with a brainstorming session comprised of interested faculty from online and on-ground campuses. The first area of focus was to develop a clear mission and vision statement that would guide the development of the academy. The following is a product of that session.

VAOGP Overview

The VAOGP is a confluence of efforts designed for overcoming poverty on a national and international level. The focus of VAOGP is to form partnerships with departments and groups both within and outside of TCSPP in order to develop best practices through synergy of multiple resources that together form solutions to global poverty that could not be achieved by a single resource.

VAOGP intends to do more than develop well-intentioned efforts to address the global issues of poverty; it also intends to form alliances between groups of people that will yield solutions that match the culture of the groups we want to impact. TCSPP is already engaged in a variety of community outreach efforts, and VAOGP can help to more efficiently coordinate and expand these efforts.

VAOGP is engaged in developing and evaluating efforts to overcome global poverty through the implementation of educational opportunities, community outreach, and research. It is time to break through the barriers that have prevented meaningful and widespread impact on this critical and chronic social issue.

VAOGP Mission Statement

VAOGP is committed to taking current knowledge into action in order to address poverty in all its forms in a sustainable manner.

VAOGP fulfills this mission by:

- Engaging in and encouraging research to determine sources and consequence of global poverty
- Assisting businesses with approaches to and development of interventions directed at alleviating poverty
- Utilizing the international assets of TCSPP to obtain local and global partners for research efforts and related activities focused on the prevention and reduction of poverty
- Implementing an interdisciplinary approach to addressing issues of poverty and incorporating this into the curricula
- Potentiating the use of technology to address poverty by addressing the related issues of mental health
- Determining solutions to economic and technologic inequities that contribute to health crises among the poor as well as the displacement of families and individuals
- Promoting efforts to break through the obstacles to ease of access to care in underserved groups
- Participating in and supporting scientific research based on the cultural needs of the population we are affecting
- Creating a database for the widespread distribution of effective interventions

VAOGP Vision Statement

VAOGP sees a world where participation in research, service, action, and innovation come together to alleviate poverty (Virtual Academy for Overcoming Global Poverty, 2015, p. 2).

VAOGP Focus

After the development of a solid mission and vision statement, a number of Chicago School Faculty began to form teams that would address the broad scope of the academy and to formulate specific, sustainable, and actionable goals.

The first of team works in the area of International and Community Partnerships. The goals of this team are as follows:

- To create and disseminate a resource database for potential partners addressing poverty
- To involve students in the efforts of the academy
- To partner with faculty and students to develop curriculum aimed at developing cultural competency
- To create Study Within courses targeted on addressing poverty issues within the United States

A second team with longer-term goals works in the area of Telehealth/Telepsychology. The goals of this team are:

- To create a virtual clinic to provide mental health services to those in at risk areas staffed by volunteer faculty and students
- To establish research efforts in the area of telehealth/telepsych and be pioneers in establishing efficient and effective delivery models

An additional team focused on the development of a journal and publication of poverty-related research. The focus of this group is as follows:

- To form a free, open access online journal aimed at encouraging and publishing research related to the reduction of global poverty
- To provide assistance for faculty and student research related to the reduction of poverty
- To establish partnerships between qualitative researchers who study the issues associated with poverty with quantitative researchers who objectively measure the results of interventions and their ability to ensure independence of the affected populations

The current editorial board includes: Chris Stout (Director of the Center for Global Initiatives), Marc Pilisuk (author of *Who Benefits from Global Violence and War*), Carroll Cradock (member of IP faculty and past President of the Chicago campus of TCSPP), Joel Federman (writer, teacher activist Saybrook University), and Paul C. Gorski (founder of

EdChange), and Patricia Perez (faculty of TCSPP's International Psychology program).

Due to the current status of the technological divide between those who can afford technology and those who cannot, we also created a Technology Team. This team is devoted to the following:

· To establish existing technologies that can be used to support the efforts of the academy

· To approach technology corporations with a mutual interest in addressing poverty to encourage the development of technology related solutions to poverty

As referred to in the CLASP newsletter (2016), there is evidence that social policy has a positive impact on the reduction of poverty. As such, a Social Policy/Advocacy team was formulated. Its goals are:

· To stay in touch with current social policy and advocacy efforts tackling issues related to poverty

· To inform faculty, staff and students of social policy and advocacy efforts

It is worth mentioning that VAOGP was listed in "Opportunities to Create Change like Never Before," a LinkedIn Take Action series in which Influencers discuss how to fight poverty and drive change that matters.

Most poverty related interventions will rely on funding from grants and corporate and individual contributors. A Grants/Funding team was developed to provide assistance to faculty and staff who wish to apply for grant support. Their goals are:

· To determine funding sources for collaboration between faculty, staff and students conducting research related to reducing global poverty

· To establish the academy as a source of sustainable outcomes, garnering interest of potential funders

Since there are opportunities for faculty, staff, and students to contribute to the poverty-related literature, departmental support is necessary in order to coordinate efforts and to match like-minded faculty and staff with similar interests. This team's goals are:

· To develop a synergistic relationship with all TCSPP campuses and departments by producing information related to global poverty to faculty and students and supporting theses and dissertations by developing a global poverty track for students interested in conducting their research in this area

· To work in conjunction with current support networks to generate curriculum related to reducing global poverty

· To join with interested faculty to incorporate cultural competency and related issues into the curriculum

·To support and develop fieldwork and practicum opportunities closely alighned with VAOGP projects

The development of our teams was based on the interest and existing projects of multiple faculty and staff. Together, they comprise a multi-pronged effort to affect social policy, to encourage the development of sustainable, evidence-based solutions to poverty, to provide service to those in need, and to coordinate people involved in existing efforts in a way that maximizes impact.

Harnessing Resources

> *"As long as poverty, injustice and gross inequality exist in our world, none of us can truly rest."*
> — *Nelson Mandela (Mandela, 2005, p. 1)*

The focus of the Academy morphed broadly across multiple fronts. As such, there was a need for the development of a detailed plan regarding how we would best function in the future. We used a version of a logic model to create specific goals and outcomes. The logic model is comprised of the following: Assumptions, Inputs/Resources, Activities/Deliverables, Symmetrical Partners, Outputs, Outcomes and Impact and is a version of the W. K. Kellogg Foundation Logic Model (2004). The definitions of the terms are listed below. An abbreviated version of the model can be found in Appendix A*.

1. "Assumptions" are accounts of circumstances upon which the outcomes and impacts depend. Altering these alters the outcomes, and therefore the impacts.
2. "Inputs/Resources" are the resources (funds, personnel, materials) necessary to conduct the activities resulting in the outputs.
3. "Activities/Deliverables" are steps that must be accomplished in order to produce the outputs or outcomes.
4. "Symmetrical Partners" are the crucial personnel engaging in the activities and accountable for the outcome.
5. "Outputs" are the effects of actions.
6. "Outcomes" are the preferred result of the plan.
7. "Impact" outlines the advantages of completing the project to the organization.

Since the VAOGP was conceptualized as part of a university, it became necessary to educate faculty, staff, and students in best intervention

---

* Appendices for this chapter can be found at: http://tinyurl.com/wghm-attachments

practices that will result in sustainable, meaningful interventions. As a virtual academy, this process is further challenged by its distance education nature and few, if any, opportunities for face-to-face interaction. Keeping the learning environment dynamic and supportive involves multiple factors. First, it is important to find and harness each individual's motivation for involvement in poverty-related work and to provide training in matching that motivation to that of the individuals or groups with whom they plan to work. Infusing the concepts of partnership and taking the position of servant in the intended community are important variables that lead to sustainability. Historically, efforts that did not take into account the unique capabilities and needs of the persons being impacted have failed. We now know that interventions of this type have not yielded sustainable results.

More often than not, the impoverished groups we intend to impact know more about what will work and what will not work than we do. Once we understand this, we can begin to see how we can facilitate empowerment through connecting with necessary resources. For example, teachers in Colombia are not provided with any teaching-specific curriculum in their course work. There is no teaching certificate required. When preparing for a teacher training in Popayán, Colombia, we asked about the specific needs of the teachers. We also planned for two weeks of follow up in the classroom to ensure teachers were given the support necessary to implement the strategies covered in training. As a result, we were able to see teachers being empowered to better serve the needs of their students.

There is much to be said about the proverb "Give a man a fish, and you feed him for a day. Teach a man to fish, and you feed him for a lifetime" (Maimonides, date unknown). The time spent learning from the group you wish to impact and matching the intervention and tools to the unique needs of the group is critical. For example, while training teachers to use technology in rural South Africa, we spent time talking to the previous trainers and to the teachers themselves to determine what obstacles they were encountering in utilizing the internet in the classroom. It became clear that, although the teachers had been trained to use the technology provided, they did not know how to use the technology to access information that could be used when teaching. This became the focus of future training followed by in-class support for initial efforts. This approach empowered teachers to access the wealth of knowledge available through the internet and to open up new avenues for learning for their students.

A distinctive aspect of a virtual academy is its ability to provide access to individuals from remote, regional, and rural areas throughout the world. A worldwide focus can encourage a broader source of creative solutions and broader understanding of the diverse needs of impoverished groups. An online presence can also be beneficial in the following ways:

446

· Creating a supportive network for feedback, problem solving, and
   sharing effective strategies
· Facilitating questions, reflections, and discussions
· Linking content to events and examples, thus creating a historical
   compilation of information and resources
· Providing a voice to impoverished groups
· Creating an environment of encouraged inquiry

Although access to the technology necessary to participate in an online
network remains an issue, there are increasingly more and lower-cost
options that have emerged in practice (Davis, 2013, Rhodan & Dias, 2014).

Measurable Results: Making a Meaningful Difference

'If it can't be expressed in figures, it is not science; it is opinion.
— Robert Heinlein (Heinlein, 1973, p. 263)

As a Board Certified Behavior Analyst, I (Cohen) am well aware that
determining the impact of an intervention focused on reducing poverty can
only be achieved though objective measurement. However, due to the
complexity of poverty, the large number of people one might intend to
impact, and the health, educational, and financial influences already in play,
what measures are meaningful, and how do we determine which ones to
use?

In 1999, Maxwell discussed how to measure poverty and differences
based on poverty models (Maxwell, 1999). He believed that poverty is best
measured through metrics related to the underlying causes of poverty. This
presents a significant challenge in our ability to determine the effectiveness
of interventions. I suggest simplification of poverty measures by
concentrating on poverty by household level, income, differentiating
chronic from transitory poverty, and considering relative poverty and
deprivation.

In 2005, the World Bank stated that poverty measures should come
from survey data that is obtained directly from households. These explicit
measures will go far to inform policy makers of the conditions of the poor,
to identify interventions, and to clearly target resources such as plans to
increase employment. This measurement strategy also helps in
understanding the relationship between education as well as gender and
poverty.

Alkire and Santos (2013) recommends building a more systematic
framework for reducing multi-dimensional poverty that is based on people's
experiences and value system. This would incorporate dimensions such as

health, education, living standards, quality of work, and more innovative elements.

The lack of agreement about and the inconsistency surrounding poverty measures create a daunting problem for the VAOGP and similar groups. Drawing from the field of psychology, VAOGP created a needs assessment that could be distributed to the group we plan to impact and potentially provide a means of measuring need and later impact of an intervention. The assessment is shown in Appendix B.

The VAOGP needs assessment focuses on factors that are important to the individual. For example, interventions that support dependency on others do not allow for empowerment of the individual or group. Poverty cannot be effectively eradicated without focus on the root causes, which can be found at an individual level (Ssekamtte, 2012). Determining community leaders who could help to collect the needs assessment data contained to form a bridge between those who are intervening and those who are receiving intervention would strengthen the social validity of the results. While other measures such as income and access to health care are also important, this assessment adds to those.

Future Directions

"Don't let complexity stop you. Be activists. Take on the big inequities. It will be one of the great experiences of your lives."
— Bill Gates (Gates, 2007, p. 6)

Our VAOGP concept was presented for the Executive Leadership Academy at the University of California, Berkeley in spring of 2016. We are appending this power presentation (Appendix C) to exemplify powerful purposefulness and exhibit potential practice of the VAOGP.

VAOGP is no longer sustained by TCSPP; however a number of faculty remain committed to its efforts. The academy seeks to find a new base from which to work and to extend collaboration to other universities, corporations, and other parties that are focused on sustainable poverty reduction. This goal will hopefully be achieved within the next few months.

Most book chapters end with conclusions and suggestions for future direction. In this case, we call for readers to add to the conversation initiated here. Suggestions for the future direction of the academy, ways in which collaborative efforts can be developed and extended, ideas for designing future research, thoughts on new initiatives and innovations are some of the concepts that could be added to our chapter as a means of addressing the complex issues surrounding poverty. This chapter does not have all of the answers. It is a start of what will hopefully lead to the elimination of poverty. In this way, we can make what might appear impossible, possible.

References

Adamu, M. & Hogan, L. (2013, October 8). Point of entry: The preschool-to-prison pipeline. Retrieved from https://www.americanprogress.org/issues/earlychildhood/report/2015/10/08/122867/pointofentry

Alkire, S. & Santos, M. E. (2013). Measuring Acute Poverty in the Developing World: Robustness and Scope of the Multidimensional Poverty Index. *OPHI Working Paper*, 59, 1-48.

Anan, K. (2002). *Marking international day for eradication of poverty* [Press release]. Retrieved from http://www.un.org/press/en/2002/sgsm8431.doc.htm

Bassuk, E. L., DeCandia, C. J., Beach, C. A. & Berman, F. (2014, November 30).

America's youngest outcasts: A report card on child homelessness. Retrieved from http://www.air.org/center/national-center-family-homelessness

Church, R. L. & Sedlak, M. W. (1976). *Education in the United States*. New York, NY: Free Press.

CLASP. (2016, September 13). Statement: Strong reduction in poverty,improvement in health insurance, but more to do for next generation's families. Retrieved from http://www.clasp.org/news-room/news-releases/statement-strong-reduction-in-poverty-improvement-in-health-insurance-but-more-to-do-for-next-generations-families

Coley, R. J. & Baker, B. (2013). *Poverty and Education: Finding the Way Forward*. Princeton,NJ: Educational Testing Service.

Crowley, E. P. (2016). *Preventing Abuse and Neglect in the Lives of Children with Disabilities*. Cham, Switzerland: Springer International Publishing.

Davis, S. (2013, March 22). Can technology end poverty? *Harvard Business Review Online*. Retrieved from https://hbr.org/2013/03/can-technology-end-poverty

Davis, W. E. & McCaul, E. J. (1990). *At-risk children and youth: A crisis in ourschools and society*. August, ME: Division of Special Education, Maine Department of Educational Services, and Orono, ME : University of Maine.

Davis, W. E., & McCaul, E. J. (1991). *The emerging crisis: Current and projectedstatus of children in the United States*. Orono, ME: University of Maine and Institute for the Study of At-Risk Students.

Editors of the Chronicle of Higher Education Almanac (1994). *The Almanac of Higher Education*. Chicago, IL: Chicago University Press.

Editors of Education Week (1993). *From Risk to Renewal: Charting a Course for Reform*. Bethesda, MD: Editorial Projects for Education.

Engle, P. & Black, M. M. (2009). The effect of poverty on child developmentand educational outcomes. Retrieved from http://docplayer.net/10679953-The-effect-of-poverty-on-child-development-and-educational-outcomes.html .

Fantini, M. D. and Weinstein, G. (1968). *The Disadvantaged: Challenge to Education*. New York, NY: Harper & Row.

Featherstone, J. (1968). Report analysis: Children and their primary schools. *Harvard Education Review, 38*(2), 317-328.

Gates, B. (2007). Change the world. *Harvard Gazette*. Retrieved from http://news.harvard.edu/gazette/story/2007/06/remarks-of-bill-gates-harvard-commencement-2007

Gandhi, M., Fischer, L. & Gandhi, M. K. (2002). *The essential gandhi: An anthology of his writings on his life, work, and ideas*. New York, NY: Vintage Books.

Graham, S. E. & Teague, C. (2011). Reading levels of rural and urban third graders lag behind their suburban peers. *Carsey Issue Brief, 28*, 1-4.

Harvey, A. (2013, August 29). ETS study examines collision of poverty andeducation. *NEA Today*. Retrieved from http://neatoday.org/2013/08/29/ets-study-examines-collision-of-poverty-and-education-2/

Heinlein, R. A. (1973). *Time enough for love.* New York, NY: ACE Books.

Herold, E. & Daley G. (2007). *Stem cell wars.* London, UK: Palgrave Macmillan.

Institute of Education Sciences. (2016). Status dropout rates. Retrieved from http://nces.ed.gov/programs/coe/indicator_coj.asp

IUCN. (2002, September 4). Sustainable development, poverty and the environment: A challenge to the global community. Retrieved from http://cmsdata.iucn.org/downloads/poverty.pdf

Jargowsky, P. A. (1998). *Poverty and Place.* New York, NY: Russell Sage Foundation.

Johnson, L. B. (1964). First State of the Union Address. Retrieved from http://www.pbs.org/wgbh/americanexperience/features/primary-resources/lbj-union64/

Lacour, M. & Tissington, L. D. (2011). The effects of poverty on academic achievement. *Educational Research and Reviews, 6*(7), 522-527.

Magrath, C. P. & Borgerstad, J. (1985). *In the future of state universities: issues in teaching, research, and public service.* Eds. Koepplin, L. W. & Wilson, D. A. New Brunswick, NJ: Rutgers University Press

Maimonides, M. (Date unknown). *Brainy Quote.* Retrieved from http://www.brainyquote.com/quotes/quotes/m/maimonides326751.html

Mandela, N. (2005, February 3). Nelson Mandela's Speech to Trafalgar Square Crowd. Retrieved from http://news.bbc.co.uk/2/hi/uk_news/politics/4232603.stm

Maslow, A.H. (1943). A theory of human motivation. *Psychological Review, 50*(4): 370–96.

Mason, S. (1990). *Three realities: Minority life in the United States.* Berkley, CA: Business Higher Education.

Maxwell, S. (1999). The meaning and measurement of poverty. *ODI Poverty Briefing, 3*, 1-4.

National Center on Family Homelessness (2016). *AIR index: Mothers in homeless and housing programs.* Retrieved from http://www.air.org/resource/air-index-mothers-homeless-and-housing-programs.

National Student Clearinghouse (2015, October 14). National college progression rates. *High School Benchmarks.* Retrieved from https://nscresearchcenter.org/hsbenchmarks2015

Picasso, P. (2000). Picasso quotes. *Pablo Picasso Paintings, Quotes, and Biography.* Retrieved from http://www.pablopicasso.org/quotes.jsp

Picasso, P. & Dorshka, R. (2000). *Metamorphoses of the human form: Graphic works.* New York: NY: Prestel.

Rhodan, M. & Dias, E. J. (2014, March 22). USAID using technology to fight poverty. *Time Magazine.* Retrieved from http://time.com/47530/usaid-technology-poverty

Roskens, Ft. W. (1985). *In the future of state universities: issues in teaching, research, and public service,* Eds. Koepplin, L. W. & Wilson, D. A. New Brunswick, NJ: Rutgers University Press.

Rothenberg, p. S. (2007). *Race, Class, and Gender in the United States.* New York, NY: Worth Publishers.

Ssekamtte, D. (2012, June). Why poverty interventions remain ineffective. *Daily Monitor,* 1-2.

Spalding, J. (Ed.). (1989). The international dimension in U.S. higher education: New directions in business school/liberal arts cooperation. Conference proceedings. Washington, DC: Association of American Colleges.

Stevenson, J. M. (2013). *Catalystics.* Bethesda, MD: Academica Press.

Stout, C. (2015, September 21). Opportunities to create change like never before. Retrieved from https://www.linkedin.com/pulse/opportunities-create-change-like-never-before-dr-chris-stout

United Nations Children's Fund. (2009). *The state of the world's children*. New York, NY: Brodock Press.

UNESCO (1995). Declaration of Principles on Tolerance. The Member States of the
United Nations Educational, Scientific and Cultural Organization, meeting in Paris at the twenty-eighth session of the General Conference, from 25 October to 16 November 199

UNICEF (2009). *Annual Report of 2009*. Retrieved from http://www.unicef.org/publications/index_53754.html

U.S. Department of Health and Human Services. (2016, June 2). National Advisory Council on the National Health Service Corps, *Federal* Register, 81 (106), 35368-35369.

Van der Berg, S. (2008). Poverty and education. Education Policy Series. Paris, France: The International Institute for Educational Planning & Brussels, Belgium: The International Academy of Education.

Van der Berg, S, Burger, C., Burger, R., de Vos, M., du Rand, G., Gustafsson, M., Moses, E. Shepherd, D., Spaull, N., Taylor, S., van Broekhuizen, H. & von Finte, D. (2011, March). Low quality education as a poverty trap. Retrieved from https://www.andover.edu/GPGConference/Documents/Low-Quality-Education-Poverty-Trap.pdf

Virtual Academy for Overcoming Global Poverty. The Chicago School of Professional Psychology. (2015). *The Virtual Academy for Overcoming Global Poverty Overview*. Chicago, IL

Wagoner, J. (2004). *Jefferson and education*. Charlottesville, Va.: Thomas Jefferson Foundation.

W.K. Kellogg Foundation. (2004*). W.K. Kellogg Foundation Logic Model Development Guide*. Battle Creek, MI: W.K. Kellogg Foundation.

Wolf, M. M. (1978). Social validity: The case for subjective measurement or how applied behavior analysis is finding its heart. *Journal of Applied Behavior Analysis, 11*(2): 203–214.

World Bank (2005). What is poverty and why measure it? *Poverty Manual*, 8-13.

CHAPTER 21

Investing in the Global Health Workforce

Zohray Talib and Lalit Narayan

Introduction

This chapter will explore the role of the health workforce in improving health outcomes globally and argues that workforce strengthening needs to be a priority for the decade ahead. We will start with an overview of the current global health workforce and its links to health outcomes as well as economic development. We will then briefly review key challenges that face the field of health workforce and suggestions for how these might be addressed.

Overview of the Health Workforce

Break Down of the Workforce

Health workers are "all people engaged in actions whose primary intent is to enhance health" (World Health Organization [WHO], 2006, p. xiv). The health workforce is a key component of the health system, the sum of all activities with the primary goal of improving health. In addition to the provision of health services, health workers play many other key roles within the system including leadership, supervision of other workers and facilities, health workforce planning, training, engaging communities, and even managing the finances of the health sector.

The WHO Global Health Workforce Statistics database breaks down the health workforce into the following broad categories (WHO, n.d.):

· Physicians

· Nurses and midwife personnel

- Dentistry personnel
- Pharmaceutical personnel
- Laboratory health workers
- Environment and public health workers
- Community and traditional health workers
- Other health workers (includes dieticians, rehabilitation personnel, medical imaging experts, and optometrists)
- Healthcare management and support workers (includes health economists, policy-makers, ambulance drivers, and building maintenance staff)

The best data available is through the WHO Global Health Observatory, which reports workforce data for 186 countries. Of the 57 countries identified in 2006 with low health worker density and low service coverage, 17 countries have no data point in the past five years (WHO, 2014a, p. vi). Current estimates indicate that in 2013, the total global health workforce was 43 million, of which nearly one quarter were physicians, half were nurses or midwives, and the remaining quarter were other health workers (WHO, 2016a, p. 40). The geographic distribution of the workforce is clearly slanted toward the upper and upper-middle income countries (the Americas, Europe, and the Western Pacific, which includes China). The smallest absolute and relative numbers are in Africa. Based on current trends, estimates of the workforce suggest that by 2030, the workforce will grow by 55% to 67.3 million (WHO, 2016a, p. 41).

Health Workforce Moves Up the Global Health Agenda

Health workforce issues became a part of the global health conversation in the early part of the 21st century. In 2006, the WHO published its annual World Health Report (WHO, 2006) and alerted the world to the status of the health workforce. The report highlighted a shortfall of 4.3 million trained health workers globally, with the worst shortages in the poorest countries (p. 12). The report became a catalytic moment for the health workforce in the global health agenda. The WHO then established the Global Health Workforce Alliance (GHWA) as a common platform for action to address the crisis. The alliance was a partnership between national governments, civil society, international agencies, finance institutions, researchers, educators, and professional associations. Over the last decade, the Alliance successfully elevated issues that relate to the health workforce.

In 2008, the GHWA published a report called "Scaling up, Saving Lives" (Global Health Workforce Alliance, 2008) which shed additional light on health workforce issues. In this report, the Alliance described how different types of health workers collaborate within the health system. They highlighted the role of community health workers, who provide the quickest way to increase access to many essential health interventions in rural and urban areas due to their geographic proximity and cultural accessibility. There is growing evidence that they can have a positive impact on health outcomes through health promotion and by delivering simple treatments after a short period of training. Mid-level providers represent a group that has been created by "task-shifting," which is defined as "any cadre being delegated tasks normally performed by more established health professionals with higher qualifications" (p. 41). They tend to be defined by their national contexts and include clinical officers, medical officers, and pharmacy assistants. The advantages of developing mid-level providers are similar to that of developing community health workers: they are cost-effective to train, they cost less to maintain (lower salaries), and they are less likely to migrate out of country as their scope of practice is typically defined nationally. As countries strive for universal coverage, the number of mid-level providers and community health workers is likely to increase. Strengthening these cadres will increase demand for high-level health workers because they will refer cases that are complex or beyond their scope. High-level health workers include physicians, nurses, pharmacists, and midwives. Nurses and doctors provide essential care and provide supervision to other cadres. As community-health workers and mid-levels increase in number, referral systems will also need to be strengthened so that those with special or advanced needs have access to necessary services. Appendix A* provides a graphic of these three categories and how they fit within the global health workforce. Information in the graphic is taken from "Scaling Up, Saving Lives" by the GHWA (2008, p. 39).

Today, attention to the health workforce and the issues of improving the quality, quantity, and retention are at an all-time high. In May of 2016, the member states of the World Health Assembly unanimously adopted the Global Strategy on Human Resources for Health: Workforce 2030 to address human resource challenges and achieve universal health coverage (WHO, 2016a). This milestone is an acknowledgement that health workforce shortages are closely interlinked with both the problems and the solutions to tackle global health issues.

The Link between Health Workforce and Health Outcomes

The link between the health workforce and health outcomes is most apparent during crises such as natural disasters and epidemics, when a lack of trained responders often leads to an alarming number of preventable deaths. The recent Ebola epidemic in West and Central Africa starkly

---

*Appendices for this chapter can be found at: http://tinyurl.com/wghm-attachments

illustrated both the vulnerability of health workers in the face of an epidemic as well the long-term consequences that health worker loss can have on a fragile health system (Evans, Goldstein, & Popova, 2015).

Linking the changes in the numbers, distribution, and quality of health workers to health outcomes in non-crises situations is harder. It is certainly difficult to untangle the contribution of the workforce from other parallel and synergistic efforts. At the macro level, there is a definite association between health worker density and health outcomes (WHO, 2006, p. xvi). At the national level, there are many examples of how investments in health workforce have led to improved health outcomes.

·According to one report, investing in midwifery education in the context of improving community-based services has been found to have a 16-fold return on investment in terms of lives saved and costs of caesarean sections avoided (UNFPA, International Confederation of Midwives, & WHO, 2014, p. 45).

·In Brazil, between 1990 and 2009, the number of nurses increased by 500% , the number of physicians increased by 66%, and the population growth grew by 31%. During the same period, neonatal mortality decreased from 26.8 to 9.7 per 1000 live births, and under-five mortality decreased from 58 to 15.6 per 1000 live births (Campbell et al., 2013, p. 855).

·In Mexico, between 1990 and 2009, the number of nurses and physicians increased by 80% and 170%, respectively, and the population grew by 30%. During the same period, infant mortality and under-five mortality decreased by more than half: from 32.6 to 14.6 per 1000 live births and from 41 to 17.8 per 1000 live births, respectively. Maternal mortality reduced by more than 50% overall (Campbell et al., 2013, p.857).

However, increasing training programs for health workers may not always yield improved health outcomes. The rise in private, for-profit training programs can sometimes be uncoupled with the health needs in a community. This can occur when there is a demand for a type of health care professional, but that type of health care professional is not aligned with the health needs of the community (from a population health perspective). Countries like India and Brazil have witnessed a rapid expansion of private medical colleges that have confounded regulatory mechanisms and have led to spiraling tuition fees and the production of low-quality practitioners (D'Silva, 2015; Scheffer & Dal Poz, 2015). Ill-informed clinical practices, such as over-testing or over-treating, can be dangerous to the population at large. Healthcare expenditures on ineffective diagnostics and therapeutics leads to mounting family debts and contributes to a medical poverty trap in low- and middle-income countries (McIntyre, Thiede, Dahlgren, & Whitehead, 2006). Inappropriate use of antibiotics by poorly trained health workers is a key factor in the development of drug resistant pathogens (Costelloe, Metcalfe, Lovering, Mant, & Hay, 2010).

The Link between Health Workforce and Economic Development

Health sector employment and a robust health workforce are increasingly recognized as contributing to economic development. The United Nations (U.N.) established the High-Level Commission on Health Employment and Economic Growth in March 2016 and tasked it to make recommendations to stimulate job growth in the health sector in order to address the projected shortfall of health workers, primarily in low- and lower-middle income countries, by 2030. The Commission's first report (WHO, 2016c) identified the health sector as one experiencing growth despite the global economic downturn. Across high-income countries that belong to the Organization for Economic Co-operation and Development (OECD), employment in health and social work grew by 48% between 2000 and 2014, a time when other sectors such as industry and agriculture were witnessing net job losses (WHO, 2016c, p. 9). The Commission's report moves away from a traditional understanding of health care spending as a "cost," towards an understanding of the ways in which the health sector, and specifically expansion of health employment, can stimulate economic activity. Health employment, the report describes, creates decent jobs and upward mobility, particularly for young people and women, which leads to economic growth and even stability. The report specifically highlighted the opportunities for women, who made up 67% of employment in the health and social sectors (compared to 41% of total employment, according to a study of 123 countries) (p. 25).

The report described six pathways which link investing in the health workforce to economic development:

1. The first pathway is the direct link between a healthier society and a more productive workforce. One extra year of life expectancy has been shown to raise GDP per capita by about 4% (p. 10).
2. Second, investments in the health sector and health workforce lead to spin off spending in other sectors like manufacturing, pharmaceuticals, and education.
3. The third pathway describes the benefit of social protection through increased employment. A job in the health sector enhances social protection systems by providing access to insurance in cases of disability, sickness, or old age.
4. The fourth pathway describes the social cohesion and reduced inequity created by strengthening healthcare access and health employment. The report highlights that health sector jobs are particularly available in rural and remote locations (unlike other sectors, in which employment is concentrated in urban settings,

thereby increasing opportunity for marginalized and geographically isolated populations).

5. The fifth pathway describes how the health sector is in some cases driving innovation, for example in genetics, engineering, and technology.

6. The final pathway describes the contribution of health employment to health security, and how investments in the health workforce can protect a country's economy from instability due to epidemic threats and conflicts.

Why is Health Workforce a Priority and What are the Goals?

At the start of the 21st century, world leaders came together at the U.N. and committed to eight time-bound goals, which were known as the Millennium Development Goals. These goals ranged from poverty reduction to universal primary education to reduction of child mortality. For many developing countries, efforts to achieve the Millennium Development Goals, by 2015 were thwarted by inadequate health workers (Lozano et al., 2011). Global leaders have now moved from the Millennium Development Goals to the Sustainable Development Goals (SDG) which provide a more elaborate set of development objectives that are to be met by 2030 (UN General Assembly, 2015). In order to achieve these goals, particularly those related to the health of populations, investments in health workforce are required. There are nine SDGs that relate in some way to health, although the most directly related is goal number three (SDG 3), which is to "ensure healthy lives and promote well being for all at all ages" (p. 14). Within this goal there are a number of sub-goals. SDG3c relates directly to the health workforce and reads that it is important to "substantially increase health financing and the recruitment, development, training, and retention of the health workforce in developing countries, especially in least-developed countries and Small Island Developing States" (p. 17).

The challenges in achieving SDG 3 are vast but can be boiled down to the following key issues – articulated clearly in the Global Strategy on Human Resources for Health: Workforce 2030 (WHO, 2016a):

Mere availability of health workers is not sufficient: only when they are equitably distributed and accessible by the population, when they possess the required competency, and are motivated and empowered to deliver quality care that is appropriate and acceptable to the sociocultural expectations of the population, and when they are adequately supported by the health system, can theoretical coverage translate into effective service coverage. (p 10)

As such, the priorities can be translated into the following specific goals:

· Availability of health workers: We have a severe shortage of health workers, and the biggest gaps are in regions with the highest burden of disease. Current global estimates put the gap at 17 million health workers (WHO, 2016a, p. 44). Ramping up production will require finding cost-effective ways of training and innovative ways of retaining to increase the total pool of health workers.

· Accessibility of health workers: Even if the total number of health workers increases, we will only meet population health goals if they are working in areas where they are needed. If health workers converge in high-density areas and serve only those with resources to pay, we will not meet our goal of universal coverage.

· Acceptability and quality of health workers: Meeting the health needs of the population in a cost-effective, appropriate, and sustainable way will require health workers who are competent in relevant skills and are motivated to provide health services.

Challenges in Improving Availability

Calculating How Many Health Workers We Need

In 2006, the World Health Report (WHO, 2006) introduced a metric to establish a minimum number of health workers a country should have. This metric was 80% deliveries attended to by a skilled birth attendant, which translated to a minimum density of 2.28 midwives, nurses, and physicians per 1000 population (p. 12). The WHO defines a skilled birth attendant as:

...an accredited health professional – such as a midwife, doctor or nurse – who has been educated and trained to proficiency in the skills needed to manage uncomplicated pregnancies, childbirth and the immediate postnatal period and in the identification, management and referral of complications in women and newborns. (WHO, 2004, p. 1)

This metric provided one of the first benchmarks in measuring and comparing the size and distribution of the health workforce. However, there are problems with using just this one metric. Countries have inconsistent definitions of skilled birth attendants, and it does not reflect the true scope of services needed to meet population health needs.

Recent efforts have introduced a more elaborate and inclusive approach to estimating the workforce needs. In October of 2016, an expert group commissioned by the WHO Global Health Workforce Alliance published a paper on Health Workforce Requirements to meet the 2030 Goals (WHO, 2016b). With the latest data available the global health workforce was estimated to be over 43 million with expectations of 55% growth by 2030 resulting in a workforce of 67.3 million (p. 17). To estimate the need for health workers, instead of the 2006 metric (which used only deliveries with a skilled birth attendant), recent calculations used a new "SDG index." This new threshold takes into consideration the top contributors to the global burden of disease. The 12 SDG tracers used in this method include family planning, antenatal care, skilled birth attendance, DTP3 immunization, prevention of tobacco use, portable water, sanitation, antiretroviral therapy, Tb treatment, cataract surgery coverage, hypertension treatment, and diabetes treatment (p. 10). These indicators represent a more comprehensive range of health services and a transition to people-centered, integrated health care.

Using this approach, 4.45 doctors, nurses, and midwives per 1000 population would be the minimum number of health workers needed (p. 10). This number translates to a shortage of 17.4 million health workers in 2013. Of these, more than half are nurses and midwives and over 2 million are doctors. The largest shortages of health workers are currently in Southeast Asia and Africa. Given the huge, disproportionate burden of disease in Africa, the workforce shortage there is most severe and has significant implications. Using the SDG index, by 2030, the global shortage of health care workers is projected to be more than 14.5 million, only 17% less than 2013 (p. 18). Increased investment in recruiting, training, and retaining a relevant health workforce will be critical in order to meet the evolving health needs of society.

Increasing the Number of Health Workers

Absolute shortages of health workers are further exacerbated by lopsided distribution of workers across the globe. High-income countries have higher numbers of health workforce and smaller deficits while low-income countries struggle with both total numbers and distribution between rural and urban areas within their borders. Sub-Saharan Africa accounts for a 4% share of the global health workforce, yet it shoulders 24% of the global disease burden. The situation is not projected to improve. According to the health workforce projections the global deficit will drop to 17%, yet Africa's deficit of health workers will actually increase by 45% between 2013 and 2030 (WHO, 2016b, p. 18-19). There is clearly a need to increase the production of health workers, especially in low-income countries.

Increasing the production of health workers will require a number of factors to align, including interested applicants, schools, teachers, books, clinical sites, exams, and then available jobs at the end of training. In order to massively increase the number of health workers, we first need adequate numbers of qualified applicants trained in the prerequisites to enter the field of health professions. Expanding the pool of qualified and interested students will require investments in primary and secondary education by ministries of education and other stakeholders.

Alongside expanding the pool of candidates who qualify for careers in the health professions, we need to ensure there is adequate interest. One study on the economics of health professions education identified three drivers for career: the personal return on investment (how much one will make after investing a certain amount of time and money), the prestige of the career (how much society values that profession), and quality of life (linked to a variety of factors including flexibility, upward mobility, and conditions of service) (Mcpake, Squires, Mahat, & Araujo, 2015). Based on country-specific health workforce targets, and depending on the types of health workers needed, efforts must be made to ensure career paths in the prioritized cadres are attractive and provide financially-sound career paths.

Assuming we can attract qualified and interested students, we then need to ensure that there are schools with expanded enrollment quotas and/or new schools to increase the capacity for training. In some countries, admissions are centralized such that governments would need to mandate expansion of enrollment. In other countries, private sector enrollment and even public sector enrollment is linked to the ability of applicants to pay tuition. Furthermore, expansion of new schools is often limited by capital investments to invest in the infrastructure and start-up costs of new training institutions.

A Framework for Health Professions Education Systems

As we look at these different attributes and goals of the health workforce, and as we examine strategies to improve the quantity, quality, and relevance of the workforce, it is important to understand the health professions education system. Figure 2 (Appendix B) is a framework that depicts the different components of the system and describes some of the stakeholders and processes within each component. The inside box is the immediate learning environment, which includes the students, faculty, learning material, training sites, curriculum, and community. When we describe a training program, this is the layer we often describe as we reflect on the teachers, learning environment, patients, or community with whom the students interact. The middle box includes the institutions that are responsible for the learning environment. Institutions establish policies and channel resources to create the learning environment. The institutional activities include developing student and faculty recruitment policies, partnerships with other institutions, evaluation of programs, and tracking of graduates. Finally, the outer box of the framework is the national (or regional) context within which the training programs exist and includes the regulatory environment, partnerships between government ministries, health workforce planning, resource mobilization, and the health service environment. The latter is both a training environment as well as the ultimate employer for graduates of training programs.

The U.S. government recently invested in the expansion of capacity of health professions training programs in Africa through a program called Medical Education Partnership Initiative (MEPI, 2015). MEPI was a $130 million investment in expanding the quality, quantity, and retention of health workers in Sub-Saharan Africa. Through a competitive process, 11 medical schools in 10 countries within Africa were awarded ten million dollars over five years to address these goals (p. 27). MEPI was the first large-scale investment in workforce in Africa and was a timely investment for the region. Medical schools in several countries in the region, including Kenya and Ethiopia, were facing government mandates to expand enrollment, yet the requisite resources to support expansion were limited. As a result, the resources from MEPI were used to support growing class sizes in innovative ways. All schools invested in leveraging technology to support better access to learning material. All schools invested in strengthening their community training sites and all schools invested in strengthening the faculty pool. (MEPI Year 5 Report, 2016)

Many of the MEPI schools were struggling to find clinical sites for their students. Expansion of programs, therefore, was triggering decentralization in training. In Nigeria, the rapid expansion of medical school class sizes resulted in tertiary care hospitals being flooded with students, who were jostling for opportunities to practice their clinical skills. This tension and strain on the clinical training sites led medical schools to send students to district hospitals for training (Talib et al., 2013). At the University of Nairobi, as class sizes increased and students were similarly saturating tertiary health facilities, the leadership used MEPI funding to invest in decentralized training sites where pharmacy, nursing, and medical students were placed at non-tertiary health facilities for clinical rotations. In order to ensure adequate supervision of their students and to incentivize staff at the health facility, the University offered supervisors the opportunity to become "adjunct faculty," pedagogy training, and access to academic resources (Kibore et al., 2014).

These types of innovative expansion models, including the decentralization of health professions education closer to the community, are necessary considerations as we expand the production of health workers.

Case Study 1: Rapid Expansion of Medical Doctors in Ethiopia

Examples of the public sector driving change can be found in Ethiopia, where governments recently mandated massive increases in enrollment in training programs. In Ethiopia, nursing enrollment increased first, followed by massive increases in medical school enrollment. In 2003, Ethiopia had only 5 health science schools but by 2009 that number had increased to 23 and annual medical school enrollment increased from 250 to 1400. Class sizes at AAU (Addis Ababa University) quadrupled in just a matter of a few years (Derbrew et al., 2014, p. s40). Students complained that classrooms that were built for less than 100 students were now being used for class sizes nearly three times that size, and students could not find space to sit. The limited number of textbooks were now being rationed by triple the number of students who described having to wake up at dawn to stand in line to borrow a textbook for a couple of hours. Students enrolled in study programs require learning resources, faculty to teach them, and in the field of health professions, they require opportunities to practice the practical skills that will transform them into competent providers. Without these critical resources, attrition rates would escalate and expansion would be compromised.

The MEPI program was timely and allowed AAU to invest in tablet devices for their students loaded with hundreds of medical textbooks. The campus of AAU was wired with Wi-Fi hotspots so students could connect (though learning material was also available offline). MEPI funding also supported the distribution of resources to newer schools throughout the country. The Ethiopia MEPI program was an example of in-country partnership of schools sharing resources to achieve a common goal of training more doctors for the country. Therefore, in addition to policy decisions to mandate increased enrollment, necessary investments include strengthening faculty recruitment, training, and retention, ensuring adequate access to textbooks and learning materials, and ensuring access to clinical training sites so all students have opportunities to practice clinical skills in a supervised setting.

Challenges in Improving Accessibility

Ensuring Adequate Distribution of Health Workers

Along with increasing the number of health workers, how do we ensure that they are distributed according to population health needs? Globally, the mal-distribution cuts clearly along income lines. Migration of high-level providers is a major challenge for the health system. These cadres cost the most, yet they are also the cadres most often trained to international standards; as such, they have opportunities to migrate out of the country. Low-income countries therefore struggle to retain talent at a huge financial cost. One study of nine African countries estimated that in aggregate, these countries lost 25-50% of their workforce at a cost of $2 billion dollars by training doctors who ultimately migrated to one of four high-income countries (Mills et al., 2011, p. 4).

Addressing geographical inequities in the density of health workers is a priority for most countries. The distribution issues within the health sectors are manifest in a number of dimensions, including the distribution of health workers who work in the public versus private system, between urban and rural areas, and between community and tertiary facilities. The poorest people with the worst access to health care tend to be in rural parts of low-income countries with limited access to secondary or tertiary care. In the Senegal, for example, the Dakar region mirrors the global disparity in that the urban area has more than half of the country's doctors but less than a quarter of the population. (Buchan et al., 2013, p. 834). Therefore, to reach those who need health care the most, we need to strengthen the primary care workforce. This is especially true for those who live in underserved or rural areas.

Approaches to improve distribution include thoughtfully selecting and recruiting students from underserved areas, locating training programs in underserved areas, providing adequate community-based experiences during training, and ensuring that the work environment and incentives post-graduation are attractive in underserved settings. Studies from developed countries have consistently shown that health professionals from a rural background are more likely to practice in rural areas, clinical rotations in a rural setting may influence medical students' subsequent decision to work in an underserved area, and appropriate educational preparation for rural service, including adapting curricula to include rural health issues, creates more interest to work in rural areas (Dolea, Stormont, & Braichet, 2010).

The WHO issued global recommendations to improve the rural recruitment and retention of the health workforce (WHO, 2010). These guidelines mapped out four key categories of interventions: first, education interventions that include targeted admissions for rural students and clinical experiences in rural areas and curricula that reflect rural health issues; second, interventions of the regulatory system that expand the scope of practice for rural practitioners and regulations that implement and enforce compulsory service in rural areas; third, financial incentives for health workers in rural and remote areas; and fourth, targeted interventions for health workers already practicing in rural and remote areas such as improved living conditions, safe and supportive work conditions, career development plans, and support for professional networks. These guidelines were based on the best available evidence at that time shown to improve retention and recruitment.

Students from rural and underserved areas are often out-paced by urban students from good high schools when applying for health professions schools. Targeted admissions and subsidized tuition help to mitigate this gap. China, for example, incentivizes rural students by waiving tuition. Similarly, the medical school in Lao People's Democratic Republic has a quota of 10% for students from the poorest districts (Buchan et al., 2013, p. 836).

There is increasing evidence of countries expanding rural and community-based health education and training. One study reported that in Thailand, the majority of medical and nursing schools were located outside Bangkok. In addition, the study reported that in Thailand, there are mandatory clinical rotations to district hospitals for all students (medical and nursing) and rural health issues are included in the curricula for all health professionals (Buchan et al., 2013, p. 836).

Compulsory service is yet another mechanism that has been shown, in some cases, to improve rural recruitment and retention. Leveraging the regulatory environment for retention is often challenging since it requires resources for policy development, implementation and enforcement. In 2010, Frehywot, Mullan, Payne, & Ross conducted the first study that looked at compulsory service requirements in all WHO countries and found that 70 of the WHO countries employed some form of compulsory service (p. 366). Factors that influence the effectiveness of compulsory service programs include alignment of expectations of the provider and the government, support for providers where they are posted (especially pay, housing and continuing education opportunities) and adequate preparation of the providers in the skills needed to work in these rural areas.

There are different models of compulsory service. Australia, for example, requires service to underserved areas for all international medical graduates. Some countries require service but provide incentives linked to education benefits, economic benefits, and/or augmentation of one's living condition. In China, short-term, compulsory service is required before health professionals can be promoted. In Laos, all new health graduates must serve rural communities for at least two years within five years of graduation (Buchan et al., 2013, p. 835). While no systematic studies have been conducted to demonstrate the impact of compulsory service, it is clear that this is a strategy used by governments both to staff underserved areas and as an attempt to groom a workforce for these areas.

The regulatory system can also influence recruitment and retention to rural and underserved areas by expanding the scope of practice of providers in these areas. Such interventions empower providers and facilitate greater job satisfaction, in some cases even improve health outcomes. In South Africa, for example, the implementation of nurse-initiated antiretroviral therapy from 2009 to 2014 was one of the contributing factors to the successful expansion of access to antiretroviral therapy (WHO, 2016c).

Financial incentives have been shown to be effective in retaining health workers once they are already working in underserved areas. One study in South Africa found that nurses in particular were incentivized to work in rural areas by the provision of financial incentives (Reid, 2004). Similarly, a financial incentive scheme in the Niger, targeted at doctors, pharmacists, and dental surgeons reported an increase of 42–44% in recruited workers (Dolea et al., 2010, p. 381).

Case Study 2: Walter Sisulu University in South Africa

The Faculty of Health Sciences at Walter Sisulu University (WSU) was established in 1985 to address inequities and to produce physicians capable of providing quality health care in rural South African communities. WSU is a government-aided institution located in a rural area of South Africa. Prior to WSU, in South Africa, admittance into medical school was based on math and physics scores, yet in black communities, there was limited capacity to teach math and physics at the high school level. WSU opened up admissions to candidates who achieved at least a "C" grade and added a personal questionnaire, which allowed an assessment of personal attributes and motivation to be part of the admissions process. In addition to the innovative admissions process, education, research, and service programs are guided by the health needs of the rural community. Education is embedded in the health system, and community health providers are recruited and trained to be teachers and mentors (Iputo, 2008). At a workshop held by the National Academy of Medicine's Global Forum on Health Professional Education in October 2016, the Dean of Walter Sisulu Medical School presented the results of their approach, indicating that the majority of WSU graduates are practicing in rural areas of the Eastern Cape within the public sector and in general practice.

Challenges in Improving Acceptability and Quality

How Do We Define a High-Quality Health Workforce?

The definition of a qualified workforce varies depending on where one looks. The WHO definition of universal health coverage includes the following description: "A sufficient capacity of well-trained, motivated health workers to provide the services to meet patients' needs based on the best available evidence" (WHO, 2014b, para. 2).

The Global Strategy on Health Workforce for 2030 (WHO, 2016a) calls for adopting strategies to transform health workforce education. Goals for the future health workforce (those in training) need to parallel goals for the existing workforce (those in service) and necessarily must include a comprehensive vision for health and health care. These goals include health workers who are competent in skills relevant for their scope of practice and for the health needs in their communities, who are able to work in inter-professional teams, who are well-versed in the social determinants of health and able to identify and address public health issues, and who are trained with a sense of social accountability so that they are committed to a public service ethic and able to provide respectful, appropriate care for the health needs of the population (WHO, 2016a).

"Well-trained" would therefore include both generic and occupational competencies. Generic competencies apply across cadres and include a health worker's ability to think critically and to be compassionate, communicative, culturally sensitive, and committed to the community. Occupational-specific competencies ensure that a health worker is competent in providing services within the scope of practice and is able to provide evidence-based care.

There is another dimension of quality that goes beyond the attributes of an individual health worker to the performance of the health workforce in aggregate. A high quality health workforce at the system-level is one that is effectively and efficiently managed. This dimension of quality requires strong leadership and stewardship of the system, robust regulatory systems, and information management systems that allow aggregate data of the health workforce to inform planning and decision making.

The difficulty of defining quality for the health workforce is identifying metrics that are universally applicable. How do we know the health workforce of a particular region or facility is high quality? Do we define quality by being better than before? Is quality defined by being adequate for the population health needs? Do we use identified local or global benchmarks to define quality? Strengthening the regulatory environment is one way of ensuring a minimum level of quality within a cadre of health workers. Regulatory bodies, through licensing exams, can require knowledge and/or experience in specific skills. Ideally, regulatory bodies should continuously, or at least periodically, assess providers and regulations to ensure that the workforce remains relevant and appropriate for the health system and the health burden.

On an individual level or facility level, the quality of care provided by health workers can be measured by tools tailored to the environment. Quality of care metrics can be developed that are context-specific (Pacqué-Margolis, Ng, & Kauffman, 2011). For example, a checklist can be developed and health workers can be observed to determine the extent to which they meet the pre-determined criteria. Similarly, guideline compliance can be observed or measured using chart-audits. Using this approach, we could measure both generic and occupation-specific skills such as compassion, communication, critical thinking, cultural sensitivity, and proficiency in diagnosing and treating.

Measuring quality is not as straightforward as measuring quantity and may explain why the global focus has been on ensuring an adequate number of health workers. However, the quality of our health workforce (individually, institutionally, and at the system-level) is important and will ultimately determine if investments in scaling up truly reduce the health burden of society.

Case Study 3: Quality of Medical Colleges in India

At the time of independence from British colonial rule in 1947, India had only a handful of medical schools. Consequently, health planners focused on increasing the number of clinical practitioners to meet the large, unmet need for health services and were less focused on developing research capacity. Teachers were saddled with the double burden of large classroom sizes and overwhelming clinical loads and found little time for other academic activity. Early growth of medical colleges in India was largely driven by the expansion of state-owned medical colleges.

By the 1980s, the Indian middle class had developed to the point at which privately owned colleges financed by student fees became viable. The shift in the Indian economy towards a neoliberal model in the early 1990s facilitated explosive growth – between 1990 and 2016, the Medical Council of India listed 287 new colleges. Of these, 186 are privately owned, bringing the total number of colleges to 426, with the capacity to produce 53,455 doctors a year (Calculated based on data available at Medical Council of India, 2016, "List of Colleges Teaching MBBS" Table). Despite this proliferation of medical colleges, research output in India has remained consistently low. Faculty advancement continues to be based on number of years of employment, and there is little professional motivation to be involved in research. Ray, Shah, & Nundy (2016) found that 57.3% of medical colleges did not have a single publication listed in SCOPUS between 2005 and 2014 (p. 50). A parallel system of centrally funded institutions contributes to the bulk of India-based research, but, with a few notable exceptions, is disconnected from the training of clinicians. A failure of regulatory mechanisms has led to both poor quality clinical training and a proliferation of unqualified clinical practitioners. Das et al. (2012) found that only 11% of available practitioners in rural districts in the state of Madhya Pradesh had an allopathic medical degree (p. 2777). When their performance was evaluated using unannounced standardized patients who presented with common ailments, they performed only marginally better than their unqualified peers. Journalist accounts of medical colleges (D'Silva, 2015; MacAskill, Stecklow, & Miglani, 2015) point to widespread failure of regulatory mechanisms to control quality in medical colleges leading to spiraling tuition fees, rampant fraud, and non-existent faculty and facilities.

Who should invest in health workforce issues?

Investing in health workforce clearly benefits health outcomes and the health system, and now we have also seen the link to a more stable, just, and robust economy (WHO, 2016c). Intuitively, when market forces drive expansion and improvement in the health workforce, the returns of investment are likely to be more sustainable. How then can we leverage market forces to bridge market failures? If demand drives supply, and supply drives the type of health workforce we produce and employ, can we truly generate demand for preventative services and population health needs? Can we generate market demand to serve underserved and marginalized populations, or should that be the responsibility of safety net sectors such as government and global health donors? Is the latter approach sustainable?

Government continues to play a key role in strengthening the health workforce, both in terms of increasing input and in reducing the brain drain. Governments have employed different strategies to improve retention as described above, but it is clear that meeting the needs of the health care workforce will necessarily require an investment in expanding the pipeline of healthcare workers through expansion of pre-service training programs by either increasing the number of schools or expanding enrollment in existing schools. Government resources, however, are limited and are unlikely to bridge the market failures, which leave us with critical shortages in low-resource settings.

The private sector plays an increasingly critical role in health workforce development. This sector includes those who are motivated by profit and those that are non-for-profit. Either way, they contribute critical resources. As government budgets continue to tighten amidst aging populations and increasing health needs of the population, the role and the opportunity for the private sector is growing. The growth of the private sector is real. According to a report by USAID (November 2014), the private, for-profit sector is responsible for the majority of new schools established in the last three decades in Sub-Saharan Africa. The challenge for the private sector is that, unlike public schools, they need to cover the cost of the infrastructure, teaching staff, and all other costs of training. In some cases, private institutions get public subsidies, but in many cases, private schools simply rely on donors, investors, and student tuition. With high operating costs and driven by the need to keep their investors happy, private schools are often not motivated by societal goals. In some instances, private schools simply produce graduates that ultimately flee the country to greener pastures. The role of the government to establish and enforce regulation is critical to ensure the quality of the health workforce produced by the private sector and to address the issue of graduate retention.

Among the private sector players are the relatively new impact investors or social entrepreneurs who are motivated as much (if not more) by the cause than the financial return on investment. An example is the social business model described by Nobel Prize winner Mohamed Yunus. A social business, his website (http://www.yunussb.com/) states, is a:

> ...company with a social mission at its core. The company is set up either by the disadvantaged population or for the population and operates exactly like a company, generating profit, but all profits are reinvested back generating sustainable social impact. (Yunus Social Business, "About" subsection, para. 1)

One example is a business that offers a franchise model for midwives in the Philippines. In this model, midwives who join the franchise benefit from access to knowledge and skills. Association with a brand increased demand for their services (Cuff, Patel, & Perez, 2015, p. 72). Those in lower-income brackets are able and willing to pay for services. The social business model leverages this financial bandwidth to create opportunities for sustained health services.

Another impact investor, the Calvert Foundation, leverages philanthropic funding for both a social and financial returns. They capitalize on the desire for social gains by investing in programs that produce both a financial and a social return. A couple years ago, the Calvert Foundation conducted an assessment to explore areas within the health system, which might appeal to their investors. In the final analysis, investing in the health workforce did not make their list. They instead chose to invest in physical delivery systems, medical devices and supplies, pharmaceuticals, payment systems, mobile devices, logistics, and distribution (Calvert Foundation, 2015). One reason investors may be reluctant to invest in the health workforce as a means to improve health is the time lag. Results are not immediate and there is difficulty in attributing improvements in the health workforce to health outcomes. The onus is therefore on those advocating for health workforce investment to develop clear, achievable, and ideally short to mid-term deliverables so that investors can measure their return on investment.

The Link between Health Outcomes and Health Labor Markets

Health workers need to be part of the innovation that tightens the link between the needs and the demand of health services. They may play a role in health promotion to educate the masses or in health policy to prioritize public subsidies for under-served populations. The scope of health services required to meet the needs of our population are vast – they include prevention and cure, and they include reaching even the marginalized segments of society (the poor, remote, and disadvantaged). To provide this vast scope of services in a cost-effective and sustainable way requires innovation and transformation in the way care is provided. Health workers are part of this innovation.

The World Bank conducted a literature review and published a report on the "Economics of Health Professions Education and Careers" (Mcpake et al., 2015). Within this report is an insightful description of the interaction between education systems, labor markets, and health systems. In essence, the report draws a link between population health needs (both curative and preventative), demand for health care (which reflects consumers' willingness and ability to pay), supply of health workforce, and health professions training programs. An example of market failure is when demand does not represent true population health needs (e.g. need for prevention and/or care for marginalized populations) translating into a workforce that is also not meeting population health needs.

The extent to which training programs contribute to supply depends on a number of factors, including the perceived personal return on investment and the social return on investment. The extent to which training programs contribute to the actual supply of the health workforce is limited by the brain drain. This includes those that leave the country to work as well as graduates who choose to stay in-country, but work in non-clinical roles.

Within this framework, one can visualize the market failures, where population health needs are not directly linked to the demand of health services. Those who purchase health services (generating demand) may not be motivated or resourced to address actual health needs. In other words, patients may not understand the need or may not be able to afford preventive services. Another market failure is the lack of health workforce to meet the present demand, either due to an inadequate number, distribution, or skill set. This framework puts the health workforce into the context of the broader health system, illustrating how health professions education programs influence the supply, how demand drives supply, and therefore how increasing demand for the right type of services (e.g., preventative services) can ultimately drive health workers that are trained in the relevant skills. If we measure the success of the health workforce by their ability to improve health outcomes, we need to bridge these gaps and ensure the market is demanding the right services and therefore, the right skills.

Academia's Role in Strengthening the Health Workforce

We have discussed the role of government, the private sector, and even impact investors in the health workforce, but we have not yet discussed the role of academia. One excellent article written by a team at the College of Health Sciences at Makerere University in Uganda nicely describes the contribution of the academic institution to health outcomes using a logic model (Pariyo et al., 2011).

They describe how the academic institution contributes through inputs (adding human resources to the health system), through improving the processes within the health system (providing students and trainees who bring rigor to decision-making), through improving the outputs of the health system (expanding populations served and/or services provided), through improving outcomes in some cases (expanding immunization coverage for academic-affiliated health facilities), and how research from the institution has contributed to improved health outcomes.

Conclusion

The global health workforce is a critical yet complex component of the health system and has become a high priority in the field of global health. With growing momentum and attention, particularly in light of specific strategies and milestones for 2030, we have reason to be optimistic. There are daunting gaps and seemingly rigid bottlenecks, yet at the same time, there are innovations that can transform the workforce, the work place, and even the pipeline for producing more health workers.

As we look at the growing shortage of health workers, can we can reinvent or re-engineer health service delivery to be more efficient? Instead of trying to fill the numerical gap, can we re-write the equation? As for quality, there remains a tension between striving for global standards and maintaining local relevance. The consequence of not addressing this tension is continued brain drain from developing countries and unmet community health needs. Can we clearly define quality so that communities in developing countries have access to relevant, affordable, high-quality care, yet avoid a double standard for low-resource settings?

We have better data now than ever before on the size and the gaps of the health workforce. We also have better data on the impact of investing in the health workforce and the benefits, not just to population health, but also to health systems and economic growth. Strengthening the global health workforce will therefore require a combination of traditional stakeholders scaling strategies that have worked and new investors re-thinking old paradigms.

References

Buchan, J., Couper, I. D., Tangcharoensathien, V., Thepannya, K., Jaskiewicz, W., Perfilieva, G., & Dolea, C. (2013). Early implementation of WHO recommendations for the retention of health workers in remote and rural areas. *Bulletin of the World Health Organization, 91*(11), 834–40.

Calvert Foundation. (2015). Opportunities and challenges for global health impact investors in India and East Africa. Retrieved from http://www.calvertfoundation.org/storage/documents/Opportunities-Challenges-for-Global-Health-Investors-GHILP-Exec-Summary-web.pdf

Campbell, J., Buchan, J., Cometto, G., David, B., Dussault, G., Fogstad, H., … Tangcharoensathien, V. (2013). Human resources for health and universal health coverage: fostering equity and effective coverage. *Bulletin of the World Health Organization*, *91*(11), 853–63.

Cuff, P. A., Patel, D. M. and Perez, M. M. (2015) 'Empowering Women and Strengthening Health Systems and Services Through Investing in Nursing and Midwifery Enterprise : Lessons from Lower-Income Countries : Workshop Summary', in *Global Forum on Innovation in Health Professional Education; Forum on Public-Private Partnerships for Global Health and Safety*. Available at: http://www.nap.edu/catalog.php?record_id=19005.

Costelloe, C., Metcalfe, C., Lovering, A., Mant, D., & Hay, A. D. (2010). Effect of antibiotic prescribing in primary care on antimicrobial resistance in individual patients: systematic review and meta-analysis. *British Medical Journal*, *340*, c2096.

Derbew M., Animut N., Talib Z.M., Mehtsun S., Hamburger E.K. (2014). Ethiopian medical schools' rapid scale-up to support the Government's goal of universal coverage. Academic Medicine. 89(8):40–44.

D'Silva, J. (2015). India's private medical colleges and capitation fees. *British Medical Journal*, *350* (January), h106.

Das, J., Holla, A., Das, V., Mohanan, M., Tabak, D., & Chan, B. (2012). In Urban And Rural India, A Standardized Patient Study Showed Low Levels Of Provider Training And Huge Quality Gaps. *Health Affairs*, *31*(12), 2774–2784.

Dolea, C., Stormont, L., & Braichet, J. M. (2010). Evaluated strategies to increase attraction and retention of health workers in remote and rural areas. *Bulletin of the World Health Organization*, *88*(5), 379–385.

Evans, D. K., Goldstein, M., & Popova, A. (2015). Health-care worker mortality and the legacy of the Ebola epidemic. *Lancet Global Health*, *3*(8), e439–e440.

Frehywot, S., Mullan, F., Payne, P. W., & Ross, H. (2010). Compulsory service programmes for recruiting health workers in remote and rural areas: do they work? *Bulletin of the World Health Organization*, *88*(5), 364–70.

Global Health Workforce Alliance. (2008). Scaling up , saving lives. Retrieved from http://www.who.int/workforcealliance/documents/Global_Health FINAL REPORT.pdf?ua=1

Iputo, J. E. (2008). Faculty of Health Sciences, Walter Sisulu University: Training Doctors from and for Rural South African Communities. *MEDICC Review*, *10*(4), 25–29.

Kibore, M. W., Daniels, J. A., Child, M. J., Nduati, R., Njiri, F. J., Kinuthia, R. M., … Farquhar, C. (2014). Kenyan medical student and consultant experiences in a pilot decentralized training program at the university of Nairobi. *Education for Health*, *27*(2), 170–176.

Lozano, R., Wang, H., Foreman, K. J., Rajaratnam, J. K., Naghavi, M., Marcus, J. R., … Murray, C. J. L. (2011). Progress towards Millennium Development Goals 4 and 5 on maternal and child mortality: An updated systematic analysis. *The Lancet*, *378*(9797), 1139–1165.

MacAskill, A., Stecklow, S., & Miglani, S. (2015, June 16). Rampant fraud at medical schools leaves Indian healthcare in crisis. *Reuters*. Retrieved from http://www.reuters.com/investigates/special-report/india-medicine-education/

McIntyre, D., Thiede, M., Dahlgren, G., & Whitehead, M. (2006). What are the economic consequences for households of illness and of paying for health care in low- and middle-income country contexts? *Social Science and Medicine*, *62*(4), 858–865.

Mcpake, B., Squires, A., Mahat, A., & Araujo, E. C. (2015). *The Economics of Health Professional Education and Careers*. Washington DC: World Bank.

Medical Council of India. (2016). List of colleges teaching MBBS. Retrieved from http://www.mciindia.org/InformationDesk/ForStudents/ListofCollegesTeachingMB BS.aspx

MEPI. (2015). Medical education partnership initiative - Year 5 report. Retrieved from http://www.mepinetwork.org/images/stories/MEPI Year 5 Report_No Appendixes.pdf

Mills, E. J., Kanters, S., Hagopian, A., Bansback, N., Nachega, J., Alberton, M., ... Ford, N. (2011). The financial cost of doctors emigrating from sub-Saharan Africa: human capital analysis. *British Medical Journal, 343*(November), d7031.

Pacqué-Margolis, S., Ng, C., & Kauffman, S. (2011). Human resources for health (HRH) indicator compendium. Retrieved from http://www.who.int/workforcealliance/knowledge/toolkit/23/en/

Pariyo, G., Serwadda, D., Sewankambo, N. K., Groves, S., Bollinger, R. C., & Peters, D. H. (2011). A grander challenge: the case of how Makerere University College of Health Sciences (MakCHS) contributes to health outcomes in Africa. *BMC International Health & Human Rights, 11*(Suppl 1), S2.

Ray, S., Shah, I., & Nundy, S. (2016). The research output from Indian medical institutions between 2005 and 2014. *Current Medicine Research and Practice, 6*(2), 49–58.

Reid, S. (2004). Monitoring the effect of the new rural allowance for health professionals. Retrieved from http://www.hst.org.za/publications/monitoring-effect-new-rural-allowance-health-professionals

Scheffer, M. C., & Dal Poz, M. R. (2015). The privatization of medical education in Brazil: trends and challenges. *Human Resources for Health, 13*(1), 96.

Talib, Z. M., Baingana, R. K., Sagay, A. S., Van Schalkwyk, S. C., Mehtsun, S., & Kiguli-Malwadde, E. (2013). Investing in community-based education to improve the quality, quantity, and retention of physicians in three African countries. *Education for Health, 26*(2), 109–114.

Medical Education Partnership Initiative Year 5 Report (2016). Retrieved from http://www.mepinetwork.org/images/stories/MEPI%20Year%205%20Report_No%20Appendixes.pdf

UN General Assembly. Transforming our world: The 2030 agenda for sustainable development (2015). Retrieved from http://www.un.org/ga/search/view_doc.asp?symbol=A/RES/70/1&Lang=E

UNFPA, International Confederation of Midwives, & WHO. (2014). State of the World's Midwifery: a universal pathway. A woman's right to health. Retrieved from http://www.unfpa.org/sowmy

WHO. (n.d.). Technical Notes - Global Health Workforce Statistics database. Retrieved October 30, 2016, from http://www.who.int/hrh/statistics/TechnicalNotes.pdf?ua=1

WHO. (2004). Making pregnancy safer: the critical role of the skilled attendant. A joint statement by WHO, ICM and FIGO. Geneva, Switzerland: WHO. Retrieved from http://whqlibdoc.who.int/publications/2004/9241591692.pdf

WHO. (2006). World Health Report 2006: Working together for health. Retrieved from http://www.who.int/whr/2006/en/

WHO. (2010). Increasing access to health workers in remote and rural areas through improved retention: Global policy recommendations. Retrieved from http://www.who.int/entity/hrh/migration/hmr_expert_meeting_dolea.pdf

WHO. (2014a). A universal truth: No health without a workforce. Retrieved from http://www.who.int/workforcealliance/knowledge/resources/GHWA-a_universal_truth_report.pdf

WHO. (2014b). What is universal health coverage? Retrieved from http://www.who.int/features/qa/universal_health_coverage/en/

WHO. (2016a). Global strategy on human resources for health: Workforce 2030. Retrieved from http://who.int/hrh/resources/pub_globstrathrh-2030/en/

WHO. (2016b). Health workforce requirements for universal health coverage and the Sustainable Development Goals. Retrieved from http://apps.who.int/iris/bitstream/10665/250330/1/9789241511407-eng.pdf?ua=1

WHO. (2016c). Working for health and growth: investing in the health workforce. Report of the High-Level Commission on Health Employment and Economic Growth. Retrieved from www.who.int/about/licensing/copyright_form/en/index.html

Yunus Social Business. (2016). Retreived from http://www.yunussb.com/

CHAPTER 22

Global Health and Ethnocentrism: Challenges in Establishing a Global Health Curriculum in Japan

Daniel Velasco

Introduction

The following chapter deals with a pertinent, yet culturally-sensitive area of global health, and that is the difficulties encountered when creating and implementing a global health-related program in a country where the majority of the population is one ethnic group. While Japan is the focus of this chapter, and a case study is used to illustrate the immense challenges that need to be overcome in order to bring education and awareness of global health topics to the people, the overarching message is that all countries experience certain levels of ethnocentrism; therefore, politicians, board members, educators, researchers, and students from all countries can benefit from the lessons presented in this chapter. Not all countries have many opportunities to engage in open, critical discussions with people from other cultures on important topics such as global health, so this chapter should not be taken as an attack on Japanese culture or the way Japanese society has progressed in its educational reform. Surely there is much to praise in Japan's efforts to educate its people; however, there are some areas that should be open for discussion and critique in order to increase efforts toward a globalized society. It is my hope that this chapter becomes a catalyst for meaningful discussions between educators, government officials, and students, so that all will benefit from learning about and from the various cultures in this diverse world.

Global Health

Definition

Although this entire book is dedicated to global health, and will therefore undoubtedly present multiple definitions of what global health is and what it means to individual countries and the global society, it would still be appropriate to offer a definition for the sake of this chapter's unique topic on global health and ethnocentrism. Global health can be defined as the "an area for study, research, and practice that places a priority on improving health and achieving equity in health for all people worldwide" (Koplan, Bond, Merson, Reddy, Rodriguez, Sewankambo, and Wasserheit, 2009, p. 1995). It highlights issues that move beyond national borders and that have a global, political, and/or economic impact (Global Health Initiative, 2014). Within the area of global health are a multitude of aspects, factors, and issues that add to the overall definition of what global health means today. While they are important, an in depth examination of each one is beyond the scope of this chapter; however, they deserve to be mentioned so that possible connections can be made to different areas of global health that have been explored in other chapters.

One of the main issues regarding the forward movement of the current global health system is the challenge of refocusing attention not on what needs to be achieved, but how to realistically achieve it. This relies heavily on the current global health system, which needs to be constantly evaluated for improvement. One framework, created by the Lancet Commission on Investing in Health (CIH), identified four essential functions of the global health system: managing cross-border health threats, supplying global public goods, providing direct country support, and exercising leadership and supervision for "facilitating negotiation and building consensus on health agendas and priorities" (Schäferhoff, Suzuki, Angelides, and Hoffman, 2015, p. 13).

With this in mind, those developing global health programs and curricula need to take into account vulnerable populations, cultural differences and needs, and diversity. Beech and Danner (2016) describe this new component of health services:

A relatively new but equally important component of workforce development is the implementation of diversity training which moves beyond the idea of enhancing underrepresented racial and ethnic minorities in the workplace but recognizes the increasing need of inclusion of gay, lesbian, and transgender students, faculty, and providers. (p. 326)

Many countries, including the United States and the United Kingdom, have done much to increase awareness for underrepresented groups, and new legislation is consistently being introduced that supports diversity and inclusion. However, others struggle with promotion due to a variety of relevant cultural and societal issues. This chapter aims to discuss some of those issues by examining a case study of a university in Japan that had decided to open a liberal arts department and, within that department, a psychology major with a focus on global health. Before moving into the details of the case study and how it serves as an example for other monocultural-heavy cultures, it would be beneficial to look at an overview of global health programs in other countries and how and why they have become successful educational programs.

Overview of Global Health Programs in Western Countries

Many well-known universities continue to lead the educational revolution toward a just society that provides support in areas like physical and mental health. We can use these globally minded programs as examples for other universities, particularly universities in countries where issues related to gender and race still permeate business and politics and threaten to further alienate large portions of the population.

One example of a well-established and transparent global health program is Princeton University's Global Health Program. Princeton (2016) is world-renowned for its educational rigor, and the Global Health Program's description is a reminder of why universities, educators, and students admire the university:

Complex policy issues directly impact the wellbeing of people worldwide. The Princeton University Global Health Program stands at the forefront of interdisciplinary health and health policy research and education. By promoting serious health scholarship with an international perspective, we work to...power change today [and] prepare the next generation of global health leaders. (About Global Health at Princeton section, para. 1)

This goal is commendable and is one that should be shared among educational institutions across the globe.

Other American universities have unique offerings that benefit students and contribute to global health. Georgetown University (2016) offers a Master of Science in Global Health program, which provides students with experiential training, Duke University (2016) claims that its Master of Science in Global Health is "one of the first programs of its kind in the United States" (Master of Science in Global Health, para. 2). Duke's program offers funded fieldwork opportunities, a tailored curriculum, and a focus on applied, relevant research and skills (Duke University, 2016).

Other countries, such as the United Kingdom, offer diverse programs in global health. In England, the University of Oxford offers a robust Master of Science in Global Health Science and focuses on pressing global issues, such as premature death and disability (University of Oxford, 2016).

In Scotland, the University of Edinburgh's Global Health Academy stresses current global health concerns, such as the Zika virus and the global Ebola crisis (University of Edinburgh, 2016).

Of course, this is just a sampling of programs in two Western countries. There are many more examples of global health educational programs that offer a modern training from a diverse faculty to multicultural student populations.

Overview of Global Health Programs in Japan

Western countries are clearly on the forefront of global health education and training for multiple reasons, including well-funded research programs and diverse faculty and student populations. However, some countries in the East continue to struggle with issues ranging from societal issues (e.g., power and privilege from socioeconomic status and class hierarchy) to institutional issues (e.g., power harassment and gender or racial discrimination).

Before examining these issues, we will consider the educational programs in Japan related to global health. Although the outlook is rather bleak at this time (late 2016), there are proverbial silver linings in the Japanese educational landscape that bear mentioning in order to gain a general (but clear) overview of global health programs in Japan. The entire overview can be broken down into three tongue-in-cheek categories: the good, the bad, and the ugly.

The Good

Japan has a long history of education. The humble beginnings of Japanese higher education can be traced to public education systems for the samurai warrior class (*terakoya*), public learning centers for commoners, and private schools that were open to anyone regardless of class. This history can now be admired in institutions like Tokyo University and Kyoto University – two of Japan's top universities (Japan International Cooperation Agency, 2005, p. 13). The upper echelon of academia leads Japan in new ways of thinking about education, and the term "globalization" is often seen on university websites or in academic journal article titles. We will review the programs at two prominent Japanese universities – Tokyo University and Nagasaki University.

Tokyo University has Master-level and PhD-level programs in global health, and its website mentions having a diverse student population, a multicultural group of professors, and international field training. Their program also appears to use primarily English as the language of instruction, which makes sense because Japanese is not used as a main language in any country other than Japan and will be of little use in international settings.

Although not as famous as Tokyo University, Nagasaki University is an educational force in Japan and excels in both research and teaching. Nagasaki University has a Master-level program in global health, celebrates diverse student and faculty members, and has international training sites. As leading Japanese universities, it would be surprising to if these two institutions did not have programs in global health.

These global health programs are a testament to the fact that Tokyo University and Nagasaki University (along with a handful of other top-ranking higher education institutions) have realized the importance of a multi-dimensional Japan participating in, if not being a leader in, global society. Although Professor Shibuya (2014) from Tokyo University admits that that the programs currently available in Japan are not ideal, they provide a good foundation for the field of global health in Japan and can serve as models for additional globally aimed programs.

The Bad

There are four negative points regarding Japanese educational institutions' attempts to incorporate global health programs. First is accessibility. Only a few higher education institutions in Japan – Tokyo University, Kyoto University, etc. – offer degree programs in global health, and acceptance into these universities is extremely competitive. Secondly, the average Japanese university (that the majority of high school students will attend) does not have a global health program at all.

Third, generally speaking, university-level curricula in Japan (regardless of whether or not the university has a global health program) lack psychological training. There is no concrete evidence that explains why the field of psychology is missing from Japanese global health studies; however, it could be connected to the stigma associated with mental health in Japan. This cultural component will be further discussed in subsequent sections.

The Ugly

Unfortunately, the lack of diverse global health programs with international training experience is not the most disheartening factor when considering Japan's attempt to update its university-level curricula. According to Shibuya (2014), the fourth negative point is that either the country of Japan is unaware of the growing importance of global health programs, or, even more frighteningly, it doesn't care about globalizing higher education curricula. The remainder of this chapter will be dedicated to a thorough discussion of this "ugly" side, which will lead to a complex solution that unravels the very core of Japanese society. This exploration begins with the country's ethnocentricity, followed by other challenges to developing and implementing a global health curriculum: racism, xenophobia, corrupt leadership, sexism and sexual harassment, infantilization of Japanese society, and population concerns.

Challenges in Establishing a Global Health Curriculum in Japan

Ethnocentrism

Merriam-Webster defines the term ethnocentrism as "having or based on the idea that your own group or culture is better or more important than others" (Ethnocentrism, n.d.). Berry, Poortinga, Breugelmans, Chasiotis, and Sam (2011) describe ethnocentrism as "a strong tendency to use one's own group's standards as the standards when viewing other groups, to place one's group at the top of a hierarchy and to rank all others as lower," or the "us better/them worse" mentality (p. 4). Ethnocentrism is not unique to Eastern countries; in fact, it is prevalent concept in all cultures. That begin said, ethnocentric ideas are often instilled in people at a very young age, and this long-term belief in one's cultural superiority can cause problems on a national scale.

The negative impact of ethnocentrism can be viewed in four different ways, which I have adapted from Berry, Poortinga, Breugelmans, Chasiotis, and Sam's (2011) assertion of ethnocentrism and its effects on cross-cultural research (p. 5-6). They include: the incorrect interpretation of behavior (e.g., in a classroom, during a research study), applying culture-specific methods to another culture (e.g., not adapting language in a classroom or social study), forming and asserting theories that may have been affected by cultural prejudices and biases (e.g., introducing a new teaching method that favors the dominant group in class), and finally, who or what researchers choose to focus on, and how they may generalize their findings to other cultures. Although Western researchers have been dominant in most areas of research, and therefore have been susceptible to criticism for biased research, this list is by no means restricted to Western countries.

This basic definition of and discussion on ethnocentrism may not seem well-connected to the topic at hand – challenges associated with establishing a well-rounded curriculum in global health – but it has critical implications when dealing with a country like Japan. In order to establish this point, we must look at Japanese history to see how the country has evolved and where it currently stands within modern global society.

Japan and Current Challenges to Global Health

According to the Central Intelligence Agency's World Fact Book (2016), Japan's population stands at 126,702,133 (estimated in July 2016), and Japanese is the majority ethnic group (98. 5% of the population) (People and Society section, para. 1 and para. 3). In his chapter on Japanese education and education reform, Goodman (2011) offers the following cultural insight:

> The 1980s in Japan were characterized as a period of great reform. Throughout the middle part of the decade, a high-status Special Committee on Education...discussed the strengths and weaknesses of the Japanese educational system and made recommendations for change. The composition of the 25-person committee itself was symptomatic of the way education was perceived in Japan: the majority of members were industrialists, bureaucrats, and professors at the leading universities, with only two members with any direct teaching experience in schools...This composition reflected the assumption...that education should serve the interests of the state rather than the individual. (p. 52)

This quotation summarizes Japanese cultural beliefs in the fields of education, politics, and society, and the disturbing reality is that not much reform has taken place since the 1980s. Goodman (2011) reveals that Japanese education specialists still cannot agree on what exactly has changed within the Japanese education system since then, and that most people in Japan "did not see the need for reform, and hence no real blueprint for reform has even been developed" (p. 61). This is a startling revelation, but the question still remains: why is Japan unwilling to promote rapid change in its education system to reflect a global society rather than solely a Japanese one?

Ethnocentrism

Ethnocentrism is the most significant obstacle to the growth of global health in Japan. Individuals who have not experienced international travel or any type of cultural immersion will find it difficult to think beyond his or her cultural borders. This lack of experience affects other areas of life, including educational choices, relationship formation, and even research conduct.

When ethnocentrism is mentioned in academic textbooks, classrooms, or forums, there is a tendency to immediately associate ethnocentrism with Caucasians. MacDonald (2007) posits an interesting approach to white ethnocentrism:

> Ethnocentric tendencies continue to influence the behavior of white people. Despite the current cultural programming, white people are gradually coalescing into what I term "implicit white communities" in multicultural America – that is, communities that reflect their ethnocentrism but that "cannot tell their name" – they cannot explicitly state that they are an expression of white ethnocentrism. (p. 8)

Although this specific observation is focused on "white" communities, it could be applied to other cultural groups. Communities with little influence from outside cultures begin to become a reflection of their own ethnocentric beliefs.

Delving into ethnocentric beliefs will never be an easy task, for controversy follows quickly behind those who expose and question cultural beliefs; however, Japanese homogeneity and the associated implied racism have already been well studied and documented. Sugimoto (2014) offers a scathing review of Japanese homogeneity:

> For decades, the Japanese leadership inculcated in the populace the myths of Japanese racial purity and of the ethnic superiority which was supposed to be guaranteed by the uninterrupted lineage of the imperial household over centuries...Many observers have attributed Japan's economic success and political stability to its racial and ethnic homogeneity. Conscious of the extent of support for racist ideology of this type, the Japanese establishment has often resorted to the argument that mono-ethnic Japanese society has no tradition of accepting outsiders. (p. 196)

Traditions and long-held beliefs are most often hardest to break, and yet the belief that Japan is safest (and purest) when outsiders are kept out (or at least controlled within) threatens to thrust Japan backwards to being the ancient, mysterious country that was closed off to foreigners for so many years.

This ethnocentrism has most certainly polluted modern Japanese education institutions. From a Western perspective, the Japanese education system often seems "unbearably uniform," and uses examples of "rebellion as signs of pathology in a social system that seems to deny the very individuality that they regard as so important" (Hendry, 2013, p. 81). To combat this view, Japanese universities sought to globalize, yet they do so in shallow ways. For example, they hire "token" foreign professors, but limit them in terms of curriculum development, student engagement, and tenure (Aldwinckle, 2016). Experts have suggested these high levels of discrimination come from a history of ethnocentric beliefs and an "inferiority complex towards the Caucasian West and the superiority complex towards Asian neighbors" (Sugimoto, 2014, p. 196). The most dangerous part of this theory is that this type of skewed cultural identity formation could lead to a new formation – a modern "global" identity that is deeply embedded in ethnocentric values, racist beliefs, and xenophobia.

Racism and Xenophobia
    "Japanese Only!"
    So read signs all across Japan warning foreigners, in English, that their presence is not wanted or allowed in certain establishments (Aldwinckle, 2014). These establishments, ranging from public baths to restaurants, are

representative of the underlying issues of racism, discrimination, and xenophobia that continue to plague the modern-day Japan.

Although Japan has anti-discrimination legislation to combat issues like hate speech, blatant racism exists. Recently, the driver of a crowded train apologized to Japanese customers for the amount of foreign passengers: "本日は多数の外国人のお客さまが乗車されており、大変混雑しておりますので、日本人のお客さまにはご不便をおかけしており ま," which is translated as, "We have many foreigners on board today. We apologize for causing you inconveniences" ("Osaka train driver apologizes," 2016). As the future host of the 2020 Olympic games, Japan, specifically Tokyo, is struggling to find solutions to the large number of foreigners who will arrive and be greeted by a seemingly inhospitable native population (Aoki, 2016).

Other incidents, such as "wasabi terrorism" (sushi restaurants purposely applying irregular, excessive amounts of wasabi to dishes), are appearing more frequently in news bulletins. This is evidence of a childish, almost bullying response to the "foreign nuisance" that continues to grow in Japan (McCurry, 2016). The Japanese Justice Ministry has finally taken notice, and will soon conduct a large-scale survey of foreign residents – a first in Japanese history ("Justice Ministry to conduct," 2016). The survey will be given to 18,500 foreign residents in Japan, and inquire about their experiences with racism and other forms of discrimination ("Justice Ministry to conduct," 2016, para. 2).

In spite of the Japanese government's acknowledgment that discrimination is becoming a social concern across Japan, critics point to the increasing number of foreigners who have been placed in leadership positions in small and large companies, businesses, and organizations throughout Japan; however, these increases in foreign management positions have led to a more serious problem than a few extra dollops of wasabi.

Leadership

Japanese companies who have chosen to "internationalize" their brand by bringing on foreign management have certainly taken a step in the right direction. However, a change in management does not necessarily equate to a change in business culture. Oftentimes, the issues that were pervasive before the management change still exist and are exacerbated by the presence of someone from outside the Japanese culture. Although this chapter is dedicated to Japanese educational institutions, it should be noted that universities in Japan are viewed very much like any other big business: "Education culture within the elite school settings has gradually come to reflect corporate culture within the enterprise environment" (Sugimoto,

2014, p. 135). Japanese universities, therefore, suffer from the same issues and challenges as businesses.

The first and second challenges that workers face are power abuse/harassment and gender issues (e.g., sexism and sexual harassment). In Western cultures, issues and evidence of power abuse are reported to the appropriate government agency. Power harassment is also documented, and either the appropriate agency is contacted or a lawsuit is filed. Some states in the U.S. make this process very transparent and convenient: The California Department of Industrial Relations (2016) has an online form to report labor law violations, as well as retaliation and discrimination complaints. Sexual discrimination is also not tolerated in Western countries. However, Japan has a different way of dealing with various forms of harassment in the workplace:

> In her research on female clerical workers in Japanese companies – who are usually known as "OLs" (an abbreviation of "office ladies") – Yuko Ogasawara (1998) finds that although OLs are unlikely to directly resist the sex discrimination that fundamentally shapes the nature of their work and limits potential for advancement, they are quite aware of workplace power dynamics. (LeBlanc, 2011, p. 124)

This tolerance has become deeply embedded in Japanese business, but an ethnocentric viewpoint allows Japanese workers to understand this way as the "right" way – the way in which Japanese society functions and maintains stability. Going against this way means going against the fabric of Japanese culture and society.

The third challenge - the infantilization of Japanese society – is a difficult topic to discuss, as it is just coming to the forefront of social issue discussions. This directly affects the Japanese education system, for Japanese students are treated in an infantilizing way from the time they are in kindergarten until they complete their undergraduate studies. For example, many foreign secondary teachers and university professors have publicly complained about Japanese students being allowed to sleep in class, not turn in assignments, or miss most (or sometimes all) classes and still receive a passing grade (Shearon, 2013). As Buruma (1984) notes:

> Everyone is the same. All are equally sweet. Individual differences are wiped out, just as they are, ideally, in the mind of womb-like group life the majority of Japanese feel most comfortable leading. And if they don't actually lead it, they dream about it. (p. 25)

Professor Yamamoto (1998) adds to this comment: "That is to say, the Japanese...are not just regressive, they are embryonic; they actively desire not only a preverbal and preconscious state but a gestational one" (p. 18). The issue of infantilization is deep-seated, and can be seen in many aspects of Japanese culture (e.g., fashion). Again, from an ethnocentric perspective, this is the best way Japan can function as a collective society, so changing this system is extremely difficult.

The last challenge we will discuss in this chapter is probably the most well-known in global forums: Japan's aging population, low birthrate, and ageism. While this challenge moves beyond the scope of this paper, it is already well-documented and debated among academic, economic, and political circles. The issue can be looked at from an ethnocentric perspective and applied to the field of education, which continues to confine faculty members and departments with counterproductive measures, such as age restrictions. For example, Japanese universities advertise openings for faculty positions, but limit applicants on the basis of age, asking for interested individuals to be, as one well-known university in Hokkaido stated, "under 40 years of age at the deadline of application" (Hokkaido University, 2017). The issue of an aging, yet ageist, population continues to persist, and Japan continues to adhere to the related beliefs, policies, and procedures because it believes this is the best way a society can maintain peace and harmony.

Overcoming the Challenges: A Case Study

Instead of outlining ways in which these challenges should be overcome, a case study will be presented in order to illustrate the deeply embedded issues within Japanese educational institutions. Through mismanagement and corruption, Japanese and foreign managers and administrators enable and perpetuate the dysfunctional ethnocentric system that is currently running throughout national and private institutions of higher education in Japan. The following case study is based on interviews, counseling sessions with faculty members (both previous and current), field observations, and knowledge of internal communications. Please note that names, dates, and locations have been changed to protect participants' identities.

In 2014, a Kanto-based university, Transparent University, decided to change its image in Japan by creating a new liberal arts program. This new department boasted an English-only curriculum, faculty members from various Western countries, a mandatory study abroad component, and exchange programs with non-Japanese universities that allowed for a more international campus. The department chair chosen to lead the department was a non-Japanese corporate businessperson, Dr. Cathartidae, hired for his management and academic experience in several Japanese universities. Dr. Cathartidae pledged to move away from traditional Japanese education systems by promoting transparent management and creating a more international environment that reflected global perspectives and collaboration.

Soon after the university launched its new program, however, problems began to surface. These problems not only revealed how corporate values conflict with collegial values, but also how Japan's ethnocentric values play a role in seemingly "global" programs. The faculty and staff working at the new department were treated unfairly and poorly – much differently than the Japanese faculty in the other university departments. While this is not uncommon in Japanese universities, the situation was exacerbated when the university president decided to grant full authority over the new department to the department chair, who promptly created new policies and procedures that restricted faculty members from freely demonstrating or voicing their opinions on how the department operated. Although filled with new rules, Dr. Cathartidae's system lacked clear policies and moved well beyond ethical boundaries as he alone had all decision-making authority.

McNay's (1995) model of universities as organizations describes four different kinds of university cultures based on their degree of policy definition and control of implementation: "Collegium" universities focus on academic freedom and liberty and "institutional freedom from external controls." "Bureaucracy" organizations focus on policies and procedures, and "committees become arenas for policy development." "Corporation" schools stress supreme executive authority to the individual or individuals solely responsible for making decisions for the entire department or institution, and are "dominant...in the treatment of people, with a consequent reaction of resentment, at times verging on anomie." Finally, "Enterprise" universities focus on making key decisions that are client-centered, meaning "the good of the client should be the dominant criterion for decision-making" (p. 106-108). Dr. Cathartidae's management system clearly fits the corporation-style university culture, which goes against the bureaucratic style to which Japanese universities tend to adhere.

During this time, Dr. Corvidae, a faculty member, proposed a global health program for the new department with a focus on global psychology. This new program would offer courses mostly in English, but some courses would be taught in Japanese, thereby making it an attractive option for both Japanese and international students. At first, the idea was welcomed, but this opportunity to open the university to a more global audience was met with hesitation and suspicion, possibly due to Dr. Cathartidae feeling threatened by a new proposal that he had little control over. At the urging of the department chair, the university president and vice president quickly withdrew support from the idea of creating a global health program and instead took the idea and quickly established a health program that focused solely on Japanese culture, athletics, and psychology.

Dr. Corvidae continued to press for a more global approach to mental health, an aspect the new department lacked, and he became more vocal as

Japanese and international students began to show signs of anxiety, stress, culture shock, and acculturation issues. Soon, though, he became the victim of power harassment, social isolation, and slander, which are common tactics in Japanese universities used for weeding out undesirable faculty members who choose to speak out against the establishment. This accepted form of power harassment is commonly associated with the Japanese proverb, "The nail that sticks out gets hammered down." Watanabe (2012) explains:

> The nail that sticks out [i.e., the undesirable person] can be hammered down for many reasons – better grades, worse grades, making a mistake in a team activity, [so] in a country where an unspoken rule of conformity is combined with a strict hierarchical structure, bullying – or *ijime* – becomes an ingrained, almost tolerated phenomenon. (para. 4)

Dr. Corvidae has become an easy target by going against both the Japanese university's perspective on group harmony/obedience and the "old boy" corporate management style that Dr. Cathartidae instilled in the new department.

Japanese ethnocentrism, combined with Dr. Cathartidae's history of power and sexual harassment in previous institutions, created the proverbial "perfect storm" within the department. As a result, several faculty and staff members left the department, and multiple formal complaints (including one sexual harassment and two power harassment claims) were filed with the university's human resources department. In turn, the human resources department made several unethical decisions to cover up these claims, which is another common procedure that Japanese universities use when dealing with foreign complaints.

This department is currently struggling to increase its student enrollment numbers, and with more faculty members and students leaving the program, it will most certainly meet its end soon, at least in its current incarnation. As McNay (1995) points out, this type of corporate-run university…

> …cannot be maintained for long periods without such consequences: it is a culture for crisis, not continuity. It is political also in its processes of bargaining and negotiation, with senior staff developing alliances and understandings outside formal decision arenas and dis-empowering committees. (p. 107)

The likeliest future scenario is for the university to replace the current department chair with a Japanese academic and move forward with a more Japanese approach to education, thus furthering the belief that the Japanese perspective on education is the only way to survive.

Clearly, it is not just a case of Japanese ethnocentrism that harmed this university's new department – the blending of Eastern ethnocentric values and Western corporate values was disastrous. Whoever replaces Dr.

Cathartidae will not be able to simply impose a Japanese approach to management and education, considering the university's high percentage of foreign faculty and international students. Therefore, there is still hope that the university will reevaluate their educational stance and consider a more global, ethical approach to its education programs.

Conclusion

This chapter should not be seen as an attack on Japan, the Japanese education system, or the Japanese identity (or "Japaneseness" [日本人論/Nihonjinron]). No country's system is perfect, and most are fraught with issues, such as power and sexual harassment and racial profiling and discrimination. That being said, many countries in the world are becoming more diverse as each year passes, either by choice (welcoming foreign residents) or by force (refugee exoduses). However, there are still some countries whose national make-up favors the majority, and with this scenario comes the inherent issue of ethnocentric values permeating politics and business.

When dealing with issues of exclusivity and prejudice, all hope is not lost. Sugimoto (2014) points to "signs that youngsters are gradually freeing themselves from entrenched prejudice and taking a more open stance" (p. 205). This open stance, although a welcome sign of change, has yet to manifest into legislation that will fundamentally change the way Japanese businesses and educational institutions operate. Therefore, until progress is made, ethnocentrism will continue to dictate who receives appropriate treatment and who is bullied and silenced.

Famed Japanese novelist Haruki Murakami recently accepted Denmark's Hans Christian Andersen Literature Award in 2016. During his speech, he had this message to deliver to Japan: "No matter how high a wall we build to keep intruders out, no matter how strictly we exclude outsiders, no matter how much we rewrite history to suit us, we just end up damaging and hurting ourselves" (Yamaguchi, 2016, para. 3). This message is not a message of rebuke, but one of hopeful optimism for the future and one that every country should listen to and learn from. Ethnocentrism is just another way of building walls to keep outsiders out, in an effort to protect and preserve the way that a society functions. The current political and economic climate throughout the world is causing more and more countries to build higher and higher walls, further cementing the belief that one country's ways are better than the rest. Until this ethnocentric way of thinking is cast aside, the walls will continue to grow, leaving future generations with little hope for a truly global, united society.

References

Aldwinckle, D. (2014). The rogues' gallery: Photos of places in Japan which exclude or restrict non-Japanese customers. Retrieved from http://www.debito.org/roguesgallery.html

Aldwinckle, D. (2016). Blacklist of Japanese universities. Retrieved from http://www.debito.org/blacklist.html

Aoki, M. (2016). The race is on for volunteer interpreters for the 2020 Olympics. Retrieved on November 5, 2016, from http://www.japantimes.co.jp/news/2016/08/10/national/race-volunteer-interpreters-2020-tokyo-olympics/#.WB1EiNwkliM

Beech, D.J., and Danner, O.K. (2016). Building diversity initiatives in academic medicine. In R. Parekh and E. W. Childs (Eds.) *Stigma and Prejudice: Touchstones in Understanding Diversity in Healthcare* (pp. 325-338). Switzerland: Springer International Publishing.

Berry, J. W., Poortinga, Y.H., Breugelmans, S.M., Chasiotis, A., and Sam, D.L. (2011). Cross-cultural psychology: Research and applications. Cambridge: Cambridge University Press. Retrieved from http://www.cambridge.org/us/academic/subjects/psychology/cultural-psychology/cross-cultural-psychology-research-and-applications-3rd-edition?format=PB&isbn=9780521745208

Central Intelligence Agency. (2016). World factbook: Japan. Retrieved from https://www.cia.gov/library/publications/the-world-factbook/geos/ja.html

Duke University. (2016). Global health institute: Master of science in global health. Retrieved from https://globalhealth.duke.edu/education-and-training/graduate/master-of-science

Ethnocentrism. (n.d.). In Merriam-Webster online. Retrieved from http://www.merriam-webster.com/dictionary/ethnocentric

Georgetown University. (2016). Master of science in global health program. Retrieved from https://globalhealthms.georgetown.edu/

Global Health Initiative (2014). Global health matters. Retrieved from http://familiesusa.org/issues/global-health/matters/

Goodman, R. (2011). Japanese education and education reform. In V.L. Bestor and T.C. Bestor (Eds.) *Routledge Handbook of Japanese Culture and Society* (pp. 52-62). New York: Routledge.

Hendry, J. (2013). *Understanding Japanese Society.* London and New York: Routledge.

Hokkaido University (2017). Jobs at Hokkaido University. Retrieved on April 18, 2017, from https://www.global.hokudai.ac.jp/about/jobs-at-hokkaido-university/

Japan International Cooperation Agency (2005). The History of Japan's Educational Development. Retrieved on April 15, 2017, from https://www.jica.go.jp/jica-ri/IFIC_and_JBICI-Studies/english/publications/reports/study/topical/educational/pdf/educational_02.pdf

Justice Ministry to conduct first major survey on racism in Japan (2016, October 30), *Japan Times.* Retrieved from http://www.japantimes.co.jp/news/2016/10/30/national/social-issues/justice-ministry-conduct-first-major-survey-racism-japan/#.WBZqxNwkliM

Koplan J.P., Bond, T.C., and Merson, M.H., Reddy, K.S., Rodriguez, M.H., Sewankambo, N.K., and Wasserheit, J.N. (2009). Towards a common definition of global health. *Lancet, 373,* 1993–1995. doi:10. 1016/S0140-6736(09)60332-9

LeBlanc, R.M. (2011). The politics of gender in Japan. In V.L. Bestor and T.C. Bestor (Eds.) *Routledge Handbook of Japanese Culture and Society* (pp. 116-128). New York: Routledge.

MacDonald, K. (2007). Psychology and white ethnocentrism. *The Occidental Quarterly, 6*(4), pp. 7-46.

McCurry, J. (2016). Japanese train conductor blames foreign tourists for overcrowding. *The Guardian*. Retrieved from https://www.theguardian.com/world/2016/oct/11/japanese-train-conductor-blames-foreign-tourists-for-overcrowding

McNay, I. (1995). From the collegial academy to corporate enterprise: The changing cultures of universities. In T. Schuller (Ed.), *The changing university?* (105-115). Buckingham, UK: The Society for Research into Higher Education & Open University Press.

Osaka train driver apologizes to Japanese passengers for 'having many foreigners' on board (2016, October 30), *Japan Today*. Retrieved from https://www.japantoday.com/category/national/view/osaka-train-driver-apologizes-to-japanese-passengers-for-having-many-foreigners-on-board

Princeton University. (2016). Global health program. Retrieved from https://globalhealth.princeton.edu/

Schäferhoff, M., Suzuki, E., Angelides, P., and Hoffman, S. (2015). Rethinking the global health system. London: The Royal Institute of International Affairs. Retrieved from https://www.chathamhouse.org/sites/files/chathamhouse/field/field_document/20150923GlobalHealthArchitectureSchaferhoffSuzukiAngelidesHoffman.pdf

Shearon, B. (2013). The infantilization of University student. Retrieved on November 5, 2016, from http://sendaiben.org/2013/11/15/the-infantilization-of-university-students/

Shibuya, K. (2014). Global health will make Japan stronger – The national strategy that many Japanese people don't realize. Retrieved from www.synodos.jp/welfare/6770/2

Sugimoto, Y. (2014). An Introduction to Japanese Society. Melbourne, Australia: Cambridge University Press.

University of Edinburgh. (2016). Global health academy: Current health challenges. Retrieved from http://www.ed.ac.uk/global-health/current-health-challenges

University of Oxford. (2016). Master of science in global health science. Retrieved from http://www.ox.ac.uk/admissions/graduate/courses/msc-global-health-science

Watanabe, A. (2012). 'The nail that sticks out gets hammered down': Bullying in Japan. Retrieved from https://asiancorrespondent.com/2012/07/the-nail-that-sticks-out-gets-hammered-down-bullying-in-japan/

Yamaguchi, M. (2016). Accepting award, Murakami warns against excluding outsiders. Retrieved on November 8, 2016 from https://www.washingtonpost.com/entertainment/books/accepting-award-murakami-warns-against-excluding-outsiders/2016/10/31/f153caf4-9f37-11e6-8864-6f892cad0865_story.html

Yamamoto, T. (1998). Masking Selves, Making Subjects: Japanese American Women, Identity, and the Body. Berkeley, California: University of California Press.

PART 4

SUSTAINABILITY

CHAPTER 23

From Surviving to Thriving:
The Role of Mental Health in Facilitating Global Health and Attaining Sustainable Development

*Roseanne Flores, Ayorkor Gaba, Rashmi Jaipal, Nelida Quintero, and Neal Rubin**

Introduction

The 2030 Agenda for Sustainable Development by the General Assembly of the United Nations (U.N.) identified health and well-being as essential targets for human progress in the 21st century. This historic insight by world leaders essentially defined mental health as inextricably related to human health and envisioned well-being as an overarching concept concerned with the human rights of all persons. The fundamental linkages among health, sustainability, human rights, mental health, and well-being articulate a new, highly integrated framework for understanding these relationships and constitute the realization of the values and goals of the U.N. for humanity. In so doing, the leaders of U.N. member nations have, for the first time in human history, committed themselves to achieving identifiable goals related to sustainable progress on health, mental health, and well-being (United Nations, 2015).

There are seventeen Sustainable Development Goals (SDGs), and they range from ending extreme poverty to promoting gender equality and from facilitating economic development to limiting the impacts of climate change (United Nations, 2015, p. 6). This ambitious global agenda follows the relative successes and shortcomings of the Millennium Development Goals

---

* Authors are listed alphabetically and have contributed equally to this work

(MDGs) that were established at the turn of this century (United Nations, 2014). From 2000 to 2015, progress on the MDGs varied by individual goals and by country and region; therefore, the SDGs were conceived of as defining new emerging issues, addressing the needs of vulnerable populations around the world where change has been insufficient, and creating support for progress that will be sustainable over time. Sustainable Development Goal 3 – to "ensure healthy lives and promote well-being for all at all ages" (United Nations, 2015, p. 14) – is associated with specific targets to be achieved. These targets include Target 3.4, which involves "promoting mental health and well-being" (p. 16), and Target 3.5, which identifies the need for the "prevention and treatment of substance abuse" (p. 16). As a consequence, this new vision for global health integrates mental health as a meaningful component of sustainability for future generations.

Health, Well-being, and Mental Health as Human Rights

Since the establishment of the U.N. in 1945, health and well-being have been enshrined as human rights in a series of foundational instruments. The Universal Declaration of Human Rights (UDHR) assures the right to "health and well-being" (United Nations, 1948, Article 25, para. 1), even in the event of sickness or disability. The Covenant on Economic, Social and Cultural Rights (CESCR) assures the "enjoyment of the highest attainable standard of physical and mental health" for all persons (United Nations, 1966, Article 12, para. 2). The Convention on the Elimination of All Forms of Discrimination against Women (CEDAW) calls on States "to eliminate discrimination against women in the field of health care" (United Nations, 1979, Article 12, para. 1). The Convention on the Rights of the Child (CRC) sets forth guarantees "to ensure that no child is deprived of his or her right of access to such health care services" (United Nations, 1989, Article 24, para. 1). The Convention on the Rights of Persons with Disabilities (CRPD) provides that "States Parties recognize that persons with disabilities have the right to the enjoyment of the highest attainable standard of health without discrimination on the basis of disability" (United Nations, 2006, Article 25, para. 1). Therefore, the idea that health and well-being are human rights has been upheld consistently by member states of the U.N. for all persons and for particular groups in need of additional protections due to traditionally having been targets of discrimination.

However, history also suggests that the inclusion of mental health as a core component of global health and well-being has been slower to receive similar attention. The progress represented in Sustainable Development Goal 3 appears to have resulted from momentum created by several sources. The CRPD has contributed to this momentum as it provides human rights protections for persons with disabilities, including mental health conditions. While the conceptualization of disabilities as deficits has receded in favor of a more proactive model of viewing disabled persons as challenged, this attention has provided an avenue for the inclusion of mental health as an integral component of a rights-based perspective on health. Another significant development in the recognition of mental health as essential to well-being is the World Health Organization's (WHO) Mental Health Action Plan 2013-2020 (WHO, 2013). Adopted at the 66th World Health Assembly, this plan for action established the unquestionable linkage between mental health and human rights. It addresses the longstanding stigma of mental health and calls for change in attitudes and policies that result in discrimination. Through a series of major objectives, the WHO plan aims to achieve greater acceptance of mental health as a part of human health and to systematically expand available mental health services in community-based settings.

Non-governmental organization (NGOs) advocacy has been a significant contributor to the momentum for including mental health as a part of global health. For example, in 2014, the Psychology Coalition at the U.N. (PCUN) (which was established in 2012 and consists of psychological organizations with NGO status at the U.N., such as the American Psychological Association [APA] and the International Association of Applied Psychology [IAAP], among others), has combined with representatives of Member States to form the Friends of Mental Health and Well-Being and has successfully lobbied for the inclusion of mental health and well-being in the SDGs.

As members of the APA's United Nations NGO Team, we have been engaged in advocacy regarding a number of issues linking mental health, sustainable development, and global health. In the sections that follow, we will illustrate those links by examining the relationship between poverty, children's mental health, and well-being from a rights-based perspective, by linking the global rise in adolescent suicide rates with the costs of globalization, and by exploring substance use across the life cycle and its impact on sustainable development. Finally we will describe the mental health ramifications of human migration, displacement, and well-being in the 21st century. Throughout, we will emphasize a strength-based framework in the face of these challenges to global mental health and will articulate how we can thrive in a context that values well-being as a part of a sustainable future for people and planet.

Poverty, Child Rights, and Child Well-being

Over the last decade, global income inequality has increased and has reached epic proportions – the top 1% of the global population has as much money as the bottom 56% of the population (Ortiz & Cummins, 2011, p. 20). Children and youth have been disproportionately affected by these disparities. As of 2007, "more than two-thirds of the world's youth had access to less than 20 percent of the global wealth" (Ortiz & Cummins, 2011, p. 21). Research has shown that economic insecurity is highly associated with housing insecurity and poor educational and health outcomes. Without adequate income, children and their families are less likely to experience a quality of life that affords them the opportunity to grow, prosper, and thrive.

The effects of growing up in chronic poverty are many. Children and their families face many barriers and challenges that make it difficult for them to move out of poverty. Many lack access to adequate food and shelter. Most are silenced with little or no access to the political process, the very process that shapes their existence. Many face social discrimination and are denied access to basic needs and services; many are exploited and have access to only low-paying jobs (Ortiz, Moreira & Engilbertsdottir, 2012). The consequences of growing up under such conditions are devastation and destruction. Living in chronic poverty ultimately forces many children and youth into prostitution, gangs, and drug use.

Children's Rights, Quality of Life, and Sustainable Development

Child well-being is a multi-dimensional construct that encompasses psychological, physical, and social dimensions. The Child Rights approach to child well-being (1) places emphasis on the rights of children as human beings, (2) seeks to explore the child's experience within the here and now, and (3) includes the perspective of children in decision making. This approach is based on the principles of the Convention on the Rights of the Child (CRC) (Pollard & Lee, 2003).

The guiding principles of the CRC include the following elements: (1) non-discrimination, (2) adherence to the best interests of the child, (3) the right to life, survival, and development, and (4) the right to participate. Survival and development rights include the child's basic right to thrive (not just to survive) and to develop to their full potential (UN General Assembly, 1989). According to Article 6 of the CRC, children have a right to live, and governments must ensure that they can survive and have what they need to reach their full adult potential (UNICEF, 2014). But what does it mean to live? Do children just have a right to survival, or is the issue one of a quality of life? One might argue that growing up in chronic poverty provides for neither survival nor access to a quality lifestyle.

In an effort to address global poverty, the concept of social protection has been raised as a high priority on development agendas (Voipio, 2012; UNICEF, 2012). According to UNICEF, social protection involves public and private actions that address economic and social inequities. The purpose of addressing both areas is to ensure that state parties develop policies that take into account economic hardship and examine the role exclusion from social, cultural, and political capital plays in maintaining the ongoing cycle of poverty across generations of children and families (UNICEF, 2012).

On May 18, 2012, UNICEF presented its first "Social Protection Strategic Framework" in New York. The purpose of the framework was to ensure that children's rights were being protected, particularly in regard to Article 26, which addresses a child's right to social security. The framework also integrates Article 27, which addresses the right of all children to have a "standard of living adequate for the child's physical, mental, spiritual, moral and social development" (p. 7) and specifies the states' responsibility to assist parents and adults who care for children and youth by providing the material support required to ensure their adequate growth and development. In addition, the framework addresses the need for states to ensure the overall well-being of children and youth by promoting global economic growth and development (UNICEF, 2012). In Brussels in June of the same year, UNICEF presented the framework during a roundtable discussion on Social Protection. UNICEF, the World Bank, and the International Labor Organization (ILO) addressed their commitment to working with countries to develop sustainable financing strategies and to providing technical support to ensure ongoing social protection for children and youth (UNICEF, 2012).

On September 25, 2015, the U.N. adopted the 2030 Agenda for Sustainable Development to ensure the establishment of human rights and well-being for all, including gender equality, access to quality health care and education, and the reduction of poverty – in short, the right to a quality of life (United Nations, 2015). The first of the 17 agenda goals is to eradicate poverty. Although Social Protection did not become one of the Sustainable Development Goals (SDGs), it is explicitly addressed as a critical element in achieving SDG1 (ending poverty in all forms) and SDG10 (reduction of inequality), and it is implicitly necessary for achieving SDG2 (ending hunger), SDG3 (ensuring healthy lives and promoting well-being across the life-span), SDG4 (ensuring inclusive and quality education), SDG 5 (ensuring gender equity and empowering girls), and SDG6 (providing safe water) (EADI Working Group Social Protection, n.d.). Thus, in order to achieve many of the sustainable development goals, state parties must address social protection. But how can states ensure that social protection takes into account the voices of children and youth? The answer: by asking them.

Children's Voices and the SDG's

In December 2012, the U.N. partnered with several organizations to develop the MyWorld global survey in order to capture the voices of youth and adults from around the world with the purpose of informing global leaders as they established the new development agenda (MyWorld Data Analytics, n.d.). The MyWorld survey provided the opportunity for children under 15 years of age to express their top five priorities for the future. The results demonstrated that in general, children desired greater access to education, better job opportunities, better health care, access to clean water and sanitation, and better transport and roads (MyWorld Data Analytics, n.d.).

Building on the success of the MyWorld survey, in June 2015, UNICEF partnered with other organizations to design an e-consultation to solicit feedback from children and youth about the SDGs. Children were asked to answer five questions concerning: (1) the importance of the SDGs to themselves and other children around the world, (2) the prioritization of the goals that would help them to achieve the world they want to see in the future, (3) the ability of the SDGs to tell them about their rights and inspire them to have their human rights valued and respected, (4) any additions they would add to the declaration to make it more child-friendly, and (5) any methods would they recommend to help raise awareness of the goals for children and young people. The consultation ran for four weeks and consisted of approximately 400 individuals from 47 countries (UNICEF, 2015, p. 3).

In general, children and youth agreed that the SDGs had a direct impact on their lives and overall well-being. According to the findings, many children felt that the SDGs provided them with both a way to find out about what was going on in the world and a hope for the future amidst overwhelming, global problems. With respect to what they felt were the most pressing goals that would lead to a better future, children and youth recognized that the SDGs were interconnected. The majority of youth advocated for ending poverty and hunger, having access to a good education and health, ensuring gender equality, living in peace and free of conflict, having access to clean drinking water, and protecting the planet. While the majority of children felt that obtaining an education and ending hunger were the top priorities, ending poverty was a close second, and many children emphasized that ending poverty was inextricably tied to achieving the other goals. In response to the questions concerning human rights, many children felt that the SDGs provided them with adequate information about their human rights and motivated them to advocate for human rights for themselves and others. With regard to the accessibility of the language of the SDG agenda for children and youth, some of the children felt that the language was overly complicated and not written in child-friendly text. They felt that if the overall goal was for more youth to engage with the document and find it useful, a more child-friendly version would need to be created. They also pointed out that their voices were not included in the original document, that they had not been invited to participate as is called for in the CRC, and that the document itself rarely mentioned children and youth.

Furthermore, the youth articulated that the framers of the SDG's had conceptualized three pillars of sustainability – social, economic, and environmental – but they requested that youth be mentioned as being important to economic growth, not just social growth. They also wanted to be recognized as being important to the environment and argued that children and youth should be included in addressing environmental damage. They requested that they have a voice in implementation, monitoring, and ongoing review of the goals. Finally, with respect to raising awareness of the goals, they felt that using social media would be helpful as many children and youth use technology. That said, youth from developing countries with limited access to technology advocated for SDG promotion through books or by placing the information in public transportation. In addition, youth suggested that SDGs be part of school curricula and that SDG information be translated into different languages and be made available for children with disabilities (UNICEF, 2015). Thus, the responses from youth from around the world support the promotion of a social protection framework that ensures the global economic, social, and environmental well-being of all.

In short, children and youth know what they need to thrive. Article 12 of the CRC calls upon adults to listen to children and to involve them in the decision-making process. The U.N. has involved children, and they have participated. The results are clear. The psychological, physical, and social well-being of children and youth is dependent upon the global community eradicating poverty, ensuring access to quality health care and education, ensuring gender equality, and upholding the rights of the child. But will we listen?

Mental Health and Youth Suicide:
The Psychological Costs of Globalization

The focus of the community of nations on sustainable development implies that previous efforts to change key global issues have not achieved sustainability. As discussed above, income inequality must be addressed in order for the 2030 global agenda to succeed. A key issue in addressing inequality and achieving progress regarding mental health and well-being is the impact of globalization. In fact, poor mental health outcomes can serve as indicators of a lack of sustainability in regards to human well-being. The unsustainability of the current model of economic development or globalization is usually discussed in terms of growing social inequality, environmental degradation, and climate change. There is, however, a psychological dimension to development which is tragically reflected in suicide rates among youth worldwide. Recent reports from the World

Health Organization (WHO, 2010, 2014) show growing mental health problems, stress related disorders, depression and the emerging trend of youth suicide worldwide, which, along with social inequality and environmental degradation, may also be indicators of unsustainable development.

Economic globalization, along with its benefits, seems to be creating a competitive, materialistic environment that has negative impacts on mental health and well-being. Faced with many challenges, governments in both low- and high-income countries tend to place mental health needs at the bottom of the list of national priorities. However, as mental illness is on the rise, it is becoming increasingly important to rearrange these priorities. According to the WHO (2016) about 676 million people suffer from mental illness globally, and over 800,000 people die by suicide every year (p. 62). Mental health problems include serious conditions like schizophrenia, but also more widespread psychosocial distress that results from poverty, human rights violations, and trauma from conflict or natural disasters. The rapid development of the last two or three decades may be creating or exacerbating these problems due to the current model of economic growth and cultural globalization. This argument will be developed further below. The cultural globalization associated with these outcomes appears to be the spread of consumer culture. As the media, internet, and other forms of technology present images and information that challenge traditional values and expectations, youth increasingly experience social pressure and identity confusion. For example, compared to results from 5 years before, a recent study by The Children's Society, UK (2016) found a sharp rise in unhappiness in 2013-2014. Among 10 to 15-year-old girls, 14% were unhappy with their lives, and 34% were unhappy with their appearance and felt ugly or worthless (Burns, 2016, p. 1). In the United States, New Jersey college students reported experiencing an increase in personal hardships and emotional distress. Furthermore, they were in need of additional support on several levels, which rendered them vulnerable to mental health problems. In response, the New Jersey State Legislature passed a suicide prevention act requiring colleges and universities to provide students with 24-hour access to a mental health professional (Madison Holleran Suicide Prevention Act, 2016). Mental health problems, including the emerging trend of youth suicide, have become so widespread that the WHO views them as a global public health problem. Therefore, it is imperative to understand the relationship between rising mental health problems and globalization.

WHO Statistics on Youth Suicide

According to the WHO (2014), suicide is ranked as the second-leading cause of death globally among young adults aged 15–29 and accounts for

8.5% of all deaths (p. 22). There are large regional variations in suicide rates. In some countries, suicide is the leading cause of death for young people. High-income countries (e.g., Japan, South Korea, and countries in North America or Western Europe) have a higher rate of suicide (12.7 per 100,000) than the lower- or middle-income countries (LMICs) (11.2 per 100,000); however, the Southeast Asia region (e.g., India, Sri Lanka, and Indonesia) has the highest rate of suicide at 17.7 per 100,000 (WHO, 2014, p. 17). The WHO reports that in both high-income countries and LMICs in Southeast Asia, suicide is the leading cause of death for men and women aged 15−29 (17.6% of all male deaths and 16.6% of all female deaths) (WHO, 2014, p. 22).

The pattern of suicide is different for developed, high-income countries than it is for developing, LMICs. In high-income countries, suicide rates increase steadily across the life span, but in Southeast Asia, suicide rates peak during young adulthood and then decreases in middle age. Young adults and elderly women in LMICs have much higher suicide rates than in high-income countries, and middle-aged men in high-income countries have much higher suicide rates than middle-aged men in LMICs. Youth in Southeast Asian LMICs have the highest suicide rates in the world. A large epidemiological study conducted from 2001-2003 reports that, "In India, suicide death rates are amongst the highest in the world for youth and women...suicide rates per 100,000 for ages 15 years and older was 26.3 for men and 17.5 for women" (Patel et al., 2012, p. 2). The WHO reported an increase since then. In 2012, the youth suicide rate for the 15-29 year age group was 35.5 per 100,000 in India (which is tragically higher than in the U.S., for example, where the rate was 12.7 in the same age group during the same time period) (WHO 2014, p. 83).

Although the suicide pattern across the lifecycle is different in high-income countries than it is in Southeast Asian LMICs, the underlying causes of recent increases in suicide may be the same. A recent surge in the suicide rates in an "advanced" country like the U.S. may be connected to the same phenomenon of economic growth also occurring in Southeast Asia. In the Southeast Asian developing world, globalization may cause acculturation stress through the pressures of modernization and assimilation to an individualistic, competitive, consumer-culture environment (particularly for youth). In contrast, in the developed world, in order to promote profit, strategies such as outsourcing have created pressures such as job loss (particularly for middle-aged men), which leads to growing inequality. It appears that economic globalization is creating these pressures, both of which can lead to an increase in psychological distress and suicide.

High-Income Countries and Effects of Economic Globalization

According to the WHO (2014), financial insecurity and the impact of the global economic downturn have contributed to an increase in stress-related disorders and mental health problems in some high-income countries. A recent study by the National Center for Health Statistics in the U.S. found that the suicide rate in 2014 had increased to the highest levels in nearly 30 years. Results indicated that the suicide rate increased by 24% from 1999 to 2014. Suicide rates across gender and all age groups increased from 10 to 74. In the middle-aged group (ages 45 to 64), whose suicide rates had changed little since the 1950s, the suicide rate for women suddenly rose by 63 percent, and the suicide rate for men rose by 43 percent. There was also a sharp increase in suicide among young girls aged 10 to 14 (Curtin, Warner, & Hedegaard, 2016, p. 2-3).

The increase in suicides may be due to job loss, financial insecurity, home foreclosures, or lack of social support, especially for middle-aged Americans or those with low education levels. In a New York Times interview, Dr. Alex Crosby, an epidemiologist from the National Center for Health Statistics, said that suicide rates seem to be connected to economic fluctuations. They rise when the economy is weak (the rate during The Great Depression was 22.1 per 100,000) and decrease when the economy is strong (10.5 per 100,000 in 1999) (Tavernise, 2016, para. 21). Populations most affected by economic downturns are likely to be citizens who are less-educated and who feel less hope for finding employment.

LMICs, Cultural Globalization, and Acculturation Stress

The WHO report (2014) also discusses community and relationship risk factors, including acculturation stress, discrimination, sense of isolation, and lack of social support. Acculturation stress refers to psychological and social changes that occur with cultural contact (Berry, 2006). High acculturation stress can lead to serious mental health problems. Cultural values and norms shape our basic social identity, build resilience, and are internalized through early childhood socialization. Changes in cultural identity and erosion of social support can be stressful. Children and youth are particularly affected when growing up in two disparate cultures with conflicting social norms and value systems. Differences in basic values can render integration into the dominant culture challenging and can cause discrimination, identity confusion, internal conflict, loss of social support, and feelings of isolation (Berry et al., 2006). Children tend to internalize negative attitudes towards and perceptions of their backgrounds from the surrounding dominant cultural environment. They try to fit in but often feel lost, as if they simply do not belong to mainstream culture. These dynamics have been documented as psychosocial processes for minority youth assimilating to the dominant culture. However, it can also be hypothesized that similar challenges exist when transitioning from traditional cultures to the modern, globalized economy as this new, socio-cultural, economic environment can virtually represent a cross-cultural experience.

Suicide Rates in Globalizing India

Thus, the much higher rates of youth suicide in Southeast Asia could be due to acculturation stress related to the rapid economic development and modernization taking place in that region. According to Indian psychiatrist L.Vijaykumar (2007), "The liberalization of the economy and privatization leading to job insecurity, huge disparities in incomes, social change from the breakdown of the joint family support system and inability to meet role obligations" (p. 5) has led to a great increase in stress and difficulty in adjusting to the new norms and values associated with modernization. Interestingly, V. Patel's (2012) epidemiological study on suicide in India found that higher rates of youth suicide occur among the more educated in society (p. 9); however, suicide death rates in high-income countries are greater among the less educated. Perhaps educated youth in India feel more pressure to assimilate to the individualistic norms and values of modernization represented to them in their education, the internet, and social media. Competing to find a job or fitting into modern workplace norms and values can be challenging, especially when there is pressure to move away from interdependent values and to assimilate to the incoming individualistic culture of globalization. Therefore, acculturation stress resulting from the challenges of globalization may be a contributing factor to the higher rates of suicide among educated youth with higher socioeconomic status in India.

However, youth with low educational levels or a lower socioeconomic status may also experience acculturation stress when exposed to rapid modernization. While trying to adjust to the modern world, they are vulnerable to identity confusion and discrimination. A study in India by Verma, Sachdeva, & Pandey (2013) found that suicides occurred among youth without a high school education but with unrealistically high aspirations and expectations for a modern lifestyle. They reported having difficulty adjusting from collectivist to individualistic norms and values as well as from the associated decrease in social support they experienced. The exposure to overwhelming amounts of information on global media can be hard to navigate for youth in these vulnerable groups and can lead to unanticipated mental health problems. Constant exposure to values of consumerism, celebrity culture, and entitlement leads to feeling pressured to assimilate. As a consequence, social comparisons engender depression and loss of self-worth, alcoholism, drug use, and suicide. Furthermore, they typically lack the social normative, linguistic, educational, and economic advantages necessary to compete in the global market place. Like other youth around the world, they are exposed to cyberbullying, pornography, and graphic images of violence on the internet, all of which can affect psychological integrity (Chisholm, 2013). With little support, these youth remain vulnerable to the impacts of globalization.

Overall, globalization seems to be linked to conditions that undermine the sustainability of mental health and well-being. The global rise in suicide rates may be associated with the impact of socioeconomic and acculturation pressures resulting from globalization and development in high-income countries and LMICs. However, the paradigm shift towards sustainable development in the U.N. 2030 agenda, especially considering its emphasis on social justice and inclusion, may protect youth with vulnerable mental health against acculturation stress and promote resilience amidst the challenges of maturing in a globalized, culturally diverse environment. Attention to the need of cultural integration supports will hopefully enhance the capacity of youths to adapt to a rapidly changing socioeconomic world.

The Impact of Substance Abuse on Global Health and Sustainable Development

Another growing mental health challenge for attaining sustainable development is substance abuse. The harmful use of substances, illicit drugs, and alcohol is a global health and public health concern that affects people of all ages. Approximately 27 million people from ages 15 to 64 are problem drug users and qualify as having a drug use disorder (United Nations Office on Drugs and Crime [UNODC], 2016a, p. 8). Globally, about 16.0% of drinkers aged 15 or older engage in heavy episodic drinking (HED), which is defined as six or more standard drinks in at least one single occasion at least monthly (WHO, 2014b, p. 34). HED is associated with detrimental consequences, even if the individual's average level of alcohol consumption is relatively low. Predictions indicate that the number of illicit drug users worldwide is likely to grow by 25% by 2050; significant increases are expected to take place among the rapidly rising urban populations of developing countries (UNODC, 2012, p. 94). About half of problem drug users (approximately 12.1 million people) are intravenous (IV) drug users and are at very high risk for contracting health conditions such as HIV and hepatitis (UNODC, 2015b, p.4). In addition, the harmful use of alcohol is a causal factor in more than 200 disease and injury conditions (Lim, et al., 2012, p. 2247). Substance abuse is not only a clear threat to health – it is also a significant threat to sustainable development and is inextricably linked to many SDGs. Global action is needed to address the impact of substance abuse on health and sustainable development.

For the first time in history, world leaders recognized mental health and well-being (including the prevention and treatment of substance abuse) as health priorities in the global development agenda. Specifically, Target 3.5 in the SDGs requests that countries "strengthen the prevention and treatment of substance abuse, including narcotic drug abuse and harmful use of alcohol" (United Nations, 2015a, para. 5). The inclusion of substance abuse in the SDGs provides a unique opportunity to understand and address substance abuse as a public health concern that impacts global sustainable development. Similar to other health issues, such as HIV, reducing rates of substance abuse and its negative impacts will require coordinated, culturally-informed, evidenced-based, multi-systemic approaches (United Nations, 2015b). As noted by United Nations Secretary-General Ban Ki-moon, it is time for "countries and communities to improve the lives of everyone blighted by drug abuse by integrating security and public safety with a heightened focus on health, human rights, and sustainable development" (UNODC, 2016b, p. 1). Following are key areas to consider as governments and NGOs begin to tackle this important issue.

Gender and Treatment

Historically, men abuse substances at much higher rates than women; however, current projections indicate that the biggest area of growth in illicit drug use will be amongst women (UNODC, 2015b). There have already been changes in female drug use patterns. For example, in India, a country where substance abuse among females had previously been almost unheard of, 20% of IV drug users in India are women (Wherley & Chatterjee, 2015, p. 1). Understanding and addressing gender differences in social and biological factors related to the initiation, maintenance, and recovery from substance use disorders will be critical as countries tackle Target 3.5.

Researchers have found that compared to men, women seem to have a higher risk of suffering from several negative health consequences of alcohol. Women tend to have a later age of onset of problem drinking than men, but they develop various problems more quickly, including liver, heart, and brain damage (Johnson, Richter, Kleber, McLellan, & Carise, 2005, p. 1139). The link between drug use and HIV amongst women is of particular concern because HIV is often considered one of the most significant threats to sustainable development worldwide. The available data show that, in many countries, women who inject drugs are more vulnerable to HIV infection than their male counterparts. Furthermore, the prevalence of HIV is higher among women who inject drugs than among their male counterparts (UNODC, 2015b).

In addition to these unique physical health risks, substance-abusing women experience a host of co-occurring, psycho-social risk factors (e.g., trauma, gender based violence, etc.), which place them at increased risk. For example, a study of women and drug use in India found that more than 75% of female substance users sustained physical injuries because of violence and had a significantly higher frequency of suicidal attempts in the previous year. Furthermore, a majority (75.2%) had General Health Questionnaire (GHQ) scores above the cut-off for diagnosable psychiatric illness (Murthy, 2008, pp. 105-110). Unfortunately, women are not getting the help they need. Women with substance use disorders are less likely to enter treatment than their male counterparts, as they are more likely to face barriers that affect their access and entry to drug treatment (UNODC, 2015b). Researchers have identified a multitude of systemic, structural, social, cultural, and individual barriers that lead to women having less access to treatment (UNODC, 2015b). The primary structural barrier is childcare. Women typically serve as primary caretakers in the family, and without childcare, many women are unable to attend treatment. In addition, across societies and cultures, substance use in women is heavily stigmatized, and cultural bias may explicitly or implicitly deter women from seeking treatment. Over the last decade, researchers have demonstrated the effectiveness of comprehensive or enhanced treatment for women. These treatment models include components such as women-only treatment, childcare, prenatal care, all-female staff members, and a focus on post-traumatic stress disorder (PTSD), intimate partner violence (IPV), reproductive health, employment (including non-stigmatizing discussion of sex-related occupations), empowerment, and the intersection of cultural and gender issues (UNODC, 2004; Thomas & Pandian, 2015; Prendergast, Messina, Hall, & Warda, 2011).

Prevention

Prevention is an essential and cost-effective strategy in the global effort to address substance abuse. The international community has worked together for many years to build the knowledge base in substance abuse prevention. These efforts can also inform the implementation of Target 3.5. To reduce substance use and abuse among young people, the United Nations Office on Drugs and Crime (UNODC) and the WHO partnered from 1998-2003 to develop and implement the Global Initiative. The Initiative supported a number of local partners in communities in 8 countries (Belarus, South Africa, Philippines, the United Republic of Tanzania, Thailand, the Russian Federation, Vietnam, and Zambia) to mobilize communities and to develop and share substance abuse best practices. The overall evaluation demonstrated positive outcomes, including decreased substance use, increased age of onset of psychoactive substance use, attitudinal shifts regarding substance use, and lowered substance use amongst adults (who were not the target population for these interventions) (WHO, 2007). More recently, UNODC (2013, p. 31) developed the

International Standards on Drug Use Prevention. These standards summarize the scientific evidence on the effectiveness of drug use prevention efforts and set forth the following key recommendations:

- Support children and youth, particularly at critical developmental stages and/or transition periods at which they are most vulnerable (e.g., transition between childhood and adolescence or from middle to high school).
- Target the population at large (universal prevention), but also support groups (selective prevention) and individuals (indicated prevention) that are particularly at risk.
- Address both individual and environmental factors of vulnerability and resilience.
- Reach the population through multiple settings (e.g., families, schools, communities, the workplace, etc.).
- Employ and expand the systematic use of evidence-based tools.
- Engage the community via community participatory research in efforts to develop culturally grounded prevention programs.
- Support practitioners and policymakers in developing their knowledge, skills and competencies in effective prevention of drug use.

Policy

On a global level, drug control policies result in serious human rights abuses such as mass incarceration and violence. For example, in the United States, approximately half a million people are currently incarcerated for drug offenses (The Center for Prisoner Health and Human Rights, 2015, para. 3). The vast majority of these drug arrests were for possession. In addition, approximately half of prison and jail inmates in the United States meet the DSM-IV criteria for substance abuse or dependence, and significant percentages of state and federal prisoners committed the crime for which they are incarcerated while under the influence of drugs (The Center for Prisoner Health and Human Rights, 2015, para 2.). In Asia and other parts of the world, governments mandate the detention of people who use drugs to compulsory drug detention and rehabilitation centers where violence, forced labor, and other human rights violations are perpetuated in the name of "treatment" (United Nations, 2012, p. 1).

Due to its criminalization, the harms associated with drug use constrain individuals' and communities' ability to thrive. Continued criminalization and stiff penalties regarding drug use will have significant impacts on the achievement of many SDGs. The criminalization of drug possession and use disproportionately impacts poor and minority individuals and communities. It often leads to trans-generational cycles of arrests, under-employment, and exclusion from housing, educational opportunities, and political participation, which forces individuals deeper into poverty (UNODC, 2015a). Unfortunately, women within these communities are disproportionately impacted. Women in Europe, Asia, and Latin America are imprisoned at a disproportionately high rate for non-violent drug offenses. Today, women incarcerated for drug offenses represent the fastest growing prison population worldwide (Inter-American Commission on Women, 2014, p. 27). The over-incarceration of women for drug offenses has a ripple effect – children left without their primary caregivers develop increased risk for a multitude of negative outcomes, including substance abuse, that hinder progress related to the SDGs. The impoverishing impacts of non-violent, drug-related incarceration have damaged individuals, families, and communities across the globe. There is mounting evidence demonstrating that it is time to challenge policies that criminalize drug use and the lack of resources available to provide effective intervention (American Public Health Association, 2016).

"Leaving no one behind" is a core human rights value embedded within the SDGs. Via the SDGs, the international community has agreed to make a concerted effort to identify and help the most vulnerable – those who are often overlooked by their societies, including individuals, families, and communities struggling with substance abuse. By addressing substance abuse the global community is better-positioned to achieve the SDGs, and individuals and communities have greater potential to thrive.

Displacement, Migration, and Sustainable Well-being

Similar to substance abuse, the current global migration crisis affects people of all ages. For the growing number of migrants in the world today, upholding human rights and achieving sustainable well-being may appear to be out of reach.

According to the 2015 United Nations International Migration Report, the number of international migrants worldwide has increased rapidly in the last 15 years, from 173 million in 2000 to 244 million in 2014 (United Nations, 2016a, p. 1). Additionally, a much larger number of people migrate within national borders, often from rural to urban areas. The 2009 Human Development Report estimates that approximately 740 million people are internal migrants (United Nations, 2009, p. 1).

The United Nations' Sustainable Development Goals and Targets address migration through calls to: eliminate human trafficking (Goal 5), protect the labor rights of migrant workers (Goal 8), facilitate orderly, safe, regular, and responsible migration (Goal 10), and disaggregate data by migratory status (Goal 17) (United Nations, 2015).

The need to migrate is elicited by widely diverse circumstances. Some migrate due to a desire to live in a place with more work opportunities or better life conditions. Others move to escape dangerous environmental conditions, war zones, or areas of widespread and extreme poverty or violence. While the experience of adapting to a new place is challenging under any circumstance, it can be particularly distressing in already-traumatic, forced migration situations. It is estimated that 65.3 million people worldwide were forcibly displaced by the end of 2015 in an effort to escape persecution, conflict, generalized violence, or human rights violations (United Nations, 2016b, p. 5).

Understanding the impact of loss from migration is complicated by the fact that for some, much can be gained, but for others, much is lost. Some find safety, health, and resources when relocating from a dangerous or low-resource area to one that is safer or resource-rich. While the conditions and outcome of migration vary widely, many migrants do find the anticipated opportunities and safety that compelled them to migrate (United Nations, 2009). However, for others, particularly those who are forced to migrate due to violence, poverty, natural disasters, climate change, or human rights violations, the challenges may be more difficult to overcome. These migrants face many difficulties throughout the migration process that can impact their mental health. During the pre-departure phase, they might face the trauma of war and violence. During flight or travel, they are vulnerable to abuse, isolation, and discrimination. Upon resettlement, they may experience legal, economic, or social exclusion (International Organization for Migration, 2013).

Research has shown that these experiences can enhance or problematize the acculturation and integration process during resettlement, including the process of developing a sense of belonging or attachment to place and identity under new circumstances (Porter & Haslan, 2005). Often, responses to immediate basic needs for survival are readily identified and provided. However, social and psychological losses and injuries are often less apparent, more complex, and may have deep and long-term impacts. Trust, safety, identity, and a sense of belonging, for instance, can all be deeply affected by displacement. Migrants often lose established social connections within and cultural knowledge of the community they left behind. Furthermore, they often sacrifice familiarity and emotional bonds associated with meaningful possessions and surroundings (Brown & Perkins, 1992).

Migration, Mental Health, and Well-being

Studies have found a higher prevalence of mental distress among those who are forced to migrate (Lindencrona, Ekblad & Hauff, 2008), particularly in the form of PTSD, depression, and anxiety (Fazel, Wheeler & Danesh, 2005). Resettlement or post-migration stressors can trigger or aggravate these conditions (Lindencrona et al., 2008). For instance, refugees who resettle into permanent, private housing tend to have better mental health than those who resettle into temporary, institutional or temporary, private accommodations (Porter & Haslam, 2005).

Refugees are exposed to multiple stressors before, during, and after resettlement. These stressors include socioeconomic disadvantage, acculturation difficulties, marginalization, and the loss of social status, social networks, and cultural fluency (Porter & Haslam, 2005).

Learning the culture and language of the host country and developing social networks can be a slow process for many migrants, particularly for those who are older and have a longer history in their country of origin (Boğaç, 2009; Ruton & Breen, 2002; Virgincar, Doherty & Siriwardhana, 2016). Older refugees may also have experienced a greater number of traumatic events over a longer period of time, which could possibly affect their psychological well-being (Virgincar et al., 2016). "Place attachment" or a "sense of place" refers to emotional and social bonds built over time to particular locations and communities (Altman & Low, 1992). Because place attachment appears to increase with familiarity and time, older migrants might have a deeper sense of loss after migration (Burton & Breen, 2002). The sense of belonging and connection with places plays an important role in psychological well-being (Fullilove, 1996; Brown & Perkins, 1992). As a consequence, adult and older migrants might find it more difficult than younger ones to develop a sense of belonging in their new communities. Research has shown that in the process of displacement and resettlement, coping with loss and rebuilding social networks and emotional attachments is important in re-establishing psychological well-being (Brown & Perkins, 1992).

In some instances, bonds with physical and social environments can be strong enough to deter migration from adverse locations. In a study of a Peruvian community in a region affected by socioeconomic marginalization and a changing climate (which limited water availability), Adams (2016) explored the barriers to migration among those who expressed dissatisfaction with the conditions in this region. Both financial and socio-psychological or affective reasons may influence the capacity and decision to relocate away from dangerous or difficult living conditions or environmentally hazardous locations. While resource barriers and low mobility potential were identified in this study as deterrents to migration, a connection to place and satisfaction with the social life in their communities were found to play an important role in influencing the decision to stay among residents.

Similarly, in a study of residents of a flood-prone area in Santa Fé, Argentina, it was found that attachment to community and place was a deterrent for relocation. Residents who had been offered new housing in one of two resettlement projects expressed dissatisfaction with the location, particularly in terms of distance from family, resources, and the old neighborhood. Only those in the project that offered better quality housing resettled there permanently (Marti Rojas Rivas, 2010).

In cases of forced migration or relocation, the building of emotional and social bonds in the host communities can be deterred by the memories and connections to former places. In a study of Turkish Cypriots forcibly relocated from Southern to Northern Cyprus after conflict between Cyprus and Turkey, the resettled refugees reported not feeling fully socially integrated into their new communities and identified with the town they had left, Paphos, more than with the town they had lived in for 34 years after relocation (Boğaç, 2009).

The compounded impact of psychological stress faced during forced migration can affect physical and mental health and is often intensified by linguistic, cultural, legal, and economic barriers that may limit access to health services in host communities (International Organization for Migration, 2013). In addition to the stresses of socioeconomic inequality that can alter the health outcomes of disadvantaged populations (Friedli, 2009), displaced persons face additional stressors linked to the migration experience, including disruptions to place attachment and community ties and the loss of social and cultural capital (Brown & Perkins, 1992). At a time when migration within and across borders affects millions of people worldwide, understanding the role of place and community in the process of resettlement is essential when addressing the mental health needs of displaced persons.

Psychological well-being influences every aspect of daily life, enhances resiliency, and enables people to reach their full potential (Friedli, 2009). Safeguarding, maintaining, and promoting well-being is an important global aspiration, as reflected SDG 3. International human rights laws have long protected the right to the enjoyment of the highest attainable standard of physical and mental health, regardless of race, religion, political belief, economic or social condition, and immigration status. This right is delineated in Article 12(1)24 of the International Covenant on Economic, Social and Cultural Rights (CESCR; Friedli, 2009). Exploring ways to address the stressors that undermine psychological well-being during the migration experience helps to ensure that this right is upheld for migrants, and thereby benefits the global community. Understanding and exploring ways to address the stressors that undermine psychological well-being during the migration experience can help to ensure that all migrants have the opportunity to enjoy this right for the benefit and in the interest of the global community.

Conclusion

In our highly inter-connected, global society, a new vision for global health matters. At the U.N., a newly conceived agenda for the world community sets an ambitious series of goals to achieve by 2030. The aim of this agenda is to promote sustainable development that will enhance the lives of all persons and protect our environment. Addressing health is integral to the U.N.'s 2030 global agenda, and, for the first time in the history of this world body, mental health and well-being are defined as essential components of human health.

Here we have presented key issues in achieving progress on SDG 3 regarding health and well-being. Addressing poverty and inequality in the lives of children is foundational to the social protection required for enhancing health. Mental health challenges are apparent for youth as research suggests a link between the parallel rise of globalization and youth suicide. Substance abuse is a related growing health and mental health issue that compromises sustainability for men and women of all ages. As the community of nations grapples with responding to the global migration crisis, the transitions that migrants face introduce challenges to their adaptive capacities. If U.N. member states realize the targets associated with the 2030 agenda goals, vulnerable populations will not only survive, but will thrive in a new era of human well-being.

References

Altman, I. & Low, S. (Eds.). (1992). *Place attachment*. Boston, MA: Springer.

American Psychiatric Association. (1994). *Diagnostic and statistical manual of mental disorders* (4th ed.). Arlington, VA: American Psychiatric Publishing, Inc.

American Public Health Association. (2016). Defining and implementing a public health response to drug use and misuse. Retrieved from https://www.apha.org/policies-and-advocacy/public-health-policy-statements/policy-database/2014/07/08/08/04/defining-and-implementing-a-public-health-response-to-drug-use-and-misuse

Assembly, U. G. (1989). *Convention on the rights of the child: United Nations, treaty series*. New York: UN.

Berry J. W. (2005). Acculturative stress. In Wong, P.T.P and Wong, L.C.J (Eds.), *Handbook of multicultural perspectives on stress and coping*, New York, NY: Springer, pp. 287-298.

Berry, J. W., Phinney, J. S., Sam, D. L. and Vedder, P. (2006), Immigrant Youth: Acculturation, Identity, and Adaptation. *Applied Psychology, 55,* 303–332.

Boğaç, C. (2009) Place attachment in a foreign settlement, *Journal of Environmental Psychology* 29(2), 267–278.

Burns, J. (2016, August 31). UK girls becoming more miserable-study. *BBC News Education and Family*. Retrieved from http://www.bbc.com/news/education-37223063

Burton, A. & Breen, C. (2002). Older refugees in humanitarian emergencies. *The Lancet, 360,* 47–48.

Chisholm J.F. (2013). Cyberbullying among and against girls, female adolescents, and women: National and international trends. In F. Denmark & J. Sigal (Eds.), *Violence against girls and women: International perspectives,* Vol 1 (pp. 175-210). Women's Psychology Series, Santa Barbara, California: Praeger, an imprint of ABC-CLIO LLC

Curtin S.C., Warner M., Hedegaard H. (2016). Increase in suicide in the United States, 1999–2014. NCHS data brief, no 241. Hyattsville, MD: National Center for Health Statistics. Retrieved from https://www.cdc.gov/nchs/products/databriefs/db241.htm

EADI Working Group Social Protection (n.d.). Social protection and the sustainable development goals SDGs. Retrieved from http://eadi-nordic2017.org/2016/08/30/social-protection-and-the-sustainable-development-goals-sdgs-working-group-social-protection/

Fazel M., Wheeler J. & Danesh, J. (2005). Prevalence of serious mental disorder in 7000 refugees resettled in western countries: a systematic review. *Lancet, 365,* 1309–1314.

Friedli, L. (2009). Mental health, resilience and inequalities. Copenhagen, Denmark: WHO Regional Office for Europe. Retrieved from:
http://www.euro.who.int/__data/assets/pdf_file/0012/100821/E92227.pdf

Fullilove, M. T. (1996). Psychiatric implications of displacement: Contributions from the psychology of place. *American Journal of Psychiatry, 153*(12), 1516.

Inter-American Commission on Women. (2014). Women and drugs in the Americas: A policy working paper. Washington, DC: Inter-American Commission on Women. Retrieved from https://www.oas.org/en/cim/docs/WomenDrugsAmericas-EN.pdf

International Organization for Migration. (2013). International migration, health and human rights. Geneva, Switzerland: International Organization for Migration. Retrieved from: http://www.ohchr.org/Documents/Issues/Migration/WHO_IOM_UNOHCHRPublication.pdf

Johnson, P., Richter, L., Kleber, H., Mclellan, A., & Carise, D. (2005). Telescoping of drinking-related behaviors: Gender, racial/ethnic, and age comparisons. *Substance Use & Misuse,* 40*(8),* 1139–1151.

Lim, S. S., Vos, T., Flaxman, A. D., Danaei, G., Shibuya, K., Adair-Rohani, H., …, & Memish, Z. A. (2012). A comparative risk assessment of burden of disease and injury attributable to 67 risk factors and risk factor clusters in 21 regions, 1990-2010: A systematic analysis for the Global Burden of Disease Study 2010. *Lancet, 380,* 2224-2260.

Lindencrona, F., Ekblad, S. & Hauff, E. (2008) Mental health of recently resettled refugees from the Middle East in Sweden: the impact of pre-resettlement trauma, resettlement stress and capacity to handle stress. *Social Psychiatry and Psychiatric Epidemiology, 43*(2), 121-131.

Madison Holleran Suicide Prevention Act, N.J. S. 557 (N.J. Stat.2016). Retrieved from ftp://www.njleg.state.nj.us/20162017/S1000/557_I1.HTM

Marti Rojas Rivas, B. (2012). Is better housing an incentive for people to relocate from disaster prone areas? The case of post-flood outcomes from Santa Fé, Argentina, In G. Lizarralde, R. Jigyasu, R. Vasavada, S. Havelka & J. Duyne Barenstein (Eds.), *Participatory design and appropriate technology for disaster reconstruction. Conference proceedings. 2010 international i-Rec conference* (pp. 147-158). Ahmedabad, India. Montréal: Groupe de recherche IF, GRIF, Université de Montréal.

Perera, B. & Torabi, M. (2009). Motivations for alcohol use among men aged 16-30 years in Sri Lanka. *International Journal of Environmental Research and Public Health, 6,* 2408-2416.

Mels, C., Derluyn, I., Broekaert, E., & Rosseel, Y. (2010). The psychological impact of forced displacement and related risk factors on Eastern Congolese adolescents affected by war. *Journal of Child Psychology & Psychiatry, 51*(10), 1096-1104.

Murthy, P. (2008). Women and drug use in India: Substance, women, and high-risk assessment study. New Delhi, India: United Nations Office on Drugs and Crime Regional Office for South Asia. Retrieved from https://www.unodc.org/documents/southasia/reports/UNODC_Book_Women_and_Drug_Use_in_India_2008.pdf

MyWorld Data Analytics. (n.d.). Retrieved from http://data.myworld2015.org/

Ortiz I. & Cummins, M. (2011) .Global inequality: Beyond the bottom billion-a rapid review of income distribution in 141 countries. Retrieved from SSRN: https://ssrn.com/abstract=1805046 or http://dx.doi.org/10.2139/ssrn.1805046

Ortiz, I., Moreira Daniels, L., & Engilbertsdóttir, S. (2012). Child poverty and inequality: New perspectives. Retrieved from SSRN: https://ssrn.com/abstract=2039773 or http://dx.doi.org/10.2139/ssrn.2039773

Patel V., Ramasundarahettige, C., Vijayakumar, L., Thakur, J.S., Gajalakshmi, V., Gururaj, G., Suraweera, W. and Jha, P. (2012). Suicide mortality in India: A nationally representative survey. *The Lancet, 379*, 2343–2351.

Pollard, E. L. & Lee, P. D. (2003). Child well-being: a systematic review of the literature. *Social Indicators Research, 61*(1), 59-78.

Porter, M. & Haslam N. (2005). Predisplacement and postdisplacement factors associated with mental health of refugees and internally displaced persons: a meta-analysis. *The Journal of the American Medical Association, 294*, 602–612.

Prendergast, M. L., Messina, N. P., Hall, E. A., & Warda, U. S. (2011). The relative effectiveness of women-only and mixed-gender treatment for substance-abusing women. *Journal of Substance Abuse Treatment, 40*, 336-248.

Tavernise, S. (2016, April 22). U.S. suicide rate surges to a 30 year high. *New York Times*. Retrieved from http://www.nytimes.com/2016/04/22/health/us-suicide-rate-surges-to-a-30-year-high.html?_r=0

The Center for Prisoner Health and Human Rights. (2015). Incarceration, substance abuse, and addiction. Retrieved from http://www.prisonerhealth.org/educational-resources/factsheets-2/incarceration-substance-abuse-and-addiction/

The Children's Society, UK. (2016). The good childhood report 2016. Retrieved from www.childrenssociety.org.uk/what-we-do/research/the-good-childhood-report

Thomas, R. & Pandian, R. D. (2015). Need for women-specific psychosocial intervention for women with substance use disorders: The Indian scenario. *Kerala Journal of Psychiatry, 28*, 174-179.

UNICEF (2012, November). Social protection strategic framework. Retrieved from http://www.unicef.org/socialprotection/framework/index_61844.html.

UNICEF (2014, May). Fact sheet: A summary of the rights under the Convention on the Rights of the Child. Retrieved from http://www.unicef.org/crc/files/Rights_overview.pdf

UNICEF (2015, July). A post-2-15 agenda understood by and inspiring to children and young people: Final report of the e-consultation with children and youth on the SDGs draft declaration. Retrieved from: http://www.unicef.org/agenda2030/files/SDGDeclaration_ChildConsultationSummary.pdf.

United Nations. (1948). Universal declaration of human rights. New York, NY: UN Department of Public Information. Retrieved from www.un.org/en/documents/udhr

United Nations. (2012). Joint statement: Compulsory drug detention and rehabilitation centers. Vienna, Austria: United Nations. Retrieved from https://www.unodc.org/documents/southeastasiaandpacific/2012/03/drug-detention-centre/JC2310_Joint_Statement6March12FINAL_En.pdf

United Nations (2015). Resolution adopted by the general assembly on 25 September 2015, Transforming our world: The 2030 agenda for sustainable development. Retrieved from http://www.un.org/ga/search/view_doc.asp?symbol=A/RES/70/1&Lang=E

United Nations. (2015a). Mental health included in the UN sustainable development goals. Vienna, Austria: United Nations. Retrieved from http://www.who.int/mental_health/SDGs/en/

United Nations. (2015b). Transforming our world: The 2030 agenda for sustainable development. A/RES/70/1. Vienna, Austria: United Nations. Retrieved from https://sustainabledevelopment.un.org/post2015/transformingourworld

United Nations. (2014). Millennium development goals and post-2015 development agenda. Retrieved from: http://www.un.org/en/ecosoc/about/mdg.shtml.

United Nations, Department of Economic and Social Affairs, Population Division. (2015, December). Integrating migration into the 2030 Agenda for Sustainable Development. *Population Facts, No 2015/5*. Retrieved from: http://www.un.org/en/development/desa/population/migration/publications/popula tionfacts/docs/MigrationPopFacts20155.pdf

United Nations, Department of Economic and Social Affairs (DESA), Population Division (2016a). International migration report 2015: Highlights. New York, NY: United Nations. Retrieved from: http://www.un.org/en/development/desa/population/migration/publications/migrat ionreprt/docs/MigrationReport2015_Highlights.pdf

United Nations, United Nations Development Programme. (2009). Human development report 2009: Overcoming barriers: Human mobility and development. New York, NY: Palgrave Macmillan. Retrieved from: http://hdr.undp.org/sites/default/files/reports/269/hdr_2009_en_complete.pdf

United Nations, United Nations High Commissioner for Human Rights. (1966). The international covenant on economic, social and cultural rights. Retrieved from http://www.ohchr.org/EN/ProfessionalInterest/Pages/CESCR.aspx

United Nations, United Nations High Commissioner for Human Rights. (1979). The convention on the elimination of all forms of discrimination against women. Retrieved from http://www.ohchr.org/EN/ProfessionalInterest/Pages/CEDAW.aspx

United Nations, United Nations High Commissioner for Refugees (2016b). Global trends: Forced displacement in 2015. Retrieved from: http://www.unhcr.org/576408cd7.pdf.

United Nations, United Nations High Commissioner for Human Rights. (1979). The convention on the rights of the child. Retrieved from http://www.ohchr.org/EN/ProfessionalInterest/Pages/CRC.aspx

United Nations, United Nations High Commissioner for Human Rights. (2006). The convention on the rights of persons with disabilities. Retrieved from http://www.ohchr.org/EN/HRBodies/CRPD/Pages/ConventionRightsPersonsWith Disabilities.aspx

United Nations Office on Drugs and Crime. (2004). Substance abuse treatment and care for women: Case studies and lessons learned. Vienna, Austria: United Nations. Retrieved from https://www.unodc.org/pdf/report_2004-08-30_1.pdf

United Nations Office on Drugs and Crime. (2012). World drug report 2012. Retrieved from http://www.unodc.org/documents/data-and analysis/WDR2012/WDR_2012_web_small.pdf

United Nations Office on Drugs and Crime. (2013). International standards on drug use prevention. Vienna, Austria: United Nations. Retrieved from https://www.unodc.org/documents/prevention/UNODC_2013_2015_international_s tandards_on_drug_use_prevention_E.pdf

United Nations Office on Drugs and Crime. (2015a). Drug policy and the sustainable development goals: Why drug policy reform is essential to achieving the sustainable development goals. London, Britain: Health Poverty Action. Retrieved from https://www.unodc.org/documents/ungass2016/Contributions/Civil/Health_Poverty _Action/HPA_SDGs_drugs_policy_briefing_WEB.pdf

United Nations Office on Drugs and Crime. (2015b). World drug report 2015 (United Nations Publication, Sales No. E.15.XI.6). Vienna, Austria: United Nations. Retrieved from http://www.unodc.org/documents/wdr2015/World_Drug_Report_2015.pdf

United Nations Office on Drugs and Crime. (2016a). World drug report 2016 (United Nations Publication, Sales No. E.16.XI.7). Vienna, Austria: United Nations. Retrieved from https://www.unodc.org/doc/wdr2016/WORLD_DRUG_REPORT_2016_web.pdf

United Nations Office on Drugs and Crime. (2016b). UN Secretary General Ban Ki-Moon: Message on the international day against drug abuse and illicit trafficking. Retrieved from https://www.unodc.org/listenfirst/en/WDD/sg-statement.html

Verma S.K., Sachdeva, S. A., & Pandey, V. (2013). Suicide among Sikkim's Youth: An Exploration. *Shoryabhumi, 1*(1), 147.

Vijaykumar L. (2007). Suicide and its Prevention: The Urgent Need in India. *Indian Journal Psychiatry, 49*(2): 81–84.

Virgincar A., Doherty, S. & Siriwardhana C. (2016). The impact of forced migration on the mental health of the elderly: a scoping review. *International Psychogeriatrics, 28*(6), 889–896.

Virupaksha, H. G., Kumar, A., & Nirmala, B. P. (2014). Migration and mental health: An interface. *Journal of Natural Science, Biology & Medicine, 5*(2), 233-239.

Voipio, T. (2012). Social protection for all-An agenda for pro child growth and child rights. In Ortiz, I., Moreira Daniels, L., & Engilbertsdóttir, S. (Eds.), *Child poverty and inequality: New perspectives* (pp.118-124).

Wherley, S. & Chatterjee, S. (2015). India's growing problem of injecting drug misuse. *The British Medical Journal, 350,* h397. Retrieved from http://www.bmj.com/content/350/bmj.h397

World Health Organization. (2007). Outcome evaluation summary report: WHO/UNODC global initiative on primary prevention of substance abuse. Geneva, Switzerland: World Health Organization Press. Retrieved from http://www.who.int/substance_abuse/publications/global_initiative_summary_report.pdf

World Health Organization. (2010). Mental health and development: Targeting people with mental health conditions as a vulnerable group. Retrieved from http://www.who.int/mental_health/policy/mhtargeting/en/

World Health Organization. (2013). Mental health action plan 2013-2020. Retrieved from http://www.who.int/mental_health/action_plan_2013/en/

World Health Organization. (2014). Preventing suicide: A global imperative. Retrieved from http://www.who.int/mental_health/suicide-prevention/world_report_2014/en/

World Health Organization (2014b). Global status report on alcohol and health 2014. Retrieved from http://apps.who.int/iris/bitstream/10665/112736/1/9789240692763_eng.pdf

World Health Organization. (2016). World health statistics 2016: Monitoring health for the SDGs. Retrieved from http://www.who.int/gho/publications/world_health_statistics/2016/ en/

CHAPTER 24

Primary Care in Global Health: A Sustainable, Integrative Approach

Genomary Krigbaum, Gretchen Johnson, and Amma Boakye

Primary Care

In recent years, global health initiatives have increased in order to address the worldwide health gap in primary (medical/mental health) care and to account for environmental and bio-psycho-social factors. There is a vested interest in supporting host (native) countries healthcare systems' efficiency in providing primary healthcare services and sustaining the practices/provisions provided through the healthcare initiatives. 23% of global deaths (an estimated 12.6 million), as well as 26% of deaths among children under the age of five are a result of environmental factors and can be addressed by sustaining these health care initiatives (as cited in Prüss-Ustün, Wolf, Corvalán, Bos, & Neira, 2016, p. x). Furthermore, 60-80% of cases presenting to a primary care provider (PCP) have significant psychosocial components. Hence, it is important to adopt primary care practices as an integrative enterprise (Vannieuwenborg, Buntinx, & De Lepeleire, 2015, p. 3; Prüss-Ustün, Wolf, Corvalán, Bos, & Neira, 2016, p. x; White, Imperiale, & Perera, 2016).

The word "primary" can be defined as first occurrence, basic or essential, early stage or first in time, principal, and first-hand (Primary, 2016). In that sense, "primary care" is named such because the patient first presents to a primary health care provider (e.g., physician, psychologist, mental health clinician, etc.) who decides if the patient requires the secondary and tertiary care of specialists and sub-specialists. These definitions imply that a PCP is often the most-consulted member of the patient's health care team. The nature of primary care in health care is broad. Depending on the location and context, PCPs triage and manage chronic and acute illness across various ages, developmental stages, and socioeconomic status (SES). PCPs tend to see the most common health problems, and they manage chronic health conditions.

In the United States of America (U.S.), PCPs include physicians who are board-certified in family medicine, pediatrics, or internal medicine. There are instances in which a physician in a specialty like obstetrics and gynecology would serve as a PCP and focus on women's acute/chronic care and health maintenance needs. Globally, some psychologists, mental-health clinicians, community health workers (CHWs), and physicians can be considered PCPs because they are the first providers to whom patients present, they coordinate care, and they treat a broad set of problems in a diverse patient population. PCPs become the "gate keepers" responsible for facilitating available services for patients and connecting them with needed services, as is contextually possible (Andersen, Tørring, & Vedsted, 2014, p. 7; Kok et al., 2015; Primary Care -- AAFP Policies, 2016). In many instances, PCPs will care for a high number of underserved patients. Many global health concerns arise from a lack of access to well-trained PCPs who can address the physical and mental health concerns of a given population.

Thus, the World Health Organization's (WHO) global and national efforts to meet the health Millennium Development Goals (MDGs) have been refocused to address the quality and the level of integration (e.g., both physical and mental health, inter-professional health collaboration, Complementary and Alternative Medicine [CAM]) of the health care provided. The intent is to, among other things, manage illnesses more effectively and promote health. The WHO staff and partners are tasked with fostering the same level of health in low- and middle-income countries that is found in high-income countries. This has been categorized as a priority/sustainable development goal; it is critical that services are assessed for efficacy and efficiency due to the level of complexity in health services provided (Akachi, Tarp, Kelley, Addison, & Kruk, 2016). It is particularly important to purposely strengthen the provision of acute care, which could support the sustainability of a developing health system. In this context, acute care also includes mental health concerns (e.g., trauma care and crisis management), "emergency medicine, trauma care, pre-hospital emergency care, acute care surgery, critical care, urgent care and short-term inpatient stabilization" (Hirshon et al., 2013, p. 386). Therefore, a critical element of global health sustainability is not only to provide primary care and health preventive interventions in low- and middle-income countries, but also to encourage and foster contextual, efficacious, and efficient practices to benefit the patients and the work-life balance of providers. To this effect, Frenk and Moon (2013) noted the importance of taking into account both the dimensions of health (which include risk factors that are psycho-social [e.g., environmental, behavioral, or trauma-related] and illnesses) and the ways in which a given community addresses health concerns. Furthermore, Jamison et al. (2013) noted, "The returns on investing in health are impressive. Reductions in mortality account for about 11% of recent economic growth in low-income and middle-income countries as measured in their national income accounts," even though the specifics and the value of improved health are not targeted (p. 1898).

In order to support the strengthening of health care deliver in low- and middle-income countries, medical communities in the U.S. and other countries have partnered to address shortages in health care (e.g., through medical missions). At the same time, the U.S. faces its own health care deficit (Fields, Bigbee, & Bell, 2016). Over the past several years, the U.S. has been facing a growing health care shortage and has been trying to address it in various ways. Among the proposed solutions are new models of care, educational initiatives, patients reaching out to CAM providers, and patients implementing self-management skills. As the results of these efforts are monitored, insight can be gained as to what is effective and what is not. Certain insights gained via trial and error in the U.S. are applicable in other places around the world.

For instance, the deficit in the U.S. primary health care is due, in part, to the increasing needs of an aging population coupled with the aging and retirement of currently practicing physicians (Fields et al., 2015). There is also a contributory element of disparity between different geographic areas. A study completed in 2008 projected that population growth will result in a shortage of 44,000 adult care generalist (primary care) physicians by 2025 (King, Holloway, & Walker, 2013, p. 42). Another study approximates a shortage of 39,000 family physicians by 2020 (King, Holloway, & Walker, 2013, p. 42). Fields et al. (2015) notes that the most rural areas of the U.S. have the lowest health care provider-to-population ratio, which in many ways is similar to the situation in rural areas globally. There are 7,512 ZIP (Zone Improvement Plan) codes, representing a combined population of 5.8 million, with no PCPs (including dentists, physician assistants, nurse practitioners, and certified nurse midwives) (Fields et al., 2015, p. 235). Since much has been written about the need for primary health care worldwide, there is a tendency to assume that more physicians in a given area is always better than less. However, simply having a greater number of physicians in an area is not associated with higher levels of population health because many of those physicians may be specialists. Higher specialist physician-to-population ratios do not improve population health and, in some cases, there has been shown to be overtreatment and counterproductive effects when there is excess supply of specialists. In contrast, higher primary care physician-to-population ratios are associated with improved population health (Fields et al., 2015).

In many countries, there is a shortage of physicians (both PCPs and specialists) (Kok et al., 2015; Kruk et al., 2016; Yong Kim, Farmer, & Porter, 2013). The information given above suggests that the most positively impactful investment into the health of a given population is to promote the training of PCPs for that population. If a country is going to put communication efforts and resource spending on training higher numbers of physicians, it would greatly benefit from focusing on primary care fields rather than specialty fields. Once PCPs are trained, it is important to retain them within areas of need for as many years as possible because high turnover rates of PCPs threaten the sustainability of the system. For a system to be sustainable, it must maintain a certain degree of consistency, so it is essential to address PCPs needs of work-life balance, safety and security, suitable compensation, and so forth (Kok et al., 2015). PCPs may experience burnout from working in an area that has a low provider-to-population ratio and that lacks resources for the provision of their personal and professional needs. King et al. (2013) reported on the various models of primary care within rural areas of the U.S., and suggest that creating cooperative community between PCPs can increase the desire of physicians (and other PCPs) to stay in the area of need. The outcomes of studies performed in the rural areas of the U.S. can be applied in areas across the globe where the shared feature of low provider-to-population ratios is present.

The Medical Home Model

An example in the U.S. of an underserved, low- and middle-income area with a low provider-to-population ratio of primary health care service is West Virginia. This is one rural area of the U.S. in which a family physician would often provide a broad spectrum of care without the support of other nearby health care providers (e.g., advance practice nurses, physician-specialists, physician assistants, psychologists, and mental health clinicians). This situation is reminiscent of the plight of many doctors worldwide who find themselves without the support of their colleagues while facing daunting medical needs. As PCPs find themselves over-worked and under-supported, they become disenchanted with working in their geographic area. This creates challenges for PCPs, patients, and communities. There is a high rate of physician turnover in such cases, which makes health care less sustainable in that geographic area. In an effort to address high turnover rates, new models of providing primary care are being introduced to West Virginia and other similar areas. Some of these models offer promising solutions to the challenges of solo, unsupported practices in a geographic area with a low provider-to-population ratio (King et al., 2013). A promising model is the rural interdisciplinary *medical home model* noted in King et al. (2013). In this model, several basic services are provided in the same building. In addition to a PCP, patients have access to a part-time or full-time pharmacy, as well as mental, dental, and public health services, including social work. Under the medical home model, health care workers gain a sense of community, and they each make the work of the others more effective. This approach to primary health care and related models has yielded positive results as well as sustainable integrative practices; in fact, the WHO staff advocates similar approaches (e.g., the integrated mental health care plan [MHCP]). A core emphasis to the integrated approach is holistic, patient-centered care and preventive interventions, as emphasized in the Osteopathic premise of care (Grace, Orrock, Vaughan, Blaich, & Coutts, 2016; Shidhaye et al., 2016; Sweetland, et al., 2014; White, Jain, & Giurgi-Oncu, 2014).

Thus, the medical home model (and similar approaches) could be adapted to the needs of any underserved community worldwide in a way that respects the community's values, culture, and approaches to responding to health concerns (Frenk & Moon, 2013). Some geographic areas might be best served by a combination of physicians, agricultural education providers, nutritionists, midwives, spiritual health providers, local herbs experts, mental health providers, CHWs, and nurses in charge of handling minor injuries. There are virtually endless combinations of health care workers that can be placed in the same physical location in order to best serve the needs of that particular community. The benefits to the patient are many, including eliminating the need to travel to multiple locations in order to access different facets of health care, and the provision of resources to address nutritional needs through sustainable agricultural practices, which can assist in preventive health care (Grace et al., 2016; King et al., 2013; Shidhaye et al., 2016; Sweetland et al., 2014). Furthermore, Aboud and Yousafzai (2015) reported that nutritional education plus psycho-education are integral for maximizing parental health behavior, which mediates the positive results on reaching developmental milestones (including language and cognitive abilities).

Imagine that a 35-year-old male patient presents to a community PCP with physical complaints of thiamine deficiency secondary to chronic alcoholism. His physical complaints stem from a lack of nutritional education, a lack of a solid support network, and a lack of mental health care. In solo practice, the physician would be forced to try to address the patient's lack of nutritional education and mental health care by handling it all alone or by sending the patient to a different location to see another provider (which the patient may or may not actually do). Contrast this situation with the medical home model, in which the physician would simply send such a patient down the hallway to the appropriate providers (in this case a nutritionist and a mental health provider) who could address the root of the problem and prevent the physical symptoms from returning. By delegating treatment of this particular patient to other providers, the physician is able to see the next patient of the day without delay. The work of the physician, nutritionist, and mental health provider is now integrated. All those involved in this process gain a sense of community support, which increases both the quality of care for the patient and job satisfaction of the providers; thus, they become more likely to continue serving in their current location, which increases system sustainability (Akachi et al., 2016; Collins, Insel, Chockalingam, Daar, & Maddox, 2013; Patel et al., 2013; Sweetland et al., 2014).

Although the medical home model could work well in many situations, it does not include a plan for a physician to partner with a local hospital (King et al., 2013). Naturally, a single model cannot be expected to be the best for every situation. In some communities around the world, a hospital may be the sole source of health care, and therefore the first place a patient would go if they had a medical need, major or minor. In that situation, there is no option to go to a PCP for a more minor condition that does not require hospitalization. When the hospital is the only place in the community that a PCP can be found, it may be under overwhelming strain of a large patient load. If PCPs can be established in clinics (such as those under a medical home model) separate from the hospital, they could reduce the burden on the hospital by treating minor illnesses in the clinics and triaging patients who are in need of hospitalization. If some of their patients became hospitalized, the PCP would need to travel to the hospital to see them on a daily basis while maintaining the patient load at the clinic. This would require the physician to travel long distances every day, and such a schedule could easily cause burnout (King et al., 2013). One noteworthy approach to address this kind of situation is the *spoke and wheel model*, which has also been put into practice in rural U.S.

The Spoke and Wheel Model

In the spoke and wheel model, there is a central hospital with associated branches of family practice physicians (which could be PCPs), each serving their own small community (King et al., 2013). Typically, family practice physicians in small community settings would be working solo and would have to be constantly on call for their set of patients in addition to traveling to and from the hospital to round. However, this model counters that demanding schedule by connecting all the physicians in a cooperative network and adding at least one mobile physician. For example, if there were four small communities serviced by the same hospital, there would be a fifth mobile physician. Every five weeks, the mobile physician would work every day at the hospital. Over the next four weeks, he or she would spend a week at each of the four family practice sites so that the family practice physician at that site could work at the hospital for that week. This ensures that no physician has to travel to both the office and the hospital in one day. It provides a sense of community and a professional support system for the physicians who would otherwise be working alone as the only PCP in their community (King et al., 2013). The spoke and wheel model could theoretically be applied in any location, provided that a hospital is present. With the hospital supported by the PCPs and the PCPs supported by a mobile physician, patients receive better quality of care that is tailored to their needs. Additionally, a mobile provider reduces the burden carried by each of these PCPs. The sickest patients would go to the hospital, the minor illnesses would be treated on an outpatient basis by the PCPs, and the mobile physician would ensure that neither the sickest patients nor those with minor illnesses remain without care.

The Medical Group Visit Model

A creative solution to address time-constraints in patient contact hours is the *medical group visit model* (Crespo & Shrewsberry, 2007). In this model, several patients have their annual health visit at the same time in a group meeting space, allowing the physician to focus on medical concerns while other staff members work on lab results, self-management plans, etc.; therefore the time that would usually be spent waiting in an exam room is well-used (Crespo & Shrewsberry, 2007). This can be adapted to underserved areas and war zones (including refugee camps). Consequently, interdependent health systems are needed in order to address the emergent and evolving health care needs of underserved communities (Frenk, & Moon, 2013; King et al., 2013).

The models discussed above are promising ways to retain PCPs in areas of greatest need. However, if population growth exceeds the number of PCPs entering the workforce, the primary care deficit will continue to grow not only in the U.S., but worldwide. Much has been written about a declining interest in primary care and family medicine amongst medical students. Family practice is the cornerstone specialty of primary care. A family practice physician can provide a broad spectrum of services including patient education, preventive and health promotion, health maintenance, counseling, diagnosis, and treatment of acute and chronic illnesses (Primary Care -- AAFP Policies, 2016). To effectively address the primary care shortage, it is important to identify factors that influence medical students' choice of specialty so that they can increase student interest in primary care practice,

Gill, Mcleod, Duerksen, and Szafran (2012), reported that certain factors were identified as being significantly associated with medical students choosing family practice. Those who chose family practice expressed an emphasis on continuity of care, their preference for working in a rural location, and their desire for shorter length of residency. They also expressed that their choice had been influenced by family, friends, or community (Gill et al., 2012). In contrast, medical students who chose a specialty other than family medicine were influenced by a variety of identified factors including a desire for a higher average income and a preference for working in an urban location. They were also influenced by a perception of higher prestige and higher intellectual content within specialties other than family practice (Kirchhoff, Hart, & Campbell, 2014). Also present was a desire to do research and a desire to master a small set of procedural skills (Gill et al., 2012). Thus, medical students are less inclined to choose family practice if they believe the myths that family physicians have lower intellect and lack procedural skills or opportunities to work on challenging cases (Gill et al., 2012).

Nonetheless, Gill et al. (2012) indicated that across the medical student population, interest in family medicine rose as students started having clinical experiences in their third and fourth year, perhaps due to students completing their family medicine rotation in the third year. It has been suggested that working with medical educators and physician mentors who practice family medicine is critical to dispelling the myths that drive students towards choosing other specialties. Increasing the number of family medicine-related clinical experiences in the first and second years of medical school could increase student interest in the specialty. The same could apply to other health disciplines that could potentially lead to primary care. An increase in clinical experiences would mean an increase in the number of family physicians educating and mentoring medical students. Even though it may hard for a busy physician in an underserved area to find time to mentor and educate medical students, it is an important facet of health care sustainability. By mentoring the medical students, the PCP can inspire the students to work in similar, underserved areas.

Since rural areas are most significantly underserved, and because growing up in a rural area is an identified factor that motivates health care students to choose primary care practice, it makes sense to increase health students' recruitment from rural areas (Gill et al., 2012). In addition, it is important to take into account that training for primary care practice should involve cultural and contextual understanding of values, practices, and environmental factors (Korhrt et al., 2015; Kruk et al., 2016; Patel et al., 2013; Shidhaye et al., 2016). Therefore, recruiting health care students from underserved areas could increase sustainability of primary health care practice in those areas, as continuity of care is increased when PCPs remain in the same place long-term. In order to maximize the success of the recruitment process, the truths about the nobility of primary care practice should be shared. For example, family physicians in rural settings are dispelling myths about their specialty by rising to meet the daily challenges that come with their job. Rural family physicians tend to maintain a particularly broad scope of practice compared to their urban colleagues (Peterson, Blackburn, Peabody, & O'Neill, 2015). This difference may be due to the rural geographic situation of having fewer sub-specialists, emergency medicine physicians, and internal medicine hospitalists. In a rural area, a family physician might provide emergency services, inpatient care, obstetrics and gynecological care, counseling and mental health care (including crisis management and trauma-related interventions), dermatological care, pediatric care, and palliative care that would be provided by seven or more sub-specialists in an urban setting (Peterson et al., 2015). Maintaining a broader scope of practice led rural family physicians to be more likely than their urban colleagues to be multifaceted in their skills and maintain them throughout their practice time. In doing so, these PCPs (like osteopathic physicians, allopathic physicians may choose to be further trained in this perspective) approach patient care holistically and in a patient-centered way (Grace et al., 2016; Licciardone, 2015). It is not surprising, then, that in the U.S., rural primary care physicians have higher passing rates for boards than their urban counterparts (Peterson et al., 2015, p. 265).

After studying approximately 3,602 physicians, Holmboe et al. (2008) confirmed that a broader scope of practice (that includes CAM and non-pharmacological interventions) was associated with higher exam scores and greater continuity of care (p. 1397). For instance, in the U.S., PCPs trained from an osteopathic framework also practice non-pharmacological interventions and may manage some conditions, like lower back pain. In a national study of primary health care, osteopathic physicians were more likely to maintain greater continuity of care by treating patients with Osteopathic Manipulative Treatment (OMT) where somatic dysfunction was diagnosed, and they were less likely to prescribe medication to manage the condition (Licciardone, 2015). This suggests that this distinctly osteopathic approach to treating low back pain in primary care settings could be an important aspect of medical education for family physicians and PCPs (Licciardone, 2015). So, while medical education is important for a country in order to address its primary health care shortage, patient education and provision of resources is equally essential. However, educating more PCPs is only part of the solution. Patients are also key members of the health care team, and collaborating with them is vital in health delivery, improvement, maintenance, holistic care, and patient outcomes.

Integrative Care

Since healthy behaviors and health improvement are key in well-being maintenance, supporting an integrative approach in patient care aligns with the WHO's MDG stance that "there can be no health without mental health" (as cited in Coventry et al., 2015, p. 2). The use of integrative primary care, which could include PCPs, CHWs, CAM providers, psychologists, psychiatrists, etc., could further close the treatment gap in low- and middle-income countries (Akachi et al., 2016; Coventry et al., 2015; Mohan, Seedat, & Pradeepa, 2013). This is important because mental health, behavioral concerns, and neurological disorders account for 10% of the global disease burden, and this statistic is projected to increase to 15% in the next five years (as cited in Prüss-Ustün et al., 2016, p. 51). The disease burden is often the result of diverse bio-psycho-social factors, including environmental, social, and behavioral risk factors; thus, a holistic approach to primary health care is essential (Gureje et al., 2015). Patients are interested in being healthy and in holistic care, which includes mental health. For instance, in Africa, patients understand health as physical, mental, and spiritual. They also see health as including the stability of the self, the family, and the community (Gureje et al., 2015). This implies that patient self-management results in best outcomes when patients engage in behaviors that help them manage their health concerns and prevent complications (Crespo & Shrewsberry, 2007; Gureje et al., 2015); thus, it is important to include primary care mental health professionals trained at a master's degree level (e.g., psychologists, behavioral health consultants) and CAM providers (World Health Organization, 2010a, b, c, d).

The rate of CAM usage ranges from 10-76%, depending on the population. In countries subscribing to Western cultural norms, CAM prevalence is 20-50%, with the U.S. and Australia on the high end of the spectrum (Gureje et al., 2015, p. 3). Gureje et al. (2015) also noted that The African Union proclaimed 2001–2010 as the "Decade of Traditional Medicine." Most patients reported improved health when using CAM modalities, and also indicated that most CAM providers would take a deposit as initial payment, but the rest of the payment would be contingent on patient improvement (Gureje et al., 2015). Furthermore, in some health systems (such as in India and China), the importance of holistic care and collaboration with the patient is acknowledged. Thus, CAM (such as Ayurveda and Traditional Chinese Medicine [TCM]) modalities have been integrated into mainstream health care systems. These modalities are considered cost-effective because, as it is possible, all variables that could be contributing to a given disease process are addressed holistically, and disease maintenance is prevented (Patel et al., 2013; Shidhaye et al., 2016). Gureje et al. (2015) noted that in Africa and similar cultures, health is thought of holistically, and thus integrative primary care, including CAM, is emphasized. In addition to the integration of CAM modalities, it is critical that health care staff is trained and mentored as services are provided (World Health Organization, 2010abcd); for instance, if the PCPs and health care staff practice self-management, they would be supportive of their patients' self-management and resiliency process. Furthermore, if they were sensitive to the value of integrative care, they would be able to partner more effectively with their patients in health seeking behaviors and health improvement (Kok et al., 2015).

CAM providers are an important source of primary care; however, they are not necessarily accounted for in the statistics quoted about the growing primary care shortage (Leach, 2013). CAM providers include TCM acupuncturists, Tuina massage therapists, naturopaths, hypnotherapists, massage therapists, TMC/Ayurveda herbalists, and more (Leach, 2013). These distinct practices are embraced by many worldwide, especially when facing chronic conditions not treated adequately under conventional medicine (Gureje at al., 2015). For instance, Leach (2013, p. 364) indicated that 62% of the U.S. population reports using CAM at least once over a twelve-month period. In 2007, U.S. adults made 253.2 million visits to CAM providers, and the trend has increased over the years. The out-of-pocket cost for these visits was estimated to be $11.9 billion (Leach, 2013, p. 365). Recent reports indicate that there has been an increase in CAM use associated with patients aspiring to actively participate in their health care, cultivation of holistic practices, greater disease chronicity and severity management, and increases in health-awareness behavior (Leach, 2013). In the U.S., a great number of patients are using CAM as a source of primary care, in addition to (or in place of) allopathic and osteopathic physicians. The most prevalent CAM occupation is massage therapy, and the CAM occupation in shortest supply is naturopathy (Leach, 2013). Due to the importance and demand for CAM providers, encouraging further CAM training and engagement in CAM practices could prove to be efficacious.

In war-stricken zones, a health care staff member might come across a patient with high blood pressure (HBP); however, the war-related psychosocial trauma could exacerbate the HBP. Hence, the staff membercould discuss self-management and native evidence-informed CAM treatments with the patient while taking his/her vitals at the start of the physical examination. Although it may be difficult to address nutritional management with available resources, the patient could be instructed to monitor salt intake and to be as active as possible, thus implementing lifestyle modifications (Mohan et al., 2013; Rotheram-Borus, Swendeman, & Chorpita, 2012). In conjunction with medical treatment, the patient could engage in biofeedback (psychological) self-management techniques including diaphragmatic breathing, Cognitive Behavioral Therapy (CBT), Motivational Interviewing (MI) to target behavior modification, and prayer (which could be a value practice endorsed by the patient). Witten, Jansen Van Vuuren, and Learmonth (2013) found that CBT paired with MI was effective in fostering behavior change and treatment adherence when working with a peri-urban population in South Africa. Since Zambia's cultural context is similar in many ways to South Africa, this approach may account for Zambia's cultural nuances (White et al., 2016).

Perhaps a patient with generalized anxiety disorder self-manages by practicing mindfulness and nourishing relationships that give him/her a sense of support or by engaging in CAM-Traditional Chinese Medicine via acupuncture treatments, which could help in reducing tension. A patient with diabetes might limit his/her sugar intake and monitor his/her blood sugar regularly or he/she might engage in CAM-Ayurveda by consuming evidence-based herbs known to maintain adequate blood sugar levels. A patient with gout might eat less red meat and drink less alcohol.

Additionally, PCPs could use several tangible tools to successfully promote self-management, customize care, and practice principles of personalized medicine (Crespo & Shrewsberry, 2007; Patel et al., 2013). Crespo and Shrewsberry (2007) noted that they could keep pads that resemble prescription pads, dedicated to prescribing behaviors. The health care staff could use social marketing pamphlets called "Choose to Move," "Balance Your Plate," and "Kick the Habit." They could also utilize pamphlets with drawings to help patients with low literacy skills. Patients without access to a gym or park could find the home exercises in the "Choose to Move" pamphlet helpful. These pamphlets were more effective when the health care staff handed them directly to patients (as opposed to having them available in a stack in the waiting area) (Crespo & Shrewsberry, 2007). Rotheram-Borus et al. (2012) reported that lifestyle influences physical and mental health morbidity and mortality. Coventry et al. (2015) noted that patients who participated in integrative care reported decreased symptoms of depression and anxiety (1.45 points pre-post) and increased lifestyle modifications and self-management (p. 6). Therefore, if patients engage in self-management behaviors, they could avoid numerous acute exacerbations of chronic conditions and could delay or prevent the development of certain prolonged conditions. Family, friends, and other sources of care for a patient can help the patient succeed in self-management efforts. Empowering patients and their families with this kind of psycho-education allows them to prevent exacerbations of health problems and decreases their need to travel to access health care. Thus, having an array of integrative interventions available helps patients to embrace therapies that could yield positive outcomes (White et al., 2014). White et al. (2014) noted that integrative interventions that include CAM account for the higher rate of recovery from serious mental illnesses and/or mental health difficulties in low- and middle-income countries vs. high-income countries (Sweetland et al., 2014).

Patient self-management and the direct involvement of mental/behavioral health professionals in primary care and staff training can increase PCPs' effectiveness and efficiency in the delivery of services. This also promotes preventive strategies, which translate into improved health and a cost-effective system (Crespo & Shrewsberry, 2007). Therefore, it is necessary to implement integrated, sustainable primary care practices that respect values, culture, and country-specific CAM practices. Integrative care is collaborative and cultural in nature. Collaboration between different providers is needed, and cultural context plays a role on how health is addressed in those communities (Frenk & Moon, 2013; MacLachlan, 2014). Integrative, collaborative care should be sensitive to bio-psycho-social concerns of the patient and should strike a meticulous balance between institutional practices and high-quality services (Andersen et al., 2014). Gureje et al. (2015) indicated that successful integrative primary care practices have been introduced in Puerto Rico, Ecuador, Brazil, Kenya, and in the Maori tribes of New Zealand.

Other interventions that were reported as being efficacious, efficient, and respectful of institutional/country guidelines include psychotherapy frameworks (e.g., CBT, MI, etc.), self-care practices, self-monitoring, patients' religion/spirituality, and pharmacological treatment (Patel et al., 2013; Prüss-Ustün et al., 2016; Sweetland et al., 2014; White et al., 2014; White et al., 2016). In countries where the environmental factor of pesticide toxicity is prevalent, such as Sri Lanka, a helpful intervention has been psycho-education regarding the negative effects of pesticides (e.g., induced deaths, depression, anxiety) and the proposal of the removal of those pesticides (as cited in Prüss-Ustün et al., 2016). In order to implement and sustain integrative primary care practices, different levels of intervention need to be taken into account, including: primordial prevention (noticing/decreasing risk factors), primary prevention (preventive practices/life-style modifications), secondary prevention (prevention of complications), and tertiary prevention (limiting the effects/progression of physical/mental disability) (Mohan et al., 2013). Likewise, practicing from a contextually-informed perspective offers greater opportunities for sustainable, optimal management and health promotion practices (Collins et al., 2013). Therefore, in order to facilitate the success of previously presented models and integrative practices, it is important to foster sustainability and to respect the culture, values, and health approaches of the health system of a given community.

Sustainable, Integrated Primary Care

As has been noted, PCPs are often the first contact point in the intervention of disease or health concerns, and they enjoy a unique social standing in many communities. They are often seen as integral parts of family life and the community, which allows them to witness patient experience first-hand and to address a wide range of health concerns. To integrate all of these components effectively is to manage health optimally. One way to support these endeavors is through medical missions.

While the word "mission" has historically held a religious context, medical missions as we refer to them are not necessarily faith-based. Rather, they describe organized, purposeful ventures to accomplish a goal (Lasker, 2015). Initially, international development was relegated to the realm of governments, non-governmental organizations, and the private-sector. However, as technology created opportunities for the everyday person to be informed, more people, including academic institutions and faith-based organizations, have become involved in international development, particularly with regards to global health (and even tele-health when the opportunity arises). It has been said that the number of domestic and international volunteers contributing through volunteer organizations in thirty-six countries would compromise the world's ninth largest country in terms of population. That estimate was calculated between 1995 and 2000, and the numbers have drastically increased in following years (Lasker, 2015, p. 1). Therefore, it is increasingly important to evaluate the effectiveness and sustainability of these medical missions, as well as the best way to execute them.

One thing to consider is the structure of the mission, particularly its duration, which is commonly critiqued. Two terms used to describe the duration of medical missions are "short-term" and "long-term." While there is no universally accepted timeframe for short-term missions, long-term missions are generally considered to be at least 6 months long. The majority of medical missions are short-term, and the vast majority of those last two weeks or less (Lasker, 2015). Since ideally, medical missions provide sustainable, effectively-integrated medical care while fostering long-lasting relationships between the host country and the medical mission team, short-term medical missions draw a lot of scrutiny. Short-term medical missions are typically best for addressing immediate, short-term health problems with simple fixes. While there are some advantages to this approach, it can lead to symptoms-based treatment, rather than holistic treatment of the source of the problem. This practice has been described as "slapping a Band-Aid on a gaping wound" (Martiniuk, Manouchehrian, Negin, & Zwi, 2012, p. 4). Furthermore, poorly designed, short-term medical missions teams can cause the host country to be dependent on their services and thereby hinder growth of both infrastructure and the economy.

After all, why would local businesses invest in a service that is provided for free by another entity? For example, a large number of well-intentioned volunteers travelled to help displaced Haitians after the 2010 earthquake. While the volunteers were able to provide much-needed supplies, assistance, and medical care in the short-term, these efforts (which were not always well-planned for the long-term) paralleled both local efforts and the efforts of non-governmental organizations (NGOs). This created a redundancy in aid; problems were not addressed in a focused, effective way (Loh et al., 2015).

Of course, long-term medical missions can fall prey to similar problems. If, prior to the mission, the team is inadequately educated regarding local norms, medical practices, and expectations, ineffective communication between the host country and medical mission team is more likely. This could hinder the development of sustainable medical care in the host country, regardless of how long the medical mission team works there. The situation could be further exacerbated by inadequate education of the host country's citizens, inadequate knowledge of the host country's health care providers, or an overabundance of medical missions teams (Loh et al., 2015). Additionally, long-term progress is often slow and requires a great investment of time, volunteers, and money. Because of this, typically only a few problems can be addressed at once.

Logistics of delivering care to patients serves as another point of comparison between long- and short-term medical missions. There are a variety of medical procedures performed during the trips. These procedures differ in complexity and difficulty and require different types of follow-up care. Pediatrician Nguah (2014) describes how access to initial treatment and follow-up care varies from patient to patient at the Komfo Anokye Teaching Hospital (KATH) in Kumasi, Ghana. Patient care can hinge on many factors which determine whether treatment will harm a patient more than it will benefit him/her. These include financial means, availability of transportation to the site of care, and ability of the patient's family to assist in care. Of particular interest is transportation to the site of care. This seemingly simple issue is a common barrier to treatment, as patients often travel from areas that are not central to the site of care. For instance, Nguah (2014) treated patients that had travelled over 200 miles to receive care. He describes a situation in which a patient developed potentially life-threatening complications after a surgery, but was too far away to return to the hospital. Fortunately, the issue was resolved with long distance communication (tele-health), but Nguah wondered: "What happens to the other children who might also have complications like these, but whose parents cannot afford to come back to the clinic for financial reasons for because they live so far away?" (Nguah, 2014, p. 316)

Provided that there is good communication between the host country's health care team and the medical missions' team, it is possible to set up a good framework for providing patients with easy access to initial and follow-up care. This is a feat that is executed more effectively with long-term missions, which can be helpful in avoiding the complications that Nguah (2014) described.

This task looks different in short-term medical missions. There is a shorter time frame in which the medical mission team can perform a procedure and provide follow-up care. Because of this, access to initial or follow-up care can determine who receives care and who doesn't. Some patients may be automatically disqualified due to the complexity of their case or ability to receive follow-up care. The situation becomes even more tenuous when determining the parameters that would deem a potential patient eligible for care. Nguah (2014) stated this ethical dilemma during his experience at KATH, where the order in which patients were to be screened for eligibility was determined by the distance they had traveled. The patients that had traveled the farthest got screened first, creating an ethical dilemma in which he could not guarantee that the first patient seen was the one who would benefit most from the surgery. Nonetheless, it is imperative to provide the necessary services and to put all effort into attending to the patients' needs with available resources while supporting the host team.

The Impact of Using Foreign (not Local) Resources

The use of foreign resources, while convenient, can alter a host country's economy and thus alter the manner in which health care is delivered long after the visiting providers have left. In this way, the health of the host country's economy is tied to how effectively a medical mission is executed. Ideally, medical missions are geared towards sustainability in that they generate a program of which the host country can take ownership and that involves and bolsters the local community (Berry, 2014; Lasker, 2015; Loh et al., 2015; Phillips & Watson, 2011).

During medical missions, it is often attractive to use foreign physicians and other health care personnel, as their care is presumably high-quality (Rockwell et al., 2015). However, using foreign health care personnel could undermine the transition from the short-term health care system to a self-sufficient, sustainable model. The same risk is present for long-term medical missions that do not involve local health care personnel. Additionally, it is possible that volunteers select sites based on their preference or expense, rather than the need of each site (Rockwell et al., 2015).

Regardless of site preference, health care volunteers must be educated on the customs and cultural nuances of the host country. Additionally, they must be familiar with the host country's health care practices, the hierarchy of the healthcare system, and the people involved in the mission. Many mission volunteers believe that some care is better than no care. This belief, combined with the idea that medical goals can only be set by the visiting country's perception of the host country's needs, can be detrimental to meeting the true needs of the host country and to the formation of a healthy partnership between the visiting country and the host country. This is especially applicable to medical/health care students who typically do not have expertise in managing projects of this nature. They are often unaware of underlying political or social issues that nuance the execution of an effective mission (O'Donnell, McAuliffe, & O'Donovan, 2014). Without pre-departure training, well-meaning visiting medical teams can hinder the mission's efforts, pose a risk to patients, and obstruct potential partnerships. In other words, a misunderstanding of local medical practices, a paucity of local health personnel or resources, or the perception that medical polices in host countries are lax can tempt students to take uncalled action by acting outside of their scope of practice.

Furthermore, while it may be cost-effective for a team to bring all necessary resources with them, this risks the creation of an artificial, temporary environment. Such an environment is not sustainable because the visiting team eventually leaves. If the visiting team provides equipment that is not routinely used in the host country, the host team should be shown how to operate the equipment. It should be easy to use and easy to maintain (Rockwell et al., 2015). This is a part of fostering sustainable practices.

Sustainable Practices

In order to encourage sustainable, integrative practices, Loh et al. (2015) suggested the recruitment of local health care staff. This practice mitigates logistical, linguistic, and cultural barriers and therefore facilitates partnership formation. Local medical personnel are already well aware of the medical needs of the community. This knowledge is a valuable tool for visiting teams, especially since interventions and programming should be tailored to the needs of the host community, not the visitors' perceptions of its needs (Berry, 2014; Loh et al., 2015). The efforts of any mission should be supported by local resources and should be suitable for the duration of the trip.

To be sustainable means to be maintainable at a certain level or rate (Sustainable, 2016). While this is certainly foundational to sustainability in the context of a medical mission, there are several factors unique to health care delivery that contribute to the definition of sustainability in global health care. Ethical considerations and proper education of the medical mission team and local health care personnel are both key elements of generating sustainable health care.

In order to sustain the provision of adequate health care, the host country should have capable, trained personnel. When possible, host country health care educators or tele-health should be utilized. When there are not enough personnel with university degrees, capable, skilled, lay individuals should be trained as CHWs (Coventry et al., 2015; Kohrt et al., 2015; Kok et al., 2015). Optimally, medical missions' goals should include training a host country health care team based on their training needs. For example, U.S. volunteers to the Dominican Republic from the Operation Walk Boston mission noted the learning preferences and practice styles of the Dominican staff. They also noted that the hierarchal structure of the local organization may impede changes that they were trying to implement. One U.S. physical therapist on the mission stated, "For me, it's respecting somebody else's culture and their beliefs and their way of doing things" (Bido, et al., 2015, p. 947). In another example, during a mission at the KATH in Kumasi-Ghana, faculty from the University of Utah partnered with faculty from the KATH to teach residents from both countries together. This was done via virtual education and with adequate translation to ensure proper understanding of the concepts. Both of these examples show dedication to forging partnerships and respect of one another's learning processes and modes of operation in providing quality care for patients (McGinnis, 2016).

It is also essential to evaluate the needs and goals of the host country. This evaluation should not be overly influenced by the visiting country's perceptions (Loh et al., 2015). Expectations must be set for all involved parties, and an appropriate amount of flexibility should be allowed during the mission to address any unforeseen developments. The same is true in the evaluation of the effectiveness of the medical mission. Evaluations are often structurally biased. In other words, the very questions that comprise the content of the evaluation are created by the providers, and therefore patient feedback is limited to what the providers think is important. For complete assessment of the success of a medical mission, it is important to consider topics that patients consider necessary to their health. Sustainable, integrative primary care delivery should be a collaborative, patient-centered enterprise.

Community-Supported Agriculture

An often-neglected topic in integrated primary health is nutrition (specifically, preventive nutrition) (Aboud & Yousafzai, 2015). Nutrition is fundamental for sustainable health care. Health maintenance starts with the health care team and continues in homes and communities. Community Supported Agriculture (CSA) is a collaborative effort in which a community partners with a local farmer to buy shares in the crops. When it is time for harvest, each community member receives a portion of the crop and pays an affordable fee for a share. Each community member assumes responsibility for the crop and accepts its benefits and risks. Share participation varies – some CSAs require volunteer time, and others require no hands-on work at all.

CSA started in Japan and Chile in the 1970's. In Japan, it is known as a "teikei system." There are similar systems in Europe and the U.S. CSA has numerous benefits, including: a sustainable farming system with local produce, a partnership between supplier and consumer, stewardship and self-sufficiency in relation to local ecosystems, support of the local economy, nutritious food at a reasonable cost, and a sense of accomplishment. In turn, this supports preventive practices and health maintenance (Kelley, Kime, & Harper, 2013). This also facilitates an environment in which community members are aware of where their food comes from and how it is grown.

By partnering with local farmers, medical organizations could strengthen their relationship with the host community in a way that considers additional determinants of health that are traditionally overlooked (e.g., the economy, spiritual/mental health, nutrition). Medical missions should also consider supporting CSA, which can alleviate some of the burden of poverty and improve food security. In countries where these issues are present, such support would improve health in the long-term (Phillips & Watson, 2011).

Conclusion

In sustainable, integrative primary care, the local partner (host team) could act as the "wheel" in the spoke and wheel model, and the visiting medical mission teams could be the "spokes" that serve host country communities. Ideally, this method would remove some of the barriers to care (e.g., location, lack of native providers, etc.). Therefore, clear communication is of utmost importance, particularly regarding the expected outcome of the relationship between visiting medical teams and host country health care providers.

The medical home model could be a starting point for CSA integration, as it would allow for a variety of medical services to be provided in one building (which would preferably be central to the community and the site of care). Having a variety of medical services available in a central location facilitates more effective and consolidated follow-up care because it eliminates the need of transportation. Furthermore, other concerns unrelated to the initial reason for travel (e.g., mental health care, pharmaceutical needs, physical therapy, CAM, nutrition, etc.) could be addressed at the same location. Adding a CSA opens an opportunity for nutritional counseling and the availability of produce at an affordable price. Also, since the produce would be centrally-located, it would be accessible to a larger group of people.

By implementing models of integrative primary care into medical missions, it is possible to create a viable model of sustainable global health programming that addresses immediate medical concerns and moves communities towards health via preventative practices and patient empowerment (Jamison et al., 2013). This requires careful consideration of the needs of the host country (as outlined by the host country), education of local health providers and the visiting medical teams, deliberation of cultural and ethical nuances surrounding the delivery of health care, and practical contemplation regarding logistics.

References

Aboud, F. E., & Yousafzai, A. K. (2015). Global health and development in early childhood. *Annual Review of Psychology, 66*, 433-57. DOI: 10.1146/annurev-psych-010814-015128

Akachi, Y., Tarp, F., Kelley, E., Addison, T., & Kruk, M. (2016). Measuring quality-of-care in the context of sustainable development goal 3: A call for papers. *Bulletin of the World Health Organization, 94*, 160–160A. DOI: http://dx.doi.org/10.2471/BLT.16.170605

Andersen, R. S., Tørring, M. L., & Vedsted, P. (2014). Global health care–seeking discoursesfacing local clinical realities: Exploring the case of cancer. *Medical Anthropology Quaterly, 29*(2), 1-19. DOI: 10.1111/maq.12148

Berry, N. S. (2014). Did we do good? NGOs, conflicts of interest and the evaluation of short-term medical missions in Sololá, Guatemala. *Social Science & Medicine, 120*, 344–351. DOI: 10.1016/j.socscimed.2014.05.006

Bido, J., Singer, S. J., Diez Portela, D., Ghazinouri, R., Driscoll, D. A., Alcantara Abreu, L., …& Katz, J. N. (2015). Sustainability assessment of a short-term international medical mission. *The Journal of Bone & Joint Surgery, 97*(11), 944-949. DOI: 10.2106/JBJS.N.01119

Collins, P. Y., Insel, T. R., Chockalingam, A., Daar, A., & Maddox, Y. T. (2013). Grand challenges in global mental health: Integration in research, policy, and practice. *PLoS Medicine, 10*(4), e1001434. DOI: 10.1371/journal.pmed.1001434

Coventry, P., Lovell, K., Dickens, Ch., Bower P., Chew-Graham, C., McElvenny, D., … Gask, L. (2015). Integrated primary care for patients with mental and physical multimorbidity: Cluster randomized controlled trial of collaborative care for patients with depression comorbid with diabetes or cardiovascular disease. *BMJ, 350*(h638), 1-12. DOI: 10.1136/bmj.h638

Crespo, R., & Shrewsberry, M. (2007). Factors associated with integrating self-management support into primary care. *The Diabetes Educator, 33*, 126S-131S. DOI: 10.1177/0145721707304138

Fields, B.E., Bigbee, J.L., & Bell, J.F. (2015). Associations of provider-to-population ratios and population health by county-level rurality. *The Journal of Rural Health, 32*(3), 235-244. DOI: 10.1111/jrh.12143.

Frenk, J., & Moon, S. (2013). Governance challenges in global health. *New England Journal of Medicine, 368*, 936-942. DOI: 10.1056/NEJMra1109339

Gill, H., Mcleod, S., Duerksen, K., & Szafran, O. (2012). Factors influencing medical students' choice of family medicine: Effects of rural versus urban background. *Canadian Family Physician, 58*(11), e649-e657. PMCID: PMC3498039

Grace, S., Orrock, P., Vaughan, B., Blaich, R., & Coutts, R. (2016). Understanding clinical reasoning in osteopathy: A qualitative research approach. *Chiropractic & Manual Therapies, 24*(6), 1-10. DOI: 10.1186/s12998-016-0087-x

Gureje, O., Nortje, G., Makanjuola, V., Oladeji, B., Seedat, S., & Jenkins, R. (2015). The role of global traditional and complementary systems of medicine in treating mental health problems. *Lancet Psychiatry, 2*(2), 168-177. DOI: 10.1016/S2215-0366(15)00013-9. P. 2 18

Hirshon, J. M., Risko, N., Calvello, E. J. B., Stewart de Ramirez, S., Narayan, M., Theodosis, Ch., & O'Neill, J. (2013). Health systems and services: The role of acute care. *Bulletin of the World Health Organization, 91*, 386–388. DOI: http://dx.doi.org/10.2471/BLT.12.112664

Holmboe, E.S., Wang, Y., Meehan, T. P., Tate, J. P., Ho, S. Y., Starkey, K. S., & Lipner, R. S. (2008). Association Between Maintenance of Certification Examination Scores and Quality of Care for Medicare Beneficiaries. *Archives of Internal Medicine, 168*(13), 13961403. DOI: 10.1001/archinte.168.13.1396

Jamison, D. T., Summers, L. H., Alleyne, G., Arrow, K. J., Berkley, S., Binagwaho, A., ... & Ghosh, G. (2013). Global health 2035: A world converging within a generation. *The Lancet, 382*(9908), 1898-1955.

Kelley, K. M., Kime, L. F., & Harper, J. K. (2013). Community Supported Agriculture (CSA). Retrieved from: http://extension.psu.edu/business/ag-alternatives/marketing/community-supported-agriculture-csa

King, D.E., Holloway, L., & Walker, R. (2013). Expanding models for rural primary care in West Virginia. *West Virginia Medical Journal, 109*(4), 38-43. PMID: 23930561

Kirchhoff, A.C., Hart, G., & Campbell, E.G. (2014). Rural and urban primary care physician professional beliefs and quality improvement behaviors. *The Journal of Rural Health, 30*(3), 235-243. DOI: 10.1111/jrh.12067

Kohrt, B. A., Jordans, M. J. D., Rai, S., Shrestha, P., Luitel, N. P., Ramaiya, M. K., ... Patel, V. (2015). Therapist competence in global mental health: Development of the Enhancing Assessment of Common Therapeutic factors (ENACT) rating scale. *Behaviour Research and Therapy, 69*, 11-21. DOI: http://dx.doi.org/10.1016/j.brat.2015.03.009

Kok, M. C., Kane, S. S., Tulloch, O., Ormel, H., Theobald, S., Dieleman, M., ... de Koning, K. A. M (2015). How does context influence performance of community health workers in low- and middle-income countries? Evidence from the literature. *Health ResearchPolicy and Systems, 13*(13), 1-14. DOI: 10.1186/s12961-015-0001-3

Kruk, M. E., Yamey, G., Angell, S., Y., Beith, A., Cotlear, D., Guanais, F., ... Goosby, E. (2016). Transforming global health by improving the science of scale-up. *PLOS Biology*, 1-16. DOI: 10.1371/journal.pbio.1002360

Lasker, J. N. (2015). *Hoping to help: The promises and pitfalls of global health volunteering.* United States: ILR Press.

Leach, M. J. (2013). Profile of the complementary and alternative medicine workforce across Australia, New Zealand, Canada, United States and United Kingdom. *Complementary Therapies in Medicine, 21*(4), 364-378. DOI: 10.1016/j.ctim.2013.04.004

Licciardone, J. C. (2015). A national study of primary care provided by Osteopathic physicians. *The Journal of the American Osteopathic Association, 115*, 704-713. DOI: 10.7556/jaoa.2015.145

Loh, L. C., Cherniak, W., Dreifuss, B. A., Dacso, M. M., Lin, H. C., & Evert, J. (2015). Short term global health experiences and local partnership models: A framework. *Globalization and Health, 11*(50), 1-7. DOI: 10.1186/s12992-015-0135-7

MacLachlan, M. (2014). Macropsychology, policy, and global health. *American Psychologist, 69*(8), 851-863. DOI: http://dx.doi.org/10.1037/a0037852

Martiniuk, A. L., Manouchehrian, M., Negin, J. A., & Zwi, A. B. (2012). Brain gains: A literature review of medical missions to low and middle-income countries. *BMC Health Services Research, 12*(1), 134. doi:10.1186/1472-6963-12-134

McGinnis, J. M. (2016). Income, life expectancy, and community health: Underscoring the opportunity. *Journal of the American Medical Association, 315*(16),1709-1710. DOI: 10.1001/jama.2016.4729.

Mohan, V., Seedat, Y. K., & Pradeepa, R. (2013). The rising burden of diabetes and hypertension in Southeast Asian and African regions: Need for effective strategies for prevention and control in primary health care settings. *International Journal of Hypertension, 409083*, 1-14. DOI: http://dx.doi.org/10.1155/2013/409083

Nguah, S. B. (2014). Ethical aspects of arranging local medical collaboration and care. *The Journal of Clinical Ethics, 25*(4), 314-316. PMID: 25517569

O'Donnell, P., McAuliffe, E., & O'Donovan, D. (2014). Unchallenged good intentions: A qualitative study of the experiences of medical students on international health electives to developing countries. *Human Resources for Health, 12*(49), 1-8. DOI: 10.1186/1478-4491-12-49

Patel, V., Belkin, G. S., Chockalingam, A., Cooper, J., Saxena, S., & Unützer, J. (2013). Grand challenges: Integrating mental health services into priority health care platforms. *PLoS Medicine, 10*(5), e1001448. DOI: e1001448. doi:10.1371/journal.pmed.1001448

Peterson, L. E., Blackburn, B., Peabody, M., & O'Neill, T. R. (2015). Family physicians' scope of practice and American board of family medicine recertification examination performance. *Journal of the American Board of Family Medicine, 28*(2), 265-270. DOI: 10.3122/jabfm.2015.02.140202.

Phillips, E., & Watson, D. (2011). *Miami rice in Haiti: Virtue or vice? In food policy for developing countries: The role of government in the global food system.* Ithaca: Cornell University.

Primary. (2016). In Oxford English dictionary. Retrieved from http://www.oed.com/view/Entry/151280?rskey=KtSzV0&result=1#eid

Primary Care -- AAFP Policies. (2016). Primary care. Retrieved from http://www.aafp.org/about/policies/all/primary-care.html

Pruss-Ustün, A., Wolf, J., Corvalán, C., Bos, R., & Neira, M. (2016). *Preventing disease through healthy environments: A global assessment of the burden of disease from environmental risks.* Geneva, Switzerland: World Health Organization.

Rockwell, W. T., Agbenorku, P., Olson, J., Hoyte-Williams, P. E., Agarwal, J. P., & Bradford, R. (2015). A model for university-based international plastic surgery collaboration builds local sustainability. *Annals of Plastic Surgery, 74*(4), 388–391. DOI: 10.1097/SAP.0000000000000222

Rotheram-Borus, M. J., Swendeman, D., & Chorpita, B. F. (2012). Disruptive innovations for designing and diffusing evidence based interventions. *American Psychologist, 67*(6), 463–476. DOI: 10.1037/a0028180.

Shidhaye, R., Shrivastava, S., Murhar, V., Samudre, S., Ahuja, Sh., Ramaswamy, R., & Patel, V. (2016). Development and piloting of a plan for integrating mental health in primary care in Sehore district, Madhya Pradesh, India. *The British Journal of Psychiatry, 208*(s56), s13-s20. DOI: 10.1192/bjp.bp.114.153700

Sustainable. (2016). In Oxford English dictionary. Retrieved from http://www.oed.com/view/Entry/195210?redirectedFrom=sustainable#eid

Sweetland, A. C., Oquendo, M. A., Sidat, M., Santos, P. F., Vermund, S. H., Duarte, C. S., ... Wainberg, M. L. (2014). Closing the mental health gap in low-income settings by building research capacity: Perspectives from Mozambique. *Annals of Global Health, 80*, 126-133. DOI: http://dx.doi.org/10.1016/j.aogh.2014.04.014

Vannieuwenborg, L., Buntinx, F., & De Lepeleire, J. (2015). Presenting prevalence and management of psychosocial problems in primary care in Flanders. *Archives of Public Health, 73*(10), 1-6. DOI: 10.1186/s13690-015-0061-4

White, R. G., Imperiale, M. G., & Perera, E. (2016). The capabilities approach: Fostering contexts for enhancing mental health and wellbeing across the globe. *Globalization and Health, 12*(16), 1-10. DOI: 10.1186/s12992-016-0150-3

White, R., Jain, S., & Giurgi-Oncu, C. (2014). Counterflows for mental well-being: What high- income countries can learn from low and middle-income countries. *International Review of Psychiatry, 26*(5), 602-606. DOI: 10.3109/09540261.2014.939578.

Witten, J., Jansen Van Vuuren, A., & Learmonth, D. (2013). Psychological intervention to address hypertension in South Africa's peri-urban settlements. *Online Readings in Psychology and Culture, 10*(1), 1-18. DOI: http://dx.doi.org/10.9707/2307-0919.1123

World Health Organization (2010a). *Benchmarks for training in traditional/complementary and alternative medicine: Benchmarks for training in Ayurveda.* Geneva, Switzerland: World Health Organization.

World Health Organization (2010b). *Benchmarks for training in traditional/complementary and alternative medicine: Benchmarks for training in Naturopathy.* Geneva, Switzerland: World Health Organization.

World Health Organization (2010c). *Benchmarks for training in traditional/complementary and alternative medicine: Benchmarks for training in Osteopathy.* Geneva, Switzerland: World Health Organization.

World Health Organization (2010d). *Benchmarks for training in traditional/complementary and alternative medicine: Benchmarks for training in Traditional Chinese Medicine.* Geneva, Switzerland: World Health Organization.

Yong Kim, J., Farmer, P., & Porter, M. E. (2013). Redefining global health-care delivery. *The Lancet, 382*(9897), 1060–1069. DOI: http://dx.doi.org/10.1016/S0140-6736(13)61047-8

CHAPTER 25

Planting Seeds, Growing Docs in Kenya

Kathleen B. Harrison and John A. McNulty

This chapter tells the story of how a small non-government organization (NGO) is making a significant impact in global health through focused community development and education. Within the larger framework of the global health community, our story is mostly a personal account, a blend of academic issues and anecdotes, a combination that provides a narrative on the development of human resources with compelling local and global implications.

Introduction

Our thoughts on global health reflect a very personal concern. The title of this book, "Why Global Health Matters," begs the question "Why does anything matter; what meaning and value are present in my life?"

With exposure to the larger world, two insights emerge relevant to this question. First, we are all more alike than we are different. Second, a significant difference among the world's peoples – one amenable to change – is the inequitable distribution of resources.

In addressing the first, some iteration of the Golden Rule lies at the center of religious and humanistic belief systems the world over: Islam: "No one of you is a believer until he desires for his brother that which he desires for himself" ("Islam," 2017, para. 2). Christianity: "Do to others what you would have them do to you" ("Christianity," 2017, para. 9). Judaism: "Whatsoever you do not wish your neighbor to do to you, do not unto him" ("Judaism," 2017, para. 1). Buddhism: "One should seek for others the happiness one desires for one's self" ("Buddhism," 2017, para.

1). And so on… This directive underlies Baha'I, Sikhism, Janism, even Wicca: "An' it harm no one, do what thou wilt" ("Wicca," 2017, para. 1). In a secular context, it is expressed in the Universal Declaration of Human Rights (United Nations, 1948) as well as the United Nations Millennium Development Goals (United Nations, 2016).

Compassion and sharing are common to all caring people and cut across colors, creeds, and cultures. Given the unequal distribution of resources in the world, this is the essence of why global health matters. We share concern for the well-being of all our brothers and sisters in the human race. In our digital age, when global communication is ubiquitous, communities are connected worldwide. People of even very limited means access the internet and readily learn that, indeed, we're all more alike than we are different. At the same time, however, they become aware of vast distributive injustices. This underscores the urgency behind the goals of sharing and equitable access to resources, particularly those involving the fundamental right to health care.

> *"I believe that, as long as there is plenty, poverty is evil."*
> — *Robert F. Kennedy ("Robert F. Kennedy," 2017, para. 15)*

What Then Must We Do?

Project Harambee (Swahili for "all pull together"), a registered 501c3 non-profit organization, answers this mandate for action with a practical response. We have been working for the last twelve years in sub-Saharan Africa implementing our mission to support sustainable development projects in education, health care, and economics – projects that are not "charitable" but empowering. Addressing these fundamental and intertwined needs holistically in a community enables reversal of the downward spiral of poverty and hopelessness in places where resources are scarce or inaccessible. Moreover, this approach draws on strengths within communities and offers a "hand-up" rather than a "hand-out." Our partnership programs promote sustainability because all Project Harambee beneficiaries are required to give back in some way. This fosters not only growth, but neighborliness. What, after all, is more empowering than the ability to help another? When neighbors share with neighbors, the entire community is strengthened.

In locations where Project Harambee is engaged, we have projects that focus on each of the three areas mentioned. Here we concentrate on a program that builds capacity in education and health care in Kenya.

Figure 1: © Logo for Project Harambee

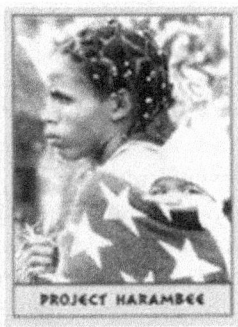

The Founding of Project Harambee (by KBH)

Project Harambee (www.projectharambee.org) originated as a result of an unlikely, serendipitous chain of events. I never particularly wanted to go to Africa. Ever. But in 2001, while I was a faculty member in the Semester at Sea shipboard education program (www.semesteratsea.org), I found myself dockside in Mombasa, Kenya. My plan was to escape the ship, go off on safari, and enjoy a hot-air balloon ride over the romantic African savannah. Instead, I was asked to lead a group of students on a service mission in Nairobi. Together we spent several days at Nyumbani Home, an orphanage for HIV-positive children (www.nyumbani.org). There was a serious shortage of antiretroviral drugs in Kenya at that time and most of the children were dying.

Figure 2: Cemetery, Nyumbani Home, 2001

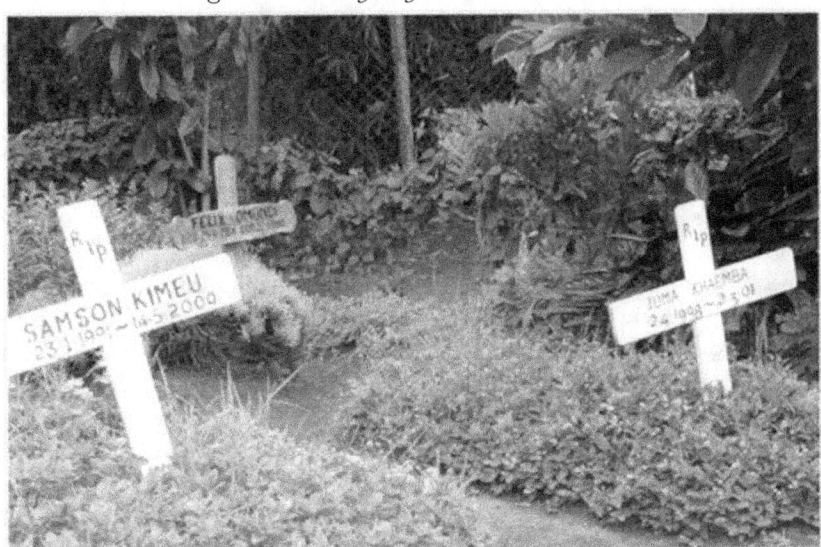

The experience was a game-changer for many of us, and I returned home with a plan to leave my genetics position at Columbia University, relocate to Kenya, and run the diagnostic laboratory at the orphanage. But a few months later the events of September 11 short-circuited many plans, including mine. For security reasons, no volunteers could travel to the orphanage in Kenya; however, I returned as a visitor in 2004 and travelled alone throughout the country, gaining firsthand experience of the HIV pandemic that was decimating entire nations. Even a geneticist could see that socioeconomic factors largely determined the health of a region and that if the disease burden of HIV in Africa were to be solved, a primary strategy must address improving the economic status of those who were hit the hardest – the poor. As I flew home across the Atlantic, I pondered all I'd witnessed, and I knew that I couldn't walk away without responding in some way to the desperate conditions in a country – in a continent – caused by a vicious disease rooted in poverty. I had to do something. What could I do – a clinical geneticist with no training in organizing, development, finance, or global issues? How could I avoid doing more harm than good? Yet act I must.

Initially, I was questioned about working in Africa. Some said, "I believe in helping, but we should take care of our own here at home first." My response: In this century, there's no denying that we're now part of a global village. There is no more "them" and "us." It's all "us." This work is what was placed in front of me and the need I saw was unquestionable; I merely accepted. When others see challenges here in the U.S., I hope they do the same. The important thing is to share from the bounty in our lives and to reach out to those less fortunate.

Even a cursory search of charity efforts reveals example after example of well-meant but uninformed efforts to provide resources without due attention to the dignity of the recipients. This has led to a manifestation that has been termed the "White Savior Complex." Teju Cole (2012) described this when he wrote "The White Savior Industrial Complex is not about justice. It is about having a big emotional experience that validates privilege" (p. 1).

Right from the start, I believed I could do more and do it better.

A single phone call to a professor at Loyola University Chicago to ask for advice on starting a microeconomics project began a remarkable journey that has continued for twelve years. Though small, Project Harambee has a big impact in the places it's most needed. Through fund-raising, sale of handcrafted wares from organized African support groups, and cooperation with other non-profit organizations in several countries, we have developed a number of programs that assist several thousand families affected by HIV. Most relevant to global health is our PLANT A SEED, GROW A DOC project, which is just one thread in a tapestry of responses to community needs.

The project originated in 2008. While working in a village in southeastern Kenya, we were frustrated in failed attempts to hire a physician from Nairobi to come and evaluate the health of the children, most of whom had never been seen by a health care worker. We'd previously traveled with U.S. medical student volunteers to Kenya, and although they all recognized the need for a more permanent health care project, managed by Kenyans, there was little at the time we could do to effect it. An impulsive thought arose: "If we can't hire a doc, we'll just have to grow our own!" The more I considered the idea, the better it looked.

> *"Remember, failure is just a dress-rehearsal for success!"*
> *— Stanley Waudo (2014, p.3)*

Why not provide a university medical scholarship for one or more promising Kenyan students with the goal of cultivating "home-grown" professionals to serve a community's health care needs? Why not, indeed! We could turn our efforts into a project to plant a seed and grow a doctor. The only obvious obstacles were: lack of money ($5,000/year/student), lack of resources to organize a sustainable program remotely from a distance of 6,000 miles, lack of knowledge of the Kenyan university system, and no way to evaluate suitable candidates. What could stop us?

> *"You do not need to know what is happening, or exactly where it is all going. What you need is to recognize the possibilities and challenges offered by the present moment and embrace them with courage, faith and hope. In such an event, courage is the authentic form taken by love."*
> *— Thomas Merton (1966, p. 206)*

Building Capacity

Education is arguably the most effective avenue for building capacity in any culture, and international organizations have consistently pointed out that to be sustainable, a country must create and continuously improve human and physical resources for education (Neufeld, 2001; Pang et al., 2003). The Kenyan government has notably increased efforts to provide education at all levels (Kenya Vision 2030, 2007) and, between 2012 and 2014, doubled enrollment in university programs (Clark, 2015, p.1, para. 1).

Building capacity in the health arena addresses a variety of concerns. For example, it enhances and prolongs access to health care in the communities, especially in underserved areas of the country. The need is obvious. One out of fourteen children born in Kenya do not reach their fifth birthday, and children in rural areas are three times as likely to die between their first and fifth birthdays as children in urban areas. In 2015, the death rate of children in the U.S. was 7/1,000; in Kenya it was seven times greater: 49/1,000 (World Bank, 2015, Table 1).

Kenya is a country with a large NGO presence and is a favored destination for volunteers and aid workers because English is a national language, the country is relatively stable, and the climate is temperate. However, as was recently reported (Kuo, 2016), the Kenyan government, through its NGO Coordination Board, has been pressuring NGOs in Kenya to justify the high number of expatriates who are employed in place of Kenyans. The debate on the role of NGOs is complicated by the breadth and number of NGOs in Kenya as well as by political intrigues (Kuo, 2016), but there is little doubt that forces are moving away from the "White Savior Complex" (Cole, 2012).

It was within this context of the "White Savior Complex" and concerns of the Kenyan government regarding NGOs that Project Harambee developed the infrastructure for PLANT A SEED, GROW A DOC (and indeed all of our service programs). We work directly with Kenyans and employ no expatriates. Our policy is not to dispense charity, but to contract mutual agreements by which we supply assistance; in return, our African partners share their successes by giving back to their communities. Our Kenyan students and graduates are fulfilling this obligation by responding in diverse ways to both the need for enhanced and prolonged access to health care and the need for research.

> *"There are those that look at things the way they are, and ask why? I dream of things that never were, and ask why not?"*
> — *Robert F. Kennedy*
> *("Robert Kennedy in His Own Words," 2017, para. 1)*

As our vision and plan slowly emerged, we traversed Kenya in 2009 and visited several universities (Moi University, Kenya Methodist University, Kenyatta University, Egerton University, Jomo Kenyatta University, and Mount Kenya University) to learn the educational system and begin the process of forming sustainable networks with faculty and administrators. Travel, scheduling, and communication were sometimes challenging, but we maintained our broad vision and open minds. Some of the contacts proved invaluable later as we embarked on another venture central to development of the program: adjunct lecturing in Kenyan medical schools. In order to obtain a clearer understanding of health education in Kenya, we immersed ourselves in the system. We were fortunate to have an opportunity to spend ten days lecturing and teaching in laboratories at Mount Kenya University Medical School in Thika, Kenya and to deliver guest lectures at other universities.

Figure 3: Concrete encouragement
at the Blue Post Hotel, Thika, Kenya

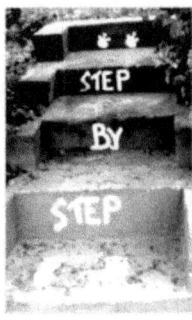

The next challenge required faith that our limited budget could sustain a commitment of $5,000 per student over several years of university medical training. At Project Harambee, rather than asking outright for donations, we prefer to give something back to donors. For our GROW A DOC funding, one idea was to purchase crafts and artwork made by members of African support groups and market them here in the U.S. We also devised the equally effective "alternative gift cards" for holidays, birthdays, and other gift-giving celebrations (see Figure 4). When someone donates, he or she receives a handmade card in return. This alternative gift idea has worked very well, particularly among those in age groups where material gifts are not needed. Further, our program is highly cost-effective because our overhead expenses are almost nil. Potential donors are confident in giving when they learn that 100% of their donation goes to Africa.

Figure 4: Sample gift card

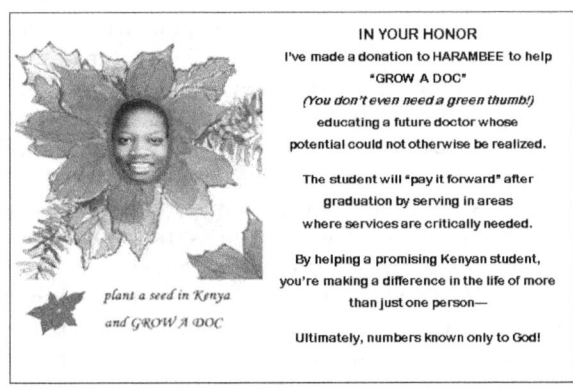

The next task was finding potential students. Once again, our contacts in Kenya proved invaluable in our goal of selecting candidates who met the following somewhat stringent requirements:

1. Good scholarship standing and study habits (faithfulness to commitment)
2. Highly motivated to study health care
3. No other means of obtaining higher education
4. Willing to give back to the community and "pay it forward"

The last point is particularly important to the sustainability of GROW A DOC. We want not only to build human potential and increase health care delivery to people in underserved areas, but also to foster values that will positively influence the future of a country.

Although we collaborate with faith-based institutions, Project Harambee itself is not faith-based. In our experience, religious organizations in Kenya work hand-in-hand with both government and secular agencies to most effectively provide social services. To our knowledge, neither clients nor students are asked about church affiliation, nor does Project Harambee inquire about religious identity or health status from any of those we support. We ask that suitable GROW A DOC candidates, screened by our collaborators, write a letter of application about their life and why they want to enter a health care profession. Remarkably – or perhaps not – every single applicant to date has lost one or both parents to HIV/AIDS. They all have seen a loved one die a horrendous death – a powerful motivator to enter medicine and help others.

A Typical Application Letter

My name is KJ aged 19 years old. I was born in 1995 and brought up in a family of nine at Homa-Bay my homeland. Two of my siblings departed. I am a total orphan.

I started schooling at the age of six in 2002. Life has been hard since I was young. All my parents were jobless and only did some small-scale farming. We struggled with life until the year 2008 when my father departed. By then I was in class seven. After the departure of my beloved father, life became much harder as he was the bread winner in the family. Too much struggling to earn a living made me to lose hope in education.

I was going to school and helping my mum to get something to eat. She encouraged me to continue working hard so as to have a better life in future. From then onward, I added more effort to my studies.

In the year 2009, I did my national examination; Kenya Certificate of Primary Education (K.C.P.E). I had a lot of hope in passing the exam and in December I found I had passed. But I was still worried for I was not sure of pursuing secondary education.

The following year, 2010, still in my world of wondering, I received good news from my uncle in Nairobi. He called and affirmed that I could get a chance to pursue my high school education. I was so excited to hear this. He thought I could secure a vacancy at St. Aloysius. Unluckily, on arriving to the school, we were told that all places had been taken. Being ashamed of sending me back to the village, he took me to a private school in Kibera slum. At that school, 20,000 Kenya shillings ($240) was paid as fee per academic year. This marked the beginning of another hell. He was not ready to pay the school fee. I therefore most a time stayed back and only go to school during exams.

In Form two, it was even worse for he could not even provide the basic needs such as food and clothes. This moved to a point that he sent me out of his house. Having nowhere to go to, I joined the street children and I was set to start another life in the street. For six months I was a street boy. Then my uncle looked for me to inform me of my mother's death in August of 2011. After the burial, I was back to Nairobi. A friend pleaded with me to go and try if I could get a chance at St. Aloysius so that I could continue with my education. At the back of my mind, I knew that it was difficult but I took courage and said that I must try. After a long talk with the school principal, I was given an interview of which with God's mercy I passed. This is how I ended up in St. Aloysius Gonzaga secondary school.

In form three, I went back to stay with my uncle. Though I had no problem with school fee, but home chaos were too much. My uncle is an alcoholic. He could come home and order me to do all the chores. This denied me time to undertake my personal studies. I had only my limited time at school to study. This continued till I sat for my final exam at form four.

Despite this I still managed my time well. I waited my results with great hope. In March this year, I received my results. I was in third position. I am now looking forward to join university to pursue a degree in medicine and surgery as it has been the course of my dream. (Personal communication, KJ, April 14, 2014).

Every applicant tells a similar story. The letters may seem melodramatic, but within the context of African life they are not; the difficulties described are everyday realities for a large percentage of children growing up in Africa. During the global HIV epidemic, an estimated 17 million children lost one or both parents to AIDS. 90% of those children live in sub-Saharan Africa. Currently, in Kenya, health and development problems related to poverty are common. These include stunted growth (>25%), acute malnutrition (4-23% depending on region), and low weight for age (11%) (National Bureau of Statistics-Kenya and ICF International, 2015, p. 11).

*Figure 5: KJ and MK, currently third-year medical students
at Mount Kenya University*

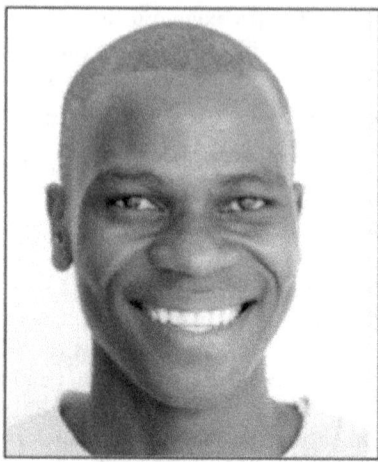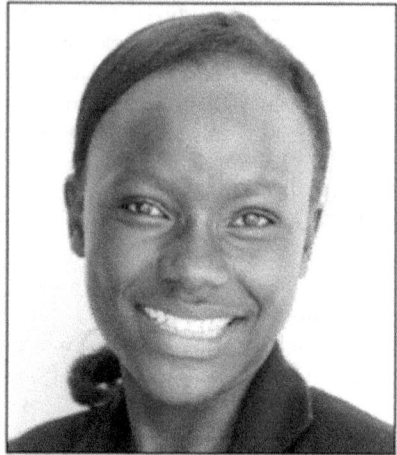

Initially we committed to support students in a four-year baccalaureate program in any science related to health care. The reasons behind this decision were:

1. GROW A DOC was an experimental program. We were taking a risk regarding both outcome and funding sustainability; we were hesitant to commit to more than four years of support.
2. Because the majority of health care in developing countries is provided by clinical officers (comparable to physician assistants in the U.S.) and nurses, PLANT A SEED, GROW A DOC would likely have the largest impact with graduates in these professions, requiring a four-year (or less) degree.

"You've got to jump off the cliff...and build your wings on the way down."
— Ray Bradbury
("Moonlightened Way," 2012, para. 2)

In 2010, we jumped off the cliff and sent our first three GROW A DOC students off to Mount Kenya University in Thika, Kenya. We all committed to grow wings together. Each year we interviewed and cautiously accepted a few more candidates, looking particularly for qualified young women. The women confided concerns to us regarding the possibility of exploitation by male authority figures on campus. A proposed solution for this problem resulted in a successful student support organization.

Progress of the Program

As of this writing, we have seven graduates with eight students still in training, representing a 100% success rate. Among the graduates are clinical officers, nurses, and one pharmacist. They all participate in volunteer service projects, mentor incoming students, and work in medically underserved areas before and after graduation. In 2013, we felt confident enough to accept our first student for a six-year medical doctor (M.D.) degree program. He is now entering his fourth year and doing very well at Kenyatta University. Five additional students are in M.D. programs. Three of them are young women, one of whom is the highest scoring student ever from her secondary school and has begun studies at the University of Nairobi, the highest-rated medical school in Kenya.

Building Community

We wanted to build a sense of relationship among the students and to make GROW A DOC a close-knit family. We also needed help with pragmatic tasks such as distribution of funds, tracking progress, coordinating student volunteer initiatives, and maintaining communication with students. In addition to regular internet communication and meetings with students when we are in Kenya, we require that they participate in community activities, meet regularly, and report to our coordinator Thomas Nyawir at St. Aloysius Gonzaga Secondary School. We are indebted to Father Terry Charlton, S.J. for his support and to Thomas Nyawir for coordinating student communication and administrative work. This is another example of a faith-based organization working closely with a secular NGO to serve students without regard to religious affiliation. At St. Aloysius, boys and girls learn values of compassion, discernment, and service in solidarity with the poor – entirely consistent with our own values. Because these values extend across religious lines, there has been no conflict stemming from diverse religious affiliations of students.

Each year while in Kenya, we interview candidates who have been screened by our partnering NGOs (i.e., St. Aloysius Gonzaga Secondary School, Upendo Village) and explain the contractual nature of our scholarships. For a young person coming from a life of poverty and street life, adjusting to the culture of a middle-class university campus is daunting and lonely. The help of a "big brother" or "big sister" is valuable and further promotes a sense of family. Thus, we stipulate that students must mentor and be mentored by future and prior GROW A DOC students.

Required service work has been one of the most enjoyable facets of the GROW A DOC experience. We have sent several students to puppeteer training school in Nairobi and have outfitted them with puppets and a portable stage and sound system. During university break periods, they perform health care educational shows for children in schools and churches. Because girls are at particular risk of discrimination, special girl puppeteer groups perform interactive puppetry plays on behavior change and gender sensitivity issues to help girls gain self-confidence and avoid exploitation. Thomas Nyawir coordinates this student volunteer activity.

Figure 6: GROW A DOC puppeteers

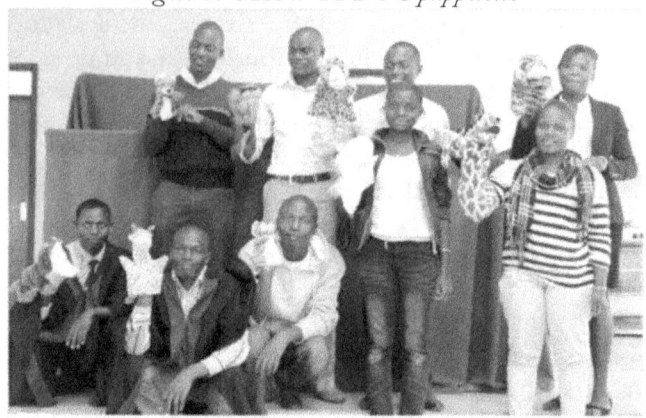

Figure 7: Puppet show audience at a Kibera school

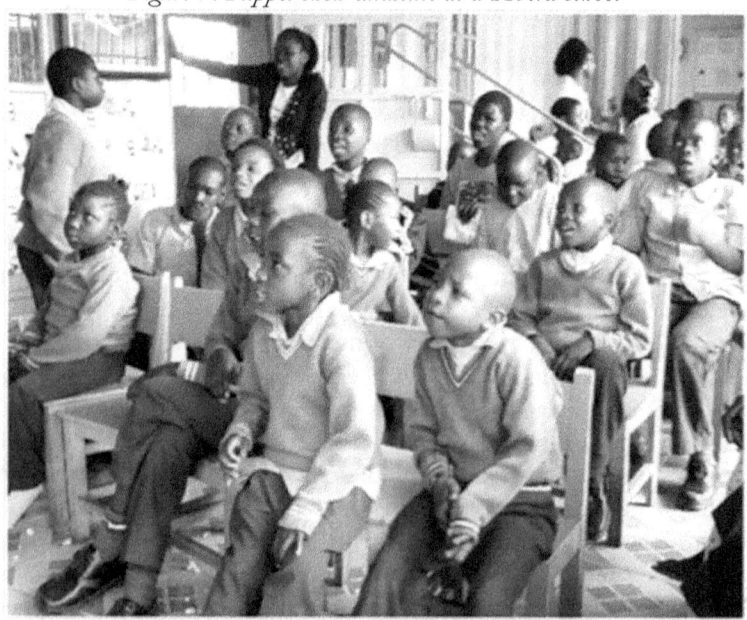

The requirement of regular reporting to us both promotes community and alerts us to individual needs of students. We share their letters with our supporters. They offer insight to a world vastly different from our own and build bridges that we hope will continue to expand and strengthen.

A Student Letter from F.M.

Hallo! Dr. Keen and John.

Allow me to say that your support to me with my education is highly appreciated. What you did for me to securing this golden chance in my life, I assure you that I will not forget it. I cannot really express all my gratitude in this mail but what I can say is, thank you very much. I am doing well with my education, I finished my 1st semester and did end of the semester exams. When the results are out I shall update you. It is so tough with a lot of sacrifice as you know. However, I am not complaining I like being busy and I have a passion for my course. I am more tough than it is and I promise not to disappoint your effort in supporting me. Again, allow me to wish you a very blessed and strong health. Love you all...Thank you, yours, F.M. (Personal communication, F.M., January 20, 2015).

A Student Letter from E.O.

I am now in my second semester of my junior clerkship in my first clinical year. The experience in the hospital is encouraging for me to even study more I have to admit that it is not all merry, sometimes I feel bad when I see very young men and women succumb to different forms of cancer and sexually transmuted infections because of seeking treatment very late. I am in the gynecology section and in the last 2 weeks we have admitted 15 women ages 29-60 with cervical cancer most of whom are in the advanced stages that have already metastasize.

I would like to thank you for everything and most of all seeing us as your own children whom you wish the very best for. I have to admit that every time you come and we interact you always spark rays of hope and determination to achieve the very best especially when you tell us of the stories of those who donate whole heartedly to this project. I can never thank you all for the opportunity you granted me to help people in the way that I always dreamed of. Chao for now. Truly, E.O. (Personal communication, E.O., May 3, 2015)

A Student Letter from L.O.

So far am doing mainly anatomy; that is gross anatomy, embryology and histology. Besides these, We were also introduced to cell biology, physiology and other three common units.

My first experience with the cadavers was a bit scary but as per now, am very comfortable with them. It is really nice and great fun doing what one loves. Indeed I love the course with passion.

Thanks to you for making my dream come reality, may God bless you more and more....AMEN. May I tell you that am always happy and counting myself as one of the few luckiest persons in Africa.

I once mention for you that I have a mission of not only going to make the hardware (body) healthy, but also making sure that my client's (patients) software (soul) is equally healthy. All pulling together, I believe I will make it despite of the associated challenges. I and you, Kenya, Africa and the world at large must be healthy in all dimensions!

Further, I have a dream of one day becoming a neurologist! Am pushed to this because many lose their lives here in Kenya not that they should, but just because of lack of such practitioners. I therefore hope I'll live to become one. Yours Sincerely, L. (Personal communication. L.O., November 11, 2015)

A Student Letter from F.J.

I really do not know what I would be looking like if compassion had not touched my life, when I was at the age of 14 starved, almost naked and frustrated with no hope. I cried in my neighborhood, but no one listened to me. But not far from God's hands a sponsor, a parent, came to me from the far country that is beyond the sea where my eyes could not imagine through what a blessing and love.

Your generous HARAMBEE contributions helped making my dream a reality by helping with all my fees.

Presently I am a mature adult and above all it's through St. Aloysius secondary school and Harambee that I grew up to become an adult with a mission to change my family, my community, my country and world at large. What can I give you and what can I say if it had not been your incomparable love you extended to me, I believe in the next day that I always count as a day of grace and new hope. By God's love I am whom I am today because of what you have done to my life, where my parents were unable to support me in all the aspects of life.

Life has meaning when someone touches it at a tender age. someone stood out and shaped my life. I now believe in life of fullness. I extend my sincere gratitude to everyone who contributed through this journey, and ask for God's blessings in their lives. Regards, F.J. (Personal communication, F.J., August 19, 2013)

We're often not only gratified, but surprised at reports from the students. One student, after a single term in medical school, described himself as "less than half a doctor."

Additional Letters from L.O.

Am happy to share with you how I encountered a choking child in the countryside during the holiday and was able to save him by using my knowledge of Heimlich's maneuver which I learnt last semester. I hope I will learn more and put them to practise when need arises. (Personal communication, L.O., January 23, 2016)

And later:

Hello mum, I want to share with you that I started my community service on Monday this week. I am helping at a local hospital within Kibera. My duties include receiving patients, directing them to various consultation rooms and at times measuring blood pressure. I do this simple tasks since I am not even half a doctor yet.

It is quite challenging as some patients come very ill and I at times feel scared to handle them but am overcoming my fears.

All this is possible because of your support. Thank you so much God bless you abundantly. Your loving son, L. (Personal communication, L.O., April 22, 2016)

A Student Letter from A.O.

USHIRIKA MEDICAL CLINIC, where I worked were greatful and delighted with the work I was doing and the vast knowledge and skills I possess. Working at this local clinic has really helped me in understanding many things about our society and their attitude towards health. I love my patients so much and they love me too.

The reception I get from my community KIBERA is very superb. Since a lot of them know me or have seen me grow really appreciated my presence. I act like an inspiration to them, their children and the future generation at large. Some guys tell me when they come to the clinic "Are you the small boy I saw growing up here in this community? How comes you are a Doctor?" Others say, "Did you know I carried you while you were young, are you sure you are going to treat me until I feel better?"

I just look at them then give a bright smile and tell them, "No matter where you come from, no matter your current situation, things change. You can become what you want to become."

I love this place and the people around so much. The result they get from my services are awesome. This is what keeps me moving. I have also done several radio health talks at (PAMOJA FM), one of the most popular radio stations in Kibera. This is done to educate the people of Kibera & give them information about aspects of community health. A.O. (Personal communication, A.O., June 14, 2015)

Students often referred to me as "Mum." Initially this was unsettling; however, it occurred to me that they reside in a culture where family is everything, and their families had been fractured or lost. It should be no surprise that they eagerly accept a benefactor as a parental figure. They rely on us not only for financial assistance, but often for guidance in life situations.

Figure 8: Three of the first GROW A DOC graduates, 2014

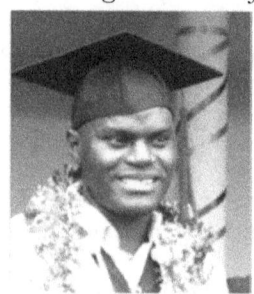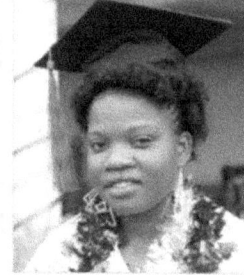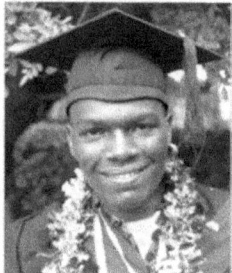

Outcomes of the Program

"As you travel on through life, brother (& sister),
whatever be your goal,
keep your eye upon the donut,
and not upon the hole."
— Edward Abby (1988, p. 502)

In addition to our 100% academic success rate, current and anticipated graduates are working in various underserved areas of Kenya. However, several other significant outcomes have also resulted. Foundational to them all has been formation of the International Healthcare Student Association (IHSA), conceived and initiated by our first young female student, F. J., as an effort to meet the challenges of female students. When we first interviewed her, she was asked, "Are there particular difficulties faced by young women students, and if so, what would you suggest as a solution?" Her response was dramatic and indicated the same problems faced by girls in many countries and cultures. There is both overt and covert discrimination and exploitation – particularly for sexual favors – by those in power over them. Her solution: formation of a networking system to provide mutual support and to give a public face for group strength and equality. She felt that collectively, students would have a voice for change. While beginning her medical studies, F.J. worked diligently to gain support among students and faculty for such an organization. Joined by students of both genders, the group has grown in number and is now represented by thirty-nine students at five universities. As a group they have written a constitution and by-laws and elected officers. The IHSA also provides a good platform for conducting student research, some of which was presented at the 2013 Catholic University of East Africa Conference on Justice and Peace.

Figure 9: International Healthcare Student Association, 2013, Catholic University of East Africa

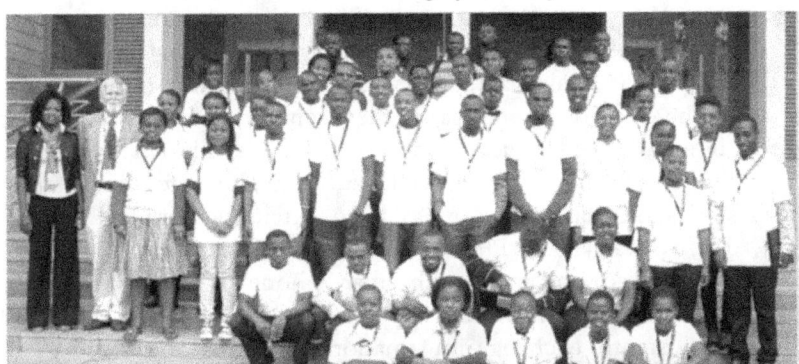

The biggest success of the IHSA has been the strong sense of community among the students, which is reflected in their mentorship of new students, their professional development resulting from publications, their development of community programs, and their international collaborations.

The goodwill and motivation of the students served as catalysts, but technology was the facilitator of the IHSA. As Lansang and Rodolfo (2004) emphasized, enhancement of health care research and services depends critically on information access and dissemination. The exponential growth of information technology in Kenya in the last decade coincided closely with development of GROW A DOC. This growth, especially in cellphone use, has been a major factor in the rapid successes of the program.

One of the initial research programs undertaken by the GROW A DOC students was a survey of the status of information and communication technologies (ICT) in health profession education in Kenya (Otieno et al., 2014). This landmark study of 310 health profession students from five universities reported that 73% of students owned a computer, 60% owned a smart phone, and almost 50% owned both (Otieno et al., 2014, p. 635, para. 1). Rapid increase in the level of technology use by health education students in Kenya contrasts with earlier studies which showed that only a small subset of students used computers at the University of Nairobi in 2009 (Gituma et al., 2009) and that only 12% of medical students owned computers in English-speaking countries of East Africa in 2010 (Williams et al., 2010, p. 486, Table 1).

A second research project involved a genetics survey, the results of which indicated the need for increased clinical genetics teaching and provision of genetic services (Harrison et al., 2010). This is another salient example that professionals in developing countries, because of widespread internet access, are aware of resources available in other parts of the globe and expect equitable access to them to better serve their patients.

Technology in health and education took another major leap with arrival of the "smart phone" and the digital capabilities that became available in a hand-held device (images, video, audio files). The importance of cell phones to the economies, education, health, and social fabric of countries in sub-Saharan Africa has been extensively studied (Aker and Mbiti, 2010; Kaplan, 2006; Prensky, 2005; Czerniewicz and Brown, 2010). The effectiveness of the media-rich smart phone in medical education is demonstrated in the use of the app "WhatsApp" by GROW A DOC students to instantly exchange information on clinical cases and to reach out to remote resources. Cases typically include images, videos, and occasional audio files. This exchange of material promotes convenient, timely information that is useful to education and clinical practice. For example, a baby was born with *ectopia cordis*, an extremely rare condition that few health care providers ever have occasion to experience and understand. There is no question their viewing of the posted video and the related discussion significantly broadened their comprehension of the disorder and of important issues in medicine (e.g., privacy and ethical issues associated with family interactions and treatment). Another case involved an American health care worker who posted a photo of an unusual skin lesion to query a possible diagnosis of a tropical epidermal disease common in Africa but rarely seen in the U.S.

Participation in the GROW A DOC "WhatsApp" group extends to faculty and medical professionals worldwide, which further promotes information exchange and awareness of health care and educational needs. For instance, there is an ongoing project in which students in the IHSA are collaborating with colleagues at Stanford University (Palo Alto, CA) to investigate the effectiveness of an innovative tool, the Foldscope ™, for use in health care delivery and research in resource-poor areas of Kenya. The scope is an ingenious origami-based print and fold paper microscope that is simple to use and convenient to carry and that includes an adapter that allows attachment to a smart phone camera to record images (Foldscope, 2016).

The future of technology in health and education for these students is certainly bright. In 2015, Mark Zukerberg (the founder of Facebook) announced a collaboration with Eutelsat to place a satellite into a geostationary orbit to provide internet coverage to large parts of sub-Saharan Africa. Accordingly, smart phones and other Internet-capable devices will continue to narrow the "digital divide" between Africa and other parts of the world through the diffusion of ideas and information (Baliamoune-Lutz, 2003). Clearly, technology has been responsible for highlighting and addressing many distributive justice issues.

Figure 10: IHSA meeting, Nairobi, 2016

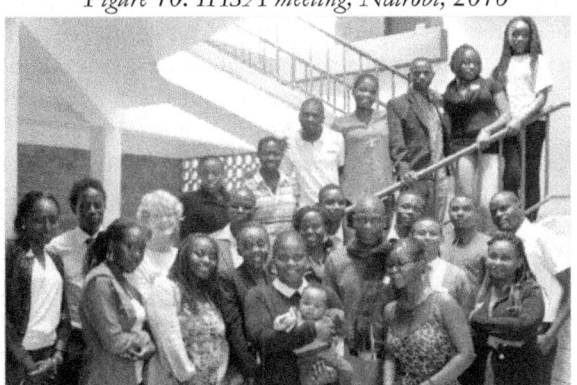

RESILIENCE

In the cockpit of a 747 plane bound for Hawaii is a little black box--a computer called "Fred." Every time the plane goes off course, Fred, who serves as the navigator, can tell how many degrees the plane's off. Fred then communicates to another computer called "George" who steers. When Fred communicates a necessary correction in course, George adjusts the plane's steering in the right direction.
The 747 is "off-course" about 90% of the time during the 5 1/2 hour flight to Hawaii. But Fred and George keep doing their job, and the plane lands safely on target in Hawaii--which isn't bad.
In learning something new, or in trying to transcend our habitual limits, we are always going to be a little off-course, just like the 747. Correction, either through feedback from the environment or another person, is a necessary part of the process of learning and living.
— R. *Fields in* Chop Wood, Carry Water *(1984, p. 23-24)*

Lessons Learned to Prepare for the Future

1. We have as much to learn from Kenyans as they have to learn from us. Americans are well known for problem-solving, an eager "can-do" outlook, and pro-active generosity, but this can prove a risky combination when encountering others with limited material resources. It is common to assume that "the American way is the best way," or that those in another culture lack expertise to solve their own problems. Experience has taught us first to observe, ask questions, and investigate local knowledge for answers to local problems. Africans don't need a neo-colonial handout, but a hand up. We've learned – sometimes the hard way – to examine our own habitual premises of reality. Contrary to our ethnocentric leanings, Americans aren't experts on everything! And, indeed, we are not called to be "white saviors."

2. Careful planning with foresight is needed to minimize unintended consequences. In Africa, we've encountered programs conceived in altruism that have failed due to a nearsighted approach to helping those in need. Specifically, nearsightedness can take the form of:

   a. Unfounded assumptions about the people, living conditions, and behavior patterns in a community.

   b. Lack of local engagement in or "ownership" of a project.

   c. Ineffective communication. We're at great risk of this when working in an English-speaking country. Our presumption is that, because we speak the same language, we grasp the meaning of what's being said and that others understand us.

   d. Unforeseen consequences. For instance, a well-constructed, well-equipped, new secondary school in a village was built by a prominent charity and hailed as a significant step forward in education. But we observed children fainting at their desks because they had walked several miles to the school having eaten nothing – teaching was futile in this situation. A better plan might have been to build a less impressive physical structure equipped with a porridge program to ensure that children begin the school day ready for learning. This demonstrates the need for problem-solving within a human context and the benefit of using a holistic approach that addresses more than one targeted need in a community. Good intentions and charity alone don't lead to realistic solutions; capacity-building with foresight and flexibility does.

3. Technology is not the most important instrument in the success of GROW A DOC and the IHSA, but it certainly ranks high because

a virtual community resulted from its rapid and frequent communications among the students and with us. All of the students rely on ICT for daily activities, so there is little doubt that ICT will continue to influence GROW A DOC's evolution and contribute to its sustainability. In the future, technology could include expanded international collaborations and education through continually improving virtual networks planned for all of Africa.

4. GROW A DOC is succeeding because it is part of an intertwined support and growth network of students, faculty, administrators, donors, and community members realistically looking at needs in communities and pragmatically sharing resources. Women's craft groups from Nairobi slums sell us items to market in the U.S., the profits of which all return to Africa. Additionally, the craft group leaders are collaborating with medical students to develop campus shops to help support their education. The metaphor of planting seeds is quite apt because once the seeds of networks are planted and nurtured, participants see results, develop new ideas, and continue to flourish. In the words of one GROW A DOC student: "I believe that the seeds you are planting in us will grow to very big trees with branches that will be home to many fine birds" (K.J., personal communication, June 10, 2015).

Benefits of networking within the university include faculty, administrators from private foundations, and students collaborating to develop grants, educational programs, international associations, and research projects. Another networking benefit of our holistic development strategy is the engagement of our newly minted professionals with other Project Harambee program sites. We are currently planning a "medical camp" for children's health evaluation and care at a dairy goat project supported by Project Harambee in rural Kenya.

5. Two factors are important to the sustainability of GROW A DOC. The first is funding. To date, the program has been maintained through the generosity of many small donors and sales of crafts and alternative gift cards. Assuming the status quo, funding will be sufficient for the present, but future growth is limited. This is a challenge for small NGOs. They are extremely efficient – the vast majority of funds go to projects – but they lack resources to attract larger funding for growth. A possible solution is an NGO co-operative where multiple smaller operations are organized under a larger umbrella organization that has the resources and development personnel needed to help secure more funding.

However, this raises a topic regarding small NGOs that can be delicate. Because a non-profit usually has been conceived and developed through the vision and dedication of an individual, there is a risk of exclusiveness or narrow focus. The view of an organization as one's "baby" is understandable, but could be counterproductive in the long run. We subscribe to the notion that, even in a competitive market, there are sufficient resources for all and we stress cooperative sharing whenever possible.

The second factor important to sustainability of any NGO is the replacement of its primary champion, the founder. Regardless of other factors important to sustainability, transition to new leadership from the visionary founder is critical and can be a significant challenge to a small NGO.

"Few will have the greatness to bend history itself; but each of us can work to change a small portion of events, and in the total of all those acts will be written the history of this generation."
— *R. F. Kennedy (1966, p.12,430)*

Our seven graduates, eight students, future candidates, and members of the International Healthcare Students Association will have careers that touch the lives of thousands. Because of their solidarity, commitment, and shared values of compassion and service, we expect the students and graduates to positively influence the future of their country. There are many well-qualified young people whose great potential will be lost because relatively modest funding is unavailable. We continue to identify them and honor their capability by advocating on their behalf.

Acknowledgements

Project Harambee has as its business model the story of the widow's mite. Our work has flourished for several years with the help of innumerable small investments in social justice by our donors, and we acknowledge and value equally a $5 donation and a more substantial gift. Nonetheless, several larger contributions have allowed us to confidently continue our work. We are particularly grateful to the following:

·St. Raphael Parish, Naperville, Illinois, Social Concerns Ministry
·A faithful annual anonymous donor
·St. Giles Family Mass Community, Oak Park, Illinois
·The John McGleam Family
·S.I.S.T.E.R.S., from St. Thomas More Parish, Glendale, Arizona

Additionally, we are indebted to a number of individuals who pass along medical tools, books, and supplies for GROW A DOC students. These greatly help in their education and are cherished resources in the areas where they work.

Contact Information

Address: PROJECT HARAMBEE, POB 1724, North Riverside, IL 60546
Email: keen@projectharambee.org
Facebook: Project Harambee, NFP

> *'Just what makes that little old ant*
> *think he'll move that rubber tree plant?*
> *Everyone knows an ant*
> *CAN'T*
> *move a rubber tree plant.*
> *But he had high hopes. High hopes!*
> *High apple pie in the sky hopes!*
> *So every time you're feeling low,*
> *instead of letting go, just remember that ant...*
> *Oops! There goes ANOTHER rubber tree plant!*
> *— Sammy Cahn (1959, stanza 1)*

References

Abbey, Edward. (1988). *The Fool's Progress: An Honest Novel.* New York, Henry Holt & Co.

Aker, J. C. & Mbiti, I. M. (2010). Mobile phones and economic development in Africa. *Journal of Economic Perspectives 24*(3): 207-232. doi=10.1257/jep.24.3.207

Baliamoune-Lutz, M. (2003). An analysis of the determinants and effects of ICT diffusion in developing countries. *Information Technology for Development 10*,151-169.

Buddhism. (2017). Retrieved May 12, 2017 from http://goldenruleproject.org/buddhism/.

Cahn, S. (1959). "High Hopes" (Recorded by Frank Sinatra). Los Angeles. Capitol Records.

Christianity. (2017). Retrieved May 12, 2017 from http://goldenruleproject.org/christianity/.

Clark, N. (2015, June 2). Education in Kenya. *World Education News and Review.* Retrieved from http://wenr.wes.org/2015/06/education-kenya

Cole, T. (2012, March 12). The white-savior industrial complex. *The Atlantic.* Retrieved from http://www.theatlantic.com/international/archive/2012/03/the-white-savior-industrial-complex/254843/?single_page=true

Czerniewicz, L., & Brown, C. (2010). Born into the digital age in the south of Africa: the reconfiguration of the "digital citizen". In Dirckinck-Holmfeld L., Hodgson V., Jones C., de Laat M., McConnell D. & Ryberg,T.. (Eds.). *Proc. 7th Int. Conf. Network Learning.* pp. 859-865. Retrieved from http://www.lancaster.ac.uk/fss/organisations/netlc/past/nlc2010/abstracts/PDFs/Czerniewicz.pdf.

Fields, R. (1984). *Chop Wood, Carry Water.* New York: Penguin Group.

Foldscope (2016). Retrieved from http://www.foldscope.com

Gituma, A., Masika, M., Muchangi, E., Nyagah, L., Otieno, V., Irimu, G., … English, M. (2009). Access, sources and value of new medical information – views of final year medical students at the University of Nairobi. *Tropical Medicine & International Health. 14,* 118-122. doi:10.1111/j.1365-3156.2008.02209.x.

Harrison, K., May, K., McNulty, J., & Ng'ang'a, Z. (2010). Genetics as a Component of World Health: Computer Networking With Medical Schools in Kenya for Education, Service, & Health Care. (Abstract) *American College of Medical Genetics Annual Clinical Genetics Meeting A329.*

Islam. (2017). Retrieved May 12, 2017 from http://goldenruleproject.org/islam/.

Judaism. (2017). Retrieved May 12, 2017 from http://goldenruleproject.org/judaism/.

Kaplan, W. A. (2006). Can the ubiquitous power of mobile phones be used to improve health outcomes in developing countries? *Globalization and Health, 2*(9). Doi: 10.1186/1744-8603-2-9.

Kennedy, R. F. (1966). Day of Affirmation. *Congressional Record, 112,* 12430.

Kenya Vision 2030. (2007, July-August). Retrieved from http://theredddesk.org/sites/default/files/vision_2030_brochure__july_2007.pdf

Kuo, L. (2016, July 19). Kenya is pressuring thousands of expat NGO workers and volunteers to go home. *Quartz Africa.* Retrieved from http://qz.com/716518/kenya-is-pressuring-thousands-of-expat-ngo-workers-and-volunteers-to-go-home/

Lansang M.A., & Rodolfo, D. (2004). Building capacity in health research in the developing world. *Bulletin of World Health Organization 82*(10), http://dx.doi.org/10.1590/S0042-96862004001000012

Merton, T.(1966). *Conjectures of A Guilty Bystander.* New York, Doubleday & Co.

Moonlightened Way. (2012). Retrieved May 12, 2017 from https://moonlightenedshelves.wordpress.com/2012/06/30/favorite_quote_by_ray_bradbury/.

National Bureau of Statistics-Kenya and ICF International. (2015). 2014 KDHS Key Findings. Rockville, Maryland, USA: KNBS and ICF International. Retrieved from https://www.dhsprogram.com/pubs/pdf/SR227/SR227.pdf

Neufeld V. (2001). Fostering a national capacity for equity-oriented health research. In Neufeld V, Johnson N (Eds.), *Forging links for health research: perspectives of the Council on Health Research for Development* (pp. 151-178). Ottawa: International Development Research Centre. p. 141-78. Retrieved from https://www.idrc.ca/en/book/forging-links-health-research-perspectives-council-health-research-development

Otieno, A., Gachoka, S., Hillary, E., Juma, F., Maingi, M., Mugire, S., … McNulty, J.A. (2014). Status of information and communication technology (ICT) in health profession education in Kenya. *International Journal of Research Education Methods 5*(2), 633-640.

Pang, T., Sadana, R., Hanney, S., Bhutta, Z., Hyder, A., & Simon, J. (2003). Knowledge for better health – a conceptual framework and foundation for health research systems. *Bulletin of the World Health Organization, 8,* 815-820.

Prensky, M. (2005). What can you learn from a cell phone? Almost anything! *Journal of Online Education 1*(5), 2.

Robert F. Kennedy. (2017). Retrieved May 12, 2017 from https://www.goodreads.com/author/quotes/98221.Robert_F_Kennedy.

Robert Kennedy in His Own Words. (2017). Retrieved May 12, 2017 from https://www.goodreads.com/work/quotes/332487-robert-kennedy-in-his-own-words-the-unpublished-recollections-of-the-ke.

United Nations. (1948). Universal declaration of human rights. Retrieved from http://www.un.org/en/universal-declaration-human-rights/index.html.

United Nations. (2016). Retrieved from http://www.un.org/sustainabledevelopment/

Waudo, S.W. (2014). Mount Kenya University Commencement Address, Thika, Kenya.

Wicca. (2017). Retrieved May 12, 2017 from http://goldenruleproject.org/wicca/.

Williams, C. D., Pitchforth, E. L., & O'Callaghan, C. (2010). Computers, the internet and medical education in Africa. *Medical Education, 44*, 485-488.

World Bank. (2015). Mortality rate, under-5 (per 1,000 live births). Retrieved from http://data.worldbank.org/indicator/SH.DYN.MORT

CHAPTER 26

Global Health and HIV/AIDS:
Yesterday, Today, and Tomorrow

Laura Reid Marks, Madeline Stenersen, and Shondolyn D. Sanders

In 2013, the Robert Wood Johnson Foundation named the acquired immunodeficiency syndrome (AIDS) the deadliest epidemic in world history, with a total of over 25 million estimated fatalities worldwide (para. 4). Sub-Saharan Africa, Asia and the Pacific, and the Caribbean are among the chief regions affected by the human immunodeficiency virus (HIV) and AIDS and contain 1.4 million, 340,000, and 13,000 newly infected individuals in 2014, respectively (The Henry J. Kaiser Family Foundation, 2015, para. 2). These statistics highlight that HIV/AIDS is an important global health concern that continues to persist in the modern world. Psychologists are ideally positioned to assist in the prevention and treatment of HIV/AIDS. Thus, in this chapter, we give an overview of: (a) what is HIV/AIDS, (b) global statistics of HIV/AIDS, (c) the role of psychologists in prevention, treatment, and research, (d) current advances and challenges in the treatment of HIV/AIDS, and (e) future directions for psychologists working in the HIV/AIDS field.

What is HIV/AIDS?

HIV is a virulent virus. It attacks the body's immune system, specifically CD4 cells, commonly known as T cells. These T cells help "fight off" infection in the body. Once infected by HIV, an individual's T cells begin to die and reduce in number. When an individual's T cell count falls to 200 cells per cubic millimeter of blood or lower, they are considered to have progressed to AIDS. AIDS is the fatal, late stages of HIV, during which the body is vulnerable to opportunistic infections (AIDS.GOV, 2014a).

There are two different strains of HIV: HIV-1 and HIV-2. The HIV-1 strain is generally what people refer to when talking about HIV. This strain has approximately four different groups: M, N, O, and P. The M group contains at least nine different subtypes (A, B, C, D, F, G, H, J, and K). HIV-1 group M is the strain of HIV that is responsible for the epidemic of the virus across the world (Campbell-Yesufu & Gandhi, 2011; Smyth, Davenport, & Mak, 2012). The vast majority of research on the HIV epidemic has been done on subtype B, most prevalent in the Americas, Western Europe, and Australasia (Hemelaar, 2012). However, this subtype only represents approximately 12% of the HIV infections globally (Hemelaar, 2012). Furthermore, although less research is available, subtype C accounts for roughly half of those living with HIV, with a higher prevalence in areas of Southern Africa and the horn of Africa and India (Fox, Castro, Kaye, Weber, & Fidler, 2010; Hemelaar, 2012). Some studies have found that certain subtypes of group M have a greater or lesser risk of transmission and a varied rate of progression when compared to the other subtypes (Pant Pai, Shivkumar, & Cajas, 2012). Conversely, the HIV-2 strain is relatively uncommon, appears to be concentrated in the region of West Africa, and is seen very rarely in other countries (Campbell-Yesufu & Gandhi, 2011; Ekouevi et al., 2014; Sharp & Hahn, 2011). Overall, this strain of HIV is less infectious and has a slower progression than its counterpart (Ekouevi et al., 2014).

It is widely believed that HIV developed from the simian immunodeficiency virus (SIV), a virus that attacks the immune system in monkeys and apes (Worobey et al., 2010). In 1999, scientists identified a specific strain of SIV (called SIVcpz) found in chimpanzees that proved to be almost identical to that of HIV in humans. The researchers who discovered this connection determined that this similarity meant that chimpanzees were the source of HIV-1 and that the virus must have, at some point, crossed from chimpanzees to humans (Gao et al., 1999; Sharp & Hahn, 2011; Worobey et al., 2010). The most popular theory among scientists as to how this happened is considered the "hunter" theory. According to it, SIVcpz was transferred to humans as a result of the hunting, killing, and eating of chimps in the wild, or as a result of their blood getting into hunters' cuts and wounds during the hunting process. The fact that there are multiple strains of HIV-1 supports this "hunter theory" in that every time SIV was passed from a chimp to a human, it would have likely developed in a different way within the hunter's body of and would have therefore produced a different strain (Sharp & Hahn, 2011). Other theories posit that the different strains likely came from chimps that had hunted and eaten different species of monkeys and thereby created a different strain of HIV-1 (Gao et al., 1999; AVERT, n.d.). In an article by Chen et al. in 1997, the authors hypothesize that unlike HIV-1, HIV-2 likely comes from an SIV strain identified as SIVsmm, which is found in sooty mangabey monkeys rather than chimpanzees. Despite the crossover to humans happening in a similar way to HIV-1 (i.e. the consumption and killing of monkeys), HIV-2's slowly progressive nature is much more rare and is currently only found in a few countries in West Africa (Chen et al., 1997; Sharp & Hahan, 2011).

Despite the widespread belief that HIV originated around 1920, information regarding the prevalence, symptoms, and progress of HIV/AIDS was not researched until the 1980s (AVERT, 2016). In 1981, the first cases of a severe immune deficiency disorder were discovered in gay men both in California and New York (AIDS.GOV, 2016, para. 2).These discoveries were widely considered by relevant researchers of the time to be the beginning of the HIV/AIDS global epidemic (AVERT, 2016). By the end of 1981, there were 270 reported cases of this severe immune deficiency among gay men, 121 of which were already deceased (AVERT, 2016, para. 7). In September of 1982, the United States Center for Disease Control and Prevention (CDC) first used the term AIDS to refer to the virus, defining it as "a disease at least moderately predictive of a defect in cell mediated immunity, occurring in a person with no known case for diminished resistance to that disease" (CDC, 1982a, para. 7). This declaration was followed by new discoveries of the virus in regions across the globe, as well as decades of new research, support, and prevention efforts to stop the virus.

With approximately 38,401 new cases of AIDS reported to the World Health Organization in 85 different countries by the end of 1986, the first approved antiretroviral drug, zidovudine (AZT), appeared in March 1987 (AIDSinfo., 1987, para. 8). AZT was the first available treatment for HIV. Regardless of this new treatment, in 1993, the United States voted overwhelmingly to maintain the ban on individuals living with HIV entering the county (AVERT, 2016). Despite new knowledge and treatment of the HIV/AIDS disease, stigma and persecution of those living with the virus continues today.

Global Statistics of HIV/AIDS

Since the beginning of the epidemic and its reporting in 1981, 78 million people have become infected with HIV, and approximately 35 million of them have died from AIDS-related illnesses (Joint United Nations Programme on HIV/AIDS; UNAIDS, 2016, para.1). Although HIV/AIDS does not discriminate based on race, sexual orientation, or gender, there are regions of the world that experience HIV/AIDS at a significantly different pace and prevalence when compared to other regions.

Further, within these regions, different groups appear more at risk (e.g., gay men, women, etc.), which makes HIV/AIDS a global health disparities issue.

Sub-Saharan Africa

According to the AVERT (2013), the Sub-Saharan region of Africa currently houses almost 71% of the world's HIV-positive population, and a total of an estimated 25.8 million people (more than half of whom are women) are living with the virus (para. 1). Of the countries in this region, Nigeria, South Africa, and Uganda account for more than half of all new HIV infections (UNAIDS, 2015, p. 116). In 2015 alone, 960,000 individuals became newly infected with HIV, and 470,000 people died of AIDS-related causes that year (UNAIDS, 2015, p. 7). According to UNAIDS, although this area continues to remain the region most heavily affected by HIV, it is also the one with many advances in the field of HIV prevention and treatment (UNAIDS, 2015). Of note, in these regions, HIV/AIDS has decreased when compared to previous years (UNAIDS, 2015). Additionally, since 2009, efforts to increase access to antiretroviral therapy (AVT) have prevented 1.1 million new infections in the region (UNAIDS, 2015, p. 120). In regards to sex workers in this region (a specific at-risk population for contracting HIV), the median number of deaths related to AIDS and HIV has declined by 42% since its peak in 2004 (UNAIDS, 2015, p. 118).

Despite progress, individuals living in this region of Africa remain more at-risk for contracting HIV than any other population globally. Sub-Saharan Africa's high prevalence of HIV may be, in part, traced back to its designation as the site of the first transmission of SIV to HIV in humans, which is estimated to have taken place around 1920 in the Democratic Republic of Congo (Faria et al., 2014). The first cases of AIDS were also reported in this same area (Faria et al., 2014). Sadly, this region now has the highest diversity of genetic strains of HIV, and this reflects the likely high incidence of SIV that was passed from chimpanzees to humans and that mutated into different strains in the process (Faria et al., 2014). These different strains add additional complexities to treatment of individuals who are positive for the virus.

The Caribbean

The Caribbean holds the second-highest HIV rate globally with an estimated 280,000 people living with HIV in the Caribbean in 2014 (UNAIDS, 2015, p. 124). This number includes an approximate equal number of men and women living with the virus and 13,000 children (UNAIDS, 2015, p. 124). However, there have been improvements in the incidence of new HIV infections in the Caribbean. In 2014, there were 13,000 individuals newly infected with the virus, which was a 50% decrease since 2000 (UNAIDS, 2015, p. 124). The Caribbean's success in prevention and treatment has a large connection to its continued and comprehensive efforts targeting HIV-positive pregnant women, with the goal of eliminating mother-to-child transmission of HIV (UNAIDS, 2015). This effort was possible, in part, due to the increased access to AVTs for the population of HIV-positive pregnant women on the islands, 89% of whom received the medication in 2014 (UNAIDS, 2015, p. 124).

However, there is disproportionality in the prevalence of HIV/AIDS between islands. Haiti accounted for approximately 50% of all new HIV infections in the Caribbean in 2014 (UNAIDS, 2015, p. 125). Haiti's large contribution to HIV infections in the Caribbean may be partially due to its high prevalence of the HIV-1 subtype B. This subtype appears to have made its way into the country in the 1960s when many Haitian professionals who were working in the colonial Democratic Republic of Congo returned to Haiti, bringing the virus with them (Faria et al., 2014). The HIV-1 subtype B is now the most geographically spread subtype of HIV around the world, with a total of 75 million infections reported to date (University of Oxford News, 2014, para. 2).

Asia and the Pacific

While the prevalence of HIV/AIDS in Asia and the Pacific in light of population size is much lower than that of Sub-Saharan Africa and the Caribbean, this area is home to the second-largest number of people living with HIV (an estimated five million in 2014) (UNAIDS, 2015, p. 127). Unlike Sub-Saharan Africa, the individuals living with HIV in this area are overwhelmingly male – there are 3.1 million males 15 years of age or older living with HIV, compared to the 1.7 million women in the same age range (UNAIDS, 2015, p. 127). Like other regions, however, the number of newly infected people in this region declined by 31% in 2014, with an estimated 340,000 people newly infected during that year (UNAIDS, 2015, p. 128).

The Middle East and North Africa

The Middle East and North Africa is one of only two regions where the annual number of new HIV infections is increasing. New infections rose by 26% from the year 2000 to 2015 (UNAIDS, 2015, p. 132). In 2014, approximately 22,000 new infections were reported in the area, and combined, the Islamic Republic of Iran, Somalia, and Sudan account for nearly three quarters of all new infections (UNAIDS, 2015, p. 132). Among high-risk populations in this area, gay men and men who have sex with men (MSM) bear a large burden of the new infections yearly and currently measure a prevalence of over 5% in 2014 in Algeria, Lebanon, and Tunisia (UNAIDS, 2015, p. 132). One reason for the increase in new HIV infections in these regions is probably lower rates of safe sex practices.

Condom coverage among sex workers in the Middle East remains high in both Algeria (96%) and Lebanon (84%), while the use of condoms remains below 35% in Egypt, Sudan, Somalia, and Yemen (UNAIDS, 2015, p. 132). As for North African countries, HIV prevalence among sex workers ranges from no infections found in Egypt to 10% in Algeria (as reported in 2014) (UNAIDS, 2015, p. 132).

Latin America

In Latin America during 2014, 1.7 million people, including 33,000 children, were living with HIV (UNAIDS, 2015, p. 135). Similar to the Middle East and Northern Africa, HIV in this region is significantly higher in men (1.1 million) than in women (UNAIDS, 2015, p. 135). In 2014, there were 87,000 people newly infected with HIV, which represented a decrease of 17% between then and 2000 (UNAIDS, 2015, p. 136). However, there has been little change in the number of new infections in the past five years (UNAIDS, 2015, p. 136). Of note, Brazil accounts for roughly half of the new HIV infections in Latin America (UNAIDS, 2015, p. 136).

Treatment of HIV in Latin America is among the highest in the world (UNAIDS, 2015, p. 139). In 2014, an estimated 47% of people living with HIV received AVT (UNAIDS, 2015, p. 139). The prevalence of HIV among high-risk populations has decreased to below 10% for all countries between 2011 and 2014, with the exception of Guyana and Uruguay in 2011 (UNAIDS, 2015, p. 136). This lower prevalence of HIV may be, in part, due to an extremely high level of condom coverage by sex workers such that in 13 out of the 15 countries, 84-99% of sex workers reported using condoms in their last client interaction (UNAIDS, 2015, p. 136).

Western and Central Europe and North America

Western and Central Europe and North America house the vast majority of the research released regarding HIV and its prevention and treatment. Despite the higher prevalence of HIV-2 elsewhere, the research frequently focuses on the HIV-1 strain, which is most prevalent in these regions. Of the 2.4 million people living with HIV in these regions, 1.9 million (nearly 80%) are men, and 140,000 are young people ages 15-24 (70% of whom are men) (UNAIDS, 2015, p. 139). Despite the prevalence of academic and medical research in the United States, these regions account for more than half of the new HIV infections in this region (UNAIDS, 2015, p. 140).

Eastern Europe and Central Asia

Eastern Europe and Central Asia contain an estimated 1.5 million people living with HIV (as determined by analyses in 2014; UNAIDS, 2015, p. 143). This 1.5 million is comprised of 900,000 men, 600,000 women, and

17,000 children (UNAIDS, 2015, p. 143). Despite having the lowest number of people living with HIV, this area continues to see a sharp increase in their number of HIV infected individuals. 140,000 people were newly infected in 2014, and there was a 300% increase from 2000 to 2014 (UNAIDS, 2015, p. 143). Of note, the Russian Federation accounted for the vast majority of new HIV infections in 2014 (UNAIDS, 2015, p. 143).

Summary

Overall, statistics from these regions highlight that whether or not a country is considered "developing" appears to contribute significantly to its ability to prevent and treat HIV/AIDS. Countries with more readily available access to condoms and nationwide education seem to see more success when attempting to lower the annual amount of new cases of HIV, as well as more success with treating the existing cases. In contrast, developing regions of the world, such as Sub-Saharan Africa, have, by far, the largest population of individuals living with HIV/AIDS, but demonstrate some of the most restricted access to prevention (e.g., condoms, education) and treatment (e.g., medication) methods.

The Role of Psychologists
in Prevention, Treatment, and Research

Psychologists have a crucial role to play in HIV prevention and treatment and in creating and implementing a research agenda for addressing psychological factors related to both living with an HIV/AIDS diagnosis and HIV/AIDS-related health disparities. Psychologists are equipped for these roles due their unique history of understanding how social systems interact with individual behavior to impact health, which is an expertise that has been critical in creating theory-driven and evidence-based strategies (Grossman, Purcell, Rotheram-Borus, & Veniegas, 2013).

Prevention and Treatment

Psychologists are well-positioned to work in the area of HIV-prevention and treatment. In 2015, the Office of National AIDS Policy (ONAP) released the "National HIV/AIDS Strategy for the United States: Updated to 2020" and highlighted four goals: (1) reducing new HIV incidence, (2) increasing access to care and optimizing outcomes, (3) reducing HIV-related health disparities, and (4) achieving a more coordinated response to the HIV-epidemic. Although developed for use within the United States, these strategies are useful on a global level. Further, addressing HIV/AIDS along the continuum should include biomedical, behavioral, and societal interventions, and psychologists are perfectly positioned to the assist with behavioral and societal interventions.

The first goal of reducing new HIV incidence involves an

acknowledgement that some groups are at a greater risk than others for HIV (ONAP, 2015). For example, in the United States, men who have sex with men (MSMS), Black women and men, Latino women and men, people who inject drugs, youth aged 13 to 24 years, people who live in the south, and transgendered women are disproportionally affected by the virus. Groups that are at most risk should be assessed and targeted for prevention. Psychologists can provide psychoeducation on HIV and AIDS and how it is contracted to populations at risk. Psychoeducation should have an emphasis on safe sex practices and the discouragement of injection drug use (the two most common ways in which HIV is contracted). Psychologists can also provide information on pre-exposure prophylaxis (PrEP), which is a new once-daily drug that can prevent HIV if taken consistently. Psychologists may have to provide referrals to medical providers who are likely to prescribe the drug to patients.

The second goal of increasing access to care and optimizing outcomes could be more challenging than the first as it involves more systemic changes (ONAP, 2015). This goal involves providing health care coverage for individuals living with HIV, improving outcomes at each stage of the HIV-continuum, and developing models to treat individuals holistically. Psychologists' holistic approach involves an acknowledgement of the psychological factors that keep people from seeking a diagnosis and/or treatment. These psychological factors could include fear of positive test results, perceived behavioral control/self-efficacy, and prejudiced attitudes towards people living with HIV (Evangeli, Pady, & Wroe, 2016), so psychologists should address these factors in outreach activities and in individual/group counseling. In addition to these factors, providers must address issues of stigma and prejudice against those who are HIV-positive, which may affect patient behaviors (e.g., medication adherence and decisions to tell social and familial networks). Further, psychologists are uniquely trained for interdisciplinary work and can aid in the development of holistic treatment models for patients in collaboration with medical providers. Integrated care settings are ideal for the treatment of HIV as they allow multiple providers to practice in a single location, which puts less stress on patients who often struggle with going to different providers at different agencies who may or may not communicate with each other.

The third goal of reducing HIV-related health disparities includes an understanding that HIV-related disparities exist at every step along the HIV testing-to-care continuum (ONAP, 2015). An integral part of ending the HIV epidemic is addressing HIV/AIDS-related health disparities (Clay, 2012; Grossman, Purcell, Rotheram-Borus, & Veniegas, 2013). In addition, it is important to address structural approaches that can reduce HIV transmission at community and societal levels and that can reduce stigma and discrimination that can hinder HIV prevention, testing, and care

(ONAP). Psychologists may advocate for structural changes within their organizations and communities – this has the potential to ultimately lessen health disparity gaps. Further, as mentioned above, psychologists can address issues of HIV stigma and discrimination in individual and group therapy with clients and educate those not living with the virus about the realities of HIV. Ultimately, through education about the virus, stigma and discrimination may decrease.

Finally, the fourth goal of achieving a more coordinated response to the HIV-epidemic involves psychologists working with other health and service providers on the prevention and treatment of HIV/AIDS (ONAP, 2015). Efforts should not occur in a vacuum but should be collaborative across all professions and should involve advocacy and reporting of data related to HIV/AIDS to track changes that occur annually in different regions.

Research

Following the decade in which AIDS was first diagnosed, behavioral research has focused intensively on risk reduction change processes (i.e. recognizing and labeling of one's sexual behaviors as high-risk for contracting HIV and making a commitment to reduce high-risk sexual contacts and increase low-risk activities) and, to a lesser extent, on mental health needs of persons living with HIV (Catania, Kegeles, & Coates, 1990; Kelly & Murphy, 1992). Psychology has contributed to the understanding of these needs with the help of scientific research in the form of descriptive studies of behavioral change or, less frequently, studies of behavioral outcomes of controlled intervention trials (American Psychological Association, n.d.).

In 2015, the APA made recommendations to the National HIV/AIDS Strategy that included that federal agencies, in addition to supporting research on structural factors, should specifically encourage research on current mental health and substance abuse issues that may play a role in HIV-risk behaviors and that may act as barriers to engagement and retention in care for individuals living with HIV/AIDS (American Psychological Association, 2015). Behavioral research can aid in HIV/AIDS prevention and care by examining ways in which to optimize medication adherence, to document real-world decision making processes associated with biomedical interventions, and to better understand the possible unintended and/or undesired consequences of biomedical interventions. To accomplish this, psychology must remain mobilized in conducting research on strategies for improving health outcomes and in continuing basic and applied research to identify and disseminate effective universal and selective prevention strategies (American Psychological Association, 2012). The optimal goal of behavioral research in regards to the treatment of HIV/AIDS is highlighted in the following statement by the APA:

> The epidemic, in turn, provides an opportunity to expand our research on behavior change, on the needs of people and families who are coping with a long-term disease, and on multicultural approaches to meeting the needs of populations affected by the AIDS epidemic. We have the opportunity to contribute the results of decades of behavioral research as well as to extend our understanding of the problems associated with initiating and maintaining behavior changes. (APA, n.d., para. 2)

Current Advances and Challenges in the Treatment of HIV/AIDS

Over the past few decades, there have been medical advances in the treatment of HIV/AIDS that have allowed many children and adults diagnosed with the disease to live longer and better-quality lives. Despite these advances, there continue to be significant challenges.

Advances

Today, a positive HIV diagnosis does not have to equate to a death sentence. The discovery of antiretroviral therapy (AVT) has allowed many diagnosed with the virus to live healthier and longer lives (AIDS.GOV, 2015). For AVT to be successful, positive individuals must take a combination of medications daily. The medication works by preventing the HIV from duplicating in the body, and it ultimately decreases the amount of the virus in the body. When the prevalence of the virus in the body is decreased, the immune system is supported, thus reducing the likelihood of developing fatal infections or cancer. Without AVT, an HIV-positive individual will experience a compromised immune system, which results in numerous negative health outcomes and eventually death.

There are six different drug classes with more than 25 different medications that can be used to fight HIV. These are: (1) non-nucleoside reverse transcriptase inhibitors (NNRTIs), (2) nucleoside reverse transcriptase inhibitors (NRTIs), (3) protease inhibitors (PIs), (4) fusion inhibitors, (5) CCR5 antagonists (CCR5s; also called entry inhibitors), and (6) integrase strand transfer inhibitors (INSTIs). Although these drugs allow patients to live longer, like all medications, there are short- and long-term side effects that can affect patients' ability or willingness to continue taking the medications as prescribed. In terms of short-term side effects, individuals may experience symptoms such as anemia, diarrhea, dizziness, fatigue, headaches, pain and nerve problems, and nausea and vomiting (AIDS.GOV, 2015). In terms of long-term side effects, individuals my experience symptoms such as insulin resistance (a condition that can lead to abnormalities in blood sugar, which may lead to diabetes), lipid abnormalities (i.e., increases in cholesterol and triglycerides), and a decrease in bone density (which can lead to an increase in injury and broken bones) (AIDS.GOV, 2015). The choice of drugs is thus something that should be discussed thoroughly between patient and medical provider. Some considerations may include comorbid conditions, potential drug interactions, and side effects of the medication.

Previously, an HIV-positive diagnosis in an expecting mother would have also meant an HIV-positive diagnosis for her baby (AVERT, 2016). Today however, the effects of AVT are also beneficial to babies in utero. By taking daily AVT, pregnant women decrease the chances of passing the HIV virus on to their babies. This benefit continues once the baby is born and whether or not the mother chooses to breastfeed her child. By taking AVT, the chance of passing on the virus to their newborn through breastfeeding is reduced. However, it should be noted that formula feeding is safest and that once a baby reaches six weeks old, he or she should take once-daily nevirapine (NVP) to lessen the chances of contracting the virus. With these medications and precautions, mothers living with HIV can give birth to healthy babies without the virus.

The most recent advancement in the medical treatment of HIV/AIDS has been the development of pre-exposure prophylaxis (PrEP). PrEP is a once-a-day pill. PrEP can prevent an individual from contracting HIV (CDC, 2016). The pill is meant to be taken by individuals who are at higher risk of contracting the virus due to risky behaviors such as unprotected sex and injection drug use. PrEP is only effective if taken consistently and requires close monitoring by a medical provider. Although PrEP provides significant implications for prevention, the drug is controversial, and some suggest that the PrEP option leads people to practice risky behaviors as they may feel less concerned about negative health consequences (Byrne, 2015).

Challenges

Despite advances in the medical treatment and prevention of HIV/AIDS, there continue to be numerous challenges, including: continued practice of risky behaviors (e.g., sexual behaviors and injection drug use), medication adherence concerns, issues around testing, stigma and poverty (among other factors that influence the prevention and treatment of HIV/AIDS) (Schwarcz et al, 2011). These challenges lead to thousands being diagnosed with HIV annually, including babies born with the virus. These challenges highlight the need for continued efforts in the area of prevention and treatment of HIV.

First and foremost, risky behaviors continue to be a huge challenge in reducing the prevalence of new HIV/AIDS cases. "Risky behaviors" include having sexual encounters without the use of a condom, having sexual encounters with multiple simultaneous partners, and sharing syringes for the purpose of injected drug use (CDC, 2016). Individuals who are unaware they have the virus may accidently pass the virus on to someone who is HIV-negative. In addition, some still practice behaviors that facilitate HIV's transmission even though they are aware they have the virus. The majority of new HIV-positive cases in the United States are the result of sexual behaviors between MSMs. Less than 10 percent of new cases in the United States are the result of injection drug use (CDC, 2015, para. 2). To address this problem, agencies such as the CDC provide funding to local agencies to provide HIV-prevention services, to support interventions services to decrease risky behaviors, to increase funding for PrEP, to publish guidelines to assist in treatment and prevention, and to administer surveys to keep abreast of new risk factors and groups affected by HIV (CDC, 2015a). However, progress is not as it should be.

Medication adherence is a significant problem for those living with HIV. Medication adherence refers to taking the necessary AVT daily for the management of HIV viral loads (AIDS.GOV, 2016). Factors associated with medication adherence include: (1) the patient's social situation and clinical condition, (2) the prescribed medication, and (3) the patient-provider relationship (Department of Health and Human Services, 2015). Situations that may lead to patient nonadherence include behavioral, structural, or psychosocial barriers. For example, patients may struggle with depression and other mental illnesses, neurocognitive impairments, low literacy, poverty, inadequate social support, alcohol or substance abuse and dependence, or stigma. In regards to the prescribed medication regiment, patients who are on a one-pill-a-day schedule and medications with lower side effects tend to be more medically adherent. Some HIV medication regimens require individuals to take medications throughout the day and specify whether the patient should take the medication on an empty or full stomach. Finally, those who report a positive relationship with their medical provider tend to be more medically adherent.

HIV-testing, or more specifically, a lack of HIV-testing also continues to be a huge factor in the prevalence of new HIV infections. Many adults living with the disease are unaware of their positive-HIV status. For example, in the United States, more than 150,000 individuals are unaware that they have the virus (AIDS.GOV, 2014b, para. 10). As a result, when these individuals have unprotected sex or share drug-related syringes, they spread the virus. Once individuals know they have the disease, they can begin treatment to extend their life and take steps to reduce chances of spreading the disease to others. However, although the CDC recommends that patients between the ages of 13 and be tested for HIV/AIDs, in reality, this recommendation is not being followed due to barriers in medical facilities and decisions on the side of the patient (Department of Health and Human

Services, 2015).

Another significant challenge in the prevention and treatment of HIV/AIDS is stigma and fear. Stigma and fear is a barrier to both HIV-testing and medication adherence. Many people fear that they will be discriminated against if they have an HIV-positive diagnosis (Schwarcz et al., 2011). Thus, out of fear, individuals do not get tested. Further, if individuals do have a positive HIV-test, they fear that if they take AVT, others may discover that they are living with the virus. Thus, they are non-adherent to medications. Further, due to fear and stigma, HIV-positive individuals are less likely to share their positive status with their friends and family, which makes them less likely to receive the emotional support they need (UNAIDS, 2014a).

Poverty is another challenge that complicates the treatment and prevention of HIV/AIDS. For the most part, those living in poverty are disproportionally affected by the virus. For example, in the United States, those living with HIV seem to be located in poor urban cities (CDC, 2015). Further, developing countries are also disproportionally affected by the virus. However, the inverse is true in some countries in Africa (Parkhurst, 2010). Poverty might be positively related to HIV diagnosis because, with basic levels of sustenance not met, individuals are more likely to practice unprotected sex and share drug-related needles. Individuals living in poverty are also less likely to be tested for HIV, and if tested and given a positive HIV result, they are less likely to take medications, which can be costly (amfAR, 2016; Office of Women's Health, 2011).

Future Directions for
Psychologists Working in the HIV/AIDS Field

As mentioned previously, psychologists have an important role to play in the prevention efforts and treatment of HIV. According to "Guidelines for the Use of Antiretroviral Agents in HIV-1-Infected Adults and Adolescents," developed in 2016 by the Department of Health and Human Services, it is important to employ a multidisciplinary approach to HIV prevention and care, of which psychologists should be a part.

In terms of prevention, psychologists will continue to have an important role in educating individuals about HIV-testing and HIV-risk factors. In their clinical and research roles in community clinics, hospitals, and other agencies, psychologists should continue to provide psychoeducation on how HIV is transmitted by offering workshops and trainings about the virus. Psychologists should also continue to provide psychoeducation in individual sessions with patients, especially patients who are at risk for contracting HIV. It is also appropriate for psychologists to have conversations with patients about PrEP if they are practicing HIV-risk behaviors. Further, psychologists should continue to provide information on having a healthy baby despite an HIV diagnosis and should connect pregnant women with medical providers. Last, psychologists should advocate more for attention to HIV-prevention in their local and regional communities and on a national level. Advocacy can lead to increased prevention interventions (e.g., free HIV-testing through local clinics and in high risk areas, free condoms, and free information on safe sex).

Psychologists will also continue to have an important role in HIV-treatment. Psychologists should continue to provide individual counseling to patients recently diagnosed with HIV. The process of accepting that one has HIV is difficult and can take time to overcome in therapy. Psychologists may need to help patients process feelings of guilt with regards to how they contracted the disease and work with patients on self-forgiveness. Psychologists can also coach patients about "breaking the news" to loved ones so they have the necessary support of family and friends as they learn to live with HIV. Moreover, they can continue to discuss stigma with patients. Finally, psychologists can work more in collaboration with other medical providers to assess a patient's readiness to start AVT and to identify a patient's possible barriers to engaging in AVT.

Conclusion

With more than 35 million fatalities worldwide (WHO, 2016, para. 1), HIV/AIDS continues to be a global health issue. Psychologists have an important role in research and prevention and treatment efforts. By reducing new HIV infections, improving access to care and health outcomes for HIV-positive individuals, reducing HIV-related health disparities, and achieving a more coordinated response to the epidemic, we may see tangible global improvements. Psychologists are ideally positioned to help reduce HIV/AIDS on a global scale by contributing to progress in these areas.

References

AIDS.GOV (2009). Just diagnosed with HIV AIDS: Treatment options: Side effects. Retrieved from https://www.aids.gov/hiv-aids-basics/just-diagnosed-with-hiv-aids/treatment-options/side-effects/index.html

AIDS.GOV (2014a). What Is HIV/AIDS? Retrieved from https://www.aids.gov/hiv-aids-basics/hiv-aids-101/what-is-hiv-aids/

AIDS.GOV (2014b). U.S. statistics. Retrieved from https://www.aids.gov/hiv-aids-basics/hiv-aids-101/statistics/

AIDS.GOV (2015) Just diagnosed with HIV AIDS: Treatment options: Overview of HIV treatments. Retrieved from https://www.aids.gov/hiv-aids-basics/just-diagnosed-with-hiv-aids/treatment-options/overview-of-hiv-treatments/

AIDS.GOV (2016). A Timeline of HIV/AIDS. Retrieved from https://www.aids.gov/hiv-aids-basics/hiv-aids-101/aids-timeline/

AIDSinfo. (1987). Approval of AZT. Retrieved from https://aidsinfo.nih.gov/news/274/approval-of-azt

American Psychological Association (n.d.). The role of the psychologist in responding to the HIV/AIDS epidemic. Retrieved from http://www.apa.org/pi/aids/resources/role.aspx

American Psychological Association. (2012). Combination biomedical and behavioral approaches to optimize HIV prevention. Retrieved from http://www.apa.org/about/pwhatolicy/biomedical-hiv.pdf

American Psychological Association. (2015). Recommendations on federal agency national HIV/AIDS strategy for the United States: 2020 implementation plans. Retrieved from http://www.apa.org/about/gr/pi/news/2015/hiv-aids-strategy.pdf

AmfAR (2015). Statistics: Women and HIV/AIDS. Retrieved from http://www.amfar.org/About-HIV-and-AIDS/Facts-and-Stats/Statistics--Women-and-HIV-AIDS/

AVERT. (n.d.). Origin of HIV & AIDS. Retrieved from http://www.avert.org/professionals/history-hiv-aids/origin

AVERT (2013). HIV and AIDS in Sub-Saharan Africa: Regional overview. Retrieved from http://www.avert.org/professionals/hiv-around-world/sub-saharan-africa/overview

AVERT (2016) Fact sheet: HIV and pregnancy. Retrieved from https://www.avert.org/learn-share/hiv-fact-sheets/pregnancy

AVERT (2016). History of HIV and AIDS overview. Retrieved from http://www.avert.org/professionals/history-hiv-aids/overview

Byrne, J. (2015). When condoms aren't enough. Retrieved from http://www.theatlantic.com/health/archive/2015/12/truvada-hiv-prep-stigma/418119/

Campbell-Yesufu, O.T. & Gandhi, R.T. (2011). Update on human immunodeficiency virus (HIV)-2 infection. *Clinical Infectious Diseases, 52*, 780-787. doi: 10.1093/cid/ciq248

Catania, J., Kegeles, S., and Coates, T. (1990). Towards and understanding of risk behavior: An AIDS risk reduction model (ARRM). *Health Education Quarterly, 17*(1), 53-72.

Centers for Disease Control (CDC; 1982a). Current trends update on acquired immune deficiency syndrome (AIDS)- United States. *MMWR Weekly, 31*, 507-508,513-514.

Centers for Disease Control (CDC; 1982b). Opportunistic infections and Kaposi's Sarcoma among Haitians in the United States. *MMWR Weekly, 31*, 353-354.

Centers for Disease Control and Prevention (CDC; 2015a). HIV and injection drug use in the United States. Retrieved from http://www.cdc.gov/hiv/risk/idu.html

Chen, Z., Luckay, A., Sodora, D.L., Telfer, P., Reed, P, Kanu, J.M., … Marx, P.A. (1997). Human immunodeficiency virus type 2 (HIV-2): seroprelavence and characterization of a distinct HIV-2 genetic subtype from the natural range of simian immunodeficiency virus-infected sooty mangebeys. *Journal of Virology, 71*, 3953-3960.

Clay, R. (2012). The psychology of HIV/AIDS prevention. *Monitor on Psychology, 43*(7). Retrieved from http://www.apa.org/monitor/2012/07-08/hiv-aids.aspx

Department of Health and Human Services (2015). Guidelines for the use of antiretroviral agents in HIV-1-infected adults and adolescents. Retrieved from http://aidsinfo.nih.gov/guidelines

Ekouevi, D,K., Tchounga, B.K. Coffie, P.A., Tegbe, J., Anderson, A., Gottlieb, G.S., … Eholie, S.P. (2014). Antiretroviral therapy response among HIV-2 infected patients: a systematic review. *BMC Infectious Diseases, 14*, 461. doi: 10.1186/1471-2334-14-461

Evangeli, M., Pady, K., and Wroe, A. (2016). Which psychological factors are related to HIV testing? A quantitative systematic review of global studies. *Aids Behavior, 20*, 880-918. doi: 10.1007/s10461-015-1246-0

Faria, N.R., Rambaut, A., Suchard, M.A., Baele, G., Bedford, T., Ward, M.J., … Lemey, P. (2014). The early spread and epidemic ignition of HIV-1 in human populations. *Science, 346*, 56-61. doi: 10.1126/science.1256739

Fox, J., Castro, H., Kaye, S., Weber, J.N., & Fidler, S. (2010). Epidemiology of non-B clade forms of HIV-1 in men who have sex with men in the UK. *AIDS, 24*, 2397-2401. doi: 10.1097/QAD.0b013e32833cbb5b

Gao, F., Bailes, E., Robertson, D.L., Chen, Y., Rodenburg, C.M., Michael, S.F., . . . Hahn, B.H (1999). Origin of HIV-1 in the chimpanzee Pan troglodytes troglodytes. *Nature, 397*, 436-441. doi:10.1038/17130

Grossman, C. I., Purcell, D. W., Rotheram-Borus, M. J., & Veniegas, R. (2013). Opportunities for HIV combination prevention to reduce racial and ethnic health disparities. *American Psychologist, 68*, 237-246. doi:10.1037/a0032711

Hemelaar, J. (2012). The origin and diversity of the HIV-1 pandemic. *Trends in Molecular Medicine, 18*, 182-192. doi: 10.1016/j.molmed.2011.12.001

Joint United Nations Programme on HIV/AIDS (UNAIDS; 2014a). The gap report. Retrieved from http://www.unaids.org/sites/default/files/media_asset/UNAIDS_Gap_report_en.pdf

Joint United Nations Programme on HIV/AIDS (UNAIDS; 2014b). Reduction of HIV-related stigma and discrimination. Retrieved from http://www.unaids.org/sites/default/files/media_asset/2014unaidsguidancenote_stigma_en.pdf

Joint United Nations Programme on HIV/AIDS (UNAIDS; 2015). How AIDS changed everything: Mdg 6: 15 years, 15 lessons of hope from the AIDS response. Retrieved from http://www.unaids.org/sites/default/files/media_asset/MDG6Report_en.pdf

Joint United Nations Programme on HIV/AIDS (UNAIDS; 2016). UNAIDS Fact Sheet 2016 – Global Statistics 2015 [Fact sheet]. Retrieved from http://www.unaids.org/sites/default/files/media_asset/UNAIDS_FactSheet_en.pdf

Kelly, J., & Murphy, D. (1992). Psychological interventions with AIDS and HIV: Prevention and treatment. *Journal of Consulting and Clinical Psychology, 60*, 576-585. doi: http://dx.doi.org/10.1037/0022-006X.60.4.576

Office of Women's Health (2011). Barriers to care for HIV/AIDS. Retrieved from http://www.womenshealth.gov/hiv-aids/living-with-hiv-aids/barriers-to-care-for-hiv-aids.html

Pant Pai, N., Shivkumar, S., & Cajas, J.M. (2012). Does genetic diversity of HIV-1 non-B subtypes differentially impact disease progression in treatment-naive HIV-1-infected individuals? A systematic review of evidence: 1996-2010. *Journal of Acquired Immune Deficiency Syndromes, 59*, 382-388. doi: 10.1097/QAI.0b013e31824a0628

Robert Wood Johnson Foundation (2013). The five deadliest outbreaks and pandemics in history. Retrieved from http://www.rwjf.org/en/culture-of-health/2013/12/the_five_deadliesto.html

Schwarcz, S, Richards, T.A., Wenzel, C., Hsu, L.C., Chin, C.S., Murphy, J. & Dilley, J. (2011). Identifying barriers to HIV testing: Personal and contextual factors associated with late HIV testing. *AIDS Care, 23*, 892-900. doi: 10.1080/09540121.2010.534436

Sharp, P.M. & Hahn, B.H. (2011). Origins of HIV and the AIDS pandemic. *Cold Spring Harbour Perspectives in Medicine, 1*, 1-22. doi: 10.1101/cshperspect.a006841

Smyth, R.P., Davenport, M.P., & Mak, J. (2012). The origin of genetic diversity in HIV-1. *Virus Research, 169*, 415-429. doi: 10.1016/j.virusres.2012.06.015

The Henry J. Kaiser Family Foundation (2015). The global HIV/AIDS epidemic. Retrieved from http://files.kff.org/attachment/fact-sheet-the-global-hivaids-epidemic

The Office of National AIDS Policy (ONAP; 2015). National HIV/AIDS strategy for the United States: Updated to 2020. Retrieved from https://www.aids.gov/federal-resources/national-hiv-aids-strategy/nhas-update.pdf

University of Oxford News (2014). HIV pandemic's origins located. Retrieved from http://www.ox.ac.uk/news/2014-10-03-hiv-pandemics-origins-located

World Health Organization (2016). HIV/AIDS. Retrieved from http://www.who.int/mediacentre/factsheets/fs360/en/

Worobey, M., Telfer, P., Souquière, S., Hunter, M., Coleman, C.A., Metzger, M.J., . . . Marx, P.A. (2010). Island biogeography reveals the deep history of SIV. *Science, 329*, 1487. doi: 10.1126/science.1193550

CHAPTER 27

Capacity Strengthening Defined by Local Organizations

Neena S. Jain and A. Maya Casagrande

Introduction

The principle that seems clear is that each individual's journey is sacred and each individual's freedom is sovereign — regardless of their circumstances. This is in contrast to the paternalistic mentality of "aid" that imposes a solution on people instead of empowering them in support of what the people themselves sense they need. - Steve Melville, CEO and Founder, Evolutionary Enterprises LLC (S. Melville, personal communication, July 14, 2002).

Figure 1: Our team's global work
©emBOLDen Alliances

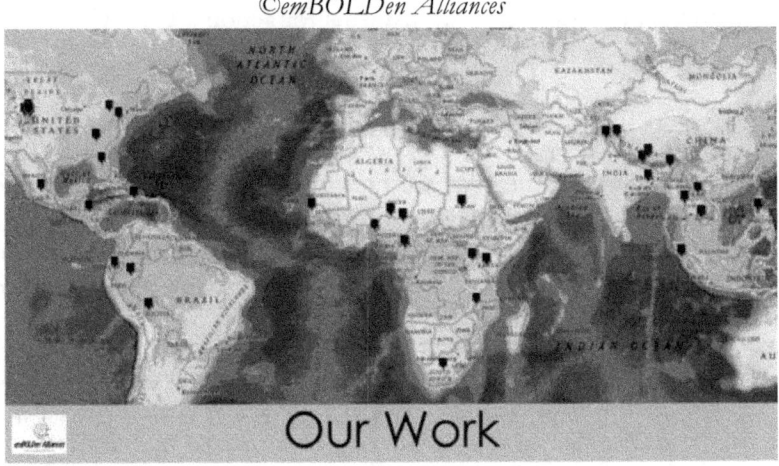

emBOLDen Alliances' humanitarian assistance and international development professionals have collectively spent over 65 years working directly with communities in locations, organizations, and contexts spanning the globe – each situation dramatically different from the last. During times of crises or development, we have witnessed common themes: communities knowing best for themselves, community-based organizations with can-do attitudes, successful and novel grassroots-driven approaches, and meaningful relationships at multiple levels of community and society.

But we have also seen firsthand many top-down models that fostered inefficacy and drowned out community voice. Between the traditional "charity" approach of handouts, the common "one size fits all" model, and insufficient resources and understanding for translating good intentions into meaningful action, we witnessed the limitations of existing methods in the field for far too long.

> *"Local NGOs are taking the risks, are the first responders, are the innovators. But we are persistently sidelined – in Nepal, in Philippines and in a grotesque way in Haiti."*
> — *Degan Ali, Head of Adeso Africa (van der Zee, 2015, para. 9)*

Programs are not completed and funding is misdirected, not tracked, and often wasted. Community voice and locally-based solutions are overlooked. Highly intelligent, capable, and dedicated people with wonderful skills and talents are disregarded. Resources are diverted from those most in need. "Sustainability" is laced with organizations' intentions to prolong their interventions indefinitely. Local systems and knowledge are ignored and parallel, duplicate mechanisms for action are created.

Listening Locally

Various methods are emerging to improve traditional models and patch the sectors' holes. Based on our experience with the glaring shortcomings of aid and development, emBOLDen Alliances is taking a different approach. As a registered 501(c)3 organization, we have created and continue to implement an innovative model whereby we serve as an "incubator" of sorts for other NGOs, specifically those embedded in their own communities throughout the developing world.

> *"In my opinion and experience, aid is most effective when it is delivered with local training and carried out with local people…I believe that we should not see it as aid but start seeing it as investment"* (Alford, 2015, para. 8).

Through hands-on partnerships specifically fashioned to solve operational and programmatic challenges that partners self-identify, we function as a catalyst for these locally-based partners to measure impact and maximize resources (whether they be human, capital, financial, or physical). Our model has already proven to be successful in various contexts globally and has earned global awards and the interest of development professionals, NGOs, and various humanitarian institutions. The response we receive most frequently is "Oh, that is so needed," followed by, "No one else is doing this."

emBOLDen Alliances is firmly committed to fostering durable impact with (not for) communities and knows that this can only be achieved when organizations have support customized to their unique context and needs. This requires putting listening at the center of our iterative methodology. It also requires:

· Learning to be prioritized,

· Skills and tools to be adapted and tested in real-time, and

· Community-driven solutions to be the focus at all times.

> *"Less than 2% of all humanitarian funding goes directly to local NGOs, despite them taking the lion's share of the risk and often being better placed to deliver, according to aid insiders" (van der Zee, 2015, para. 1).*

Figure 2: emBOLDen Alliances' Methodology
©emBOLDen Alliances

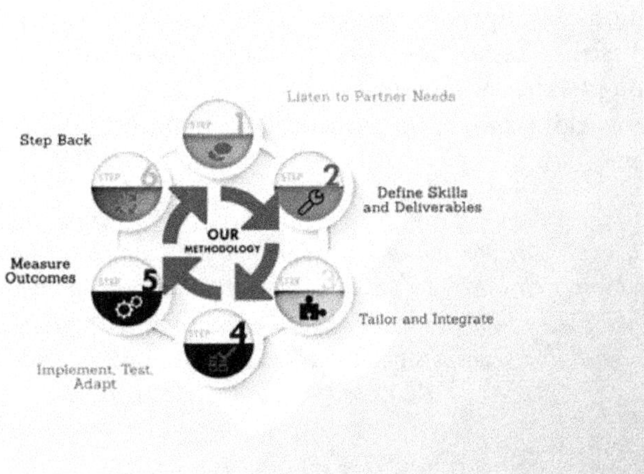

The people who are concerned most intimately with humanitarian action – those who are personally affected by a crisis – tend to be marginalised by current approaches to evidence generation in two important ways. First, they do not get to ask the questions: evidence is generally collected to meet the needs of international organisations, rather than those of affected people. Assessments, for example, tend to obtain evidence for what sort of aid is needed, rather than for whether aid is needed in the first place. Second, their answers are often not seen to be important: this review has suggested that even when gathering evidence to understand whether a situation is a crisis, or whether a particular intervention 'worked', the knowledge and opinions of those most directly affected tend to receive only limited attention. In future, international organisations should be clear about why they are collecting evidence and who it is for; should consider the degree to which they can collect evidence that is of use to civil society organisations in affected areas, and should make strenuous efforts to include the voices of affected people in their evidence collection. International organisations should identify the information and evidence needs of civil society organisations in disaster-affected areas and provide information to meet these needs. Where relevant, they should also provide training and resources to allow national and local organisations to collect information. (Knox Clarke & Darcy, 2014, p. 69)

Building from the grassroots up, we use our first-hand experience to create, implement, and build success together with communities who, with the right support, are often best-positioned for success. They know themselves best, are often ready to scale or enhance, and are passionately driven to improve the lives of their own members. We address organizations' self-identified challenges in any and every area in both operations and programming. In short, we assist local organizations in going farther faster, and we ultimately maximize funders' dollars so that continued external investment may, one day, no longer be needed. Change in the world does not come from investing in things, but from investing in people.

> *"I would love not to be doing my job and for aid no longer to be needed. But in this imperfect world, we first need to ensure that aid is as effective as possible. To do that we need to ensure that it is delivered without strings attached, with a targeted and grassroots approach that seeks to empower people to take control of their lives" (Alford, 2015, para. 10).*

Proof Points

The unanimous feedback that we have received from our partners to date – that they are all better able to positively impact their communities as a direct result of our partnerships – is, for us, the overarching measure of our model's efficacy. As we dig deeper, we see its success in different development and crisis contexts.

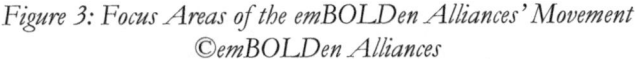

Figure 3: Focus Areas of the emBOLDen Alliances' Movement
©emBOLDen Alliances

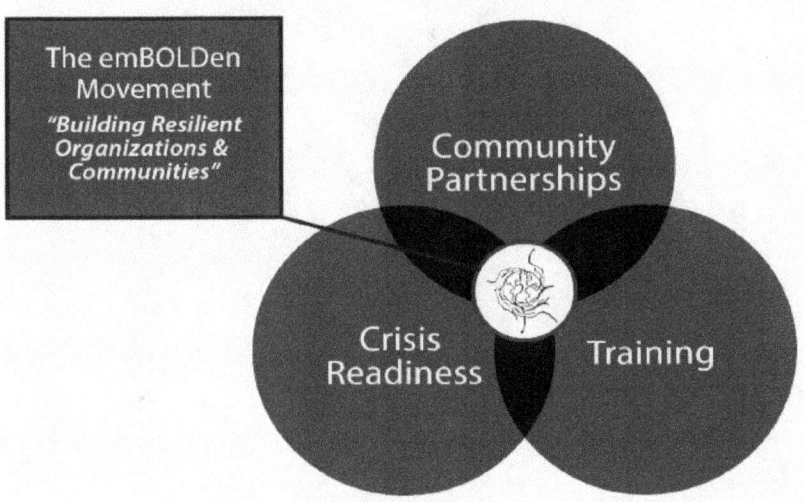

Here, we share case studies and selected stories that highlight the expertise, dignity, and profound resilience of our local, community-based partners as well as the efficacy and flexibility of our proven methodology. These serve to illustrate how, but moreover, why we put each partner in the "driver's seat" to define their own needs, meet those needs, and reach their next level.

Dignity

A young girl living on the edge of the Sahara Desert lives in a land that rarely sees rainfall and where temperatures regularly range from 86°F to 122°F (Briney, n.d., para. 9). Her family lives off what little land they own and has to survive on less than $2 per day. Should her family be able to send and support her, the girl may be able to attend school intermittently for a few years. Here, the legal age of marriage is 15 years old, and the chances of her being married before she is 18 years of age are nearly 75% (UNICEF, 2013, para. 9).

Figure 4: "Dignity" by Bill Rohs
©Bill Rohs

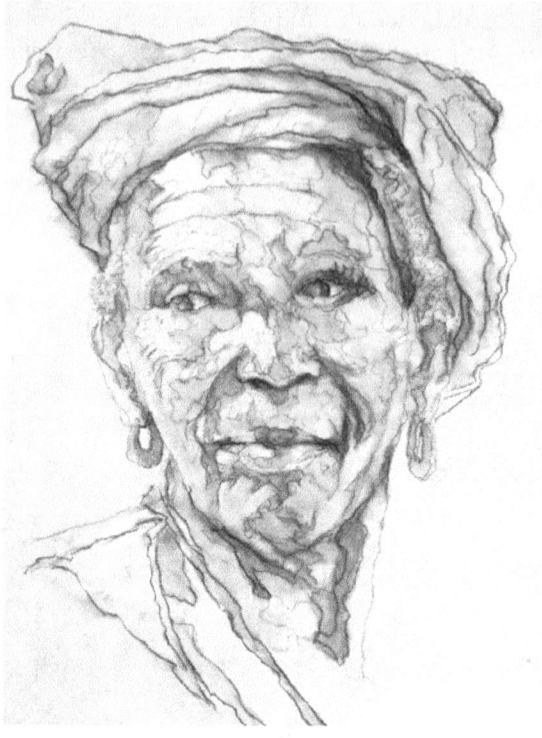

She marries at this young age, before the growth of her bones and her nutrition are able to sufficiently and safely carry a child, yet she becomes pregnant. Living far from a health facility and unable to access health care quickly enough or to afford appropriate care, she can lose one, two, three, or more of her pregnancies. During one of her pregnancies, the baby gets stuck in the birth canal and is unable to be born. She cannot access help in time and is left with a dying fetus as well as pressure from that fetus resting on her vagina, bladder, and rectum. This sustained pressure can cause destruction of the tissues and create an abnormal passage, or an obstetric fistula between these organs, causing her to leak urine or feces continuously.

Smelling of the urine that is constantly leaking onto her clothes and the ground around her, the girl is left outside her home to live with the animals. At times, the destruction of her tissues leaves her with nerve damage to her lower limbs. Being left immobile and afraid to go out, her limbs can contract and atrophy. She feels alone and isolated, scared for herself and her surviving children.

emBOLDen Alliances had the fortune to meet one such girl – Halimatou. Halimatou had had eight pregnancies, of which she had lost four. During her ninth pregnancy, the baby was stuck in the birth canal. This baby also died, and she developed a severe fistula causing her to continually leak urine. Halimatou had sought help at local health facilities where they were unable to repair her condition surgically. She had come to this new fistula center in search of hope – one last attempt to regain a "normal" life.

What she found was a comprehensive fistula center run entirely by West African staff, where women just like her were able to gather together, share their stories, and find a home amongst each other. They cared for each other's children when a mother went in for surgery. The older women, like Halimatou, comforted the younger women, and the younger women, in turn, helped the older. While at the center, they were taught how to read and write; some learned how to knit and sew. Most of all, they could envision a better life and learned to dream again.

On examination, Halimatou's damage was unfortunately beyond repair, yet the hospital director immediately saw how helpful and kind she was to the other patients. Finding herself in a new role as a staff member, she was welcomed and treated with respect. With pride, she worked tirelessly to help others. This woman, who was considered "incurable" after 7 surgeries and who would leak urine for all her days to come, found her new home and regained her dignity. Halimatou had found her hope, and was helping those around her find it too.

Niger has one of the highest rates of child marriage in the world, and women often lack access to timely and adequate maternal care (EngenderHealth, 2003). The low education completion rates for girls, high rates of child pregnancy, and lack of access to health care equate to high rates of obstetric fistula, a preventable condition (EngenderHealth, 2003; World Bank, 2015).

The West African staff of this obstetric fistula care facility was doing a terrific job with their clinical and basic literacy programs, but saw the need to improve their hospital operations, logistics, programming, and inventory. They wanted to do more with their resources, be sustainable, and scale up their work to increase their reach and impact.

emBOLDen Alliances partnered with the staff on their administrative needs, including human resources, tracking of expenses, and a three-year budget to match a programmatic scale-up. We worked with them to inventory all medical supplies and implemented a customized system to track supplies across all areas of the center and therefore avoid stock-outs. Together, we analyzed and integrated data and reporting from all programs, starting with clinical and basic literacy, and then outreach, prevention, and social reintegration/livelihoods.

In short, our partnership helped this team do what they were already doing in a way that fostered sustainability so that they could reach more women like Halimatou. They could now also measure and demonstrate that their programs were impacting knowledge and awareness among communities, helping to convince village elders to keep girls in school, and promoting job possibilities for the patients to support themselves and their families. The patients at the fistula center then had a better chance to keep their own girls in school and break the cycles of poverty, lack of education, early marriage, and obstetric fistula.

Halimatou's story is a humbling lesson. The power of individuals and local communities to change their own lives can be limitless. Labels of "shunned" or "pariah" can be changed to "contributor," "role model," or "leader." The work with this fistula center serves as one profound example of why, as a global nonprofit organization, emBOLDen Alliances works with communities most in need of assistance. Rather than arriving with pre-formed strategies created in a distant land, we arrive prepared with questions, experience, and plans to create tailored tools together and then step back.

Fighting for Freedom and Justice

Freedom of expression is something we engage in every day. We talk to our friends, we listen to various talk shows or music, we doodle, we create. But, for many around the world, having the ability to use these art forms is a luxury and can even be life-threatening.

Figure 5: "2P" by Bill Rohs
©Bill Rohs

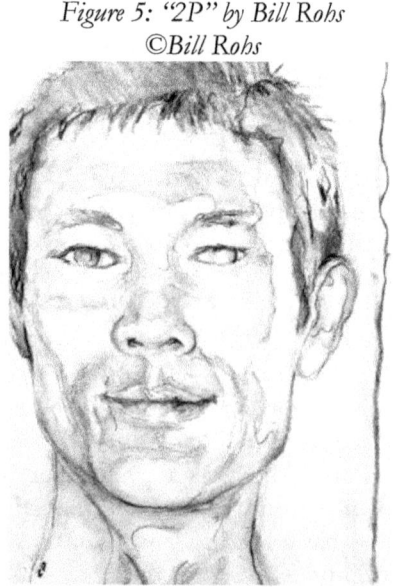

One man, 2P, expressed his political views through street art and music. He and his peers used their visual and verbal creativity to tell stories, inspire, motivate, and activate. For these actions, they were frequently arrested, jailed, tortured, and separated from family. The persecution forced them underground and, for many like 2P, out of their home country of Myanmar.

But they did not yield. They were not silenced. Their pens and spray paint did not run dry, and their guitars did not go quiet. They regularly traveled back to Myanmar, under cover, to disseminate the message of power to the people via CDs and visual art campaigns. He, like the others, never used his real name, but adopted "2P" as his identity.

One of emBOLDen Alliances' team members was fortunate enough to work with 2P and his peers to help them enhance skills in visual art, public speaking, and organizational management. Together, they listened to speeches by the greatest world leaders and dissected their tone, word usage, and ability to captivate. They practiced speaking to each other and delivering messages effectively. They worked through problems of organizational management like budgeting or program development so that they could use their resources more effectively and track their progress.

Consequently, 2P created more impactful materials and campaigns and was equipped with the skills and tools to more effectively lead his organization. 2P's gentle nature coupled with these improved skills made him and his organization stand up even taller for freedom and for justice.

2P is one of so many around the globe who possesses the inspiring combination of passion, talent, and determination. And even more impressive than their skills is their selfless devotion – working tirelessly to achieve betterment for their fellow citizens in the face of tremendous personal sacrifice.

From Driver to Manager

Ayouba had been working for many years as a driver for a foreigner living in Niger. During a period of time when his employer was away, Ayouba was hired by the director of the nearby obstetric fistula hospital to assist with construction of a new building. emBOLDen Alliances team members were also there working shoulder-to-shoulder with the West African staff to improve the hospital's operations and logistics. While Ayouba was involved in the construction side of the hospital, emBOLDen Alliances' Operations and Logistics Specialist, Bill Rohs, couldn't help but notice the keen interest and commitment Ayouba showed.

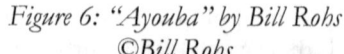

Figure 6: "Ayouba" by Bill Rohs
©Bill Rohs

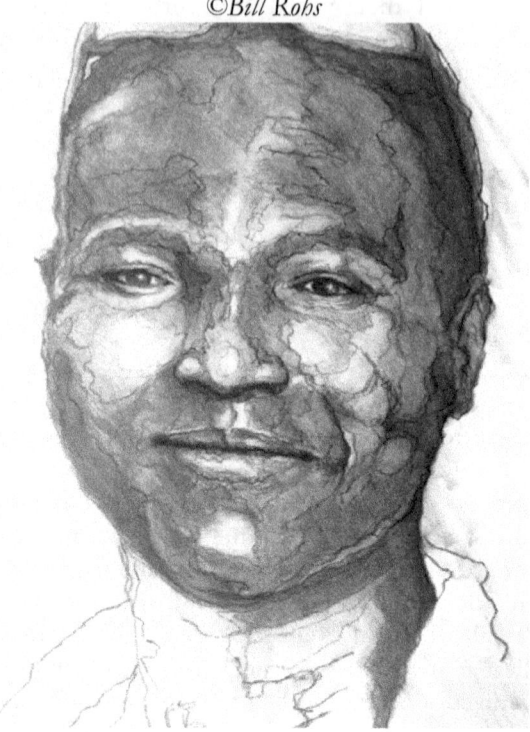

Bill began involving Ayouba in various aspects of hospital operations and logistics and realized that Ayouba had skills and talents that far surpassed those of his role as a driver. Bill was impressed by his ability to solve problems quickly and thoroughly – all with a smile and that "can-do" attitude that reminded him of only the best logisticians. Diving deeper into conversations together, Ayouba shared that he had not only been a plumber, but an electrician as well, earlier in his life! Once again, Bill was impressed.

Ayouba was intelligent, quick to learn, and adept at solving difficult problems using simple, locally-available materials. Bill began to nurture Ayouba's interest in operations and logistics and trained him on all that he could. Ayouba seized the opportunity to learn as many new skills as possible in a variety of areas, including inventory management and computer literacy. Though Ayouba had started out as an apprentice of sorts, Bill quickly came to view him as his counterpart and began engaging with the hospital director about Ayouba's potential and the need to keep him on staff. She not only supported this idea, but also suggested having Ayouba pursue additional education so he could achieve higher goals and contribute even more to the hospital and surrounding community. Before long, Ayouba was promoted to Head of Operations and Logistics.

With this new role and salary, Ayouba is able to further his own children's education and opportunities. In addition, this new position, combined with his status as a trusted and integral member of his community, Ayouba more effectively advocates for girls' education and subsequently, fistula prevention.

Ayouba's story is a testament to his remarkable character. But it also serves as a strong reminder of the power of listening. With an open mind and open ears, you never know who you might meet – your counterpart, a mentor or teacher, the next generation of leaders. And, with just a bit of support, you may be able to open doors together that no one even knew existed. You may be able to make a huge difference in their lives, an entire community, or who knows – maybe even the world.

Case Study 1: Implementation and Sustainability

Summary

An organization providing access to healthcare in East Africa had an excellent program model, implementation plan, and community connections, but recognized that they did not yet have the necessary experience, resources, or tools to pilot and scale an organization with maximum impact. With help from emBOLDen Alliances with regards to operations, programs, partnerships, grant writing, and geographic information system (GIS) mapping, the organization is successfully completing its first phase and is now looking toward expansion.

Situation

A new, well-integrated organization had a strong mission, vision, model, and implementation plan. It had also completed a comprehensive needs assessment for its program. Additionally, leadership had laid the groundwork with community members, strengthened existing ties and fostered new ones, and secured critical community ownership. However, the organization self-identified areas for improvement: program design, operational efficiency, monitoring and evaluation, grant writing, and leadership. This organization approached emBOLDen Alliances for assistance in those areas and asked, "What tools, resources, and guidance can we utilize to develop an effective and efficient pilot program that will allow us to maximize impact and scale well?"

Questions from Our Partner

· How do we write up our program framework in a useful and meaningful way?
· How do we write our next grant more effectively?

· What should we consider in data collection and analysis for our program as well as for reporting and visual presentation of results and impact?

Methodology

As with every partner, emBOLDen Alliances began by listening to this organization talk about its self-identified strengths, weaknesses, and challenges. Following an initial face-to-face discovery meeting, emBOLDen Alliances and its new partner outlined an action plan with deliverables and timelines for both parties. As this partner was a very motivated and committed organization, the partnership with emBOLDen Alliances was very effective in reviewing, revising, and implementing new frameworks, policies, and practices in a timely, progressive, communicative fashion. In addition, emBOLDen Alliances lent its skills and expertise to address other organizational desires such as methods of creating institutional memory, networking with peer individuals and organizations, and evaluating partnerships.

Outcomes

With this support, the partner organization launched the new program in 2015 with the confidence that all of the necessary elements were in place, including:

· Strategic and programmatic frameworks for years 1 and 2
· A comprehensive monitoring and evaluation plan designed to be a working, living guide used in coordination with program frameworks and grant writing
· An understanding of how to analyze data from the local ministry of health and supplement it effectively
· Plans for scaling across the region
· Clear financial alignment with budgets
· Multiple grant application submissions

Figure 7: emBOLDen Alliances' Triad of Better Data, Programs, and Mapping
©emBOLDen Alliances

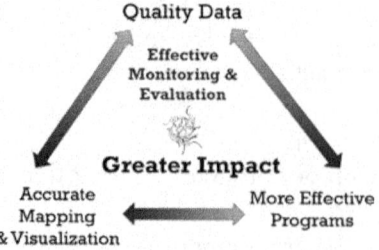

Moreover, our partner reports that the strategic planning process helped them to frame their program goals in a more productive way. They said that staff now have a clearer idea of what they are trying to achieve and how best to monitor progress toward those goals. They also feel more confident in their ability to measure impact and improve outcomes – demonstrable results that will attract more funding moving forward. Ultimately, all of these new and improved skills and resources have enabled our partner to launch its program – and its organization – and they are now effectively facilitating access to lifesaving healthcare in remote areas of East Africa.

Case Study 2: Transition of Leadership

Summary

A community-based organization working in West Africa wanted to shift leadership, program management, and decision-making from its origin and base in the United States to in-country staff, but it was very uncertain how to proceed. With support and guidance from emBOLDen Alliances, they were able to thoroughly assess the viability of this change, successfully begin the transition process, and effectively support local leadership along the way.

Situation

The organization self-identified a number of challenges:

- The board was fatigued by long-distance management and constant fundraising.
- Funds were dwindling.
- Board members were uncertain about the way forward (e.g., whether to invest more in the organization and, if so, how much and for how long).
- The board felt strongly that programs should be run locally, with the U.S. entity re-organizing to provide awareness, fundraising, and support.
- The board had identified an in-country executive director with a strong academic background and significant experience. In addition, he lived in one of the organization's community of operations, and thus understood local needs and community members well. However, this skilled individual needed more project management skills and resources.

The combination of these complex challenges prompted the organization to seek assistance from emBOLDen Alliances with the goal of creating and implementing a clear path of progress and stability.

Questions from Our Partner
- ·Can we survive this transition? If so, how? Over what timeframe?
- ·How much funding and what types of additional direct support are necessary to help the local leadership?
- ·What are the priorities in managing an effective transition?

Methodology

emBOLDen Alliances began by listening to both the U.S.-based and in-country leaders to understand their concerns, needs, and challenges. From these discussions, emBOLDen Alliances was able to outline and implement tailored starting points, including a 3-year transition plan with defined inputs, essential ingredients needed for an effective grant application, and an evaluation of the organization's current strategic plan.

Outcomes

The organization began its transition to local leadership and programs are still running. Using a transition plan as a guide, the board, staff, and integral volunteers have established priorities, roles, and responsibilities for moving forward within the new structure. The staff is also utilizing emBOLDen Alliances' guidance around essential ingredients for grants and programs in order to build local capacity to the level required for sustainability.

Case Study 3: Revamping Short-term Medical Missions

Summary

A U.S.-based hospital organization running short-term volunteer medical trips to developing countries self-identified a need for greater clarity around objectives, community engagement, and demonstrated impact. Through partnership with emBOLDen Alliances, the organization has been able to revamp its program to meet these goals and will be able to operate with greater accountability and efficiency.

Situation

Our partner was operating short-term medical mission trips in five low-income countries, but learned that stakeholders at all levels – from volunteers and donors to the CEO – were requesting a deeper understanding of the long-term objectives and a greater demonstration of their impact. In addition, leadership asked that these programs operate more strategically and clearly demonstrate the core values of the hospitals involved. The organization approached emBOLDen Alliances to assist in refining one of its country programs, identifying and progressing toward a targeted direction, and demonstrating/aligning goals.

Questions from Our Partner
- How do we re-structure our program to be more meaningful and accountable? How can we adapt a program to meet the needs of all stakeholders: volunteers, hospital administration, executive staff, clinical staff, community members, and partner hospital facilities? What tools do we need to achieve this?
- How can we operate more accountably and effectively?

Methodology

emBOLDen Alliances believes in listening and understanding before acting. As such, emBOLDen Alliances began this partnership with stakeholder engagement by bringing all interested actors to the table and listening to the experiences and perspectives of each. From there, emBOLDen Alliances was able to help the organization formulate and implement the direction forward with a concrete scope of work, appropriate deliverables, and regular follow up.

Outcomes

There were notable outputs and strong outcomes as a result of our partnership. The partner reports having created and/or improved:
- Strategic and programmatic frameworks
- Volunteer management tools
- Monitoring and evaluation, including data collection and analysis
- Definition of program scope and objectives and responsiveness to current and ongoing incidents
- Internal communication and reporting mechanisms

Additionally, emBOLDen Alliances helped the organization to develop deployment documents and corresponding communication tools for participating volunteers, improve team structure, and enhance reporting and communication processes. Moreover, emBOLDen Alliances helped to develop a structured response within the program in order to respond to patient outcomes, build sustainability, enhance community engagement, and elevate standards of care. Ultimately, emBOLDen Alliances was able to help this partner professionalize operations and programs and increase organizational structure and meaningful impact.

Case Study 4: Train-the-Trainer

Summary

Prompted by the 2015 earthquake, a Nepalese organization wanted to integrate safety and basic first aid into their work on education, but it did not have the expertise to do so. Through a partnership with emBOLDen

Alliances, both organizations were able to successfully implement a "train-the-trainer" program for teachers in remote areas to learn and practice first aid.

Situation

Following the 2015 earthquakes in Nepal, a local organization that supported education in remote areas recognized that children's health and safety is a critical part of quality education. Under normal circumstances, local health posts are sparse and difficult to access, and thus, healthcare is extremely limited. This situation worsens in times of crises. To enhance the ability of communities to address their own health and safety needs, the organization wanted to create and deliver basic first aid and preventive health education. As the organization had little experience in these topics, the leaders approached emBOLDen Alliances for assistance in creating and implementing an appropriate plan to train teachers.

Questions from Our Partner

- How can we devise and implement a first-aid "train-the-trainer" program for teachers in remote areas?
- How can we build this sustainably?
- How do we incorporate monitoring and evaluation to ensure follow through and continuation of the training?

Methodology

emBOLDen Alliances began the partnership with our first principle – listening. By working to understand the background context, the current situation, and the vision, emBOLDen Alliances was able to formulate a culturally appropriate plan that addressed the organization's self-identified needs. The partnering organization was highly motivated and open to ideas. Consequently, the partnership was truly collaborative – the organization and emBOLDen Alliances shared resources and created several components together, including the training curriculum itself. emBOLDen Alliances also assisted in developing a detailed implementation plan, clear and accurate budgets, a monitoring and evaluation framework, and a reporting structure.

Outcomes

Together, the local partner organization and emBOLDen Alliances equipped 75 teachers and 9 student assistants from 16 schools serving 4,500 students with first aid, preventative health, and hygiene training. A particularly unique aspect of this training was the emphasis on practical skills and assessment labs for participants to roll up their sleeves, demonstrate their knowledge, share with others, coordinate within a team, and practice newly-learned skills. In addition to the training, each school received a first-aid kit, a portable stretcher, health education posters, a log book to record first-aid kit use, notebooks containing health and hygiene education information, a curriculum translated into Nepali, and a certificate of completion.

Even while the program was still in progress, the partner and emBOLDen Alliances began receiving feedback on their training series. It was reported that this was the best training teachers had received in more than 25 years and that teachers were eager for additional training for themselves and for their peers across the region. In addition, information and knowledge was shared far beyond the circle of training participants. First-aid principles and health and hygiene practices were adopted widely among teachers, students, families, and communities. Moreover, emBOLDen Alliances was delighted to learn that the local partner went on to utilize these skills to provide refresher trainings for 28 participants from 11 different schools.

In reflecting on the organization's work with emBOLDen Alliances and its ability to extend the program beyond the scope of our partnership, the organization's education development manager noted:

I am personally proud and thankful to emBOLDen for successfully leading [us] during the Post Earthquake First Aid Training Program and encouraging us that the program could be carried out in long run with a better and sustainable approach on our own lead. Truly, the value that emBOLDen [Alliances] carries on assisting the partner organization to achieve their local mission is highly praise worthy. I still recall how nervous I had personally been before the training...But [their] motivation and guidance filled all the enthusiasm in me and made me believe I could facilitate [it]. (S. Sherpa, personal communication, September 19, 2006)

Since emBOLDen Alliances has had experience with "train-the-trainer" programs in many countries and contexts, we are thrilled to see evidence that this work is effecting widespread impact and positive change in Nepal and that local organizations are able to proactively replicate and adapt programs as they see most appropriate.

Conclusion

Local organizations are the first, last, and always for their own communities. Empowering locally-led solutions is a dramatic shift from paternalistic aid and should be considered "normal" instead of "innovative." Humanitarian needs and the complexity of subsequent responses are at an unprecedented high. This necessitates more informed, efficient, resourceful, and durable responses to crises. In order to meet current challenges, we must redesign and implement foundationally novel, human-centered approaches as well as evidence-based methodology and measured impact.

It is time to do better. When the lives and livelihoods of humans are at risk, there is no choice – the stakes are simply too high.

References

Alford, R. (2015). Bad aid: Should all NGOs close down? *The Guardian.* Retrieved from https://www.theguardian.com/global-development-professionals-network/2015/nov/12/aid-should-ngos-close?CMP=ema-1702&CMP=

Briney, A. (n.d.). Sahara desert. Retrieved from http://geography.about.com/od/locateplacesworldwide/a/saharadesert.htm.

EngenderHealth (2003). Obstetric fistula needs assessment report. Retrieved from https://www.engenderhealth.org/files/pubs/maternal-health/report/section/niger.pdf

Knox Clarke, P. and Darcy, J. (2014). Insufficient evidence? The quality and use of evidence in humanitarian action. Retrieved from http://www.alnap.org/resource/10441

UNICEF. (2013). At a glance: Niger. Retrieved from https://www.unicef.org/infobycountry/niger_statistics.html.

van der Zee, B. (2015, October). Less than 2% of humanitarian funds 'go directly to local NGOs'. *The Guardian.* Retrieved from https://www.theguardian.com/global-development-professionals-network/2015/oct/16/less-than-2-of-humanitarian-funds-go-directly-to-local-ngos?CMP=ema-1702&CMP

World Bank. (2015). World development indicators. Retrieved from http://databank.worldbank.org/data/reports.aspx?source=2&country=NER

CHAPTER 28

Promoting Sustainable Change
so that Communities Thrive with and without Us

Efosa Guobadia

Sustainable change is fundamental to the pursuit of making this world a better place. It demands that in addition to learning from yesterday and acting for today, we plan for a better tomorrow. Sustainable change is the promotion of the continuation of positive effects that a person or group may have – effects that accumulate over time rather than dissipate, even if the stimulus of external support is removed. In the variable realm of global health, sustainable change needs to be an invariable tenet to our approach.

In the 21st century, the world is more interconnected than ever before. Due to the progressions that we have seen in technology and travel, there is an increased interest to know more about the world around us and an increased capacity to participate in it. That increased interest is partly due to the understanding that in today's world, what occurs in one corner can (and often does) have an effect in another.

In the global health sector, at rates hitherto unseen, this increased interest has led to opportunities, ventures, and projects around the world. The threshold for participation has been lowered, and the portals for entry have grown. Organizations welcome volunteers of different backgrounds from different regions of the world to support their missions in different capacities.

Rapid growth in any sector has been known to come with challenges, yet it is always accompanied with opportunities for leadership, innovation, and positive progress. The same is true for global health in modern times. The growth that we have seen reveals that there are those who are willing to commit their talents, time, and energy to improving underserved areas and the lives of those who reside there. It is up to those in leadership to ensure that our strategies and programs are positive, responsible, and sustainable and that we are matching the appropriate participant and resource to each activity and need.

In this chapter, I share some experiences that I have had while volunteering as a doctor of physical therapy, and I share how those experiences have shaped my thinking and guided my actions. I then provide instructions that can be used in the development and deployment of humanitarian programs.

Experiences

Colombia

Dr. Tony Rinella is a spinal surgeon who founded a nonprofit organization called Global Spine Outreach. Every six months, Dr. Rinella leads a group to Colombia to work with pediatric patients who have complicated presentations and conditions and don't have the means to procure the necessary treatment. In November 2011, I was part of a multidisciplinary volunteer group led by Dr. Tony Rinella that travelled to Cali, Colombia. During the early part of the week, our volunteer group performed evaluations on the patients, and then determinations were made regarding for whom surgery was appropriate. Those not selected for surgery were instructed to begin or continue conservative care with the potential of an operation at a later date after additional assessment. Patients who had already been operated on also came so that their progress could be monitored and measured. Each patient had a file, and their current state was measured to their preoperative state. This allowed the medical team to make any necessary operative adjustments and rehabilitative and management recommendations. It mitigated the challenges that the realities of time and distance accentuate in global health. It was my first look at the importance of measurement and the establishment of a continuum between an organization's efforts.

Later that week, the surgical group, which was composed of physicians, medical equipment specialists, and neuro-technology clinicians from the United States and Colombia, performed surgeries on the selected patients. Following the surgery, our group worked with the rehabilitation department in the hospital to develop a postoperative physical rehabilitative plan. Overall preparations, decisions, and activities that usually would take months to be effectuated were done in one week. It was my first exposure to the power of collaboration and teamwork in global health, and how it allows a group to increase the amount, speed, and quality of what can be done.

I spent several full days working with clinicians in the rehabilitation department. As we co-treated patients, I was struck by how much we were able to learn from each other. I learned new styles and techniques from them and was able to share some as well during our treatment sessions together and during a presentation that I gave late in the week. I was moved and encouraged by the fact that even if we were continents apart, we all had the same hopes for our patients and wanted to help them maximize their health and life in any way that we could. I saw that when we came together, we became stronger, and we could use that strength for those that were in our care. It was made clear to me that knowledge transfers well across cultures and that you can have a continuous impact with the ideas that you leave behind.

Throughout the week, I spent much time observing Dr. Rinella and conversing with him. I took note of the preparation and planning that went into the micro and macro activities, the executions of established objectives, the integration of the team's efforts, and the communications that ensured that everyone was plugged into the overall vision. His passion and joy for medicine were contagious. The importance of leadership and how it can accentuate individual and overall efforts in an unpredictable environment was palpable when near him, and his examples have resonated with me ever since.

There was a case during the trip that made a lasting impression on me. It happened early in the week while the medical team was performing assessments and making decisions. A young mother came in with her young daughter who was in a wheelchair. The girl had a diagnosis of cerebral palsy and presented with extensor spasticity. She was twelve, yet had the cranium size of a seven-year-old. As the assessment progressed, it was determined that it would not be appropriate or safe to operate on the young girl. Complete information was acquired from the patient and her family, and they were instructed to return when the group was in Colombia next. When the girl's mother heard this, tears began to flow silently down her face. They were not tears of anger. They were a mother's tears: tears of pain, tears of hope, and tears of love. She wanted the best for her daughter and had just realized that it was not going to happen in the way or at the time that she had been imagining. I read in her face a look of love and anguish, strength and hurt. I saw a look that transcends race, culture, and time. Even now I see it. As the mother was leaving, two team members and I tacitly communicated and promptly followed her into the hallway. We then spent time with her, showing her transfer techniques, postural positions, stretching, and strengthening activities that she could do with her daughter in the days to come. We did our best to share with her what we hoped would help. At the end, we hugged her. At the end, I said to her, "Be strong." I was in awe at the strength that this mother possessed, and I felt that at that moment, she was the strongest person in the whole country. I knew then that I would never forget that mother and daughter, and I know now that they have continued to inspire me to serve and to go back to places of need. That moment confirmed my belief that there is always something we can do, even if it doesn't come in the expected form. There is always something we can give. Utilizing our hands, hearts, and words constitutes an incredible capacity that can be harnessed for good all around the world.

The following skills provided an early context for operating in the realm of global health:

· Measurement and working along a sustainable continuum
· Collaboration and working as a team
· Sharing knowledge and resources with local counterparts
· Leading effectively in new environments
· Giving what is appropriate and what you can

Since I was outside of my usual, U.S.-based practice environment, it was important for me to see the impact that could be had in an unfamiliar land and the meaningful improvements that could be made when people are given otherwise unavailable support and services. At that time, the idea of sustainable change began to take root.

ATI MissionWorks

Shortly after my return from Colombia, I was given the green light by my employers to develop an international volunteer program for our company, which would complement our already-established, domestic, philanthropic efforts. I knew that many of my colleagues had the same desire to use their hearts, hands, and words wherever they could. The program, called ATI MissionWorks, teamed our rehabilitation clinicians (physical therapists, physical therapist assistants, occupational therapists, and athletic trainers) with different organizations and their initiatives around the world.

In the early development of the program and before the first group embarked abroad, I was able to have many conversations with my mentor and friend, Dr. Chris Stout. Dr. Stout has a long history in global health and currently leads the nonprofit organization, Center for Global Initiatives. We discussed the importance of proper entry into an unknown or unfamiliar region, with the acknowledgement that it is difficult to have a sustainable impact if you don't have an auspicious start. We discussed the importance of having an open mindset and avoiding jingoism when traveling to a new place that is identified as being "in need." Outsiders can never know more about a place than the people who spend all of their days there, so it is best to learn from local persons to increase the chance of having a positive impact. Some of the questions that were formulated in these conversations are below:

- What do you know about the history of the people you are trying to help and the barriers you are trying to overcome?
- Are you dispensing services that would create a vacuum of need once you leave?
- Are you bringing in certain resources from an outside area when instead you could be working with local vendors?
- Are you aware of a similar group whose presence has preceded yours, and do you know if your efforts supplement or contradict theirs?

These questions and others were taken into consideration as I entered into my next phase of participation in the realm of global health.

Phase One: Getting to Know Global Health

The first phase of the ATI MissionWorks program was composed of introspection on the personal, programmatic, and professional levels and extrospection of new cultures and new environments. My colleagues and I partnered with different organizations with different missions in different places around the world. We worked in hospitals, clinics, community centers, and schools. Many of the places we visited were underserved and at over-capacity. Many of the patients that we saw had never had a health clinician deeply assess, touch, and palpate their pains. Not many knew what it was like for someone to ask them where it hurt, when it hurt, and how it hurt. We were creating moments of positivity, possibility, and potentiality. We were able to progress patients through aggregated physical impairments that had been mismanaged over time or not managed at all, and we saw patients become exponentially better after just one visit.

During trip to Guatemala in 2013, I met a particular patient who has stayed in my memory ever since. While setting up for clinic in a remote town, a man approached me and began to explain that there was an elderly lady in the village who needed rehab but couldn't make the trip to us in order to receive it. He asked if I would be willing to go to her home. Without hesitation my answer was "yes." We walked half a mile into town before heading up a hill to her house.

When we arrived, the older lady was surrounded by her loved ones, and they began to share her story with us. She was the grandmother and matron of the family, and after suffering a stroke a year before, she was taken to the hospital. Her stay in the hospital lasted several days, and then she was sent home without any medical or rehabilitative program or follow-up plan. The first six months after a stroke are very important for recovery. This lady hadn't had any directed care and had been largely inactive since the incident. She presented with significant weakness on the right side of her body, poor coordination with her fine motor skills, and poor balance when walking. Her daily routine mainly consisted of lying in bed and sitting in a chair at the front of the house. I proceeded to spend the next hour with her and her family, developed an activity routine and schedule for them, and then stressed the importance of adhering to it. They expressed their gratitude for finally being empowered with information and having a plan to follow.

Later that day, I found myself thinking of my own grandmother. She had lived in a similar town in Nigeria, and toward the end of her life, she had also suffered a serious stroke. When I think of her, I often find myself hoping that she had enough people around her who cared for her and attended to her needs. I feel that through the opportunity I had to treat and show love to the grandmother in Guatemala, I treated and showed love to my own grandmother. There are an untold number of similar cases. In towns near and far, we see places in which demand for care is high and supply is low or inadequate. This reality further punctuates the fact that program leaders have a responsibility to maximize each and every resource at their disposal. Not using a resource efficiently in one place means another place is missing out on its potential use. Prudent stewardship of what we have is crucial to making sustainable change a reality.

Phase Two: Time and Relations

There was a question still lingering in my mind: "What happens when we leave?" To answer this question, I began to return to the places I had been before. My groups and I spent most of our time in Zacapa, Guatemala with the organization Hearts in Motion, founded by Karen Scheeringa-Parra. This organization established itself in one region for over 30 years and in that time, fostered and nurtured relationships with community members and leaders. They showed that during these times of bonding, the ground for communication and collaboration develops. As my group returned over and over, we were able to see the long-term effects of our work on the area and its inhabitants. We were able to hear reports from patients whose back pain had stayed away since we last treated them and who were now able to return to work. We saw that the equipment we donated to clinics was being used and allowed clinicians to see more patients. We also saw that the skills and techniques we had shared with clinicians during prior visits were making a difference in the current quality of care. With the investment of time and the development of relationships, a community can be changed for the better, and your positive effects can be compounded.

Phase Three: Compassion into Action

Not too long after this, I had the chance to put some of the principles I was learning into practice. The opportunity came from Hearts in Motion.

They asked me to convert a section of one of their buildings in Guatemala into a rehabilitation clinic. I jumped at the chance. The town in which the clinic was being developed was Teculutan, Guatemala. At the time, Teculutan did not have a physician office, rehab clinic, or a hospital. Thus, when a person needed medical assistance, they would have to travel 45 minutes to the state capitol for care at the government hospital. Private transportation was not accessible to everyone, and the cost of public transportation was a barrier to some. Thus, important care was sometimes foregone. This negatively impacted lives, families, and, in extension, the community. I set to work with the local staff, and with a focus on sustainability we:

- Developed a documentation template through Google Drive
- Developed a scheduling system to maximize patient and the therapist time
- Strategically organized the new clinic to maximize patient comfort and efficient use of space
- Mentored a local physical therapist to run the place and manage logistics after I left

In the span of four weeks, we were able to provide the town with an accessible place to receive rehabilitative care. When I returned to the clinic 18 months later, I was happy to see that it was still thriving. The project solidified the importance of the empowerment, of education, and of building things with the intent that they last.

Prudent stewardship, investment of time, empowerment, and collaboration with local partners are non-negotiable. The ATI MissionWorks program continues to partner with different organizations around the world and provides support to places in need.

Move Together

Towards the end of 2015, I was in San Pedro near Lake Atitlan in Guatemala. I was between volunteer trips and taking time to write. One night while eating dinner at an outside vendor near the lake, I entered into conversation with a man and his daughter. After discovering that I was a physical therapist, the man began to tell me about his wife and the intense pain that she was having in her knee. He explained that they were staying up the road at a local hotel and asked if I would be willing to treat her. His ardor for his wife's well-being was moving. Without hesitation I said that I would come. It was after 9PM when we arrived at the hotel, and I began my evaluation. I learned that she had a bad fall several weeks prior and had only tried to manage her symptoms with pain medication. They explained that their town did not have a physical therapist. The evaluation revealed swelling and inflammation, loss of knee range of motion, deconditioning of the quadriceps muscle, and decreased ability to put weight on the affected leg. My treatment included education for pain and inflammation management, exercises to increase knee mobility and to improve local strength, and activities to improve balance. I also recommended that she follow up with the local physician so that her progress could be monitored. I then invited them to come to the rehab clinic that I was going to the next week.

I was happy to help that family, but I had to be eating dinner at the lake for that lady to receive the treatment and basic instructions that she needed. Between 2008 and 2016, I travelled to almost 30 countries and had similar encounters with people who have gone without necessary rehabilitative care. It is a problem that is multifaceted, structural, and systemic. Even if a person has the means for care, there may not be a place that delivers that care. If such a place exists, it may not have the resources or personnel to deliver the type of care that is needed. If the place is fully equipped and able to provide care, the person may not have the means to access the care. The cycle is vicious. Structural challenges need structural solutions. With this in mind, in 2016, I cofounded the 501c3 nonprofit organization Move Together with fellow physical therapist Josh D'Angelo. The mission of the organization is based on the principles of sustainable change: to increase access to quality rehab medicine around the corner and around the world.

By focusing on access, we acknowledge that our approach needs to be driven by structural interventions. In order to fulfill our mission, our programs and pillars of operations will be guided by the themes above and the instructions below.

Instructional

In order to maximize your effectiveness and efficiency and to promote sustainability in your efforts, your programs should follow this basic arc: development, deployment, and measurement. Converting program and policy into practical action requires knowledge of the nature of your organization as well as the environment in which you work.

Development and Deployment

Brest, Roumani, and Bade (2015) provide 18 steps to use during the development and implementation of a program. Below is a truncated and amended version.

Phase One: Defining the Problem
1. Describe the problem. Include a description of the current state of affairs and what the organization/person finds wrong with it.
2. Identify the relevant stakeholders, including beneficiaries and others who are to be affected for better or worse. The identification of these stakeholders and understanding of their

perspectives and needs can contribute significantly to defining the problem from the outset.

3. Identify whose problem it is. Who are going to be the beneficiaries of the solution? In this stage, err on the side of inclusion.

4. Describe why the problem is important to the organization/decision-maker/the program leader: This step helps to reveal the values and interests of the person(s) trying to solve the problem. Ask, "Why is the problem important to the foundation?" Follow the subsequent answer by repeatedly asking "Why does that matter?" or "Why is that important?" Do this until you arrive to the level in which the deepest goals and objectives are made explicit.

5. Describe the ideal world in the absence of the problem.

6. Reconsider your statement of the problem and ask what strategies may best achieve your goal. Don't frame the problem in light of the solutions that are most obvious to you; frame the solution in light of the clearest picture of the problem.

7. Prioritize and narrow the range of your intended beneficiaries. This step should begin to bring more focus to the upcoming pathway. The business guru Michael Porter famously said, "The essence of strategy is choosing what not to do" (Brest, Roumani, & Bade, 2015, p. 11).

8. Identify the beneficiaries' needs: Utilize social science research and ethnography. Social science research deals with human behavior and society. Ethnography is the description of the customs of individual peoples and cultures. An ethnographer observes the beneficiaries, engages them through empathy interviews, and, where useful, immerses him/herself in their experiences.

9. Learn whether other organizations are addressing the problem effectively. It is likely that your foundation or program is not the first to address your chosen problem. Learn whether or not others have designed successful approaches to solving the same problem. If so, adapt their strategies or, better yet, collaborate with them. With due diligence in this step, you can save the time and expense of many of the next steps. Be sure to test what you find to ensure that it works within your organization's particular context.

Phase Two: Framing the Problem

10. Articulate and prioritize the need(s) that you will address. Once you prioritize the need(s), the decision of strategy should ultimately be based on the strategies' comparative effectiveness and should be consistent with the foundation's values.

Phase Three: Solving the Problem

11. Revisit key stakeholders to understand their motivations, behaviors, and the needs of the systems in which they operate. Understand that there are many stakeholders in addition to beneficiaries who can affect outcomes. Oftentimes, these stakeholders are in situations that include complex bureaucracies that you will need to understand before you can progress to your maximum capabilities.
12. Identify barriers to moving from the present state to the ideal state.
13. Articulate "design mandates" and posit strategies that could transcend barriers, address needs, and facilitate change. A design mandate is a description of one particular need and its source. (Even though you may identify many barriers, it is generally best to focus on one at a time as you go through the following steps.)
14. Brainstorm questions emerging from the design mandate. Utilize a "how might we satisfy this need" sentence structure. This is the time for ideation and brainstorming. Divergence and creativity are important here. The next step will focus on selection and convergence.
15. Select several promising strategies from those generated. Select a few strategies to move forward. The fundamental selection criterion is the strategy's potential effectiveness in solving the problem, considering the foundation's capacity, the benefits achieved for the costs of implementing the strategy, and the positive and negative impacts on other stakeholders. Each strategy is, in effect, a causal hypothesis that if we do X, then Y is likely to happen, and that Y is likely to lead to the better state, Z.
16. Turn the selected strategies into logic models and compare them to one another. In the following order, a general logic model has:
    a) Inputs: what resources are committed
    b) Activities: things that you have to do
    c) Outputs: things that you count or deliver
    d) Intermediate Outcome: micro measures of what the organization hopes the activities and outputs produced
    e) Ultimate Outcome: the socially meaningful change that you hope to achieve

Phase Four: Implementing, Observing, Learning, and Evaluating

17. Prototype the selected solutions to test for their viability. Create a prototype of the parts or the whole solution and seek feedback from designers and stakeholders.
18. Implement and evaluate. If possible, carry out mini-pilots before investing in a full pilot project. Implementation is an iterative process as you work towards optimization of the solution.

The problem-solving process is multifaceted and does not guarantee an expected outcome. It is important to be nimble and willing not only to relook at the structure of the solution, but to relook at your perspective of the problem.

Measurement Mentality

Having a measurement mentality is paramount to promoting sustainable change in your project. Measuring what you do allows you to read the past and the present in order to maximize your efforts in the future. Peter Drucker famously said, "What gets measured gets improved" (Shore, 2014, para. 5). We need to continuously improve what we are doing to ensure that we are efficiently directing the correct resources to meet the needs of the global health sector.

Once you decide to adopt the measurement mentality, next is to understand the distinction between outputs and outcomes. Although outputs are important, higher value (and thus more of your focus) should be on measuring outcomes. By definition:

- Outputs are what we count – the volume of a program's actions, such as products created or delivered, number of people served, or activities and services carried out.
- Outcomes are what we wish to achieve – socially meaningful changes for those served by a program, generally defined in terms of expected changes in knowledge, skills, attitudes, behavior, condition, or status. These changes should be measured and monitored as part of an organization's work, link directly to the efforts of the program, and serve as the basis for accountability (Penna, 2011).

If we were to use an example of a non-profit organization whose mission is to address water scarcity in a certain region so that local families have better health, the following would be an example of an output versus an outcome:

- Output: The number of wells developed in 12 months
- Outcome: The number of families that have clean water to use each day over the course of 12 months

Many mistakenly prioritize outputs over outcomes. Rothschild (2012) emphasizes the importance of measuring what counts because what we measure drives what we do. Thus, clearly delineating, establishing, and prioritizing your metrics will provide the necessary focus for your organization and program and will allow you to maximize your path to fulfilling your mission.

Conclusion

There are many great needs in the realm of global health, and they will require great efforts to address them. These efforts must be infused with the tenets of collaboration and teamwork, education and empowerment, leadership and stewardship, and resource management and measurement. We owe it to those who support our various missions and to those whom our missions hope to support to ensure that we act with responsibility, effectiveness, and efficiency. It is my belief that turning compassion into action is possible, and that sustainable change is indeed necessary if we are to go about the work of making this world a better place.

References

Brest, P., Roumani, N., Bade, J. (2015). Problem solving, human-centered design, and strategic process. *Stanford Center on Philanthropy and Civil Society.* Retrieved from http://pacscenter.stanford.edu/2015/09/problem-solving-human-centered-design-and-strategic-processes/

Shore, J. (2014, September 16). These 10 Peter Drucker quotes may change your world. Retrieved from https://www.entrepreneur.com/article/237484

Penna, R. (2011). *The nonprofit outcomes toolbox: A complete guide to program effectiveness, performance measurement, and results.* Hoboken, NJ: Wiley.

Rothschild, J. (2012). *The non nonprofit: For-profit thinking for nonprofit success.* Hoboken, NJ: Jossey-Bass.

CHAPTER 29

A Guide to Developing Sustainable Global Health Projects

Tiffany Masson, Alisha DeWalt, and Philip Adu

Introduction

As we evolve as a human race, we continue to become more interconnected through innovations in technology, evolutions in media platforms, and migration movements (Flache & Macy, 2011). In present day, we can instantly be informed of worldwide current events and communicate with others from across the globe at the click of a button. These influences and intersections of connectivity have paved the way for projects that build human capacity in regions of the developing world that have long been neglected. Deciding to develop such a project comes with many questions and topics for consideration. With the multitude of non-governmental organizations (NGOs) and other initiatives already in place, the challenges facing an organization that will take on the task are many: to identify the need correctly, to ensure it matches the organization's area of expertise, and to create a project that is both successful and sustainable.

At the conclusion of World War II, the United Nations (U.N.) was formed to support international cooperation and prevent future international conflicts ("About the UN," n.d.). As the U.N. took shape, the NGO label was initially developed to support the world body directly, and now it is used in a wider and more diverse context. Establishment of NGOs has increased dramatically since the 1980s (Lewis & Kanji, 2009; Clarke, 1998), gaining momentum from a wave in people-centered vision of development action, dissatisfaction with government assistance, and growth in social movements. NGOs continued to gain a higher profile throughout

611

the decades that followed (Lewis, 2003), and by 2004, NGOs were responsible for approximately one-third of total international development aid funds (Riddell, 2008, p. 48).

Because the use of the term "NGO" varies, there is not an exact calculation of the number of established organizations. There are approximately 1.5 million NGOs within the United States ("Fact Sheet Non-Governmental Organizations (NGOs) in the United States," 2016, para. 5) and many more world-wide (Clark, 1998). These non-profit organizations and the human-capacity-building projects they have collectively undertaken have made vast contributions to our society (Lewis, 2003).

Human-capacity-building projects can take many forms. They can provide direct services, training, or needed goods to support underserved populations. They can strive for poverty reduction, support policy changes, lead conflict resolution, and engage in environmental activism. Human-capacity-building projects come in many organizational structures. They can be formal or informal, big or small, heavily funded or resourceful, and rigid or flexible (Lewis & Kanji, 2009). Organizations seeking to develop such projects are not required to apply for registered NGO status, but may choose to go through the process to obtain potential benefits such as tax exemption benefits ("Fact Sheet Non-Governmental Organizations (NGOs) in the United States," 2016).

This chapter offers an in-depth overview of best practices to be followed when developing an international human-capacity-building project. The practices are then applied to a real case study to demonstrate their importance in implementing strategies of change.

Best Practices

Review Country-Specific Literature

With over 6 billion people in the world speaking over 6,000 different languages (Bruno, Bates, Brock, & Anderson, 2010, para. 2), honing in on a country's history and culture is important. A thorough review of literature written about the country will provide an understanding of the population, the need it is experiencing, and the background and impact of that need. This information will provide the basis for a more focused assessment of feasibility, which must be completed.

A primary area to be considered when gauging project feasibility is the cultural distance between the assisting organization and the population to be served. Will language be a barrier and, if so, how will it be overcome? Is the solution feasible and sustainable? Are there areas of moral differences that need to be contemplated? Will these differences pose problems in the interaction between the organization and the country?

An organization also needs to determine if its area of expertise fits with the area of potential need. Can the need be adequately supported? Does the organization have the knowledge and skillset to implement this project? Will additional experts be needed to support the work? These questions should be addressed prior to moving forward in the project development process.

By completing a thorough review of the literature, one will not only hone in on the area of potential need, but will also better understand the population's history and culture. Often times, the identified need impacts other areas of the community such as mental health, economic disparity, and lack of access to medical care (Putnam, Lieberman, Putnam, & Amaya-Jackson, 2015; American Psychological Association, 1993). Being culturally competent can help to improve the service and reduce racial and ethnic disparities (Betancourt, Green, & Carrillo, 2002). This will support building the training model or service in a way that meets the population's need.

Draft Country-Specific Business Model

Once the need has been identified, time should be spent on developing the overall project plan that takes into account the culture and potential barriers. Dreesch (2008) notes various strategies to include in the business model to ensure that it is robust and assesses the identified need. The following steps are recommended in the creation of a culturally-specific business model:

· Outline the organization's mission and values.
· Concisely explain how the initiative will address the area of identified need and how those engaged with the project will benefit.
· Detail how the success of the initiative will be measured. For example, a successful initiative may treat a certain number of community members per year, scaling up each year.
· Explain how quality control will be monitored and corrected when needed.
· Detail who is currently involved with the initiative, their capacity to contribute to the project, and gaps that need attention.
· How will local partners work with the in-country partners?
· Provide proof of certification or training documents, if applicable.

Additionally, a major area of consideration for a sustainable project is funding. When drafting the business model, developing an initial financial support stream is essential. What are the short-term costs and long-term needs that will ensure sustainability and support the business model? Because those receiving the service or goods are rarely a source of funding in a human-capacity-building project, an organization's business plan requires a distinctly different model than that of a commercial or governmental organization (Fowler, 1991). Areas for funding to consider include, but are not limited to:

·Grants

·Fundraising

·Individual donations

·Self-generating revenue, built into the business model

·Partnerships with common interest organizations

·Loans

·Interest from investments

Technology continues to provide a critical means of connection and communication across the world. One shouldn't be afraid to integrate it into a business model. Leveraging technology can significantly reduce expenses that range from travel to printing. Can trainings and meetings be conducted through technology platforms? Will the targeted population have access to the needed technology? If not, how can this barrier be overcome? For example, investment in technology software for the partner may have a great return on investment. Contemplate whether technology-based training and communication needs to occur when in-country.

Remember that cultural understanding and sensitivity are key to a proposed model. "The Process of Cultural Competence in the Delivery of Healthcare Services" is one model that encourages the provider to continuously assess and strive to work in the cultural context of the individual (Campinha-Bacote, 2002). Take time to research, analyze the project, and gain feedback from peers who have experience in this arena. Development of the proposal determines if the initiative is feasible and something that will be sustainable over time. This is a crucial step in the success of the project.

Conduct Focus Groups

Direct communication with potential in-country stakeholders will support the assessment of the business model and contribute to project sustainability. Focus groups are more efficient than one-on-one interviews and allow for a discussion to occur among participants to generate ideas and innovations. The focus group will provide valuable feedback as to whether the area of potential need will be properly addressed and support decisions on maximizing potential impact. To conduct a focus group, the following areas should be considered, as discussed by Simon (1999):

·Define the purpose: What outcomes does the organization hope to achieve? How will you communicate this to participants?

·Identify participants: Finding an in-country leader can help that multiple professions are represented in focus groups to ensure robust and productive conversation. Identify the number of participants needed, depending on scope of feedback needed.

- Coordinate logistics: Will organizational representatives travel to the country, conduct focus groups virtually, or appoint an in-country partner to facilitate? Where will the focus group be located? How long will it run? Are participant materials needed? Are refreshments appropriate?

- Produce documents to review and questions to ask: Make the best use of the time allotted by coming prepared.

During the focus group, it is important to be mindful of the participants. Be culturally-sensitive. Be flexible in framing questions and guiding the direction of the meeting. Allowing for flexibility in the conversation may foster creativity and support innovations in the business model. Tactics to support group facilitation include:

- Create a safe space: Participants may feel uncomfortable providing feedback in a setting where they may not know everyone. Establishing ground rules for how the group will engage with each other can help others become more comfortable and will be more likely to get honest and robust insights.

- Be dynamic to support engagement: Engage with participants and set the tone for an authentic conversation.

- Ask exploratory questions: Develop questions that are open-ended, providing an opportunity for participants to expand on and discuss their feedback.

- Encourage participation from all members: Select participants for the varying perspectives they will bring to the group. To have the most robust feedback, ensure everyone is included in the discussion.

- Support discussions among participants: Encourage all the participants to discuss their thoughts with each other. Understanding where perspectives diverge can allow for greater inclusion in the initiative.

Once the focus group has been completed, incorporate all findings and feedback into the business model. Focus groups can be a large investment of money and resources. Use the valuable information gained to promote sustainability and success of the human-capacity building-project.

Gain In-Country Support

Developing a human-capacity project can be complex, with many different components to consider. A sustainable international global health project requires backing and support from stakeholders within the country. Bringing these stakeholders together as a steering committee or consultative body will provide insights and direction during proposal development and socialization. Building strong alliances on the ground can result in feedback, networking opportunities, and identification of potential pitfalls to avoid as the project takes hold. Organizations should use information gained during the research phase to identify in-country organizations that can be most impactful and supportive of the initiative. Outreach to these organizations is recommended.

When socializing the project proposal, it is necessary to gain governmental approval to undertake the proposed in-country work. The in-country social system may vary greatly from the one to which the organization is accustomed. Development of a network can help to navigate through this system. Gillies (1998) notes that involvement from the community and the program's sustainability grows to the degree the identified need is aligned with the interests of community and their leaders (as cited in Labonte & Laverack, 2010).

Conduct Initial Training/Launch Service

Once the business model has been developed, focus group feedback has been integrated, and in-country support has been secured, implementation can begin on the initial training or launch of service. Prior to arriving in-country, several logistical, mental, and emotional components should be considered to support the success of the launch (Singh, n.d.).

To ensure logistical preparation is complete, the organizational representative should become familiar with the community and know where he or she will stay and how the area will be navigated. Safety protocols should be considered, and an in-country point of contact should be established. Specifics of space and timing should be solidified ahead of time, and materials should be prepared. Additionally, cultural traditions should not be overlooked. Organizational representatives should familiarize themselves with acceptable ways of greeting one another and appropriate attire. Should gifts be exchanged? Can culturally relevant activities be planned for meeting breaks?

Mental preparations also need to be made. Whether a seasoned traveler or a first-time visitor to the country, project workers need to consider how the experience will impact them and how it will affect implementation of the initiative. Separation from family and friends and the absence of many everyday conveniences may contribute to culture shock. Building a strong understanding of the culture will help to navigate these obstacles.

Emotional challenges are also to be expected. Project workers who have dedicated time and resources to developing the planned initiative may experience feelings of insecurity and anxiety as they prepare to meet their in-country partners. To be most successful, address potential insecurities and shift these to a more productive mindset.

Flexibility will be important throughout project implementation. Be prepared to continually incorporate focus group feedback and culturally specific information as it becomes available. For example, if some culture-specific words are better understood by participants, find ways to integrate them throughout the presentation. Bring the implementation to life through media that is most appropriate for the community members. Diversify teaching methods and activities to appropriately match the culture. As the training continues, modify the schedule as needed based on feedback. Rigid methodology will negatively impact participant engagement as well as the initiative's success. Above all, respect the community and its culture.

Post-departure, depending on length of stay, another challenge will be culture shock as workers integrate back into their native culture. Experiences in implementing a global health project can impact one's perspectives and challenge one's schemas that have been developed over time. Individuals who take part in these initiatives will find themselves forever changed by the experience.

Additionally, organizations should take care to incorporate all of their learning into the continued implementation and scaling of the initiative. Activities that worked and areas for improvement should be identified based on feedback received. Organizations are advised to take their time in doing this correctly while ensuring that momentum or excitement from the in-country experience is not lost.

Build an In-Country Team

Building a team on the ground takes time, but it is a critical factor in relationship development and implementation of the project. Such a team should be prepared to support the initiative and implementation, provide feedback on what works, and suggest areas for further opportunity. Empowering the team and remaining receptive to their ideas will help to foster relationships and grow roots into the community. Research conducted by Nathan, Rotem, and Ritchie (2002) reports that developing productive relationships both with the country's government as well as in the community was found by many NGO members to be a key component of their success. A diverse network of contacts should be developed and maintained to support sustainability (Nathan, Rotem, & Ritchie, 2002).

A recruiting, training, and retaining model (Dreesch, 2008) could be utilized to build a team, provide in-depth training, and further the initiative's success and integration within the community. Partners can be recruited through networking and widening the scope of connections through initial partners. A "train-the-trainer" model (Winkelstein et al., 2006) could support initial training and provide the trainees with tools to take activities to the next level and to share training with others. Partner retention can be ensured through relationship development, maintaining team motivation, and reinforcing their contributions to the project.

A sustainable initiative is one that can continue to improve without assistance from outside support (Brown, 1991). Building a team on the ground can cultivate this level of ownership to further the initiative's sustainability beyond the originating organization. Fowler (1991) notes, "NGOs intervene temporarily but do not remain" (p. 2). The community should be positively impacted by the initiative and have a level of control on the direction of the human-capacity-building project (Scheyvens, 1999).

Empower Team

In order for the project to grow roots and be sustainable in the community, a sense of ownership and empowerment must be present among the team and among the population being impacted. The in-country community can guide the initiative and take it to new levels of impact if they believe in the project and feel authorized to do so. By being culturally sensitive and flexible, creativity and innovations within their expertise can be fostered.

Empowerment takes many forms. In general, it refers to the capacity of individuals to comprehend and take control over different forces, to be self-determined, and to improve their life conditions (Israel, Checkoway, Schulz, & Zimmerman, 1994; Scheyvens, 1999). To assess whether the team and community at large is experiencing empowerment or disempowerment from the initiative, the following model based on Friedmann's writing (Friedmann, 1992) and discussed by Scheyvens (1999) can be utilized. In this model, empowerment can be categorized into different sectors: economic, psychological, social, and political. Not all sectors apply to all global health projects.

Economic empowerment assesses whether the work provides the community financial benefit. As a result of the initiative, is the community provided sustainable jobs or a revenue stream? Are the funds making an overall positive impact in the community? Take into account signs that are evident of this impact, such as improvements of building structures, increased resources, and materials available in the community. Economic disempowerment is demonstrated when the elite benefit from the revenue stream, negatively impacting other groups in the community (Scheyvens, 1999).

Psychological empowerment evaluates the community's outlook of the initiative. Are the community members exhibiting an increase in self-esteem, a more positive outlook on their future, or displaying more feelings of happiness? Positive emotions and outlook on life are evidence in psychological empowerment. If individuals are instead displaying feelings of frustration with and disinterest in the initiative, community members may not feel empowered psychological capacity (Scheyvens, 1999).

Social empowerment looks at the community's engagement with the initiative. Is the community taking an active role in improving the initiative and growing it further to meet their needs? Working groups developed through the global health project is testament to a community that is empowered, cohesive, and bound together for the betterment of their community. Disempowerment is evident in this area when the community is not banded together and individuals are in disharmony. Economic disempowerment generally trickles down to negatively impact this sector. Competition, jealousy, and resentment among groups within the community are common (Scheyvens, 1999).

Political empowerment can take many forms. In general, the community is empowered if there is a system for them to voice their concerns and if they feel that they are heard. The community is empowered if they are able to provide input on decisions regarding project implementation. Representations should be present for all groups within the community. If this system of input is not available, political disempowerment will take hold (Scheyvens, 1999).

When the team and community are empowered, the initiative can grow in leaps and bounds. An initiative is successful when the community can own the project and the person who implemented the work can take a step back into a consulting role, thereby allowing in-country participants to take a more active role. Investment in this area produces great outcomes.

Develop Process to Evaluate and Modify

Developing and implementing an international, human-capacity-building project takes trial and error. Through the steps outlined previously, research, resources, and dedication will be heavily invested into this project. However, a project team won't always get it right the first time and will require a level of flexibility to modify the project to meet the country's identified need.

Establishing a system to analyze the work and create a process for modifications is essential to a project's sustainability. If training is being implemented, pre- and post- training measures should be used to assess the efficacy of the training. If a service is being rendered, feedback surveys should be developed to ascertain areas that require improvement. Feedback surveys should be conducted with those providing the work as well as those receiving it. Varying perspectives will further innovations in the project. Below are operational steps to consider when developing and implementing the evaluation process, as noted by Bennt, Aston, and Colquhoun (2000):

· Ensure the evaluation tools are completed by as many participants as possible.

· Use the feedback to modify the current process and guide future initiatives.

· Debrief members who are involved with the initiative development or implementation.

·Check in frequently to ensure modifications are being implemented.

·Continue performance management of those overseeing the day-to-day implementation of the work, based on evaluation feedback.

When developing a human-capacity-building project, a level of accountability is required. The initiative needs to have a positive impact and do no harm to the community (Ebrahim, 2003). For this reason, establishing a system of accountability can support an initiative's success. In some cases, accountability can take a formal path, with requirements to report on the initiative to the local government or donors. However, in many cases, accountability is informal and stems from being accountable to the partnerships developed and the community (Kilby, 2006). Potential pathways to ascertain accountability, described by Ebrahim (2003), are as follows:

·Reporting and disclosure statements: Be transparent in the project's finances, organizational structure, and data. Provide these documents to stakeholders for review.

·Performance evaluation: Establish tools to assess performance measures and if the outcomes are being met through the methods. External and internal evaluations can support accountability.

·Participation: This is a process instead of a tool. Invite others to be involved in a training, provide consultation on a proposed initiative component, or provide opportunities for others to view proposals for a planned initiative.

·Self-regulation: Develop set expectations and rules for how members of the project will behave and interact with others. Develop a code of conduct to support an ethical environment.

·Social Auditing: Develop or leverage a model that can assess the way in which the project is meeting ethical and social performance.

The development of an evaluation process and establishment of accountability tactics will provide better opportunities to gain support from partnerships and the community. The data obtained through these strategies should be used to report back to the approving bodies, donors, and key stakeholders. Keeping these stakeholders informed of the project's work and success is likely to lead to continued support. Ultimately, the success of your initiative will be evaluated by the community either accepting or rejecting the initiative (Fowler, 1991).

Self-Reflect

Developing and implementing a global initiative can have the effect of transforming an individual's outlook on life. The process will likely challenge constructs and schemas developed over time. Critical self-reflection challenges assumptions and builds new perceptions based on new experiences (Mezirow, 1990). Individuals involved in the development of an initiative should make an effort to find meaning in the experience rather than taking on the perspectives of others (Mezirow, 2000).

Questions to ask during the self-reflection process, as drawn upon from Heron (2005) and Yip (2005), include, but are not limited to:

- How are my values and perceptions being shaped as a result of this experience?
- How am I feeling toward the initiative?
- What and how am I resisting?
- What incongruences am I experiencing between myself and the experience?

Furthermore, consider how the in-country team is impacted by the initiative. Providing a space for them to reflect on their emotions and attitudes towards the work will help to identify if they are overwhelmed and to develop solutions to mitigate their feelings. Establishment of this support system will increase the initiative's potential to be sustainable and successful.

Relationship Development

At the center of developing and launching a sustainable and successful human-capacity-building project is the ability to develop and maintain positive relationships. These "soft skills" are often overlooked when building such a program, but they are critical to the initiative's ultimate success. They have the potential, in fact, to make or break the project. Having emotional intelligence, including (but not limited to) the ability to understand emotions in others and emotional meanings behind words. Refining interpersonal skills can positively impact the ability to develop, maintain, and grow relationships (Mayer, Caruso, & Salovey, 2016). The following are recommendations to support relationship development in this capacity:

- Actively listen: The individuals you will meet through developing and implementing your initiative are the experts. Understand their needs, ideas, and points of concerns through active listening.
- Communicate articulately: Communicate in a way that is engaging and generates a meaningful discussion. Consider potential language barriers and ways in which communication will need to occur, potentially with an interpreter.
- Provide a safe environment: By putting the individual at ease, this may support further engagement and honest feedback.
- Be collaborative: Foster an environment where the individual feels that their feedback and insights are being heard and contributing to the item being discussed.

- Ask questions: Ask questions that will allow for deeper discussions and building of relationships. Reflect on responses to ascertain if you understand them correctly.
- Be culturally mindful: Learn the importance of building relationships and how they are formed within a cultural context. Some cultures may take more time to build relationships and establish trust. They may build relationships through engaging in rituals, spiritual ceremonies, or enjoying food/drink together.
- Find a commonality: Building a bridge of connectivity starts with common interests.
- Be self-motivated: The project owner's determination and tenacity is the driving force to an initiative's success.
- Be authentic: Continue to be true to yourself when developing relationships with others.

Gathering feedback from colleagues or completing credible assessments could help to identify an individual's strengths as well as opportunities to develop these soft skills. By acknowledging areas of potential weaknesses, one can play to his or her strengths when developing relationships with potential partners, officials, and community members.

An additional component of developing relationships is managing cultural differences. Through the research and partnerships developed with the in-country stakeholders, continuing to understand how the culture shapes individual's behaviors, expectations, and perspectives (Bennett, Aston & Colquhoun, 2000) can support deeper and more meaningful relationships with others.

Building relationships with media contacts can also support the initiative's mission. Additional exposure to the identified need can result in new partners, resources, and ideas for innovations. Resources and support should not influence the overall direction of the initiative.

These best practices are intended to support an individual in developing a global initiative that positively impacts a community and continues to be sustainable. To conceptualize these recommendations further, the Global HOPE Training Initiative is detailed in the subsequent case study. Through the processes the developer engaged in, the initiative has been successful and continues to expand across Africa to date.

Case Study: Global HOPE Training Initiative*

The Global HOPE (Healing Opportunities through Purposeful

---

* Special thanks to the former mayor of Rulindo, Mr. Kangwagye, for his support. His insight, direction, and support allowed this project to expand strategically across the Rulindo district, which has resulted in 30 distinct and self-sustaining HOPE Clubs.

Engagement) Training Initiative is a 12-day "train-the-trainer" program that aids educators and youth workers in developing countries to effectively recognize, assess, and intervene with children who have been traumatized by genocide, war, natural disaster, illness, and extreme poverty. The project's purpose is to build a homegrown paraprofessional counseling infrastructure that exponentially increases the number of child care professionals with the skills to meet the needs of children who have experienced lifelong trauma and hardship.

Global HOPE was developed (2010) by Drs. Tiffany Masson and Mark Kassel and came to fruition in Rwanda, a country that was still reeling from a 1994 genocide perpetrated against the Tutsti. This genocide took the lives of millions and left in its wake many more orphaned and with significant exposure to trauma (Powley, 2006). Seven years later, the project is going strong, having trained headmasters and teachers at 50 schools across the country and expanded to Zambia and South Africa.

This case study provides an in-depth review of how the project was developed and how it has relied on best practices to create culture-specific training models, build in-country support, and ensure sustainability.

Psychological Impact of Genocide

The worst genocide in Africa's modern history had a devastating and long-lasting impact on the people of Rwanda. The effects of psychological trauma are often severe and manifested over generations. A UNICEF study found that 96% of Rwandan children had witnessed the massacres and 80% had lost at least one family member (Powley, 2006, p. 7). Even children who did not experience the genocide firsthand are at risk for the multigenerational consequences of trauma. According to Sezibera, Van Broeck, and Philippot (2009), approximately 71.6% of the 1994 genocide survivors exhibit symptoms of Post-Traumatic Stress Disorder (PTSD) (p. 108). Symptoms include intense fear, extreme anger, hallucinations, flashbacks, emotional detachment, insomnia, and nightmares. Children who suffer from trauma often become overwhelmed or debilitated academically and leave school at major risk for lifelong developmental and economic problems. They are more vulnerable to severe illness, lack energy to deal with situations, struggle with development, and find it difficult to control emotions and behavior. As reconciliation efforts continue in Rwanda, the mental health of children and those who care for them have emerged as a critical priority.

The First Step: Research

Rwanda was chosen as the site of the original Global HOPE Training Initiative (Global HOPE) because of the post-genocide resources needed to assist children with overcoming the impact of trauma, the resulting need for culturally relevant mental health interventions, and the expertise that Dr. Masson, the project lead, and her co-author of the Global Health Training Initiative, Dr. Mark Kassel, were able to bring to the project.

As a first step to creating Global HOPE, it was imperative that the project leader fully understood the culture and the challenges that exist in Rwanda. She and a colleague – with whom she authored the original training curriculum – thoroughly researched the psychosocial issues facing the post-genocide population and determined that the country's own resources were far too limited to address the impact of trauma and the emotional aftermath of the 1994 Rwanda genocide. This initial research led to the development of a trauma counseling program/training. The authors of the program believed the project would meet current needs and also be sustainable over time. What they soon realized after arriving in Rwanda, however, was how much they didn't know – how much they didn't understand about the Rwandan culture, its history, and the mindset of its people. They had to put aside their own experiences with trauma and the conceptions they had formed while reading the literature and learn from the people themselves. Many well-intentioned projects fail because NGOs rely on their own experience rather than tailoring it to the unique circumstances of the populations they are trying to help.

While articles and books written about the history of Rwanda yielded insight into the overarching psychosocial issues facing the people of Rwanda, it became evident that needs varied by population sector and that the development of a solid and sustainable training program required in-person, face-to-face interviews. The project team arrived in the country with ten ready-to-use modules only to quickly realize that much more work was needed. This is the essential part of self-reflection: the ability to recognize when something is not working and to change course as needed. Self-reflection, a critical best practice, was to be used throughout all phases of project development and implementation. It was in this moment – a humbling one for a project leader who had touted herself as a trauma expert and who had provided countless expert testimonies to the court on such issues – that a decision was made to discard the already-developed training modules and to start from scratch.

Use of Focus Groups to Gather Critical Information

Building an effective country-specific business model requires as much on-the-ground, in-person information as can be gathered. The project team decided to immerse themselves in the Rwandan culture, to listen to story after story, and to try to truly understand the needs described by the people who know them best – those who endured the horror and who live with the multigenerational scars that were left in its wake.

Twelve days were spent conducting focus groups, during which the project team listened, reflected back what they heard to ensure they understood, and encouraged individuals to convey their thoughts and stories in their native language. Although focus groups were primarily conducted in English (Rwandan teachers are now required to teach in English), it became apparent that many participants were more comfortable speaking Kinyarwanda, and English-fluent participants were enlisted to serve as translators. The project team was fully present for whatever they needed to hear and comprehend in the moment, ensuring that what they offered participants was a safe environment in which to tell their stories. They actively engaged with participants, encouraged authentic conversation, and often used open-ended exploratory questions to prompt dialogue. Focus groups were purposefully assembled to represent a variety of experiences and perspectives; it was the responsibility of the project team to ensure that all participants spoke, that all stories were welcomed, and that group members engaged with each other as well as the group facilitators. What they heard was almost unimaginable: stories of witnessing the deaths of family members and friends, hiding in unimaginable places to avoid death, and hearing about unfathomable grief. They discovered, to their astonishment, that there is no exact word in the Kinyarwanda language for "trauma."

It was in those moments that Global HOPE took shape, and the team's view of the world and their individual roles in that world changed forever. Upon returning stateside, they began to work on a business proposal/model that accurately addressed the identified needs. All findings from the focus groups were integrated into the curriculum; it was imperative that a wide range of perspectives, experiences, and needs be met in the evolving business model. Planning for sustainability was also a high priority. All too often, a well-intentioned plan can do more harm than good if sustainability is not built in at the ground level and does not serve as a foundation for the project. The initial vision — to train teachers to train other teachers — represented a large piece of that sustainability. Continued funding was also needed, however, and was ensured through internal university grants and external funders that valued the work and provided limited parameters so the curriculum could be shaped and owned by the people of Rwanda.

Building In-Country Support

Gaining in-country support is a critical step in creating an effective and sustainable capacity-building project. Early on, the team learned that their project could not succeed without governmental support. They approached the minister of education with a draft of the curriculum they proposed to offer. However, what was equally as important as a solid, quality, and culturally relevant curriculum was building trust. In light of Rwanda's history, it was important that the project leader demonstrate commitment to the country (consistency and follow-up on promised deliverables), show understanding about the impact of too many people coming into the country and leaving promises behind, and make certain to follow-up on the vision that the minister of education set forth. The minister of education suggested that headmasters be trained first (as the initial constituent body), followed by a secondary training specific to teachers. This specific flow of training allowed for a supportive environment in which each school would have a trained headmaster that could support the trained teachers and provide them with necessary resources. In addition, the minister of education also suggested a pre-service training component. He suggested a partnership with the University of Rwanda, Department of Education, to develop Global HOPE programming for students enrolled in courses to become a teacher as their long-term profession. Approximately three months after the initial meeting, the minister of education approved the project. The project leader felt honored that the minister of education trusted her ability to take such an important project forward.

A similar experience involved gaining the support of the mayor of Rulindo, the district in which the training curriculum was initially offered. As he was initially cautious, he allowed the project to begin small. However, he soon became an enthusiastic backer who mandated that all 30 schools in his district be accessible to the Global HOPE team. One headmaster and two teachers were trained in each school. Without the mayor's trust in this project, our efforts and outcomes in Rwanda would not have been possible. The project leader owes a great deal of gratitude to his mentorship, vision, and access to the district team. After several years of direct and sole focus on the Rulindo district to ensure sustainability, the project expanded to the Nyarugenge District, where the mayor agreed to allow the project to expand to the 20 schools in her district. One headmaster and two teachers were trained at each.

In-country support was also provided by an advisory board that was formed from the first group of focus group participants. The board offered essential feedback through the process of curriculum development and ensured that the content and delivery format (e.g., lecture, field experience, and telemedicine) was culturally relevant, evidence-based, and trauma-informed.

Project Implementation

The first training was offered to the advisory board. The curriculum – which had been continuously revised to integrate new learning – aimed to provide an understanding of how trauma impacts children's presenting problems (e.g. aggression, defiance, anxiety and depression) as well as the skills to promote healing relationships with traumatized children. The curriculum, available in both English and Kinyarwanda, supports teachers as they guide children beyond survival by building resilience and coping skills. It still stands true today that providing educators with valuable teaching tools designed to enhance children's ability to manage reactions, reduce high-risk behaviors, and promote constructive activity will help to improve the psychosocial well-being of vulnerable youth throughout the country. The training focuses on empowerment and helps teachers recognize that symptoms are often adaptive coping mechanisms rather than pathology.

Several studies indicate that well-trained, supervised, local paraprofessionals (such as the headmasters and teachers targeted in this project) can effectively deliver care to children affected by violence and war (Bolton et al., 2007; Hubbard & Pearson, 2004). These studies validate the direction the Global HOPE Training Initiative took: preparing culturally competent practitioners who can provide comprehensive services and integrate evidence-based practice with practice-based evidence. The curriculum was developed in three distinct phases:

1. Didactic lectures (since this was seen as normative in the culture) including a feedback section after each module so the curriculum can be improved over time.
2. Field experiences, which consisted of applied practice in the field to observe and to use the skills learned in the didactic portion of the training.
3. The use of telemedicine technology, which brought participants together by phone. A master trainer facilitated conversation for three months post-training to ensure skill maintenance.

In an effort to ensure mastery of the skills, pre- and post-training measures are used to ascertain the efficacy of the curriculum. The Global HOPE lectures, field days, and telemedicine components are designed to strengthen trainees' abilities to use effective and trauma-informed counseling skills with children in order to reduce problematic behaviors, increase protective factors that build resiliency, and increase overall academic performance. Together, the lectures, experiential component, and post-training telemedicine component provide comprehensive and varied ways of skill building. More importantly, repeated practice strengthens the trainees' ability to use their new counseling skills, and the continued telemedicine support helps them to gain confidence as they work with traumatized children and begin to train other staff at local secondary schools.

Post-training telemedicine is critical to ensuring sustainability. The fact that this component is delivered regularly (weekly) and for an extended period (three-months) ensures that trainees remain connected and supported. However, this component needed to be modified to meet the realities of the Rwandan culture. Dr. Masson had initially planned to use teleconferencing and computer-based telemedicine platforms in the post-training phase. What she learned was that cell phones were the only medium readily available at no cost to participants (individuals receiving calls in Rwanda are free and do not exhaust any talk-time); as a result, this phase was delivered solely by mobile phones.

After almost five years of completed trainings, three in-country master trainers have emerged as exceptional leaders. Master trainers are teachers or headmasters who have completed the Global HOPE training, observed at least two curriculum author-led trainings, and conducted at least two trainings observed by curriculum author(s). Additionally, pre- and post-assessment measures must demonstrate that the master trainer is able to achieve the same outcomes as those achieved by the project leaders. This ensures that quality control is in place, and the curriculum integrity is solid. These master trainers' commitment has been exemplary, and post-assessment measures show that there is no statistical difference between the outcomes between master trainers and curriculum authors who conducted initial trainings.

This finding has provided critical proof of the power inherent in building a well-trained, in-country team. It validates the realization that sustainability is about living beyond a project's creators and empowering those on the ground to own this curriculum and ensure that that team remains committed to this project. In a human-capacity-building project, it is difficult to let go and to trust that those on the ground can do it. However, in letting go, amazing things flourish in unexpected ways.

Looking back, the project leader identified mental preparation as a need that she had underestimated. Individuals embarking on a project of this magnitude should prepare mentally as the process of listening, day after day, to stories of the 1994 genocide, the descriptions of horror, fear, anger, and grief can be mentally exhausting. People facing this type of work should have plans in place for processing the information and identifying means of support.

Empowering an In-Country Team

Global HOPE has grown beyond the training project that was originally envisioned. It has successfully empowered the on-ground Rwandan professionals to take the project to the next level. These trainees developed the idea of HOPE Clubs, after-school expressive arts programs developed to cultivate skills and resiliency in Rwandan youth.

The clubs bring together children who have been identified by Global HOPE-trained teachers as traumatized with those who have not been identified as such, but have established themselves as student leaders. These are organically developed peer networks designed to help children work through their traumatic experiences with the support of trained, concerned, and caring educators. It is in these HOPE Clubs that children who have been orphaned have created their own "families" to reduce isolation and stigma. This innovative after-school project resulted from a telemedicine dialogue in which two teachers (now Global HOPE master trainers) recognized the desperate need of so many children and shared concerns about being the only individual in a classroom with the capacity and skillset to help these children heal. These many conversations resulted in the birth of HOPE Clubs, which are now an option offered at every school with teachers who have completed Global HOPE training.

To date, all 50 schools in two districts have instituted 50 HOPE Clubs that serve approximately 3,000 children collectively. Students in the clubs are carefully selected by their teachers to achieve a balance of student leaders and those in most need of emotional and financial support.

Expressive art activities include drawing, problem-solving dialogues, process groups, emotion-oriented exercises, prayer, dramas, song, traditional dance, and sports. These culturally-based activities are utilized in the HOPE Clubs to provide students with a platform for expressing their emotions. Other activities within the Children's HOPE Clubs, such as local trades and crafts, focus on economic development. Children take part in the breeding and selling of animals (e.g. rabbits) and the cultivation of gardens, which are used as a means of poverty reduction. Despite the advantages offered by activities of this kind, participants most often describe their Children's HOPE Club as a place that promotes resilience, develops and fosters protective factors, includes intergenterational healing, and builds a strong sense of future-orientation, all of which are essential in developing the human capital of a country (Hedglen, 2016).

Trained teachers and headmasters have also begun to develop unique and sustainable ways to improve children's academic performance, life skills, and emotional well-being through the creation of vegetable, bunny, and coffee farms (in addition to pig and goat giving). At several HOPE Clubs, the headmaster donated land for cultivation. The children grew and sold vegetables in the market and used the money to pay for their school fees. Additionally, at several HOPE Clubs, teachers pooled their money to buy a bunny, which was given to the most vulnerable HOPE Club child along with the responsibility of giving a bunny to another vulnerable HOPE Club child after reproduction. The next child would be expected to give one of his/her litter to the next vulnerable child and so on. In addition to creating a scalable solution to reduce poverty, this project built self-confidence in children, taught them the importance of community, and empowered them to assist their families and pay for school fees. Similarly, one HOPE Club was granted nearby land from the community which was used to develop a coffee farm; proceeds from coffee sales were used to pay school fees for children in this club. This sustainable solution has not only kept children in school, but it is during cultivation activities with the teachers that children feel safe enough to speak about their traumatic experiences and seek support from trained teachers. These are only a few of the many unique and sustainable ways that headmasters and teachers trained in Global HOPE are making a difference in the lives of the children they serve.

Another example of project improvement that came about as trained educators felt sufficiently empowered to offer curriculum changes is the self-help component for the teachers themselves. As they began to recognize the stress that inevitably results from working with severely traumatized children, they realized that they too could use some help. The result was training in stress reduction, healthy living, and self-care.

Relationship Building

In the Global HOPE initiative, relationships grew out of efforts to build in-country teams and to empower those teams to take ownership of the project. As described earlier, such relationships take time and require the development of mutual trust. When cultural differences are present, project leaders need to be prepared to negotiate those differences and to decide what aspects of a plan need to be sacrificed or modified in order to achieve agreement and build trust. The project leader's interactions with the ministry of education provide an example of this.

Important relationships also resulted from focus groups and from the ongoing contact between participants and the project lead. The partnership forged with the mayor of Rulindo, who had become a strong supporter of the efforts in his district, was leveraged to provide clear evidence of progress. That evidence is described in the following section.

A relationship was also fostered with the University of Rwanda, Department of Education, which led to the development of a model to follow through on the minister of education's vision to incorporate the Global HOPE curriculum into teacher training. This continues to be a work in progress and will be incorporated into the first guidance counseling program offered at University of Rwanda, Department of Education.

Assessment Strategy and Outcomes

Throughout implementation, the Global HOPE project has been rigorously evaluated in terms of both process and outcomes. The training program and curriculum have been modified as needed to improve the experiences of both trainees and the children they serve.

This willingness to revise – and revise again – a project as new information is received or new insights are offered is critical to the long-term success of a capacity-building program. Even with the most thorough pre-planning research and the use of focus groups, modifications will almost always be needed. Flexibility to adapt as needed is a key to achieving desired outcomes.

Evaluating the HOPE Clubs

The HOPE Clubs provided one area of measurement. At the mayor's urging, the Rulindo District surveyed schools involved in a HOPE Club to ascertain if academic benefits were gained and goals were achieved. In all, 20 headmasters completed the survey, which focused on whether or not students who are members of the HOPE Club improved their academic performance and whether or not other benefits were achieved. In addition, HOPE Club member testimonies about experiences and benefits of participation were sampled and analyzed.

Evaluation Design

A concurrent nested mixed methods design was used to analyze qualitative and quantitative data at the same time, and an integration of the findings at the interpretation stage was implemented (Creswell, Plano Clark, Gutmann, & Hanson, 2003). A phenomenological approach was used to examine students' testimonies about their experiences before and after joining the HOPE Club regarding the following areas:
 ·Needs before joining the HOPE Club
 ·Improvement in the activities of the HOPE Club
 ·Abilities gained and achieved
 ·Outcomes of their involvement
For the quantitative phase, a pre-experimental design was implemented – meaning participants' exams scores before joining the HOPE Club were compared to their scores after joining the HOPE Club to determine whether there was a statistically significant difference between the two conditions.

Qualitative Phase

For the qualitative strand, the focus was to analyze participants' record of testimonies across 30 secondary schools in the Rulindo District (Northern Province, Rwanda). These secondary schools included one trained headmaster and two trained teachers in Global HOPE with an active HOPE Club. The testimonies were viewed as archival data and analyzed to address the qualitative evaluation questions. In all, 50 student testimonies were accessed, of which 34 were analyzed.

Qualitative Analysis

The purpose of the qualitative analysis was to understand how the HOPE Clubs benefitted students. To address this purpose, testimonies from 50 students were qualitatively analyzed. To start the coding process, anchor codes were assigned to each of the four evaluation questions. The reason for assigning anchor codes to the evaluation questions was to help in organizing initial codes developed from the data (Adu, 2014). Below are the evaluation questions and their respective anchor codes.

· What were children's initial needs? Anchor code: Initial needs
· What are specific activities in the club that may have contributed to the abilities and benefits gained? Anchor code: Activities
· What abilities gained as a result of children's participation in the Hope club? Anchor code: Abilities
· What are the outcomes of children's participation in the Hope club? Anchor code: Outcomes

To capture participants' perception about the Hope Club's activities (and in an effort to use the students' own words to code), an evaluation and In Vivo coding method were used respectively. Within this method, an emotion coding technique was used to label participant's emotional experiences before and after joining the HOPE Club, a process coding method was used to code participants' verbal expression of behaviors, and a magnitude coding system was used to create codes that represent the intensity of behaviors, emotions, feelings, and HOPE Club's activities (Saldana, 2013). In all, 34 out of 50 testimonies were coded. Coding stopped after the 34th testimony because saturation was reached (i.e., a stage where no new information is being discovered).

At the initial stage of the data analysis, 110 relevant statements from the student testimonies were coded. The statements were then grouped into 44 codes and put under each of their respective evaluation questions (see Figure 1). The codes and their respective frequencies (i.e., the number of times specific codes were assigned to the significant statements from the testimonies) were analyzed to create a visual display of the codes. The illustration (see Figure 2) shows that most students indicated that their academic performance had improved after joining the HOPE Club. The codes were further categorized to directly address the evaluation questions.

Figure 1: The coding process

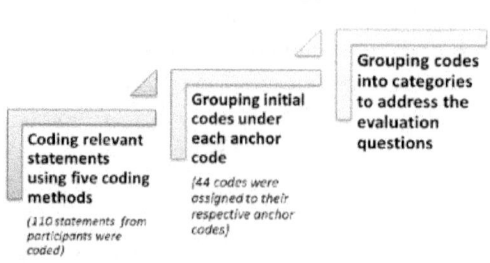

Coding relevant statements using five coding methods

(110 statements from participants were coded)

Grouping initial codes under each anchor code

(44 codes were assigned to their respective anchor codes)

Grouping codes into categories to address the evaluation questions

Figure 2: A visual display of the codes.
The higher the frequency of the code, the bigger the font.

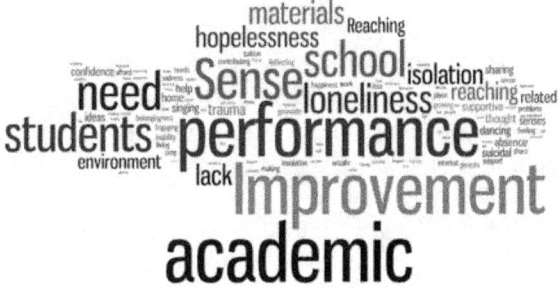

Qualitative Findings: Initial Needs.

To address children's initial needs, four main categories were identified:

· Academic difficulties and truancy

· Inability to afford education

· Experienced traumatic situation

· Exhibiting trauma symptoms

In the testimonies, students expressed the problems they faced before joining a HOPE Club. Some spoke about the traumatic situations they experienced, including rape, domestic violence, death of parents and/or family members during the 1994 Rwanda Genocide, and childhood abuse. One student expressed:

...I used to go to school with many problems at home, my father is a drunkard and my mother too and they fight at home.... I was wondering why God created me with such problems and I thought of suicide... (personal communication, June 9, 2013)

Another student said:

I have been so sad. My parents are HIV positive. My mother creates problems to my father because she says that he is the one who infected her. They fight each other day by day. There is no peace at home. I wished to die... (personal communication, May 9, 2013)

Lastly, a club member also said:

My life wasn't good before joining this club, as you see I am the eldest student in this school, the people whom we have the same age are my teachers, I have lost my parents in genocide and I felt that I lost everything. After genocide, when I was 13 years old, I was traumatized because what happened in genocide and what I faced, I was afraid of spending the night in the house, I was traumatized at the level that when a leaf of the tree fell down, I was afraid thinking that are the killers then I decided to ask for the night guard job because it was hard for me to sleep at night... (personal communication, June 9, 2013)

Students also shared their difficulties in learning and concentrating in the classroom, which led to low academic performance and truancy. One student said:

> ...I was very shy, [and] very timid, my performance in the class were reducing day by day and that was a big problem for me, but after hearing that there is Club in our school called Hope Club and also understanding the word Hope, I was excited to join the club. (personal communication, July 9, 2013)

Another student said:

> I was born my mother married another man I stayed at my grandfather's. He is very poor. He is not able to pay for me the school fees. I studied only senior one and dropped out. When the club came in this school two teachers came at home I was cultivating and they asked me to come back to school. I study for free and they give me school materials. (personal communication, May 9, 2013)

These testimonies show the effects of trauma on academic performance.

Qualitative Findings: Activities

The "activities" anchor code focused on capturing the Hope Club activities, which were carried out with the aim of questioning the activities in the HOPE Club that contributed to the abilities and benefits gained. Three categories were generated:

· Engaging in outreach program
· Supporting one another and building a community
· Engaging in recreational activities

A HOPE Club member said the following about the benefits of joining:

> I was tired of my sickness and of myself I just wanted to drop out. The teacher helped me to join the club and now I can feel that even if my headache is still here but I am happy and very happy to be in the club. (personal communication, April 9, 2013)

After joining, members provide support to each other to overcome their challenges. Some of the supports noted in testimonies were: helping in growing crops, being open with each other, sharing problems, pulling together resources to help members in need, helping each other to make good decisions, and planning for the future. One member said:

> What else I thank the club is that our leaders, the teachers trained are there for us, they help us and we share with them our problem and from there we feel comfortable. The club taught us to have love for our club members, if someone is sick we take care of him at the hospital, if someone misses the tick to go in his/her family, we contribute and we give him/her money for the ticket. (personal communication, April 9, 2013

Qualitative Findings: Abilities

With regard to the "abilities" anchor code, the focus was to code relevant information from student testimonies that reflected the skills gained as the result of being members of the HOPE Club. The main theme that emerged was a sense of confidence. Students indicated that, based on their engagement in HOPE Club activities, they gained confidence in their ability to share ideas, reach out to one another, and help those in need. One member said:

> I was happy because I heard that it will be a club which will help the students with hopeless and sadness. This time I am very happy and other children who don't know this club they are surprised when they see me laughing and even my family are surprised so I will search for other students who have the problems and sensitize them to join this club. (personal communication, June 9, 2013)

Another member recounted:

> I want to tell you how it has been closed to us the students, till now we are still working and we are very confident, after joining the club, you are like our mothers and fathers, and I would like to ask you to continue to help us for building in ourselves the hope of tomorrow. Some of us, most of the time were very shy but now we are trying to shine in front of others, when we are at school, we try to meet together and think of tomorrow and we have now the hope of tomorrow. Something which is good is that from senior four because I am in senior five, but till now I am the first of the class. (personal communication, April 9, 2013)

Qualitative Findings: Outcomes

For this anchor code, information about the impact of being part of the HOPE Club was coded to specifically evaluate the outcomes of students' participation in the HOPE Club. Four categories emerged:

- Academic support
- Optimism
- Sense of belongingness
- Improvement of academic performance (see Figure 3 in Appendix A*)

Some students expressed their appreciation for the support they received after joining the HOPE Club. They indicated that the HOPE Club improved their sense of belonging, feeling of support to share emotions, and community. A student said, "...[I] was so poor and I joined the club after [the] creation here at school, I got the school materials from the member of the club" (personal communication, July 9, 2013). Another

---

* Appendices for this chapter can be found at: http://tinyurl.com/wghm-attachments

outcome was the sense of optimism. Students expressed feeling happy and having an increased sense of self-esteem and hope for the future. The following quote from a student testimony best represents what some of the students described about the sense of belonging:

> We have other things that we do in our club for example we explain one another because we feel that the members of the club are like the brothers and sisters so we don't want anyone to fail in his/her lessons. (personal communication, April 9, 2013)

Lastly, improvement of academic performance was mentioned frequently. Out of 34 testimonies, 19 of them made reference to the fact that the improvement of their academic work was due to their involvement in the HOPE Club. The following are some of the excerpts of their testimonies. (Note that a score of 70 or higher is considered approximately a 90 plus percent in U.S. grading terms).

> ... by the arrival of Global Hope, I tried my best, I used all my effort, in O'level I had 53%, but now I get 75 marks, because Global Hope has helped me to know how I can forget my problems, how I can follow my studies... (personal communication, April 9, 2013)

> ...I am helped by other members of the club to understand the lessons and now I get 70% and before I got 56% and even my parents are proud of me. It is only the increase of the marks the club also buy for me the school materials. (personal communication, July 9, 2013)

> I dropped out for one week the club came at home to see me and they have given me school materials and I came back. I had 48 % in the 1st term on my school report but now in the 2nd term I have 61%. (personal communication, July 9, 2013)

Quantitative Phase

Twenty educators and headmasters representing 20 schools completed a survey provided by Rulindo District, which was used to better understand whether students' participation in the HOPE Club contributed to improvement in their overall academic performance. Fifty-nine HOPE Club members' exam scores were analyzed to determine whether there was a statistically significant deference of their scores before and after joining the club.

Quantitative Findings

In all, 259 club members' exam scores before joining the HOPE Club were compared to scores after joining the HOPE club. The results showed that their exam scores (M=54%, SD= 12) before joining the club were less than their scores after joining the club (M=61%, SD= 10).

To determine whether the improvement was significant, a repeated Analysis of covariance (ANCOVA) was conducted. The results show that there is a statistically significant difference of students' academic performance before and after the HOPE Club when controlling for the school to which students were affiliated ($F(1, 287) = 102.42$, p $<.05$, partial eta squared $= .26$). This means that irrespective of the school students were affiliated with, being a part of the HOPE Club significantly impacted their academic performance (see Figure 4).

There is no one, perfect approach to assessing the efficacy of a human-capacity-building project. Methodology to assess project efficacy needs to be well-thought-through and should be directly related to key stakeholders' questions about the potential impact. It is important to reflect, however, upon the value of using quantitative and qualitative data to analyze project outcomes as using both approaches can provide a more complete understanding of the project's impact. In this particular case, the qualitative and quantitative findings indicated that involving students in a HOPE Club with trained, Global HOPE teachers can have a profound, positive impact on children. HOPE Clubs have helped children gain a positive social network that provides support and a sense of community. Through expressive arts and related activities focused on helping children to heal from trauma, these children developed a sense of self-confidence, belonging, hope, and forward thinking – all of which support resiliency in children. In addition, these students developed strategies to cope with their psychological needs and became optimistic about life with a strong focus on academic achievement. Creating a space for the children to express their emotions and feelings helped them to deal with their trauma and encouraged others in similar situations to share how the felt, thereby breaking a culture of silence and allowing healing to occur (see Figure 5, Appendix B).

Figure 4. Increase in students' academic performance after joining the HOPE Club

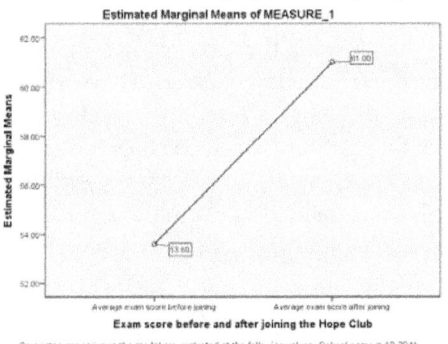

Summary

The experience of developing and implementing the Global HOPE program has been enormously positive for all involved. The initial goal of creating a "train-the-trainer" project to meet the needs of children whose lives bear the indelible scars of the Rwanda genocide was, by itself, a lofty goal – one that offered much potential benefit for the people of this war-torn African nation. The outcomes that emerged as the project came to fruition, however, exceeded the hopes and the vision of its creators. As originally planned, teachers and headmasters were trained to identify and address the symptoms of trauma in the children they taught; three went on to become master trainers who would in turn train educators across the country. But the benefits didn't stop there. Unwaveringly committed to the Global HOPE goals, trainees took the project to the next level, creating after-school HOPE Clubs that brought together student leaders with children whom teachers had identified as exhibiting the residual symptoms of trauma. In these clubs, an expressive arts curriculum was used to help children build resilience and learn economic development strategies that would help to support their families. This built their confidence and sense of empowerment.

Evaluation data showed a marked improvement in participants' academic achievement and in their emotional resilience. In addition to planting vegetable and coffee gardens, they raised bunnies — a special project that gave new meaning to the concept of project sustainability. As vulnerable HOPE Club children raised their bunnies, they took pride in sharing their wealth by passing along one of their bunny offspring to another vulnerable student who could, in turn, do the same.

The project has expanded continually since its inception in 2010. The eighth version of the training curriculum is now in use, having benefited from numerous modifications and culture-specific adaptations. While there is a demand for Global HOPE trainings in other areas of Rwanda, the project leader initially chose to stay focused on Rulindo and the commitment that had blossomed there.

In the years that followed, the project has been launched in Zambia, where child and youth care agency workers are being trained, and in South Africa, where training is being offered to psychology and social worker professionals in the Department of Education. Each country has lent its own specific needs to the project, which offers additional testimony to the need for adapting plans as needed and building culture-specific curriculums and business plans.

References

About the UN (n.d.). In *United Nations*. Retrieved October 29, 2016, from http://www.un.org/en/about-un/.

Adu, P. (2014). Qualitative Analysis: Coding and Categorizing. The Chicago School of Professional Psychology. Retrieved from http://www.slideshare.net/kontorphilip/qualitative-analysiscoding-and-categorizing-ncade-webinar.

American Psychological Association. (1993). Guidelines for providers of psychological services to ethnic, linguistic, and culturally diverse populations. *American Psychologist, 48*(1), 45-48. doi: 10.1037/0003-066X.48.1.45.

Bennett, R., Aston, A., & Colquhoun, T. (2000). Cross-cultural training: A critical step in ensuring the success of international assignments. *Human Resource Management, 39*(2,3), 239-250.

Betancourt J.R., Green, A.R., & Carrillo, J.E. (2002). *Cultural competence in health care:Emerging frameworks and practical approaches.* New York, NY: The Commonwealth Fund. doi: 10.1377/hlthaff.24.2.499.

Bolton, P., Bass, Betancourt, T., Speelman, L., Onyango, G., Clougherty, K. F., Verdeli, H.(2007). Interventions for depression symptoms among adolescent survivors of war and displacement in northern Uganda: A randomized controlled trial. *Journal of the American Medical Association, 298*, 519-527.

Brown, L. D., (1991). Bridging organizations and sustainable development. *Human Relations, 44*(8), 807-831.

Bruno, A., Bates, I., Brock, T., & Anderson, C. (2010). Towards a global competency framework. *American Journal of Pharmaceutical Education, 74*(3).

Campinha-Bacote, J. (2002). The process of cultural competence in the delivery of healthcare services: A model of care. *Journal of Transcultural Nursing, 13*(3), 181-184. doi: 10.1177/10459602013003003.

Clarke, G. (1998). Non-governmental organizations (NGOs) and politics in the developing world. *Political Studies, XLVI*, 36-52.

Creswell, J. W., Plano Clark, V. L., Gutmann, M. L., & Hanson, W. E. (2003). Advanced mixed methods research designs. In A. Tashakkori & C. Teddlie (Eds.), *Handbook of mixed methods in social and behavioral research* (pp. 209–240). Thousand Oaks, CA: Sage.

Dreesch, N. (2008). *Planning human resources development to achieve priority health programme goals* (pp. 2-16). N.p.: World Health Education.

Ebrahim, A. (2003). Accountability in practice: Mechanisms for NGOs. *World Development, 31*(5), 813-829.

Flache, A., & Macy, M. W. (2011). Local convergence and global diversity: From interpersonal to social influence. *Journal of Conflict Resolution, 55*(6), 970-995.

Fowler, A. (1991). What is different about managing non-governmental organization (NGOs) involved in Third World development. *RRA Notes, 11*, 75-81.

Gillies, P. (1998) Effectiveness of alliances and partnerships for health promotion, *Health Promotion International, 13*(2), 99–120.

Hedglen, J. (2016). *"We hear you and we help you:" A phenomenological account of resiliency in post-genocide Rwanda.* (Unpublished doctoral dissertation). The Chicago School of Professional Psychology, Chicago, IL.

Heron, B. (2005). Self-reflection in critical social work practice: Subjectivity and the possibilities of resistance. *Reflective Practice, 6*(3), 341-351.

Hubbard, J., & Pearson, N. (2004). Sierra Leonean refugees in Guinea: Addressing the mental health effects of massive community violence. In K. E. Miller & L. M. Rasco (Eds.), *The mental health of refugees: Ecological approaches to healing and adaptation* (pp. 95-132). Mahwah, NJ: Erlbaum.

Israel, B. A., Checkoway, B., Schulz, A., & Zimmerman, M. (1994). Health education and community empowerment: Conceptualizing and measuring perceptions of individual, organizational, and community control. *Health Education Quarterly, 21*(2), 149-170.

Kilby, P. (2006). Accountability for empowerment: Dilemmas facing non-governmental organizations. *The Australian National University,* 34(6), 951-963.

Labonte, R. & Laverack, G. (2001). Capacity building in health promotion, part 1: For Whom? And for what purpose? *Critical Public Health, 11*(2), 111-127.

Lewis, D. (2003). Theorizing the organization and management of non-governmental development organizations. *Public Management Review, 5*(3), 325-344.

Lewis, D., & Kanji, N. (2009). *Non-governmental organizations and development.* London: Routledge.

Mayer, J. D., Caruso, D. R., & Salovey, P. (2016). The ability model of emotional intelligence: Principles and updates. *Emotion Review, 8*(4), 290-300.

Mezirow, J. (1990). How critical reflection triggers transformative learning. *Fostering critical reflection in adulthood, 1,* 20.

Mezirow, J. (2000). Learning to think like an adult. In J. Mezirow (Eds.), *Learning as transformation: Critical perspectives on a theory in progress* (pp. 3-33). San Francisco: Jossey-Bass.

Nathan, S., Rotem, A., & Ritchie, J. (2002). Closing the gap: Building the capacity of non government organizations as advocates for healthy equity. *Health Promotion International, 17*(1), 69-78.

Putnam, F., Lieberman, A., Putnam, K., & Amaya-Jackson, L. (2015). *Opportunities to change the outcome of traumatized children: The childhood adversity narratives.*

Riddell, R. (2008). *Does foreign aid really work?.* Oxford: Oxford University Press.

Saldana, J. (2013). *The coding manual for qualitative researchers.* London: Sage.

Scheyvens, R. (1999). Ecotourism and the empowerment of local communities. *Tourist Management, 20,* 245-249.

Sezibera, V., Van Broeck, N., & Philippot, P. (2009). Intervening on persistent posttraumatic stress disorder: Rumination-focused cognitive and behavioral therapy in a population of young survivors of the 1994 genocide in Rwanda. *Journal of Cognitive Psychotherapy, 23*(2), 107–113.

Singh, D. (n.d.). Managing Cross-cultural Diversity: Issues and Challenges in Global Organizations. *IOSR Journal of Mechanical and Civil Engineering,* 43-50.

Powley, E. (2006). *Rwanda: The impact of women legislators on policy outcomes affecting children and families.* New York, NY: UNICEF.

Winkelstein, M. L., Quartey, R., Pham, L., Lewis-Boyer, L., Lewis, C., Hill, K., & Butz, A. (2006). Asthma education for rural nurses: Resources, barriers, and outcomes. *The Journal of School Nursing, 22*(3), 170-177.

Yip, K. (2006). Self-reflection in reflective practice: A note of caution. *British Journal of Social Work, 36,* 777-78

AFTERWORD
Efosa Guobadia

Exponential Love:
We Can Change the World through One Touch Point at a Time

It was October 2012, and it was a sunny afternoon. It was the fourth day that our group of healthcare volunteers was treating patients in Guatemala. After just completing a treatment session, I saw a woman heading straight for me with her young kids following behind. She moved with a sense of urgency, and her eyes were searching for hope. When she came into my treatment station, she began to share her story. Her name was Maria, and earlier in the week I treated her sister for knee pain. Her sister convinced her to come to see me as soon as possible since our group would be leaving in a few days. The evaluation started with her sharing the history of her shoulder pain, which had become progressively worse over the last several months. She had not been able to work during that time, and she was unable to lift her kids or play with them as she had before. She further shared that it had begun to affect her mood. Her family and friends would tease her to "bring the old Maria back." After continuing the evaluation and gathering objective information, it was clear that the cause of her impairment was impingement at the shoulder joint as she was unable to lift her arm higher than her shoulder. With the evaluation completed, I proceeded to treat her shoulder for the next hour. The techniques that I utilized consisted of joint and soft tissue mobilizations, general exercises, muscle re-education, and postural training. There was immediate improvement. Maria had gained full range of motion of her shoulder, and between her tears and smiles, she was able to let me know that it felt as good as it had before.

For many days after that episode, Maria was on my mind. I found myself thinking about the progress that we made in our short time together, and I found myself wondering what it would mean for her and her family. I knew that by helping to improve her shoulder, she would now be able to return to work. I visualized her picking up her kids and dancing with her husband, smiling like she had at the end of our session. I could sense that her friends and family members would be affected positively as well. I rested on the belief that helping just one family could impact a whole community. My heart tells me that by bettering one community at a time we can better the world.

That is exponential love – the notion and the belief that love and compassion can lead to seen, unseen, and unforeseen changes of positive growth. That stimulus of kindness and service to others can create ripples that can become a rising tide that changes the world for the better. That rising tide is most powerful when different people in different places offer compassion, grace, kindness, and cheerfulness to each other.

Much of what we read about in global health today looks at program paradigms, structural efforts, and sustainable change. That macro level perspective is necessary for the workings of our programs and our organizations. However, it will always be important for us to remember that the connections made at the micro level create touch points that are just as powerful and lasting. The inventor and statesman Ben Franklin would look into the mirror each morning and ask himself: "What good shall I do this day?" (Wallin, 2013, para. 2). We should ask that of ourselves. Each and every day, we have the profound

Lead By Serving, Serve by Leading
by Efosa Guobadia

I lead by serving, I serve to lead
It fulfills my honor, it fulfills my creed
With all the pain and suffering in this world
You try to play your part to fulfill the need

A mother's pain and joy in one place
Is just the same as another
It's not what I hope for myself
It's about what I hope for my brother

I lead by serving, I serve to lead
Blossoms can bloom from a single seed
There is much that can be done by every person
You can smile, hug, heal and you can feed

Be bold and go help with your helping heart
You may not be able to see the finish
But you can embrace the start

Leading and serving they are the same to me
I give courage, I gain courage, it sets the heart
free
So think about leading and think about serving
Think about helping those that you can
With all the things that can be done
I've found no better place to make a stand

capacity to do good at any moment and from any place. Love is the most powerful force in the world. It presents itself in different languages, looks, connections, and moments. It transcends time and space. It's immeasurable. It's uncontrollable. It's exponential. In our daily lives and on the front lines of global health, the world needs us to use our skills and tools for good. That's how we change it. That's how we make it a better place.

References

Wallin, Y. (2013, March 6). What good shall I do this day?' Asked Benjamin Franklin every single morning. Retrieved from https://www.good.is/articles/what-good-shall-i-do-this-day-asked-benjamin-franklin-every-single-morning

EDITOR BIOGRAPHY

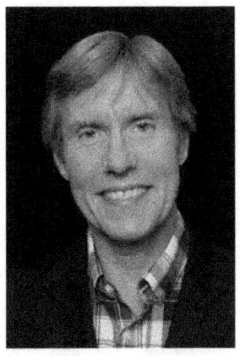

Chris Stout is a licensed clinical psychologist and has a diverse background in various domains. He is the founding director of the Center for Global Initiatives which was ranked as a Top Healthcare Nonprofit by GreatNonprofits.org (2011 -16). He also is a faculty member in the College of Medicine and Advisory Board Member to the Center for Global Health, and was a Fellow in the School of Public Health at the University of Illinois, Chicago. He served as a Non-Governmental Organization Special Representative to the United Nations. He was appointed by the Secretary of the U.S. Department of Commerce to the Board of Examiners for the Baldrige National Quality Award. He holds the distinction of being one of only 100 world-wide leaders appointed to the World Economic Forum's Global Leaders of Tomorrow 2000 and he was an Invited Faculty at the Annual Meeting in Davos. He was invited by the Club de Madrid and Safe-Democracy. He is Vice President of Research and Data Analytics for ATI, a national orthopedic rehabilitation and sports medicine organization.

Dr. Stout is a Fellow in three Divisions of the American Psychological Association, past-President of the Illinois Psychological Association, and is a Distinguished Practitioner in the National Academies of Practice. He is the Series Editor of *Contemporary Psychology* (Praeger) and *"Getting Started"* (Wiley & Sons). He produced the critically acclaimed four-volume set *The Psychology of Terrorism* and more recently, the highly praised and award–winning three volume set, *The New Humanitarians*, and is an Amazon.com Best Selling Author. His works have been translated into 8 languages. He was noted as being "one of the most frequently cited psychologists in the scientific literature" in a study by Hartwick College, and has won five Humanitarian Awards, four honorary doctorates, and is an inaugural inductee into his high school's and Purdue University's Hall of Fame.

AUTHOR BIOGRAPHIES

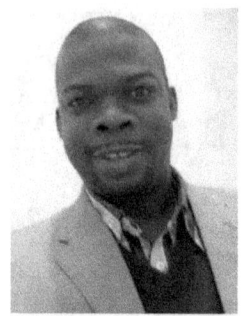

Dr. Philip Adu is currently a methodology expert at the National Center for Academic & Dissertation Excellence in The Chicago School of Professional Psychology (TCSPP). Dr. Adu was the program lead overseeing the implementation of the Doctor of Education in Educational Psychology and Technology program at TCSPP. He was an adjunct professor of educational psychology at West Virginia University. He has a bachelor's in psychology from the University of Ghana and a master's in international development studies from Ohio University. In 2011, Dr. Adu completed his doctoral degree in education with a concentration in learning, instruction, design, and technology from West Virginia University. He is specialized in program planning and evaluation, curriculum development, and technology integration. Dr. Adu was involved in diverse program planning and evaluation projects such as a National Science Foundation-funded project, "Engineers of Tomorrow," and "Quality Rating and Improvement for West Virginia Child Care," which was funded by the West Virginia Department of Health and Human Resources. He has made several presentations at the American Educational Research Association (AERA) annual conferences. He has also served as a reviewer of the *Journal of Mixed Methods Research*. He recently co-authored a book for college students, *Surviving in a Class with the "Most Difficult of Professors": A Result-Oriented Approach in Dealing with Any College Course.*

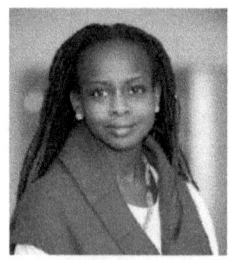

Adeyinka M. Akinsulure-Smith, PhD, is a licensed psychologist and tenured Associate Professor in the Department of Psychology at the City College of New York of the City University of New York (CUNY) and at the Graduate Center of CUNY. She has cared for forced migrants as well as survivors of torture, armed conflict, and human rights abuses from around the world at the Bellevue/NYU Program for Survivors of Torture since 1999. In addition to her teaching and clinical work, Dr. Akinsulure-Smith is the recipient of several grants, including a 2014-2015 Fulbright Africa Regional Research Program award. She is currently the principal investigator of a National Institutes of Health-funded project to examine female genital cutting among African immigrants and service providers in the United States. Drawing on her considerable experiences providing therapeutic services to diverse populations and on her ongoing research projects, Dr. Akinsulure-Smith has written extensively about forced migrants, including recent publications in the *Journal of Immigrant and Refugee Studies*, *Professional Psychology: Research and Practice*, the *Journal of Child and Family Studies*, *Human Development*, *Public Library of Science*, the *Journal of Immigrant & Minority Health*, the American Journal of Community *Psychology*, and the *Journal of Aggression, Maltreatment & Trauma*.

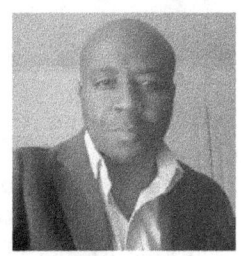

Enyi Anosike is a community psychiatrist who obtained his primary medical degree from the College of Medicine of the University of Nigeria in 1998. As well as obtaining a diploma in tropical medicine and hygiene from the London School of Hygiene and Tropical Medicine (2004) and a master of studies degree in public health medicine from Homerton College, University of Cambridge (2007), he was keen to further his training in a manner particularly useful to low- and medium-income countries. He therefore sought further studies in health systems development, quality management, and health projects monitoring and evaluation from the International Health Department of the Institute of Public Health, University of Heidelberg Germany (2009). Enyi Anosike is actively involved in work in public mental health, providing strategic support through a charity Amaudo UK (where he serves as a trustee) to Amaudo Itumbauzo, a residential and rehabilitation community psychiatry project in Southeastern Nigeria. Anosike serves as trustee of the Public Health Foundation of Nigeria, a charity which partners with the Federal Ministry of Health of Nigeria to support the health workforce and strengthen the country's health system, especially at the level of primary healthcare.

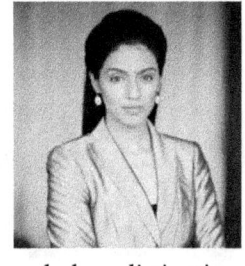

Dr. Anjhula Mya Singh Bais is an international psychologist with a specialty in trauma, a Buddhist scholar, and a feminist. Bais holds a Bachelor of Arts in psychology from Lady Sri Ram College, University of New Delhi, a Master of Science in psychoanalysis from University College London, and a Doctor of Philosophy from The Chicago School of Professional Psychology, where her doctoral research on trauma in high-SES Sri Lankan women was awarded a distinction. Previously, Bais was a researcher in the social relations and global intelligence labs of the business school and psychology departments at Columbia University. As the youngest person appointed to the board of The Institute of Semitics at Princeton, she concurrently serves as chair of languages for Division 52 of the American Psychological Association.

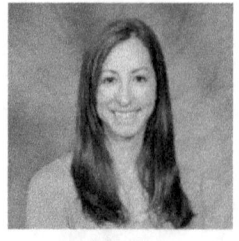

Dr. Stephanie Benjamin is an emergency medicine resident physician at University of California San Francisco-Fresno. Growing up in Long Island, New York, she always dreamt of becoming both a doctor and an artist. The September 11th attacks sparked her interest in entering emergency medicine, and her goal of working in disaster medicine developed when Hurricane Katrina hit the Gulf Coast while she was attending Tulane University in New Orleans. After obtaining a bachelor's degree in art history and studio art and a master's degree in psychology and art therapy, Dr. Benjamin went on to medical school at the University of Cincinnati College of Medicine. After medical school, she moved to California for her emergency medicine residency. Upon the completion of residency, she plans to do a fellowship in disaster medicine and hopes to make the world a safer place by working in the growing field of disaster preparedness. When she isn't at work, she can be found rock climbing, writing, making art in her studio, or at the beach with her husband and their two Rottweilers.

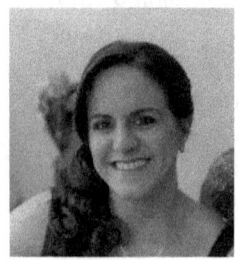

Caroline D. Bergeron, DrPH, MSc, CHES, is a program manager and evaluator at the Bexar County Community Health Collaborative in San Antonio, Texas, USA. Dr. Bergeron has a doctorate in public health from the Department of Health Promotion, Education, and Behavior at the University of South Carolina. She has gained important international experience working in aging and dementia at the World Health Organization, the Public Health Agency of Canada, and AARP (American Association of Retired Persons) International.

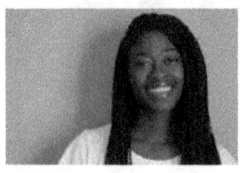

Amma Boakye is an osteopathic medical student at Marian University College of Osteopathic Medicine and a photographer-in-training. Originally drawn to medicine by a coloring book on the human body as a child, day by day, she finds that medicine is more about communities and the people living in them than about the assortment of bones, muscles, nerves, and organs of which we are made. With a love of osteopathy and a camera in hand, she hopes to tell the stories of her future patients, co-workers, friends, and family to the people all over the world. You can see her work at http://www.ammaboakye.tumblr.com.

Dr. Bruce Bongar is currently the Calvin Distinguished Professor of Psychology at Palo Alto University and previously served as a consulting professor of psychiatry and behavioral sciences at Stanford Medical School. For many years, Dr. Bongar maintained a small practice specializing in psychotherapy, consultation, and supervision specifically for difficult and life-threatening 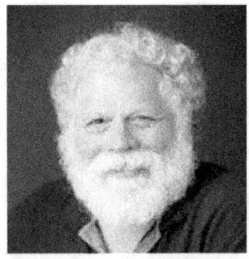 patients. Other past clinical appointments include service as a senior clinical psychologist with the Division of Psychiatry, Children's Hospital of Los Angeles and work as a clinical/community mental health psychologist on the psychiatric emergency team of the Los Angeles County Department of Mental Health. Dr. Bongar was also a recipient of the Edwin Shneidman Award from the American Association of Suicidology for outstanding early career contributions to suicide research and of the Louis I. Dublin Award for lifetime achievement in suicidology.

Lisa M. Brown, PhD, ABPP, is a professor and the Director of the Trauma Program and Risk and Resilience Research Lab at Palo Alto University in Palo Alto, California. Her clinical and research focus is on trauma and resilience, global mental health, aging, and vulnerable populations. She is a Fellow of American Psychological Association and the Gerontological Society of America and a recipient of Fulbright Specialist Award in both Jamaica and New Zealand.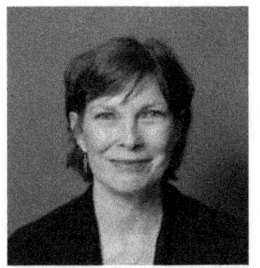

A. Maya Casagrande has worked in international development for over a decade. After serving in roles ranging from "Volunteer Manager" to "Managing Director" at various organizations, Maya spent the last several years specializing in all things grant-related. She has intimate knowledge of the grants process and the ability to transform seemingly dry financial and programmatic data into compelling narratives. Maya holds a master's degree in 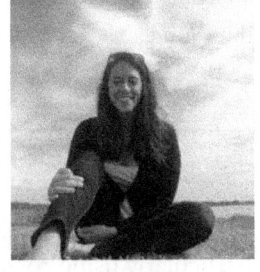 international development from the Josef Korbel School of International Studies at the University of Denver. She is currently based in Ireland by way of New Zealand, New York, and Colorado. Outside of international development, Maya is driven by a love for photography, ventures in literary editing, and being outdoors.

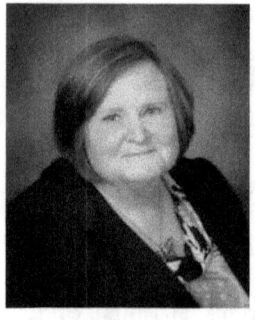

Marlene Cohen, EdD, BCBA-D, is the founder of Possibilities Consulting, LLC and has taught at The Chicago School of Professional Psychology, Rowan University, and Rutgers University. She is currently the director of the Virtual Academy for Overcoming Global Poverty. Recently, Dr. Cohen received grants to provide technology training to teachers in South Africa and Colombia. Dr. Cohen received her doctorate in educational leadership from Nova Southeastern University and is a board-certified behavior analyst at the doctoral level. Dr. Cohen has over 35 years of experience in the field of autism and developmental disabilities in private, university, and public settings. She has also worked with individuals with learning disabilities. Dr. Cohen has presented both nationally and internationally at conferences on a variety of applied behavior analysis topics. She is a co-founder and the first president of the New Jersey Association for Behavior Analysis.

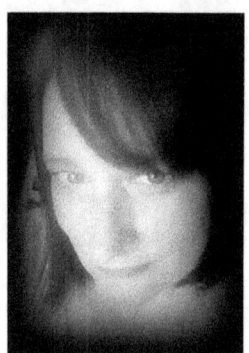

Kathleen Davis is a PhD candidate at The Chicago School for Professional Psychology and expects to graduate in December 2016. Kathleen received her master's degree in counselor education from Western Michigan University, and her bachelor's degree in business leadership from Baker College. She enjoys advocating for the rights of people with disabilities and has dedicated several years to working in rehabilitation counseling. Beyond that, Kathleen has worked i n mental health and in higher education as faculty. As part of her studies at The Chicago School for Professional Psychology, Kathleen participated in field experience internships in South Africa and Brazil. Her dissertation focused on male indigenous Mexican migrants and the effects of transnational family separation and fear of family separation with mixed-documented families. Future research interests include indigenous health concepts, disability, vocational psychology, gender studies, indigenous psychology, international psychology, and qualitative research methods, particularly using focus groups.

Alisha DeWalt holds a master's degree in clinical psychology and is currently completing her doctorate in business psychology at The Chicago School of Professional Psychology. Her dissertation is focused on exploring global competency and its impact on individuals entering the business field.

Alisha has been employed with The Chicago School of Professional Psychology for five years and has served in a variety of positions focused primarily on improving operational excellence, building efficiencies to advance online program quality, and developing infrastructure to support international initiatives. Currently, Alisha serves as the Director of Operations. She manages campus operations and 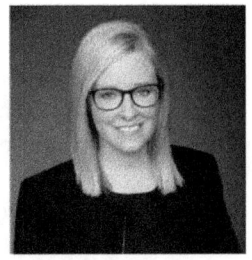 coordinates the university's strategic plan. Alisha serves as a subject matter expert facilitator and ensures that all online courses are being developed to meet university expectations and quality matters standards.

Dr. Daria Diakonova-Curtis is a postdoctoral fellow at the Department of Psychology at St. Petersburg State University in St. Petersburg, Russia, where she works on a National Institutes of Health-funded international prevention study with women at risk for HIV. Her research areas include gender issues affecting women's health and well-being, violence against women, and sexual health. She is the recipient of the Paul Werner Dissertation Award for her dissertation study of sexual assault perceptions among Russian adults and of the 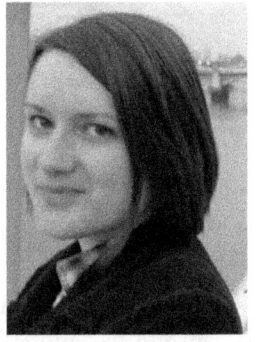 American Psychological Association's (APA) Division of International Psychology's Graduate Student Research Award. She completed her APA-accredited pre-doctoral internship in clinical psychology at the Institute for Multicultural Counseling and Education Services in Los Angeles, California, where she specialized in providing psychological services to immigrant populations from the former Soviet Union, Russia, Armenia, and the Middle East. She is an active member of the Association for Trauma Outreach & Prevention and Meaningfulworld. She is the Chair of APA's Division of International Psychology Graduate Student Research Award and an elected member of APA's Division of Psychotherapy Diversity Committee. She has served on the Editorial Student Review Board of *Psychology of Women Quarterly* and has presented at the United Nations as well as at national and regional conferences.

Myron Eshowsky, MS, is a counselor, shamanic healer, and educator. He is co-developer of the Social Health Care Program for Syrian Refugees, which provides direct services and training in trauma treatment for refugees within the Middle East. Between 1987 and 1994, he worked half-time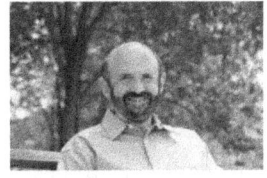

in a community mental health center specifically applying indigenous and cross-culturally influenced approaches to a wide variety of populations. He has consulted in respect to the trauma healing needs in gangs, at-risk youth, communities traumatized by violence (including historical trauma), and child soldiers in Africa. He has published dozens of articles on these topics in professional journals, his book, *Peace with Cancer: Shamanism as a Spiritual Approach to Healing*, and a chapter in *Shamanism, Ancestors, and Transgenerational Integration*. For the last thirty years, he has studied how indigenous cultures address the healing of trauma and conflict. He consults and teaches throughout the United States, Canada, Africa, the Middle East, and Europe.

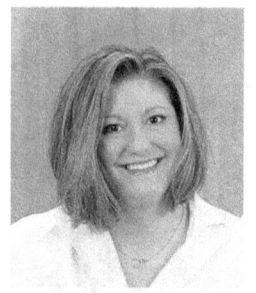

Kerrie R. Fineran, PhD, NCC, PSC, is and assistant professor and the Director of Counselor Education at Indiana University-Purdue University Fort Wayne. She is a counselor educator who specializes in school counseling and mental health training, with specific interests in suicidology, addictions counseling, and prevention and intervention using group modalities. Dr. Fineran is a nationally certified counselor and a professional school counselor. She has served on the boards of many professional organizations and is an active member of the American Counseling Association, the Association for Specialists in Group Work, the International Association of Addiction and Offender Counseling, the Association for Counselor Education and Supervision, the Indiana School Counselor Association, and Mental Health America. She is the author or co-author of numerous articles, book chapters, and is the co-editor of a handbook of group work activities. Dr. Fineran received a bachelor's degree in psychology from the College of William and Mary in Williamsburg, Virginia, a master's degree in counseling from Shippensburg University in Shippensburg, Pennsylvania, and a doctorate in counselor education and supervision from the University of Toledo in Toledo, Ohio.

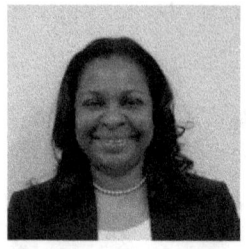

Roseanne L. Flores is an associate professor in the Department of Psychology at Hunter College of the City University of New York (CUNY). She received her PhD from the Graduate Center of the City University of New York, and more recently, an advanced certificate in public administration and public policy and a certificate in health care policy and administration, both from the CUNY School of Professional Studies. She is also a faculty associate of the Roosevelt House

Public Policy Institute at Hunter College as well as a member of the human rights faculty. She is currently serving as an ECOSOC Representative to the United Nations and as a member of the NGO Committee on Children's Rights, New York. In 2016, she served as the co-chair of Psychology Day at the United Nations, which focused on using psychology to address the global migration crisis. Her current research and scholarship focuses on environmental risk factors such as community violence, poverty, nutrition, and their relationship to the health and educational outcomes of minority children and families nationally and internationally.

Ayorkor Gaba, PsyD. Dr. Gaba is a Senior Project Director/Clinical Psychologist at the University of Massachusetts Medical School and a Representative of the American Psychological Association (APA) NGO at the United Nations (U.N.). She is the Co-Chair of the Planning Committee for 10th Annual Psychology Day at the U.N. and an Inaugural Fellow of the Dyson College Center for Global Psychology 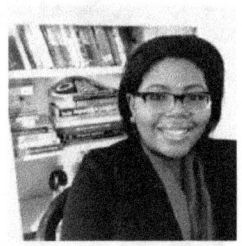 (DCCGP). Dr. Gaba's work primarily focuses on co-occurring mental health and substance use disorders (CODs) treatment research, staff training, and program implementation and specifically addresses CODs amongst criminal justice-involved populations, veterans, and women. Dr. Gaba has a strong commitment to and interest in cross-cultural psychology and international psychology. In her role at the APA NGO, she, along with a group of APA-appointed psychologists, fosters dialogue and information exchange between psychologists and U.N. community to impact U.N. policies/proceedings regarding global mental health and human rights. She has given presentations on addiction, trauma, culture, and evidence-based intervention at the U.N., national conferences, mental health organizations, and training programs.

Robert Groelsema is the Africa Justice and Peacebuilding Working Group Team Leader for Catholic Relief Services (CRS). He provides leadership for strategic programming in peacebuilding and governance in Africa, which includes the development of CRS's signature methods and approaches and the application of these to cross-sector integration. Dr. Groelsema has devoted his career to relief and development, serving as a Peace Corps teacher in Zaire, a UNHCR field 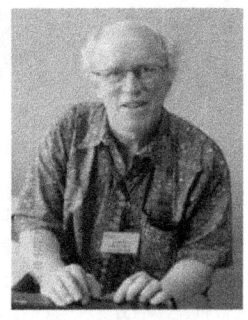 officer in the Philippines, a USAID social scientist and civil society analyst, and a Chief of Party for conflict early warning in West Africa and for resilience strengthening in northern Kenya. He has published on African history, religion and culture, geography and politics. He holds a master's of public and international affairs (MPIA) from the University of Pittsburgh, and a doctorate. in political science from Indiana University.

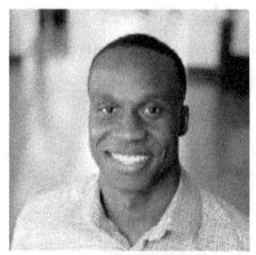

Efosa L. Guobadia, PT, DPT, is the founder of the informational website, "PT Haven," co-founder and co-director of "PT Day of Service," and co-founder, president, and CEO of Move Together, a 501(c)3 non-profit organization dedicated to improving access to quality rehab medicine around the corner and around the world. He also founded the international volunteer program ATI MissionWorks for ATI Physical Therapy. He received his Bachelor of Science in kinesiology from University of Massachusetts in 2007 and his doctorate in physical therapy from the University of Scranton in 2010.

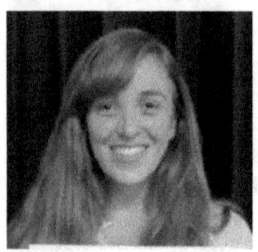

Tristan Hansell is a doctoral candidate in clinical psychology at Palo Alto University in California and is specializing in the trauma program. She completed her Master of Science in political science from the University of Amsterdam in 2011. She is currently a student therapist at The Gronowski Center in Los Altos, CA. Her research interests focus on trauma, refugee resettlement, global mental health, and resilience.

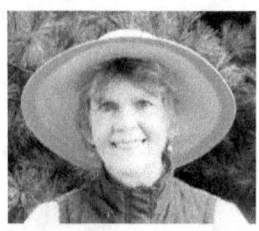

Kathleen B. Harrison received a PhD from Fordham University (Mammalian Genetics) and is a cytogeneticist certified by the American Board of Medical Genetics. While traveling and teaching, she developed an interest in global health and socioeconomic determinants of health, particularly regarding the acquired immunodeficiency syndrome (AIDS) pandemic in sub-Saharan Africa. In 2005, she founded PROJECT HARAMBEE ("all pull together" in Swahili), a non- profit organization that assists those affected by HIV in Africa. She now is a full-time social activist, public speaker, and photographer. PROJECT HARAMBEE works with in-country schools, clinics, and other organizations to sponsor education and development projects. In addition, HARAMBEE promotes global health education and conducts service trips to Kenya, Rwanda, and Zambia.

Dr. Aaron Hermann is a Visiting Research Fellow with the Law School and the School of Medicine at the University of Adelaide in Australia. He also currently holds a professorship with the Helsinki School of Business in Finland. He has worked in various fields of academia and private industry in areas such as sports, law, forensics, management, marketing, organisational psychology, cross-cultural studies, international business, archaeology, and diplomacy. Since 2007, Aaron has 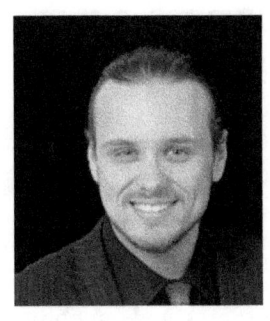 been teaching both undergraduate and postgraduate courses in many countries, including: Austria, Switzerland, Slovenia, Singapore, and Germany. In 2016, Aaron received The Executive Dean's Award for Teaching Excellence from the University of Adelaide. Aaron currently works as an international sports consultant to major international sporting bodies and sports teams in the areas of management and anti-doping policy. He is also currently an international law and counter-terrorism consultant for a number of international organizations and governments. Aaron doctoral studies at the University of Adelaide focused on an interdisciplinary study of sports criminology and doping from the perspective of international law, policy, medicine, and business. For his research, Aaron received numerous scholarships and a Dean's Commendation for Thesis Excellence and has been interviewed by various international media outlets.

Lori Holleran, PhD, MPH, is currently a Quality Scholar Fellow at the San Francisco Veterans Affairs Medical Center. She also serves as Member-at-Large, Policy and Applied Work Focus within the Society for the Psychological Study of Social Issues graduate student committee. She received her PhD in clinical psychology from Palo Alto University and her MPH in health policy from the Harvard T.H. Chan School of Public Heath, where she was a 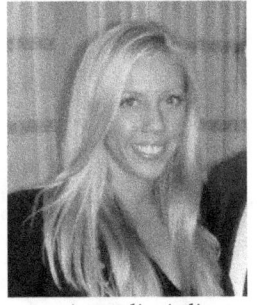 Philanthropy Advisory Fellow and completed an interdisciplinary concentration certification in humanitarian studies, ethics and human rights. Her research interests include examination of trauma related behavioral outcomes, including subsequent risk for suicide and antisocial acts. In addition, Lori is passionate about research initiatives that integrate technology with mental health interventions in order to offer more comprehensive and accessible care to a broader group of individuals.

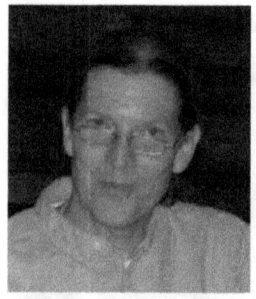

William Hoyt is a professor, the Chair of the Department of Counseling Psychology, and affiliated faculty in the Department of Educational Psychology (Quantitative Methods program) at the University of Wisconsin-Madison. His research interests are in the areas of social determinants of psychological well-being (relational processes as they relate to positive psychological functioning) and applications of these ideas to the study of process and outcome in psychotherapy and counseling (sociocultural and relational processes as they relate to effective intervention for psychological problems). Professor Hoyt has published extensively on research methods in psychology, including measurement, meta-analysis, and modeling of nested data structures, as well as research design and data interpretation. He is the recipient of distinguished teaching and mentoring awards and began his second term as associate editor for the *Journal of Counseling Psychology* in January 2016.

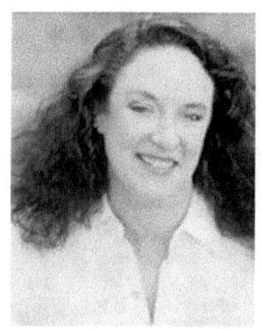

Kate Hudgins, PhD, TEP, is a certified trainer, educator, and practitioner in psychodrama, sociometry, and group psychotherapy with a doctorate in clinical psychology. She is also a certified Gestalt therapist and has developed her own integrated clinical system of experiential psychotherapy and change, The Therapeutic Spiral Model (TSM). In 1986, she was given the American Psychological Association's national Award for Graduate Student Research (Hudgins & Kiesler, 1987) and has also received three awards as a psychodramatist. While doing a National Institute of Mental Health internship at St. Elizabeth's VA Hospital in Washington, D.C. from 1980-1981, she was awarded the annual prize for the J.L. Moreno Best Psychodramatist. In 2001, the American Society for Group Psychotherapy and Psychodrama gave her the Innovator's Award for combining psychodrama with clinical psychology to produce TSM and again recognized her in 2009 with the Scholar's Award. She has written five books and 30 articles and chapters prior to the current one. She is a well-known international trainer on posttraumatic stress disorder (PTSD) and the effects of trauma. She developed the TSI International Certification in Trauma Therapy that has certified over 1000 people in 30 countries over the past 25 years. In 2004, she was invited by the government of China to be a keynote speaker for their first mandated mental health conference.

Lidija Hurni is the clinical director in the counselor education program at Indiana University – Purdue University Fort Wayne (IPFW). Though born in Bosnia and Herzegovina, her family moved to Fort Wayne, Indiana, where she attended IPFW and earned her Bachelor of Science in human services. She also holds a Master of Science in Education in counseling from Indiana University. Ms. Hurni is currently a licensed marriage and family therapist at 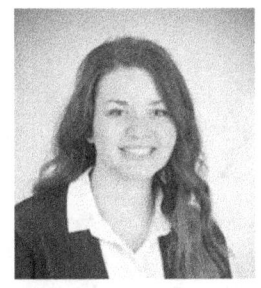 a local agency. She has served on the board of Indiana Association for Marriage and Family Therapy and is a Clinical Fellow of the American Association for Marriage and Family Therapy.

Prior to co-founding and becoming the executive director of emBOLDen Alliances, **Neena S. Jain, MD, MSTPH, DTM&H,** served in many global-health-related roles for several international non-governmental organizations throughout Africa, Asia, and the Caribbean. Dr. Jain was board-certified in emergency medicine in 2001 and practiced as an attending physician at Swedish Medical Center and 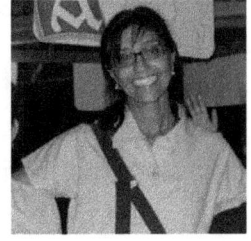 Denver Health Medical Center Emergency Department. She served as deputy director for the program in humanitarian assistance and as adjunct faculty for the global health affairs program at the University of Denver's Korbel School of International Studies. Dr. Jain co-directed the course on tropical medicine and mentored students. She completed epidemiologic studies and public health projects for the Centers for Disease Control and Prevention. Dr. Jain received a Bachelor of Arts in human biology from Stanford University, a Master of Science in tropical public health from the Harvard School of Public Health, a Doctorate of Medicine at SUNY Brooklyn Health Sciences Center, and a diploma in tropical medicine and hygiene from the London School of Hygiene and Tropical Medicine. She was clinically trained as a general surgery resident at Oregon Health Sciences University and as an emergency medicine resident at Denver Health Medical Center, where she served as a chief resident for the program.

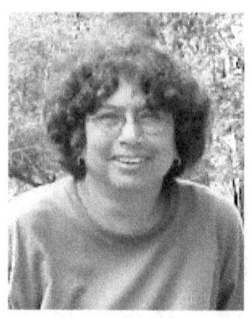

Dr. Rashmi Jaipal, PhD, is professor emeritus of psychology at Bloomfield College, New Jersey, and has been a representative of the American Psychological Association at the U.N. since 2013. In 2014 and 2016, she was the Co-Chair of the Planning Committee for Psychology Day at the U.N., and she has done mission outreach to advocate for the inclusion of mental health and well-being in the U.N. She has a doctorate in clinical and cross-cultural psychology from the New School for Social Research. While at Bloomfield College, she started a diversity training certificate program and the Center for Cultures and Communication. She also started an initiative called "Alternative Visions for the Future" to research cultures of sustainability and build bridges between the local and the global. Dr Jaipal's research is on Indian indigenous traditions, on internationalizing the psychology curriculum, and on the psychological aspects of sustainable development. She has given presentations on these topics at the U.N., at international conferences, the annual American Psychological Association convention, and the National Association of Psychology in India.

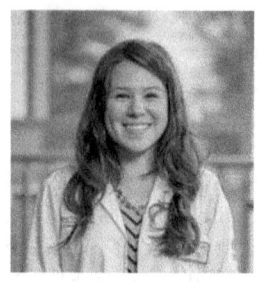

Gretchen Johnson is in her third year of medical school at Marian University-College of Osteopathic Medicine and has a particular interest in family medicine. She lives in Indianapolis with her husband, Ryan Johnson. He is a teacher. Ryan grew up in New Mexico while Gretchen grew up in New York. They met in Michigan while attending Hillsdale College. Her mother is Chinese, her father is Irish/Jewish, and she has two little brothers. Gretchen enjoys most things but especially likes crocheting, trying new recipes, taking walks, cultivating plants, playing violin, and spending time with loved ones. Although she is generally gregarious, she appreciates introvert time. The Johnsons enjoy being part of the community of Redeemer Presbyterian Church.

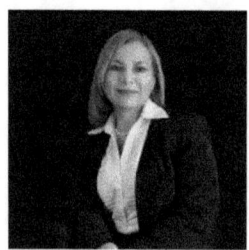

Dr. Ani Kalayjian is a psychology professor at Teachers College Columbia University and Meaningfulworld, a psychotherapist, a genocide scholar, an international humanitarian outreach administrator, an integrative healer, an author, and a United Nations representative. She was awarded both the Outstanding Psychologist of the Year

Award from American Psychological Association (2016, Trauma Division) and the University of Missouri-Columbia Humanitarian Award (2014). She is the recipient of the 2010 ANA Honorary Human Rights Award, the Honorary Doctor of Science degree from Long Island University (2001). In 2007, she was appointed Columbia University, Teacher College's Distinguished Alumni of the Year. She has published over 100 articles in international journals and books; she is an author of Disaster & Mass Trauma, the chief editor of Forgiveness & Reconciliation: Psychological Pathways to Conflict Transformation and Peace Building (Springer 2009, paperback 2010), the chief editor of two volumes on Mass Trauma & Emotional Healing around the World: Rituals and Practices for Resilience and Meaning-Making (Praeger, ABC-CLIO 2010), the author of a meditation CD called "From War To Peace," and the creator of eight films on Meaningfulworld humanitarian outreach programs around the world. Currently she is on the faculty of Teachers College, Columbia University.

Kenneth H. Kessler, PhD, is an associate professor of psychology at Rosalind Franklin University of Medicine and Science in North Chicago, IL. He has been involved in the university's global health project since 2012 and is a co-leader of "Hope of Children and Women Victims of Violence." Dr. Kessler is a 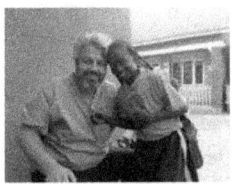 licensed clinical psychologist and a licensed clinical counselor and has been involved in the regulation of mental health practice in Illinois since 2000. He is currently the chairman of the Professional Counselor Licensing and Disciplinary Board in Illinois. He was formerly involved in local politics and served as mayor of the town of Mundelein, IL, from 2005-2013. He stepped down after a self-imposed term limit of eight years.

Brandon A. Knettel, PhD, is a postdoctoral associate in research at the Duke Global Health Institute and a licensed psychologist in the state of North Carolina. He completed his undergraduate studies at the College of St. Scholastica in Duluth, 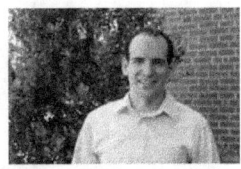 Minnesota, overlooking the shores of Lake Superior. Upon graduation, he began his path toward a career in global health, studying for a year in Australia before returning to the U.S. to finish his master's degree at the University of St. Thomas (MN), and then traveling abroad once again to teach in the guidance and counseling concentration at Mount Meru University in Arusha, Tanzania. It was there that he formulated his first international research project in partnership with Janvier Rugira, PhD. This ongoing research examines historical and modern views about mental health treatment in Tanzania through interviews with the small number of providers practicing in the country, with the goal of guiding the development of culturally-informed mental health services. From this experience in Tanzania, Brandon continues to recognize the value of community-based research and examining health systems through the eyes of the people most affected by them. Upon returning to the U.S., Brandon earned his doctorate in counseling psychology from Lehigh University, a program with strong emphases in multiculturalism and social justice.

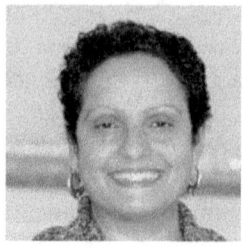

Dr. Genomary Krigbaum's, MA, PsyD, BCB, professional development started in Latin America. She migrated to the U.S. and furthered her studies by completing a BA in psychology, an MA, and a doctorate (PsyD) in clinical psychology. Dr. Krigbaum's clinical, academic, and professional experience ranges from hospital work and training healthcare professionals (e.g., medical and psychology students) to conducting research and consulting in areas of interest, such as cross-cultural neuroscience, psychophysiology, research protocols, multicultural matters, military psychology, and process consulting. She also practices as a bilingual (English/Spanish) clinical psychologist with an added focus in biofeedback and neuropsychology. She is involved in chairing dissertations, ensuring academic quality, overseeing methodology, and serving as a subject matter expert. Dr. Krigbaum is invested in scholarship and research activity, including serving on institutional review boards. With cross-cultural and developmental variables in mind, she has published in her areas of interest with inclusion of clinical and cognitive themes.

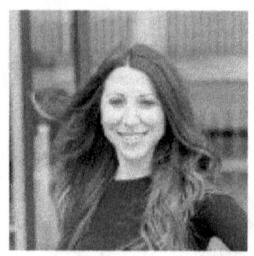

Samara Lipsky is a doctoral student in the international psychology program at The Chicago School of Professional Psychology (TCSPP). She completed her bachelor's degree in business administration at Emory University and has a master's degree in psychology. Samara has received a range of awards, including induction into the Edward Alexander Bouchet Graduate Honor Society at Yale University, the President's Scholarship at TCSPP, and the Meritorious Student Abstract Award at the Society of Behavioral Medicine's Annual Conference. She also received a National Cancer Institute/National Institutes of Health pre-doctoral research fellowship in psychiatry and behavioral medicine at Memorial Sloan-Kettering Cancer Center. She has presented at multiple conferences, co-authored a book chapter, and published in journals on public health issues. In addition, she co-founded a

501(c)3 non-profit organization dedicated to raising funds and awareness for medically oriented organizations.

Ms. Klara Lubej is an international expert in languages and cultures. She has particular interests in the convergence between culture, langauge, and marketing and has worked in localization and promotions for a number of years. She gained global experience by working for companies and organisations in three continents and numerous countries. Moreover, she gained degrees in inter-lingual communications, culture, and translation from one of the top universities in the world.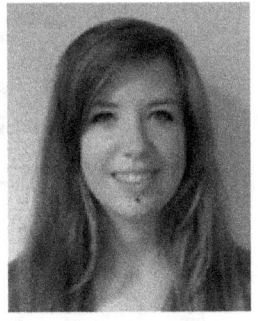
Working as a translator for some of Europe's largest firms provided Klara with unique insight into the intracacies of language and the application of linguistical skills in international business and marketing. Klara has gained work experience in a number of global firms. She has has sucessfuly applied skills working as an interpreter and public relations officer for prestigious Indian companies which provided Klara with opportunities to contribute to global trade and communications. Klara's work experience has been enhanced through volunteering for cultural groups and a number of global organisations through which she has gained deep understaning of non-governmental organizations and global cultural realities. She is fluent in several langauges which has enabled her to contribute to the development of global communication channels and business systems.

Barbara Lutz, PhD, graduated with a degree in social work in Germany in 1992, received her Master of Arts in counseling psychology from Pacifica Graduate Institute, California, in 1997, and became a licensed marriage and family therapist in 2001. She then obtained her doctorate in international psychology with a trauma focus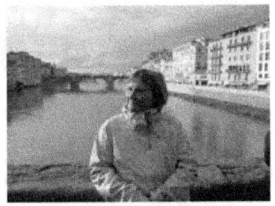
from The Chicago School of Professional Psychology (TCSPP). She has developed and instructs the course "Global Mental Health and Human Rights" at TCSPP. As adjunct faculty, she also teaches psychology to a rural and predominantly Hispanic student population at Hartnell College in California. She has provided psychotherapy in English, Spanish, and German to a wide spectrum of client populations throughout Santa Cruz County, California: children in foster care, probation youths, patients suffering from HIV/AIDS, and immigrant families. Her work experience, her own immigration history, and her marriage to a Mexican metal artist

have sparked her interest in possibilities created by commonalities and differences that affect mental and physical well-being worldwide.

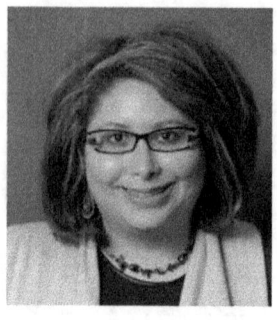

Dr. Laura Reid Marks is originally from Kingston, Jamaica. Dr. Marks's is a tenure-track assistant professor of counseling psychology at the University of Memphis in the Department of Counseling, Educational Psychology, and Research. She received her doctoral degree in counseling psychology from Purdue University. She received her bachelor's degree in psychology and her master's and education specialist degrees in school counseling from the University of Florida. She completed her pre-doctoral internship at Arizona State University Counseling Services. Her dissertation focused on the relations among discrimination, mental health, and sexual risk behaviors in Black college women. Dr. Marks's current research interests center on microaggressions, mental health, and HIV-related health disparities.

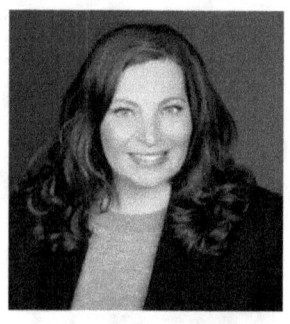

Dr. Tiffany Masson obtained her doctorate in psychology in 2002. She completed her post-doctoral training at U.C. Davis' Children's Hospital-CAARE Center, and was employed as a staff psychologist by the Cook County Juvenile Court and Northwestern School of Law. In addition to private practice and scholarship, her portfolio includes nine years of service at The Chicago School of Professional Psychology (TCSPP), where she has held several academic and operational administrative positions. Her leadership positions have included Department Chair of International Psychology, Campus Dean of Online Programs, and Vice President of E-Learning and Global Innovation. She was responsible for positioning TCSPP as a national and international leader in technology-based learning. In her current role as Chicago Campus Dean, Dr. Masson provides oversight and strategic direction for the university's largest campus location. As a global innovator, Dr. Masson develops and manages international partnerships to expand the institution's distance education market and continues to focus efforts on specific international human capacity development projects in Africa. In addition, she co-developed a country-specific, 12-day trauma training program (Global HOPE Training Initiative) that aids teachers in effectively recognizing, assessing, and intervening with traumatized children. Her work in Rwanda and her ability to develop government and private partnerships has proved successful in the expansion of the Global HOPE Training Initiative to Zambia and South Africa.

John A. McNulty received his doctorate in marine biology from the University of Southern California. He was on the faculty at the Stritch School of Medicine, Loyola University Chicago. He was a Fellow of the Leischner Institute of Medical Education for 40 years and is currently a Professor Emeritus. He was awarded research grants from the National Science Foundation, National Institutes of Health, and the U.S. Department of Agriculture for his studies of 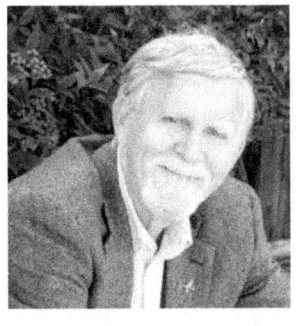 neuroendocrinology, neuroimmunology, and medical education. He was co-founder of the Loyola University Medical Education Network (LUMEN) and the Africa Medical Education Network (AMEN). Other recognitions include two first prizes in the Medical Photography Competition of the American Society of Clinical Pathologists and election as a Fellow of the American Association of Anatomists. Most recently he has actively supported the programs of the non-for profit, Project Harambee.

Lalit Narayan, MBBS, MA, is a Medical Education Fellow at the George Washington University School of Medicine & Health Sciences. He received his medical degree at St. John's Medical College, Bangalore, India in 2007. He subsequently worked as a physician in rural India for two years before moving to the 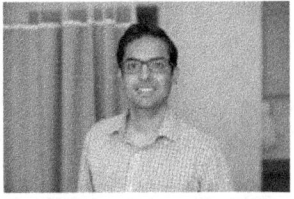 U.S. to pursue further education in social medicine. He earned a master's degree in anthropology at Syracuse University, New York in 2013 and completed his residency in primary care/social internal medicine at Montefiore Medical Center, New York in 2016. His interests include medical education systems, social medicine education, community health, and primary health care.

Amy Nitza, PhD, is the director of the Institute for Disaster Mental Health at the State University of New York at New Paltz. She is a psychologist who specializes in mental health training and group counseling in international contexts. Dr. Nitza was a Fulbright Scholar at the University of Botswana in 2008-2009, 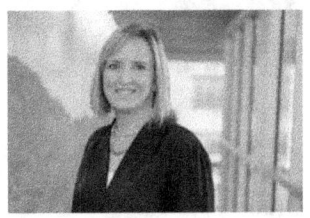 where she studied the use of group counseling interventions in HIV/AIDS prevention among adolescents. In 2014, Dr. Nitza was a sabbaticant at the National Referral Hospital in the Kingdom of Bhutan, where she provided direct service to patients and training to hospital staff and substance abuse counselors. Currently, she is consulting with the University of Notre Dame in Haiti to develop trauma-related interventions for children in domestic servitude and to provide training for teachers in dealing with traumatized children in the classroom. Dr. Nitza is president and Fellow of the Association for Specialists in Group Work. She also serves on the Executive Board of the Society for Group Psychology and Group Psychotherapy (Division 49) of the American Psychological Association. She is the author or co-author of many publications and is the co-editor of two handbooks of group work activities. Dr. Nitza received a bachelor's degree in psychology and a master's degree in mental health counseling from Purdue University. She received her doctorate in counseling psychology from Indiana University.

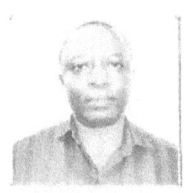

The Very Reverend **Kenneth E. Nwaubani** is from Abia State, Nigeria. He is a clergy in the Methodist Church Nigeria and the director of the Amaudo Itumbauzo Centre for Mentally Ill Destitute in Abia State, Nigeria. Along with a diploma in theology and a Bachelor of Arts in religious and cultural studies, Very Rev. Nwaubani holds both an international diploma in mental health, human rights, and law and a certificate in mental health leadership and advocacy skill.

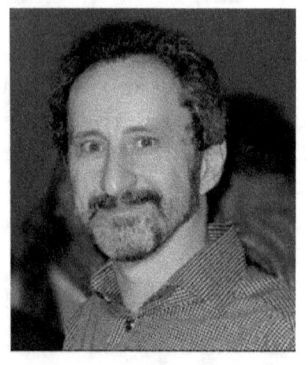

Steve Olweean is the founding director of Common Bond Institute (CBI), president of International Humanistic Psychology Association, past president of Association for Humanistic Psychology, and recipient of the American Psychological Association Charlotte and Karl Bühler Award for outstanding and lasting contribution to humanistic psychology internationally. He is a therapist with extensive experience in community-based mental health treatment, specializes in local capacity building and designing programs for treating large traumatized populations, and developed the Catastrophic Trauma Recovery model, which is the basis for the CBI's social health care training and treatment program. He speaks and writes extensively on communal and transgenerational trauma as well as fear-based belief systems.

Nausheen Pasha-Zaidi, PhD, has degrees in communications, education, and psychology and is currently working as a lecturer in psychology at the University of Houston-Downtown. Her research interests include culture, literacy, and gender studies in international populations. She recently completed a compilation of personal narratives titled "Mirror on the Veil: A Collection of Personal Essays on Hijab and Veiling," which she co-edited with her sister, Shaheen Pasha.

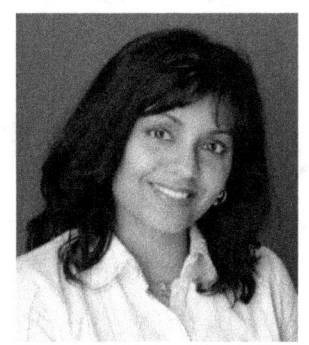

Nélida Quintero, PhD, is an environmental psychologist and licensed architect based in New York. She is an American Psychological Association NGO Representative at the United Nations, a member of the NGO Committee on Ageing/NY and Habitat III Civil Society Working Group, and a Fellow of The Center for Urban Design and Mental Health. Her project list includes commercial and residential interior architecture projects in the U.S. and Latin America as well as consulting on well-being and

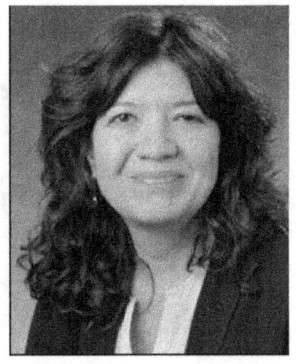

the built environment. She has taught at various colleges, universities, and certificate programs including Hunter College and Parsons School of Design. Her research interests are broadly focused on the interactions between people, behavior, and the physical environment, particularly in relationship to health, well-being, culture, new media, and gender. She holds a doctorate in environmental psychology from the Graduate Center of the City University of New York, a master's in architecture from Princeton University, and a master's in fine arts from Parsons School of Design.

Falu Rami is a PhD candidate at The Chicago School of Professional Psychology with an anticipated graduation date of October 2017. Falu received her bachelor's degree in psychology from the University of California, Irvine and her master's degree in counseling psychology from the University of San Francisco. Falu is a licensed marriage and family therapist in California, and has worked with diverse populations in various

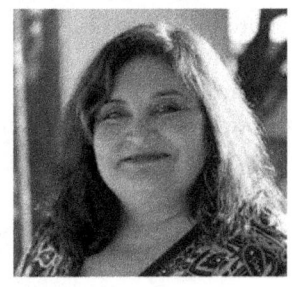

settings. Her passion is working with families and individuals that have immigrant backgrounds as well as refugees. Falu has diverse research interests which include intergroup conflict, cross-cultural counseling, acculturation, corporate social responsibility, forced migration and refugees, healthcare reform, and organization and systems interests. She is currently working as a suicide prevention coordinator in Santa Clara County at the Main Jail and Elmwood and has worked with individuals who suffer from severe mental illness. Falu is a peer reviewer for the upcoming volume of *Refugee Review* that is created by the Emerging Scholars and Practitioners on Migration Issues Network (ESPMI). Falu is also an active participant in Division 52, International Psychology, of the American Psychological Association as a student membership representative through the Early Career Program. In addition, she is also involved in the Fast Connect Committee and Task Force 5: Engaging Partners.

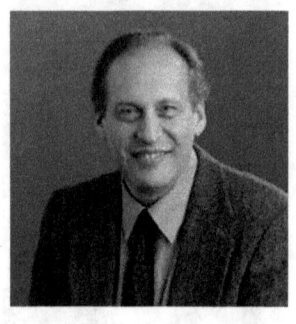

Neal S. Rubin is a professor and University Fellow at the Illinois School of Professional Psychology at Argosy University, Chicago and was formerly an assistant professor of clinical psychology in the Department of Psychiatry, College of Medicine at the University of Illinois at Chicago. Dr. Rubin has been certified as a Diplomate in Clinical Psychology by the American Board of Professional Psychology (ABPP) and is a Fellow of the American Academy of Clinical Psychology (AACP). He is also a Fellow of the American Psychological Association (APA, D39 & 52) and the Eastern Psychological Association (EPA). Since 2003, Dr. Rubin has served on the American Psychological Association's United Nations NGO Team at the U.N. Headquarters in New York City. In this role, he works to contribute to psychologically informed global policies while utilizing research-based psychological information and resources pertinent to the behavioral dimensions of human rights issues worldwide. Dr. Rubin is past president of Division 52 (International Psychology) of the APA and currently represents Division 52 on the APA Council of Representatives. He also sits on the American Association for the Advancement of Science's (AAAS) Committee on Scientific Freedom and Responsibility (CSFR), which promotes the use of science and the work of scientists in the service of human rights.

Alissa Rubinfeld, a fourth-year doctoral student, studies clinical psychology at The Chicago School of Professional Psychology. Her interest in health psychology was shaped by her master's degree in nutrition, which was completed at McGill University in Montreal. Her research in sleep medicine enhances her training in psychology and mind-body approach to treatment.

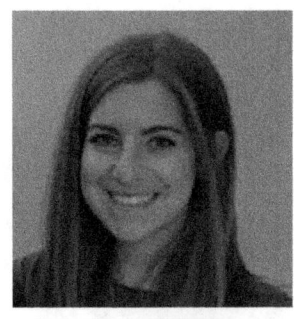

Shondolyn Sanders is originally from West Memphis, Arkansas. She is currently a doctoral student in the counseling psychology program at the University of Memphis in the Department of Counseling, Educational Psychology, and Research. She received her master's degree in counseling with a specialization in clinical rehabilitation from the University of Memphis in Memphis, TN. She received her bachelor's degree in psychology from the University of Arkansas in Fayetteville, AR. Shondolyn has worked clinically

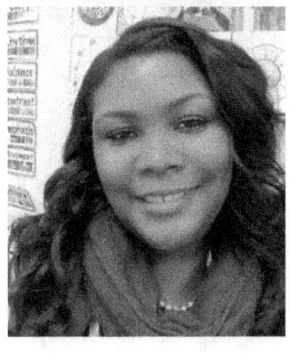

with individuals with physical and intellectual disabilities and individuals living with chronic illness and disease. She has worked in community mental health, integrated healthcare, and state vocational rehabilitation. Shondolyn's current research interests include rehabilitation psychology and health disparities, biopsychosocial adjustment to illness and disability, and the needs of those individuals during major life transition, specifically, transition to adult care and transition to employment/independence.

Octavio A. Santos, MS, is a predoctoral intern in neuropsychology at the South Texas Veterans Health Care System in San Antonio, Texas, USA. Mr. Santos is completing his doctorate in clinical psychology at the University of Wisconsin-Milwaukee. His long-term career goal is to become a board-certified clinical neuropsychologist and an expert in cross-cultural neuropsychology.

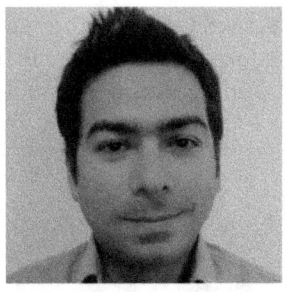

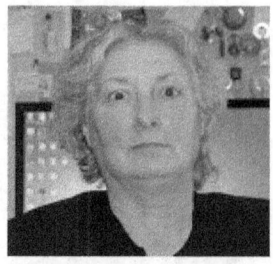

Kathy Sexton-Radek, PhD, CBSM, has over twenty-five years of private practice work in a primary care practice, with specializations in sleep medicine, health psychology, and depression cases. She is the author of over fifty peer-reviewed presentations and publications in behavioral medicine areas. Her recent publications and presentations have focused on global sleep health.

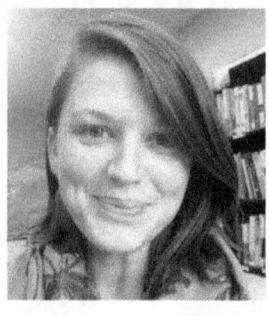

Shay E. Slifko, MA, is a program manager, leader, and educator at the University of North Carolina at Chapel Hill in the Medical School's Office of International Activities. She also serves as a researcher straddling the academic and nonprofit sectors. She pursued her master's degree from Lehigh University in international education with a focus in global health. Slifko is a practitioner in global health education, having conducted research with Dr. Sothy Eng through the organization Caring for Cambodia, located in Siem Reap, Cambodia. They examined the effectiveness of a water, sanitation, and hygiene (WASH) curriculum in influencing healthy behaviors among primary school children. In addition, Slifko has developed partnerships with nonprofit organizations to offer equitable and ethical training programs for medical learners. This includes curricula aimed at developing and recognizing ethical awareness and best practices as a short-term learner in a global health environment. Slifko also consults with community, academic, and nonprofit groups to support the creation of reciprocal global health educational activities and programming. In addition to her work in international education, Slifko collaborates with a nonprofit organization in Haiti to support their community health worker training program.

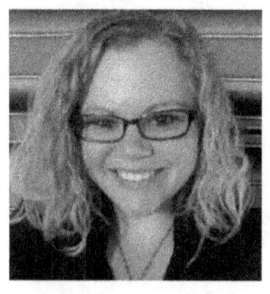

Madeline Stenersen is originally from Marion, Iowa. She is currently a doctoral student in the counseling psychology program at the University of Memphis in the Department of Counseling, Educational Psychology, and Research. She received her master's degree in clinical mental health counseling with a specialization in addictions from Marquette University in Milwaukee, WI. She received her bachelor's degree in psychology from the University of Northern Iowa in Cedar Falls, IA. Madeline has worked clinically with women in the sex trade industry, victims of human trafficking, and individuals with substance addiction. She has worked in both community mental health and correctional settings. Madeline's current research interests include international psychology and health disparities, human trafficking, and the needs of those in the sex trade industry.

As provost and Chief Academic Officer, **Joseph Martin Stevenson** lead the oversight of all academic activities for The Chicago School of Professional Psychology (TCSPP) campuses in Los Angeles, Chicago, Washington, D.C., Online, and New Orleans in collaboration with Xavier University. While in this position, he also Co-Chaired the Academic Leadership Council for the 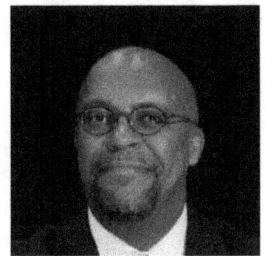 Chief Academic Officers at Saybrook University, Colleges of Law in Santa Barbara and Ventura, the Dallas Nursing Institute, and Pacific Oaks College. An advocate for fighting poverty, particularly in the deeply impoverished Mississippi Delta, Joseph has presented and published many academic works on global poverty. Prior to joining TCSPP, Joseph served as a provost and professor in New York, California, Washington, D.C, and twice in Mississippi. He has been recognized by many academic institutions and is presently a visiting scholar for the new creative leadership doctoral program at the University of the Virgin Islands. Joseph received a Global Service Award nearly two decades ago in Rio de Janeiro for his concept of an online academy on global poverty – prior to the present proliferation of MOOCs (Massive Open Online Courses). Most recently in 2016, he re-introduced the concept at University of California at Berkeley for the Executive Leadership Academy.

Shufang Sun is a doctoral student of the Department of Counseling Psychology at the University of Wisconsin-Madison. Prior to her doctoral study, she obtained a master's degree in counseling from East Tennessee State University. Her areas of research interests are psychotherapy in the global and multicultural context, global mental health, and health disparities of sexual and 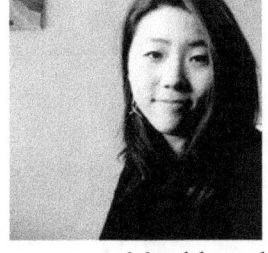 gender minorities in the U.S. and Asia (particularly on mental health and sexual health outcomes). She is a recipient of the Global Health Institute Graduate Student Research Award and the University of Wisconsin-Madison Rothney Research Award. After doctoral study, Shufang hopes to continue her research endeavor in global mental health and health disparities research via an academic career.

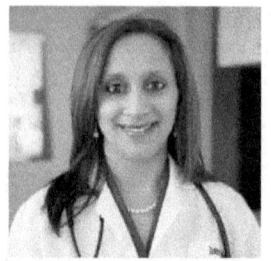

Zohray Talib is associate professor of medicine and of health policy at the George Washington University Medical School in Washington, D.C. Dr. Talib is a practicing physician and educator and leads research in the field of the global health workforce. Dr. Talib's focus is on strengthening education systems within the context of broader global health and development goals. Dr. Talib was co-investigator for the Coordinating Center for one of the largest investments in health professions education in Sub-Saharan Africa, the Medical Education Partnership Initiative. She led efforts to build a community of practice around medical education research in the region. She led a study across 10 countries in Africa to examine the impact of bringing academic rigor to community health facilities. She is a member of the National Academy of Medicine's Global Forum for Innovations in Health Professional Education and has published and presented globally on community-engagement, eLearning, faculty development, graduate tracking, accreditation, financing, and strategic partnerships between academic institutions in low-resource settings. Dr. Talib served as Associate Program Director for George Washington University's Internal Medicine Residency Program for eight years. At GWU, she has led efforts to design curricula for both the medical school and the residency program. She actively advises students, residents, and junior faculty at GWU and at a number of academic institutions in Africa.

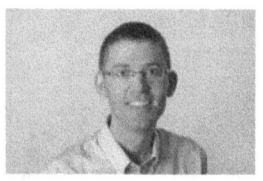

Dr. Loren Toussaint is a psychology professor at Luther College in Decorah, Iowa. He is the associate director of the Sierra Leone Forgiveness Project. He is a consultant to the Mayo Clinic, the Department of Pastoral Care at Cancer Treatment Centers of America, and the Center for Health Policy at Boise State University. He is a former visiting scientist at Mayo Clinic. Dr. Toussaint's research examines religious and spiritual factors, especially forgiveness, and how they are related to health and well-being. He has published scientific journal articles and book chapters and has given conference presentations and invited talks. Recently, he and colleagues published a comprehensive compendium of research on forgiveness and health. Dr. Toussaint directs the Laboratory for the Investigation of Mind, Body, and Spirit at Luther College and has mentored over 75 students studying in this laboratory. Dr. Toussaint's research has been highlighted in a number of print, online, and radio media outlets, including (but not limited to): *The New York Times*, *The Los Angeles Times*, *TIME Magazine*, *CNN*, *Psychology Today*, and *The Associated Press*.

Maryke Van Zyl, MA, is currently working on her doctorate in clinical psychology with an emphasis in diversity and community mental health at Palo Alto University. Maryke earned her bachelor's degree from Stellenbosch University in South Africa and her master's degree in marriage and family therapy from Pepperdine University in Los Angeles. In her work with underserved populations in South Africa, India, and Los Angeles, Maryke 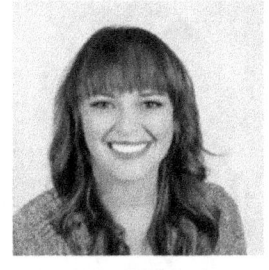 has worked to address HIV/AIDS, leprosy, and substance abuse. Maryke has served extensively in Native American tribes, focusing on suicide prevention through community empowerment. Maryke serves as coordinator of a special interest group on risk, resilience, and reasons for living within the International Association for Suicide Prevention.

Dr. Daniel Velasco earned his bachelor's degree from The University of California, Los Angeles (UCLA) and the a Master of Education from National University. He spent the first part of his career as an instructor, administrator, student counselor, and academic director at a variety of post-secondary institutions. His role as an international student counselor prompted him to diversify his education and professional experience. 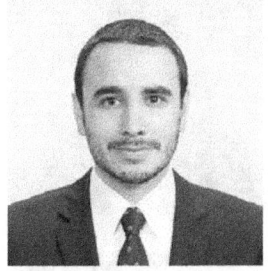 He earned a Master of Arts in psychology from Antioch University and started a private practice specializing in positive psychology. He attended The Chicago School of Professional Psychology, where he earned a doctorate in international psychology. Dr. Velasco currently resides in Japan, where he is a professor, mental health therapist, researcher, and public speaker. He regularly lectures on intercultural communication, teaching strategies, positive psychology, and counseling strategies (with a focus on adaptation and acculturation). He is an active member of the Japanese Psychological Association (JPA), the American Psychological Association (APA), the International Council of Psychologists (ICP), the International Mental Health Professionals Japan (IMHPJ), The Society for Intercultural Education, Training, and Research (SIETAR), The California Coalition on Sexual Offending, The International Society for Existential Psychology and Psychotherapy, The Global Organisation for Humanitarian Work Psychology (GOHWP), the Japan Association for Language Teaching

(JALT), and Teachers of English to Speakers of Other Languages (TESOL).

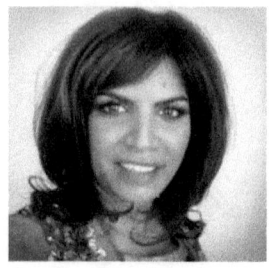

Marissa Vishnu-Mack is currently a professor of psychology at Western Wyoming Community College in Rock Springs Wyoming. Marissa, a native from Trinidad and Tobago, completed her undergraduate education in psychology from Monmouth College, and her graduate studies in human development counseling at Bradley University. She is currently a doctoral student in the international psychology at The Chicago School of Professional Psychology. Marissa has an extensive background in child development as she worked in pediatric oncology in Chicago, IL. She is also interested in immigrant acculturation experiences, migration patterns, and international travel.

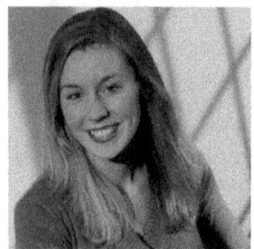

Grace Wang is a writer and editorial assistant for Dr. Chris Stout at ATI Physical Therapy and regularly authors pieces on health care, technology, and humanitarian aid. She graduated summa cum laude from North Central College, where she studied communication, global studies, and sociology. Her senior thesis explored the portrayal of human trafficking in Western media.

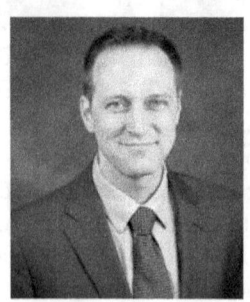

Ryan Westergaard is a physician and epidemiologist specializing in HIV, viral hepatitis, and other sexually transmitted infections. He provides clinical care for people living with HIV at the University of Wisconsin Hospital and at the AIDS Resource Center of Wisconsin, both located in Madison. He is an assistant professor in the Departments of Medicine and Population Health Sciences at the University of Wisconsin-Madison. Dr. Westergaard's research program focuses on implementation and evaluation of interventions to improve treatment outcomes for traditionally underserved patient populations, including people with substance use disorders and people who are incarcerated.

Jenifer L. White is an international psychologist, an arts-based researcher, and the founder of Project 1948. Her career in the social impact sector has contributed to her extensive work in Rwanda, Brazil, Italy, South Africa,

Germany, France, and Bosnia and Herzegovina. The heart of her work – a photo-voice for policy change – lies in Sarajevo and combines photography with human rights. Jenifer received her doctorate from The Chicago School of Professional Psychology, where she focused on international psychology and trauma. She works to make an impact in an increasingly diverse and globalized world. She is 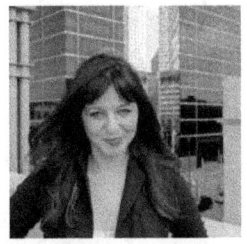 committed to empower and advocate for global social change. She utilizes monitoring and evaluation to prepare Project 1948 to achieve universal policies and procedures among civil society. She holds an international and state licensure in alcohol and drug counseling and practices as a mental health professional in Tulsa, Oklahoma.

If you enjoyed this book, you may also be interested in...

The New Humanitarians [3 volumes]: Inspiration, Innovations, and Blueprints for Visionaries

From Braille Without Borders and Unite for Sight, to Geekcorps and PeaceWorks, humanitarian groups are working worldwide largely in undeveloped countries to better the lives of the residents. Whether they are empowering people with schools for the blind, prosthetic limbs, the devices to understand and use technology, or the information to work for civil peace, the men and women of these agencies offer tremendous talent to their causes, great dedication and, sometimes, even risk their lives to complete their missions.

Working in war or civil war zones, humanitarians with nonprofits, non-governmental agencies, and university-connected centers and foundations have been injured, kidnapped, or killed. Now terrorist events and war crimes are more and more often bringing these self-sacrificing workers into the national spotlight by media headlines. Their work is, doubtless, remarkable. And so too are the stories of how they developed - including the defining moments when their founders felt they could no longer stand by and do nothing. In this set of books, founders and top officials from humanitarian organizations established in the last 50 years spotlight how and why they began their organizations, what their greatest victories and challenges have been, and how they run the organizations, down to where they get their funding and how they spend it to grow the group and its efforts. The chapters represent some of the best work from various disciplines including psychology, medicine, technology, science, politics, social work, and business.

Reviews for The New Humanitarians

This motivating set of three volumes--in the tradition of Greg Mortenson's Three Cups of Tea (2006), Harry Boyte's The Citizen Solution (2008), and other books about making a positive difference--gives what its subtitle promises: inspiration, innovation, and blueprints for changing the world...for students of health care, economics, political science, history, sociology, peace studies, and women's studies, this is a useful visionary resource. Summing Up: Recommended. Lower-level undergraduates and above; general readers.

– Choice

There is a widespread assumption, as well as growing evidence, that social environments play a key role in individuals' willingness to accept the responsibilities of democratic citizenship and participate in civic life... This message is made with compelling force throughout the three volumes of The New Humanitarians: Inspiration, Innovations, and Blueprints for Visionaries, a collection of organizational profiles reflecting a diverse range of civic commitments... Whereas many books published by psychologists are written by and designed for academics, The New Humanitarians includes the voices of people from many walks of life who collaborate in the service of specific causes.

– PsycCRITIQUES

Stout's stories of social innovators in The New Humanitarians are inspiring and instructive--helpful to anyone who wants to participate in building a better world.

- David Bornstein, Author of "How to Change The World:
Social Entrepreneurs and the Power of New Ideas"
and "The Price of a Dream." He has also written for
The Atlantic Monthly, The New York Times, and New York Newsday

Einstein taught us all that today's problems cannot be solved at the same level of thinking we were at when we created them. The convergence of a more socially conscious business community on one hand and a more entrepreneurially driven philanthropic community on the other is perhaps the greatest source of inspiration as we chart the course ahead in these interesting but yet challenging times. I have followed Dr Stout's work for several years and his passion and knowledge of the new humanitarians is as inspiring as it is important. His book is an important guide for anyone that wants to understand the emerging rules of a more humane version of entrepreneurship.

- Mats Lederhausen, Founder of BE-CAUSE,
one of Crain's Chicago Business's 40 under 40,
Chairman of the board for the not-for-profit, Business for Social Responsibility

Chris Stout has given us a glimpse into the genius, motivation, toil, frustration, and success of founding-and sustaining-humanitarian organizations in today's complex world. From the best-known to the unknown, and from the practical to the political, Chris Stout goes to the source to learn how and why 40 of these organizations were formed, how war, disease, poverty, or simply neglect created the desperate needs they fill, how these organizations serve their constituents in locations that are almost always remote and dangerous, what works, and what doesn't. These are 40 different and separate organizations, each with a founder and leader with a different vision and managerial style, but they are all driven by one goal, and that is to serve disadvantaged populations with whom they have nothing in common but their humanity.

- Harvey Langholtz, Professor,
The College of William and Mary

Poverty takes many forms, from lack of health care and the most basic education, to vulnerability to the abuse of others. Where governments and multilateral agencies are falling short, concerned individuals have been racing forward with creative solutions like white blood cells addressing infections. This is one of the most powerful movements at work in the world today and

Chris Stout is shining a bright light on their critically important work.
- *Wilford Welch, Author of "The Tactics of Hope: How Social Entrepreneurs Are Changing Our World"*

This three-volume work is a significant contribution to the commemoration of the 60th Anniversary of the Universal Declaration of Human Rights. Chris Stout and these humanitarians have dedicated themselves to global social responsibility to make a difference that counts in medical care, education, sustainable development, and social justice. Their visionary, innovative and diligent work in these various areas is educational and truly inspirational.
- *Corann Okorodudu, EdD,*
Professor of Psychology, Coordinator for Africana Studies,
Rowan University

Humanitarian Field Guide:
Ideas, Inspiration, Methods and Tools

"Change the world." It always struck me that saying that sounded a lot like grandiose hubris, or at best, a dauntingly overwhelming task. The utter impossibility of it seemed certain until I realized that it can mean helping one person at a time. That is a theme you'll see throughout this book and our websites and our work. I have added some of my LinkedIn Influencer blogs/essays that I hope may be inspirational, also.

The format of this book is inspired by Brian Eno's A Year with Swollen Appendices, not so much the diary aspect but rather the overwhelmingly large collection of information in the various appendices. Additionally, this book is an "analog" version, if you will, of the content and links found at the CenterForGlobalInitiatives.org website and the associated DropBox account.

It's long been my goal to make life easier for those working in humanitarian and volunteer endeavors, as well as those in need of help. Indeed, in one way or another, we all need help in one form or another. So, just about everything you find herein and on the Center's website, is free of charge, and a lot you could also find for yourself. What I've tried to do is speed up the search, vet what has been found, and then curate the results, making them as readily and easily available as I know how to. This is my dream of open-sourcing humanitarian work.

All proceeds from sales of this book will be donated to the Center for Global Initiatives.

§   §   §

Both titles books are available at Amazon.com or other sites and bookstores.